CLINICAL IMMUNOLOGY OF THE DOG AND CAT

Second Edition

Revised And Updated

Michael J Day
BSc BVMS (Hons) PhD DSc DiplECVP FASM FRCPath FRCVS
Professor of Veterinary Pathology
University of Bristol
Langford, Bristol, UK

CRC Press
Taylor & Francis Group
Boca Raton London New York

CRC Press is an imprint of the
Taylor & Francis Group, an **informa** business

Dedication

To Christopher and Natalie

Disclaimer

The authors and Publisher have made every effort to ensure that therapeutic recommendations (particularly those concerning immunomodulatory and cytotoxic drug selection and dosage) set out in the text are in accord with current recommendations and practice. However, in view of ongoing research, changes in government regulations and the constant flow of information relating to drug therapy and drug reactions, the reader is urged to check the package insert for any added warnings and precautions.

The cytotoxic drugs detailed in this book are not licensed for veterinary use. All of these agents are potentially hazardous to the patient and to persons handling or administering them. Veterinary surgeons who prescribe such drugs to patients in their care must assume responsibility for their use and safe handling. Veterinary surgeons who are not familiar with the use of cytotoxic agents should seek further information and advice from a specialist.

Softcover edition, revised and updated 2012

Clinical Immunology of the Dog and Cat, Second Edition

First published 2008 by Manson Publishing Ltd

Published 2019 by CRC Press
Taylor & Francis Group
6000 Broken Sound Parkway NW, Suite 300
Boca Raton, FL 33487-2742

ISBN-13: 978-1-84076-171-9 (pbk)

Visit the Taylor & Francis Web site at
http://www.taylorandfrancis.com
and the CRC Press Web site at
http://www.crcpress.com

A CIP catalogue record for this book is available from the British Library.

Layout: DiacriTech, Chennai, India
Colour reproduction: Tenon & Polert Colour Scanning Ltd, Hong Kong

CONTENTS

PREFACE
(First Edition)

Clinical Immunology of the Dog and Cat is a unique textbook that leads the reader from basic immunological principles to their practical application in the diagnosis and treatment of immune-mediated diseases of the major companion animal species. The book is primarily designed as a reference source for veterinary surgeons in general or specialist practice who may require easily accessible and up-to-date information on this important group of diseases. Sufficient immunological background is given to make the text of value to veterinarians undertaking residency training or preparation for specialist examination. The integrated approach to pathology, clinical pathology and clinical medicine should also be of benefit to veterinary undergraduates.

The first three chapters of the book summarize current knowledge of basic cellular and molecular mechanisms in this rapidly evolving discipline and describe the multifactorial basis and pathogenesis of the immune-mediated diseases. The following nine chapters are system-based and describe the immunological basis, clinical signs, diagnostic procedures, therapy and prognosis for those immune-mediated disorders of each system that are recognized in the dog and cat. Separate chapters deal with multisystems disease and disorders of lymphoid tissues, and the final chapter provides an insight into how current research and experimental immunotherapies may be applied to clinical veterinary medicine in future years.

One major strength of this work is the use of extensive full colour diagrams and photographs. To enhance understanding, the diagrams utilize a consistent set of symbols for various immunological cells and molecules, and these are defined in the key that follows. The range of photographic material includes examples of clinical cases, radiographs, endoscopy, cytology, gross and microscopic pathology, immunopathology and electron microscopy. The book also contains a list of abbreviations and a list of selected further reading for each chapter, mostly papers from readily accessible veterinary journals from the past five years.

Clinical Immunology of the Dog and Cat has been an exciting project to develop, but it would not have been possible without the valued input of many people. I would firstly like to acknowledge the role of my contributors in co-writing a number of the chapters. These clinical colleagues are each internationally recognized leaders within their disciplines, and it has been a pleasure to have the opportunity to work with them. They have generously allowed me to reproduce photographs from their collections and have provided the majority of information on therapy and management of the disease entities to complement my immunopathological observations.

My colleagues, graduate students and technicians within the Departments of Pathology and Microbiology and Clinical Veterinary Science at the University of Bristol have generated data and material that have been incorporated into this book, and I am grateful for their support and for the departmental infrastructure that has allowed me the facilities to produce this work. The majority of the colour photographs of clinical cases and gross pathology are the expert products of talented medical photographers: Malcolm Parsons, John Conibear and Tracy Townsend-Sweeting (University of Bristol) and Geoff Griffiths (Murdoch University).

I would like to acknowledge the contribution of Jill Northcott, who originally had the idea for this text. The finished product has been expertly and efficiently created by Manson Publishing, and I am grateful to Michael Manson for his enthusiasm for the book, and to the skilled production team of Paul Bennett (project manager), Peter Beynon (copy editor), and Sue Tyler and Kate Nardoni (illustrators), with whom it has been a pleasure to work.

In writing this preface, it is appropriate that I have the opportunity to acknowledge my three mentors (Professor John Penhale, Professor Chris Elson and Dr. Don Mason), who introduced me to this exciting discipline and shaped my early career in immunology. Finally, I am grateful for the unstinting indulgence of my parents who supported my drawn-out education, and the understanding of my own family, who tolerated my long hours of solitary confinement.

Michael J. Day

PREFACE
(Second Edition)

I was delighted by the success of the first edition of *Clinical Immunology of the Dog and Cat*, which clearly filled a niche in the veterinary textbook market and was eventually translated into six additional languages. Immunology, however, is probably the fastest moving of the sciences and, since the publication of the first edition in 1999, there have been numerous advances that readily justify the production of this second edition. In the area of fundamental immunology there has been a renewed focus on the importance of the innate immune system, with a realization that events at this level of antigen recognition determine the nature of the ensuing adaptive immune response. Additionally, there has been recent clarification of the role of regulatory (suppressor) T lymphocytes in the immune response and identification of several functional subsets of these cells. In parallel with this research has been an explosion of knowledge in the field of companion animal immunology, largely driven by the molecular revolution, which in turn is underpinned by publication of the canine (and, soon, the feline) genome. Techniques have been developed that have allowed us to explore and quantify the role of key immunological molecules in canine and feline immune responses, and this technology has rapidly translated to the clinical diagnostic laboratory with the advent of PCR-based tests for the diagnosis of infection or detection of clonality of neoplastic lymphoid populations. These advances are all discussed within this second edition.

In order to incorporate these advances in understanding, by necessity this second edition of *Clinical Immunology of the Dog and Cat* has grown. There is an additional chapter devoted to respiratory and cardiac disease and, given the continued focus of companion animal practitioners on vaccine-related issues, a new chapter is devoted entirely to the subject of vaccinology. The second edition also includes approximately 200 new photographic images, an updated list of further reading (specifically papers published since the first edition in 1999), and an extensive glossary of terms.

As ever, I am indebted to my contributors for their continued enthusiasm for this book and for providing updated information on current therapeutic aspects of the diseases covered. I was pleased to welcome Professor Cecile Clercx to this group of internationally recognized clinical specialists, and I thank them all for their insightful editing of the text.

This is now my third publication with Manson Publishing and I am pleased to acknowledge this continuing relationship. The reputation of this small publishing house is founded on the exceptionally high standards and quality of printed texts that they produce, and I am grateful to Mike Manson and Jill Northcott for their expertise in developing and marketing projects such as this. Both have also been very patient with the protracted gestation of this volume, the birth of which was promised some years before the actual event! I am very pleased to acknowledge the team that has worked on this second edition, including Paul Bennett (project manager), Peter Beynon (copy editor) and Sue Tyler and Kate Nardoni (illustrators).

Finally, it would be remiss of me not to acknowledge the continued patience and support of my family who, when welcoming visitors to the house, point out 'that's the study ... where we keep Dad'.

Michael J. Day

REVISED AND UPDATED 2012

Due to the continued success of this book and the need for a second print-run, an opportunity arose in 2011 to further update the content of Clinical Immunology of the Dog and Cat. Key new developments since publication of this second edition in 2008 have been incorporated into the text of each chapter, some diagrams have been subtly modified and the list of further reading that accompanies each chapter has been significantly updated to highlight the very latest research developments from this rapidly changing field. In conjunction with these updates to content, the book now appears in soft cover to enhance accessibility to our target audience.

Michael J Day

CONTRIBUTORS

Professor David Bennett BSc BVetMed PhD ILTM DSAO MRCVS
Professor of Small Animal Clinical Studies
Division of Companion Animal Sciences
Faculty of Veterinary Medicine
University of Glasgow, Glasgow, UK

Professor Cécile Clercx DVM PhD DipECVIM-ca
Professor of Small Animal Internal Medicine
Department of Veterinary Clinical Sciences
Faculty of Veterinary Medicine
University of Liège, Liège, Belgium

Professor Sheila Crispin MA VetMB BSc PhD DVA DVOphthal DipECVO FRCVS
Cold Harbour Farm
Kendal, Cumbria, UK

Dr. Jane M. Dobson MA DVetMed DipECVIM-ca MRCVS
Senior Lecturer in Veterinary Clinical Oncology
Department of Clinical Veterinary Medicine
University of Cambridge, Cambridge, UK

Professor Edward J. Hall MA VetMB PhD DipECVIM-ca MRCVS
Professor of Small Animal Internal Medicine
School of Clinical Veterinary Science
University of Bristol, Langford, Bristol, UK

Professor Andrew J. Mackin BSc BVMS MVS DVSc DSAM FACVSc DACVIM MRCVS
Hugh G. Ward Endowed Chair of Small Animal Medicine
College of Veterinary Medicine
Mississippi State University, Mississippi, USA

Dr. Susan E. Shaw BVSc MSc FACVSc DipACVIM DipECVIM-ca MRCVS
Senior Lecturer in Veterinary Dermatology
School of Clinical Veterinary Science
University of Bristol, Langford, Bristol, UK

ABBREVIATIONS

AA amyloid amyloid-associated protein
ACAID anterior chamber-associated immune deviation
ACE angiotensin converting enzyme
AChR acetylcholine receptor
AD atopic dermatitis
ADCC antibody-dependent cell-mediated cytotoxicity
AIDS acquired immune deficiency syndrome
AIEC attaching and invading *E. coli*
AIHA autoimmune haemolytic anaemia
AITP autoimmune thrombocytopenia
AL amyloid amyloid (immunoglobulin) light chain protein
ALL acute lymphoblastic leukaemia
AMD acute myeloproliferative disease
AML acute myeloid leukaemia
ANA antinuclear antibody
APC antigen presenting cell
ARD antibiotic responsive diarrhoea
ASIT allergen-specific immunotherapy
BALF bronchoalveolar lavage fluid
BALT bronchial-associated lymphoid tissue
BCG bacille Calmette–Guérin
BLAD bovine leukocyte adhesion deficiency
BMZ basement membrane zone
BUN blood urea nitrogen
CALT conjunctiva-associated lymphoid tissue
CAV canine adenovirus
CBC complete blood count
CC a chemokine in which the two amino terminal cysteine residues are adjacent
CD cluster of differentiation
CDV canine distemper virus
CGL chronic granulocytic leukaemia
CH chronic hepatitis
CH_{50} total haemolytic complement (assay)
CIC circulating immune complex
CLAD canine leukocyte adhesion deficiency
CLE cutaneous lupus erythematosus
CLL chronic lymphocytic leukaemia
CMD chronic myeloproliferative disease
CMI cell-mediated immunity
CML chronic myeloid leukaemia
CNS central nervous system
ConA concanavalin A (mitogen)
CMMM canine masticatory muscle myositis
CPM canine polymyositis
CRFK Crandall Rees feline kidney cell line
CR1 complement receptor 1

CSF cerebrospinal fluid
CSK/CSKC chronic superficial keratitis/keratoconjunctivitis
CT computerized tomography
CXC a chemokine in which the two amino terminal cysteine residues are separated by one amino acid
DAF decay accelerating factor
DAMP damage-associated molecular pattern
DEA dog erythrocyte antigen
DGGE denaturing gradient gel electrophoresis
DIC disseminated intravascular coagulation
DLA dog leukocyte antigen (canine MHC)
DLE discoid lupus erythematosus
DLH domestic longhair (cat)
DNA deoxyribonucleic acid
DOI duration of immunity
DOP duration of protection
DSH domestic shorthair (cat)
DTH delayed-type hypersensitivity
EAE experimental allergic encephalomyelitis
EBP eosinophilic bronchopneumopathy
EGC eosinophilic granuloma complex
ELISA enzyme-linked immunosorbent assay
EM erythema multiforme
EMG electromyogram
EPEC enteropathogenic *Escherichia coli*
EPI exocrine pancreatic insufficiency
Fab antigen-binding fragment (of Ig)
FACS fluorescence-activated cell sorter
FAD flea allergy dermatitis
Fc crystallizable fragment (of Ig)
FCV feline calicivirus
FcR Fc (Ig heavy chain) receptor
FeFV feline foamy virus
FeLV feline leukaemia virus
FHV feline herpesvirus
FIA feline infectious anaemia
FIE feline infectious enteritis
FIP feline infectious peritonitis
FIV feline immunodeficiency virus
FLA feline leukocyte antigen (feline MHC)
GALT gut-associated lymphoid tissue
GBM glomerular basement membrane
G-CSF granulocyte colony stimulating factor
GITR glucocorticoid-induced TNF receptor-related gene
GM-CSF granulocyte-macrophage colony stimulating factor
GME granulomatous meningoencephalitis
GP glycoprotein
GSD German Shepherd Dog
HAT hypoxanthine, aminopterin, thymidine (medium)
HEV high endothelial venule
HLA human leukocyte antigen (human MHC)
HSP heat shock protein
HUC histiocytic ulcerative colitis
IBD inflammatory bowel disease
ICAM-1 intercellular adhesion molecule 1
ICGN immune complex glomerulonephritis
IDDM insulin-dependent diabetes mellitus
IDST intradermal skin test
IEL intraepithelial lymphocyte
IEP immunoelectrophoresis
IFN interferon (e.g. IFNγ)
Ig immunoglobulin (IgG, IgM, IgA, IgD, IgE)
IGF-1 insulin-like growth factor-1
IL interleukin (e.g. IL-1)
i/m intramuscular
IMHA immune-mediated haemolytic anaemia
IMNP immune-mediated neutropenia
IMTP immune-mediated thrombocytopenia
i/p intraperitoneal
IPE idiopathic pericardial effusion
ITP idiopathic thrombocytopenia
i/v intravenous/intravascular
KCS keratoconjunctivitis sicca
KIR killer-cell inhibitory factor
LAK lymphokine-activated killer (cells)
LFA-1 lymphocyte function-associated antigen 1
LPC lymphoplasmacytic colitis
LPE lymphoplasmacytic enteritis
LPL lamina propria lymphocyte
LPR lymphoplasmacytic rhinitis
LPS lipopolysaccharide
LSEC liver sinusoidal endothelial cell
MAC membrane attack complex
MAdCAM mucosal addressin cell adhesion molecule
MALT mucosa-associated lymphoid tissue
MBP myelin basic protein
MCP macrophage chemotactic protein/membrane co-factor protein
MG myasthenia gravis
MHC major histocompatibility complex
MMP matrix metalloproteinase
MRI magnetic resonance imaging
mRNA messenger RNA
NALT nasal-associated lymphoid tissue
NBT nitroblue tetrazolium (test)
NCIWF National Cancer Institute Working Formulation
NFAT nuclear factor of activated T cells
NK natural killer (cells)
NLE necrotizing leukoencephalitis
NME necrotizing meningoencephalitis
NRIMHA non-regenerative immune-mediated haemolytic anaemia
NSAID non-steroidal anti-inflammatory drug
OspA outer surface protein A (of *Borrelia burgdorferi*)
OVA ovalbumin
PAA pancreatic acinar atrophy
PALS periarteriolar lymphoid sheath
PAMP pathogen-associated molecular pattern
PAS periodic acid-Schiff (stain)
PCR polymerase chain reaction
PCV packed cell volume (haematocrit)
PHA phytohaemagglutinin (mitogen)
PIE pulmonary infiltration with eosinophilia

pIgR polymeric immunoglobulin receptor
p/o per os
PRCA pure red cell aplasia
PRR pattern recognition receptor
PT prothrombin time
PTT partial thromboplastin time
PUO pyrexia of unknown origin
PWM pokeweed mitogen
RA rheumatoid arthritis
RAG recombination activating gene
RANTES regulated upon activation, normal, T-cell expressed, and secreted (a chemokine)
RBCs red blood cells
REAL Revised European American Lymphoma Classification Scheme
RER rough endoplasmic reticulum
RF rheumatoid factor
rHuIFNγ recombinant human IFNγ (or other cytokine)
rHuTSH recombinant human TSH
RNA ribonucleic acid
RNP ribonucleoprotein
RT–PCR reverse transcriptase–polymerase chain reaction
SAA serum amyloid-associated protein
SAARD slow-acting antirheumatic drug
SALT skin-associated lymphoid tissue
SARs suspect adverse reactions
SARSS suspect adverse reaction surveillance scheme
s/c subcutaneous
SCID severe combined immunodeficiency
SI stimulation index
SIBO small intestinal bacterial overgrowth
SJS Stevens–Johnson syndrome
SLE systemic lupus erythematosus
SmIg surface membrane immunoglobulin ($SmIg^{+}$, SmIgM, SmIgD)
SNP single nucleotide polymorphism
SPC summary of product characteristics
SPE serum protein electrophoresis
SRID single radial immunodiffusion
SRMA steroid responsive meningitis-arteritis
STAT signal transducers and activators of transcription
Tc T cytotoxic (cell)
TCR T cell receptor
TEN toxic epidermal necrolysis
TGF transforming growth factor
Th T helper (cell)
TK1 thymidine kinase 1
TLI trypsin-like immunoreactivity
TNF tumour necrosis factor
TPMP thiopurine methyltransferase
Treg T regulatory (cell)
TRH thyrotropin releasing hormone
TSH thyroid stimulating hormone
TUBA total unconjugated bile acids
UV ultraviolet (light)
VCAM vascular cell adhesion molecule
VKH Vogt–Koyanagi–Harada syndrome
VMD Veterinary Medicines Directorate
VPC Veterinary Products Committee
WBCs white blood cells
X-SCID X-linked severe combined immunodeficiency

KEY TO SYMBOLS

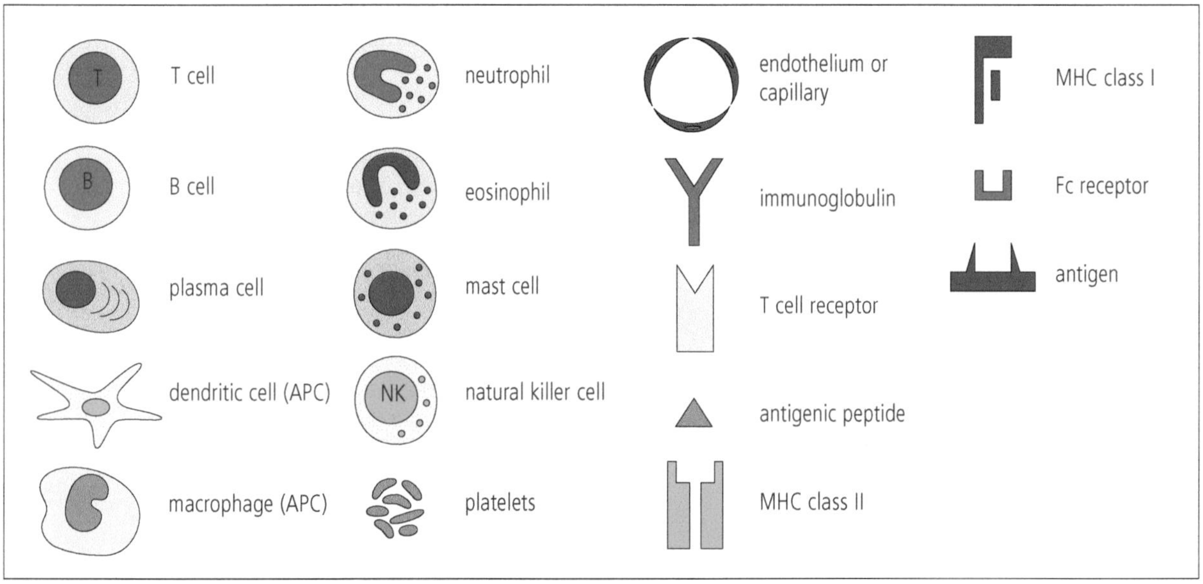

1 BASIC IMMUNOLOGY

Michael J. Day

INTRODUCTION

The immune system is one of the most complex and diverse of body components. This complexity has evolved to enable efficient neutralization of the myriad of potential pathogens that may be encountered at any site within the body during a lifetime. The same complexity, however, also provides scope for failure of the normal immunological regulatory mechanisms and the development of immune-mediated diseases.

There is a vast amount of knowledge concerning the workings of the mammalian immune system, a system which encompasses an array of cells and their surface molecules, together with soluble factors released from them and the genes which encode these substances. The basic components of the immune system have been conserved throughout evolution, and there is often a high degree of homology between similar molecules in different species. The immune systems of man and laboratory animals have been best characterized and this understanding has been extrapolated to other species.

Among domestic animals, the immune systems of the dog and cat have only been examined in detail in relatively recent times. The use of the dog as a model for transplantation surgery, and of the cat as a model for the study of virally induced neoplasia (feline leukaemia virus [FeLV]) or immunodeficiency (feline immunodeficiency virus [FIV]), has led to the application of cellular and molecular techniques to characterize basic facets of the canine and feline immune systems. The recent availability of the canine genome has revolutionized our ability to dissect the immune system of the dog and develop molecular tools for the characterization of immune-mediated diseases in this species. Alignment of the canine and human genomes has shown 75% sequence similarity, further confirming the value of investigation of spontaneously arising canine disease as a model for the human counterpart. A partial version of the feline genome is now available.

This chapter overviews the major components of the immune system at the tissue, cellular and molecular levels, where possible giving details of specific parameters as they apply to the dog and cat. Such a review cannot be exhaustive, but it forms the basis for discussion of disease mechanisms in later chapters.

THE IMMUNE SYSTEM: AN OVERVIEW

The immune system has both innate and adaptive components (**1**). The innate response is a first-line

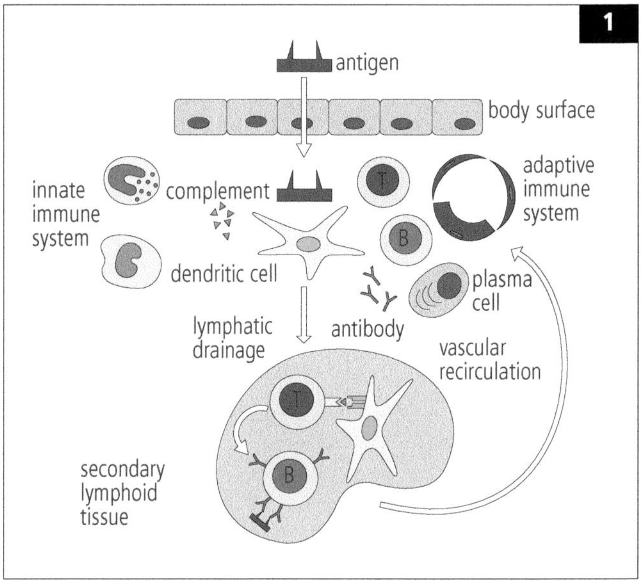

1 Overview of the immune response. When foreign antigen enters the body it first encounters the cells and molecules of the non-antigen specific, innate immune system. Antigen is taken up by dendritic antigen presenting cells and transported to the regional lymphoid tissue, where there is induction of the antigen-specific adaptive immune response. Activated cells of the adaptive immune system recirculate to the site of antigen exposure via the vasculature, where these cells and their products amplify the local immune response. The dendritic cell is the link between the innate and adaptive immune systems.

of body defence and consists of the non-specific effects of epithelial or mucosal barriers (e.g. physical structures such as cilia and secreted factors such as enzymes), together with the action of phagocytic cells (neutrophils, macrophages and dendritic cells), inflammatory mediators and the alternate pathway of the complement system. A particular subset of T lymphocytes, the $\gamma\delta$ T cells, which express a unique surface receptor, may also be considered part of the innate immune system, as they are found in high numbers at external surfaces and are particularly responsive to bacterial antigens. One of the most significant recent immunological advances has been a re-evaluation of the importance of innate immunity. It is now appreciated that the initial interaction between foreign antigen and the dendritic antigen presenting cell (APC) determines the nature of the subsequent adaptive immune response. The adaptive immune response involves the selective activation of lymphoid cells with specificity for the pathogen, and the subsequent action of pathogen-specific antibodies or effector cells. Adaptive immunity develops over time and specific immunological memory of the pathogen is retained.

ANTIGENS

An antigen is generally considered as a substance that can initiate an immune response. Technically, an 'antigen' is defined only by its ability to bind to antibody, whereas an 'immunogen' is capable of inducing antibody production. Most antigens are foreign to an individual; they include microbes, chemicals and plant-derived substances as well as tissue from genetically dissimilar individuals of the same species (alloantigen) or a different species (xenoantigen). In autoimmune disease, components of the body may also become antigenic (autoantigens).

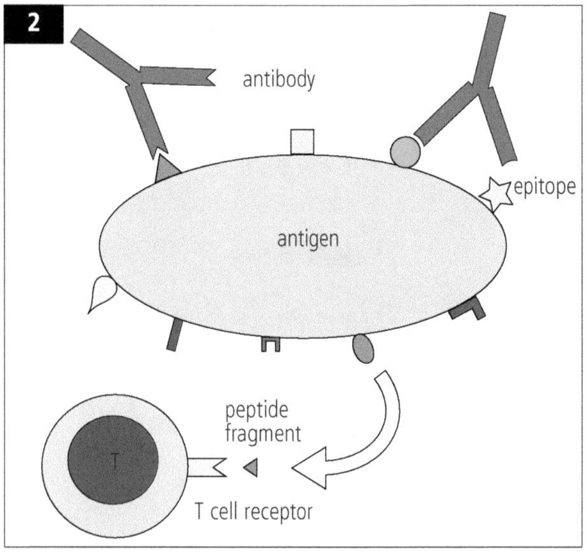

2 Antigens. Antigens have a set of antigenic epitopes (determinants) that are recognized by antibodies and TCRs of the adaptive immune system. Each antibody recognizes one epitope rather than the entire antigen, and TCRs recognize small peptide fragments derived from epitopes.

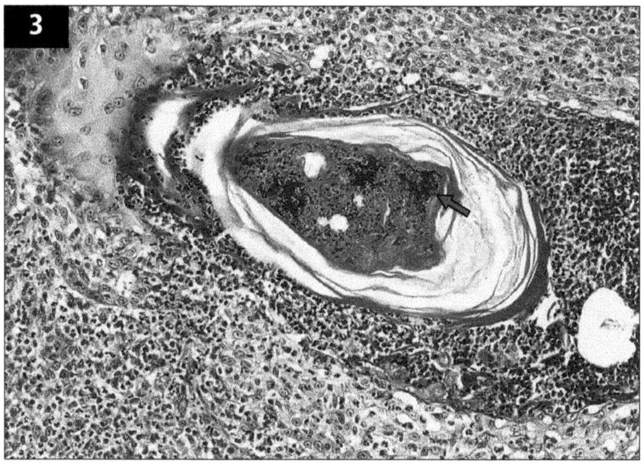

3 Antigenic epitopes. Colonies of *Staphylococcus pseudintermedius* in the lumen of a hair follicle of a dog with deep pyoderma (arrowed). Each *Staphylococcus* organism may have numerous constituent antigens.

The most effective antigenic (immunogenic) substances are large, insoluble molecules (>10 kD in molecular weight), which have chemical complexity and a stable three-dimensional structure. Biologically active substances (e.g. microbes) are particularly antigenic.

A single antigen may have numerous epitopes or determinants, each of which is capable of inducing an immune response (2–4), but some of which may be more effective in so doing (immunodominant). Some small chemical groups (haptens) are unable to induce an immune response unless chemically conjugated to a larger protein molecule (carrier protein). This mechanism is thought to underlie many adverse reactions to drugs (5).

The immunogenicity of antigens can be enhanced by incorporating them into an adjuvant (e.g. Freund's adjuvant or alum), which acts by non-specific immune stimulation and by forming a slow-release depot of antigen.

4 Antigenic epitopes. Polyacrylamide gel electrophoresis separating the components of 22 isolates of *S. pseudintermedius* by molecular weight. Each band in the gel may represent one or more epitopes. The specificity of antibody in the serum of an infected dog for these epitopes can be determined by the technique of western blotting. (Photograph courtesy D.H. Shearer.)

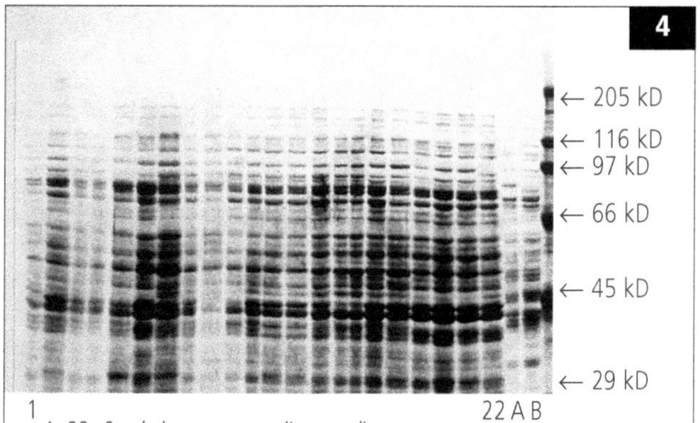

1–22 *Staphylococcus pseudintermedius*
A *S. aureus* Wood strain (low protein A producer)
B *S. aureus* Cowan strain (high protein A producer)

5 Haptens. This German Shepherd Dog was treated with ketoconazole for disseminated aspergillosis and subsequently developed lesions of the planum nasale and periorbital skin consistent with cutaneous drug eruption. In such cases the drug may act as a hapten by binding to native protein within tissue and inducing an immune response to novel epitopes thus formed.

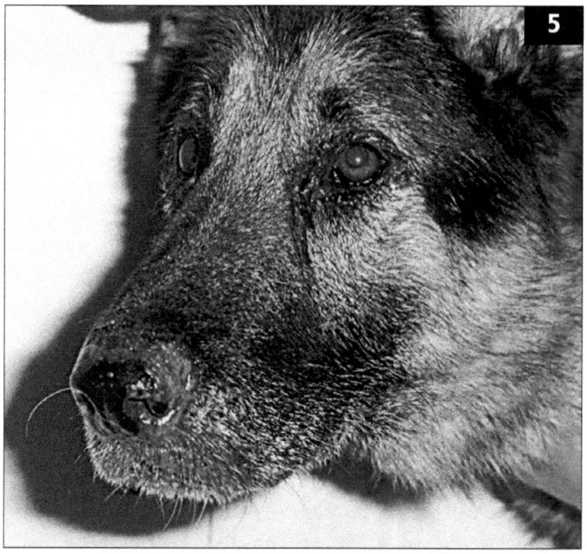

ANTIBODIES (IMMUNOGLOBULINS)

Antibodies are generated as part of an immune response and, when formed, are able to bind to antigens. Although immunoglobulin (Ig) molecules take different forms (classes and subclasses), each has a similar basic structure, consisting of a Y-shaped unit of two heavy and two light polypeptide chains (**6, 7**). There are five forms of heavy chain (α, γ, μ, δ and ε), the use of which gives rise to the five classes of Ig (IgA, IgG, IgM, IgD and IgE, respectively), and each may associate with either of the two forms of light chain (κ and λ). In the dog and cat, λ chain is more commonly utilized than κ. Subclasses of Ig are defined by subtle modifications to the sequence and structure of the constant regions.

IgG

This is the major serum Ig, which may diffuse readily to the extravascular tissue space. It comprises a single Ig unit and potentially binds two antigenic epitopes. There are four subclasses of IgG in the dog (IgG1–IgG4), defined at both the protein and gene level. Three subclasses have been recognized in the cat, but to date only a single IgG encoding gene has been characterized. The relative serum concentration of the subclasses in normal dogs is IgG1 and IgG2>IgG3 and IgG4, and there are electrophoretic similarities between IgG1 and IgG3 (cathodal) and IgG2 and IgG4 (anodal). Unfortunately, there remains much confusion regarding canine IgG subclasses due to the persistence of old nomenclature and the commercial availability of a set of antisera that purport to

6

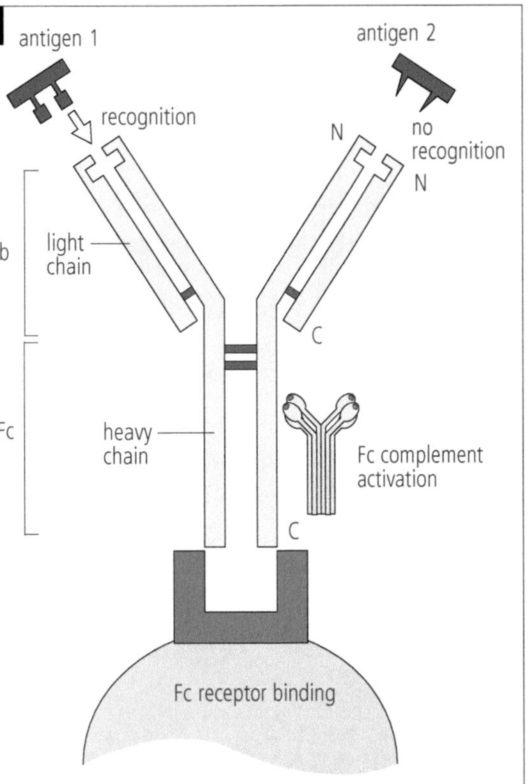

6 Basic structure and function of Ig. The Ig unit consists of two identical light polypeptide chains and two identical heavy polypeptide chains linked together by disulphide bonds (purple). The position of the amino- (N) and carboxy- (C) terminal ends of the polypeptide chains are indicated. The unit has two antigen-binding fragments (Fab) and a constant region (Fc), which interacts with crystallizable fragment receptors on cells or activates complement.

7

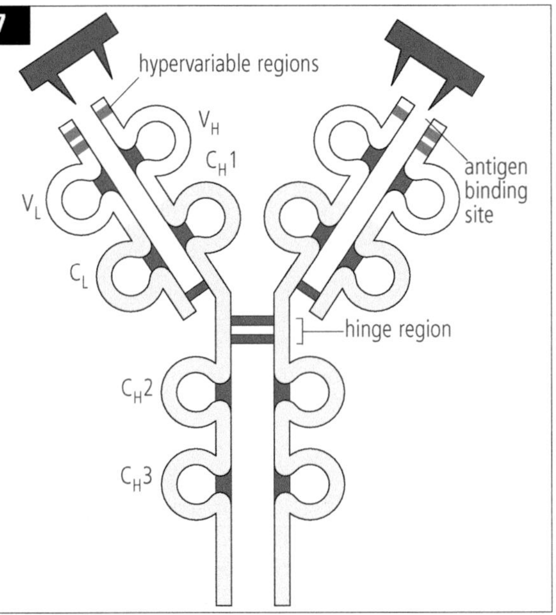

7 Domain structure of Ig. The N-terminal end of the Ig molecule is characterized by a variable amino acid sequence in both the heavy and light chains, referred to as the V_H and V_L regions, respectively. Within the variable regions are areas of sequence hypervariability. The remainder of the molecule has a relatively constant sequence. The constant portion of the light chain is known as the C_L region and the constant portion of the heavy chain is divided into three subregions known as C_H1, C_H2 and C_H3. Each subregion of the molecule has a globular 'domain' structure stabilized by intrachain disulphide bonds. The hinge region is a segment of the heavy chain between C_H1 and C_H2 that includes interchain disulphide bonds. The antigen binding portions of the molecule are flexible about the hinge region.

detect IgG subclasses, but are in fact not subclass specific. In dogs and cats, IgG is largely unable to cross the placental barrier and maternal immunity must be conferred to neonates via colostrum.

IgM

This molecule comprises five basic Ig units linked together by a joining (J) chain (8). A single IgM molecule has ten antigen binding sites and IgM is therefore very efficient at agglutinating particulate antigens. The size of the molecule generally precludes it leaving the bloodstream.

IgA

IgA may be found as a monomer of a single Ig unit (two antigen binding sites) or as a dimer with a J chain (four antigen binding sites) (9). There are species differences in the relative distribution of IgA monomers or dimers. In man, serum IgA is monomeric, while the IgA that is found at mucosal surfaces is a dimer. In contrast, both serum and mucosal IgA is dimeric in dogs and cats, which likely reflects the fact that most of this Ig is produced at mucosal sites. Because of the dimeric nature of canine serum IgA it has generally been assumed that serum IgA concentration in dogs is an accurate reflection of the level of secreted mucosal IgA. However, studies have shown poor correlation between serum IgA and salivary or tear IgA. Mucosal IgA is protected from enzymatic degradation by the secretory piece, which is attached to the molecule as it passes through the mucosal epithelium (10). It is likely that the dog has a single gene encoding the α heavy chain; however, it has recently been shown that there are four allelic variants within that part of the gene encoding the hinge region, suggesting that functional subclasses

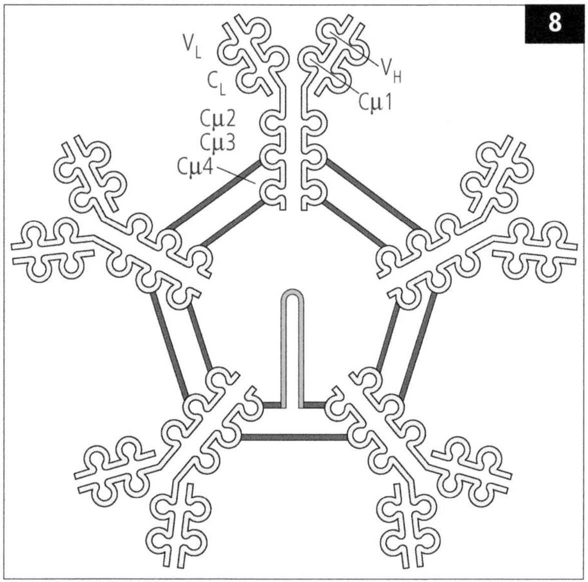

8 Structure of IgM. The IgM molecule consists of five basic Ig units linked together by a J chain. The structure shown is human IgM, which likely has similarity to the dog and cat counterpart. There is an extra heavy chain domain (C_H4) and disulphide bonds link adjacent C_H3 and C_H4 domains.

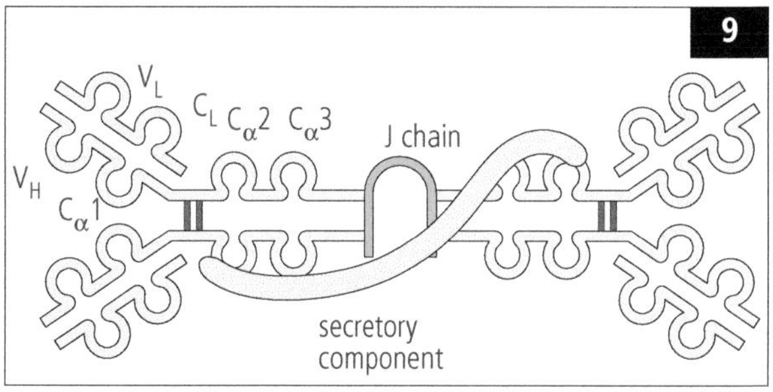

9 Structure of the IgA dimer. Dimeric IgA is found within mucosal secretions and the serum of the dog and cat. The structure shown is human dimeric IgA, which likely has similarity to the dog and cat counterpart. The two Ig units are joined by a J chain, and at mucosal sites IgA is protected from enzymatic degradation by the secretory piece, which wraps around the molecule and is linked to the C_H2 domain by disulphide bonds.

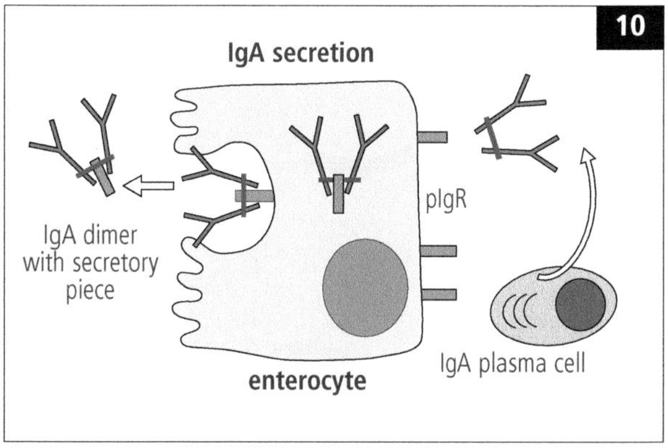

10 The IgA secretion pathway. An IgA dimer released from a plasma cell within the mucosal lamina propria is bound by the polymeric immunoglobulin receptor (pIgR) expressed on the basolateral sides of epithelial cells lining the surface. The complex of receptor and IgA is internalized and passes through the cell cytoplasm to be expressed on the external surface of the cell. The IgA dimer is released from the surface, carrying with it a portion of the pIgR, which becomes the secretory piece.

of IgA may exist. There are unique breed differences in the expression of these allelic variants and in some breeds (e.g. the German Shepherd Dog [GSD]) only a single variant has been identified.

IgD

IgD comprises a single Ig unit and is found predominantly on the surface of immature B lymphocytes. An IgD-like molecule has been characterized in the dog and the genetic sequence of the gene encoding δ heavy chain determined.

IgE

IgE consists of a single Ig unit, which is largely bound to surface receptors on mast cells and basophils, with relatively low levels in serum. IgE has been characterized in the dog and cat. Although a single gene encoding the ε heavy chain is reported, it has been suggested that there may be functional subclasses in each species that would reflect post-transcriptional changes or differences in glycosylation of the molecules.

ANTIGEN–ANTIBODY INTERACTIONS

Antigenic epitopes are bound by the N terminal end of the Ig molecule at a site formed by the apposition of the hypervariable regions (complementarity determining regions) of the heavy and light chains (**11**). The antigen binding site may appear as a cleft into which the epitope slots, or as a planar region that makes contact with a larger area of an antigen than could be accommodated within a cleft. The antigenic determinant may have a three-dimensional conformation that matches exactly the corresponding Ig binding site (high affinity binding) in what has been termed a 'lock and key' interaction, but it is possible for partial recognition of epitopes to occur (low affinity binding) and some antibodies bind linear peptides that lack conformation (**12**).

A multideterminant antigen given to an individual triggers production of antibodies that recognize a number of different epitopes (termed a polyclonal immune response). These antibodies may be detected in the serum of the immunized host. Individuals may respond differently to the same antigen, and the relative binding strength of a serum can be assessed by serially diluting it to an end point where it no longer binds antigen. The titre of a serum antibody is defined as the reciprocal of the highest serum dilution giving a positive reaction in a serological test. Antigen–antibody binding can be demonstrated *in vitro* using a range of such serological tests, which will be discussed in the following chapters.

11

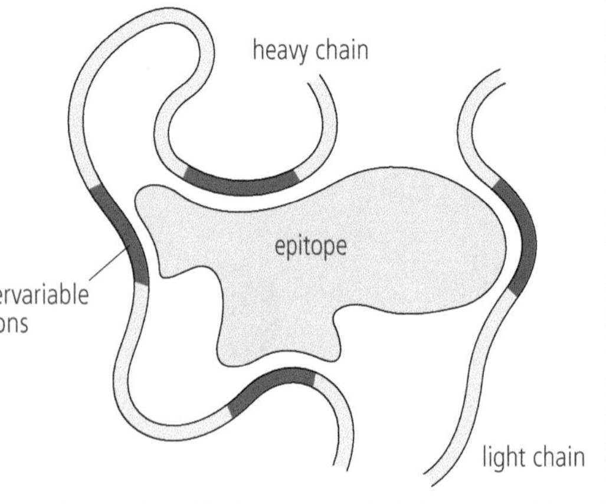

11 Antigen–antibody binding. Three-dimensional depiction of the antigen binding site seen from the perspective of the antigen. The antigenic epitope nestles in a cleft formed by the heavy and light chains. The epitope makes contact with specific amino acids in the hypervariable regions (shaded) of both heavy and light chains. The epitope is held tightly by a combination of attractive forces (hydrogen bonds, electrostatic, Van der Waals and hydrophobic).

COMPLEMENT

Complement is a series of approximately 30 proteins. When activated, they interact sequentially to form an enzymatic cascade, which has a range of end-effects important in inflammatory and immune responses. There are four complement pathways. The classical, lectin and alternative pathways have a common end product (C3b), which initiates the terminal pathway (**13**). The complement pathways have been characterized in the dog and cat, and serum levels of the individual components have been determined.

The classical pathway is triggered by the binding of antibody (IgG or IgM) to antigen or by the aggregation of these Igs (**14**). The C1 molecule contains three subunits (C1q, C1r and C1s), which are activated in sequence following binding to Ig. C1s cleaves the second factors in the pathway (C4 and C2) and two of the fragments generated (C4b, C2b) associate to form C3 convertase, which cleaves the final component of the pathway (C3). The C3b thus generated binds with the C4b and

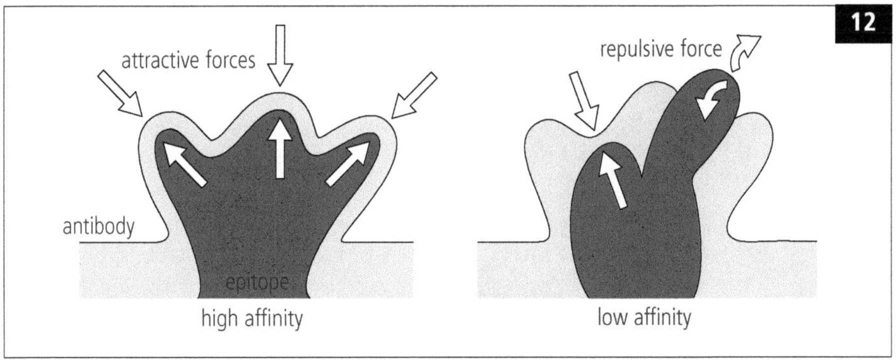

12 Antibody affinity. Antibody affinity is the sum of attractive and repulsive forces between an antibody and an antigenic epitope, and reflects how well the epitope 'fits' the antigen binding site. A high affinity interaction is depicted on the left, and a low affinity interaction on the right.

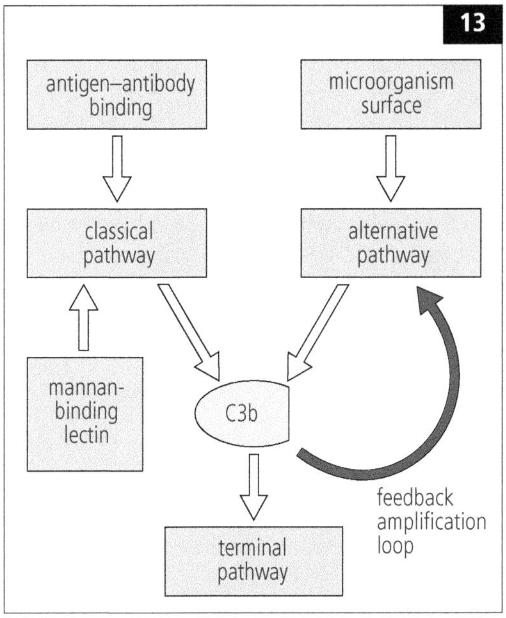

13 Overview of the complement pathways. There are four complement pathways. The classical and alternative pathways share a key molecule (C3b) and feed into a common terminal pathway. The classical pathway is largely activated following the binding of antibody to antigen, and shares components with the lectin binding pathway that is activated by mannan-binding lectin. The alternative pathway is evolutionarily older and may be activated in the absence of specific immunity (part of the innate immune system) by the presence of suitable surfaces (e.g. bacteria, yeast). The feedback amplification loop is unique to the alternative pathway.

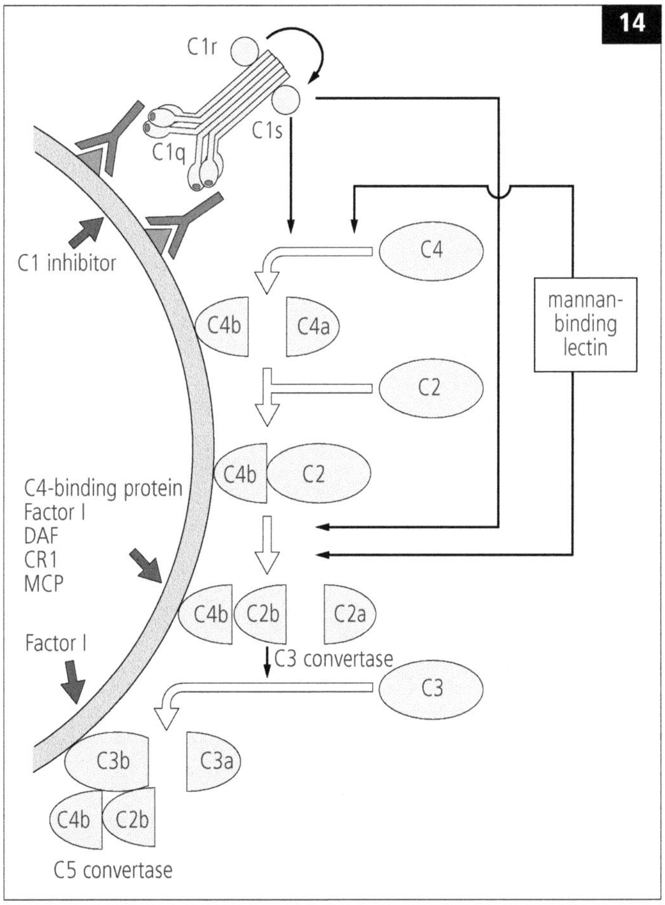

14 The classical pathway of complement. After binding of C1q to complexed antibody and antigen, C1r catalyses the activation of C1s. C1s then cleaves C4a from C4, leaving C4b, which binds to the surface of the antigen. C4b next binds C2 and C1s cleaves C2a from this complex to leave C2b. The C4b2b complex is the classical pathway C3 convertase and can also be generated by the action of mannan-binding lectin. Cleavage of C3 leads to formation of the C5 convertase (C4b2b3b). Sites of regulation of the classical pathway are shown (red arrows).

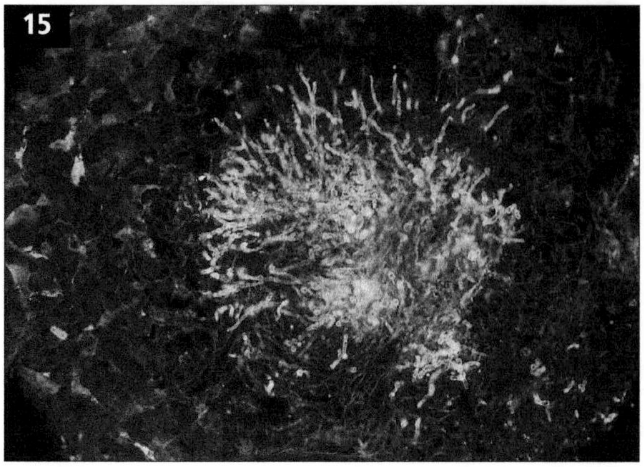

15 Deposition of complement C3 on microbial surfaces. These fungal hyphae (*Aspergillus terreus*) lie at the centre of a microgranuloma within the pancreas of a GSD with disseminated aspergillosis. The section has been labelled with fluorescein-conjugated antiserum specific for canine C3, which gives apple-green fluorescence under UV light. Complement C3 is readily demonstrated on the surface of hyphae in such lesions, but C4 is rarely found. This would suggest that complement activation via the alternative pathway dominates in such lesions. (From Day MJ, Penhale WJ (1991) An immunohistochemical study of canine disseminated aspergillosis. *Australian Veterinary Journal* **68:**383–386, with permission.)

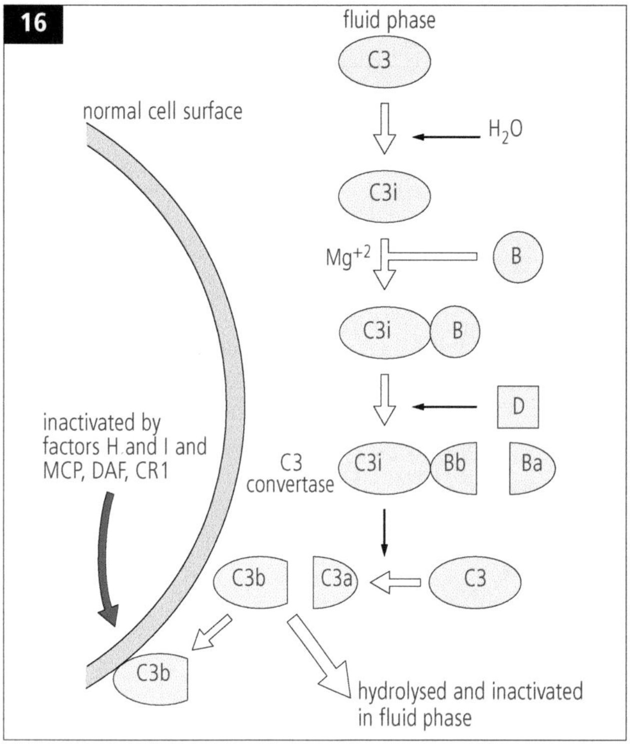

16 Alternative pathway 'tick over'. In normal individuals the alternative pathway of complement is continually ticking over at low level. Fluid phase C3 is hydrolysed by water to form C3i, which binds factor B. The action of factor D results in formation of a fluid phase C3 convertase (C3iBb), which can cleave C3 into C3a and C3b. The majority of this C3b is hydrolysed and inactivated in the fluid phase. If it should locate onto the surface of normal cells, it is bound by factor H and inactivated by factor I. Activation is further prevented by the action of the membrane complement antagonist molecules MCP, DAF and CR1.

C2b complex to form a C5 convertase, which initiates the terminal pathway. An alternative means of activating C4 and C2 involves conformational changes in the serum mannan binding lectin, following binding to bacterial surface carbohydrate (the lectin pathway). A range of regulatory factors prevents deleterious overactivity of the classical pathway:

- The short half-life of complement components.
- The C1 inhibitor, which cleaves C1r from C1s.
- The C4 binding protein, which displaces C2b from C4b with subsequent cleavage (by factor I) to inactive C4c and C4d.
- Membrane-bound factors (decay accelerating factor [DAF]; complement receptor 1 [CR1]; membrane co-factor protein [MCP]), which disrupt the C3 convertase should it be deposited on the surface of a normal cell.
- Factor I, which cleaves C3b to inactive C3c and C3d.

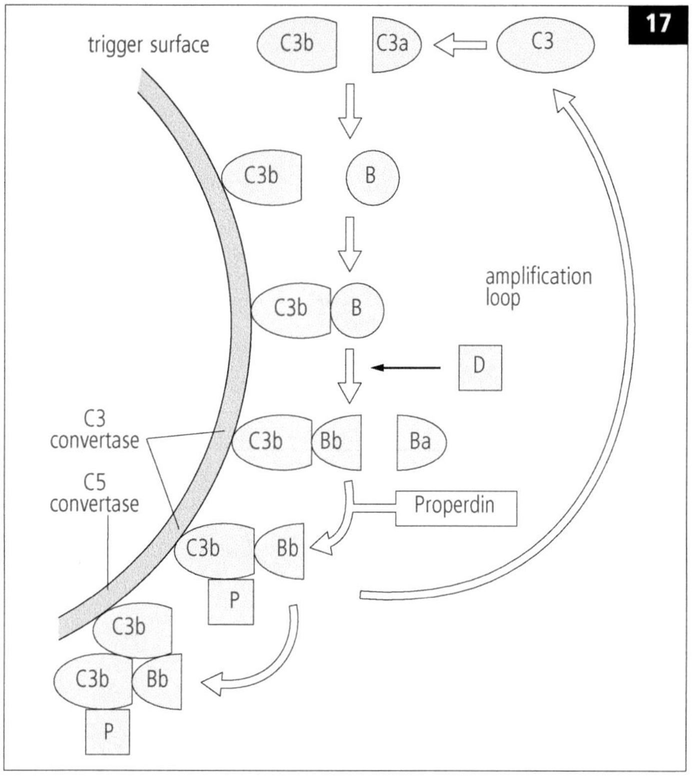

17 Alternative pathway activation. In the presence of a suitable trigger surface (lacking MCP, DAF and CR1), deposited C3b is preferentially bound by factor B, which is in turn cleaved by factor D to form an alternative pathway C3 convertase (C3bBb). The C3 convertase is rapidly dissociated unless it is stabilized by the binding of properdin (PC3bBb). The stable C3 convertase initiates the amplification loop, whereby many more molecules of C3b are generated and localized to the trigger surface. The deposition of further C3b permits formation of the alternative pathway C5 convertase (PC3bBbC3b).

The alternative pathway is evolutionarily older and can act in the absence of Ig (and is therefore considered part of the innate immune system). This pathway is active in normal individuals at low 'tick over' levels, but becomes amplified in the presence of appropriate trigger factors, which include Ig aggregates, bacterial or yeast surfaces, virally infected or neoplastic cells, or foreign particles (e.g. asbestos) (**15**). In the normal individual, plasma C3 undergoes hydrolysis to form C3i. Some C3i may bind factor B (C3iB) and then be modified by factor D to form a fluid phase C3iBb, which is a C3 convertase that may enhance C3 cleavage. Most C3b thus generated is inactivated in the fluid phase. Should any C3b be deposited on the surface of a normal cell it is dissociated by DAF, CR1 and MCP and inactivated by factors H and I (**16**). In the presence of an appropriate 'trigger surface', C3bBb becomes cell-associated and is stabilized by properdin to form a C3 convertase (PC3bBb). This initiates a feedback amplification loop to generate more C3b, which is then deposited on the trigger surface (**17**). Formation of a PC3bBbC3b complex (C5 convertase) initiates the terminal pathway. The terminal complement pathway involves the sequential deposition of C5b, C6, C7, C8 and C9 onto the surface, with eventual formation of a transmembrane pore, the membrane attack complex (MAC) (**18**).

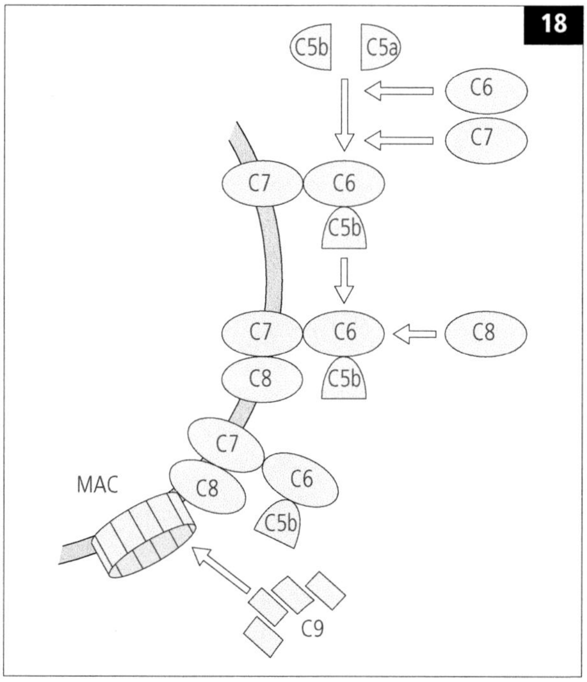

18 The terminal pathway of complement. The classical or alternative pathway C5 convertase splits C5 into C5a and C5b. The C5b binds C6 and C7 to form C5b67, which attaches to the cell membrane. C8 binds to this complex and penetrates the membrane, where it polymerizes a number of C9 molecules to form the transmembrane pore known as the membrane attack complex (MAC).

19

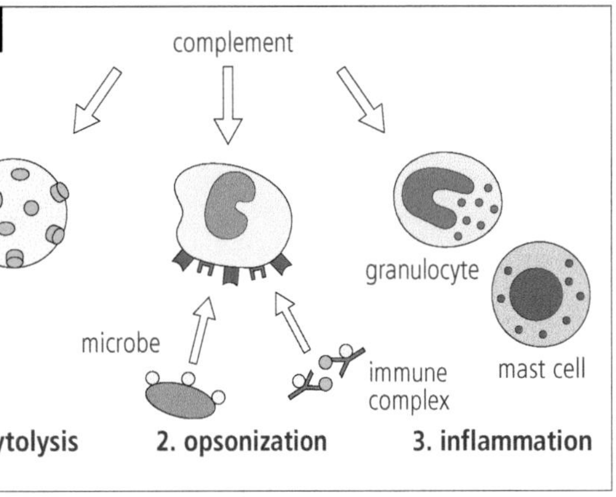

19 The major biological functions of the complement system. Activation of complement results in (1) lysis of target cells via formation of the membrane attack complex, with osmotic imbalance and a net influx of water causing cytolysis; (2) opsonization of microorganisms and immune complexes so that they are recognized by receptors on the surface of phagocytic cells; and (3) inflammation with activation of WBCs. The role of complement in opsonization and inflammation is more fully described in **20–23**.

20

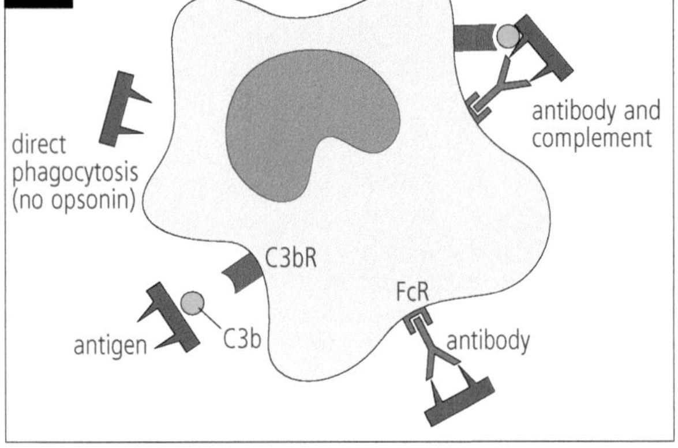

21

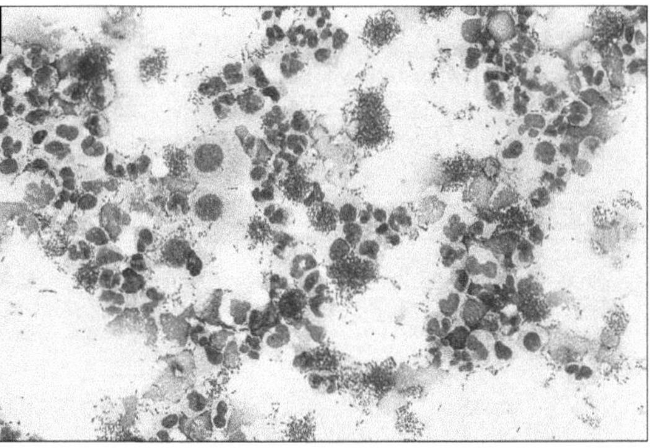

20, 21 Opsonization. (**20**) Phagocytic cells may bind directly to microorganisms, but binding can be enhanced by coating the organism with antibody and/or complement (opsonization). Molecules of IgG or C3b on the surface of the organism are recognized by FcRs and C3b receptors, and the most efficient phagocytosis of organisms occurs following opsonization by both antibody and complement. (**21**) Cytological preparation of a mucopurulant nasal discharge from a dog. There are large colonies of bacteria together with epithelial cells and neutrophils. Phagocytosis of bacteria in this case could be enhanced by the binding of opsonins such as antibody and complement.

22

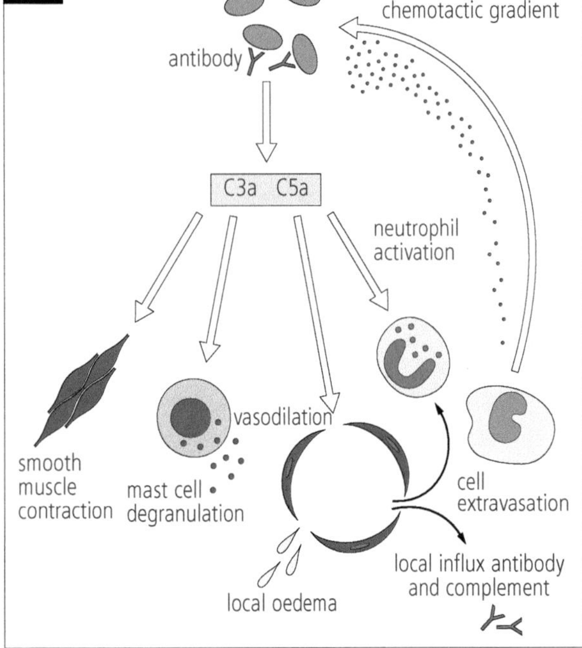

22 The role of complement in inflammation. Activation of the complement pathways leads to production of the biologically active molecules C3a and C5a (anaphylotoxins). These molecules mediate a similar range of end effects, which amplify inflammation. C5a is more potent in effect than C3a, but greater quantities of C3a are generated. The inflammatory effects include (1) smooth muscle contraction; (2) vasodilation with local tissue oedema and extravasation of protein (antibody and complement) and WBCs; (3) mast cell degranulation with amplification of the effects on smooth muscle and vessels; (4) white cell (neutrophil and macrophage) activation and release of other inflammatory mediators; and (5) establishment of a chemotactic gradient of complement molecules to cause localization of white cells. Additionally, some complement factors interact with other major inflammatory pathways, including the coagulation, kinin and fibrinolytic pathways.

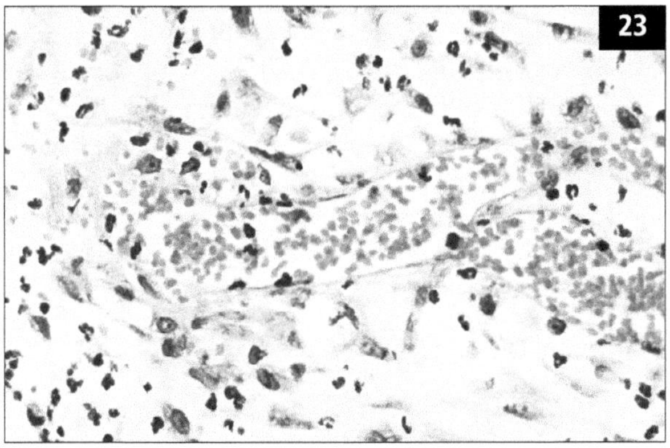

23 Tissue inflammation. Acute inflammation within this section of canine dermis is characterized by hyperaemia, local tissue oedema and extravasation of neutrophils from the vascular lumen. Such changes can result from complement fixation following bacterial infection.

The major end-effects of complement activation are cytolysis, opsonization and inflammation (19–23).

CELLS OF THE IMMUNE SYSTEM

Lymphocytes and plasma cells

The most important immunological cell is the lymphocyte. There are two major subpopulations of lymphocytes (T and B lymphocytes) (24). The majority are small lymphocytes (6–9 μm); these have a large, round nucleus with condensed chromatin and minimal cytoplasm with few organelles. Small lymphocytes may be either T or B cells and they are either immunologically naïve cells ('virgin' cells that have not been previously exposed

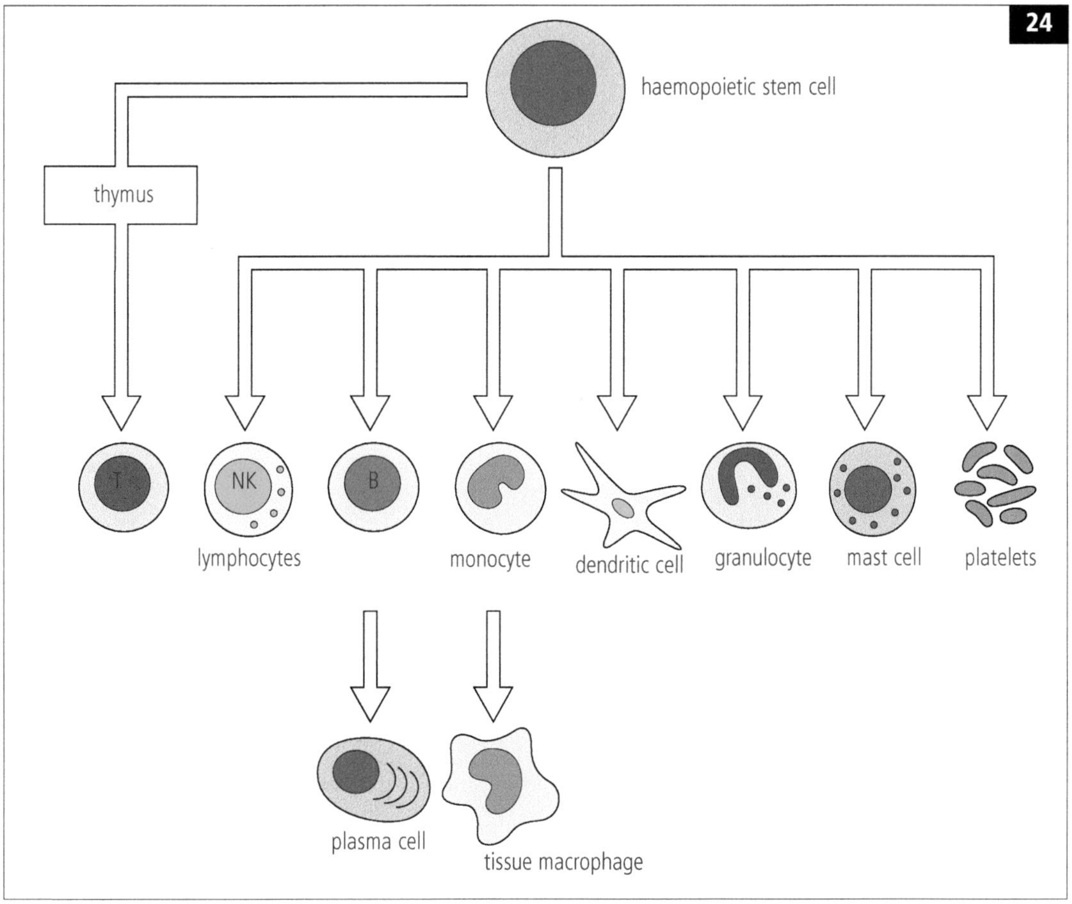

24 Cells of the immune system. All haemopoietic and immunological cells arise from the bone marrow stem cell. Circulating platelets are produced by megakaryocytes. Granulocytes and monocytes exit the circulation into the tissues, where the latter develop into tissue macrophages. Mast cells are found in many tissues. B cells mature in the bone marrow and intestinal tract in mammals, while T cells mature in the thymus. Large granular lymphocytes (NK cells) also likely originate in the bone marrow. Lymphocytes and APCs can recirculate around the body.

to antigen) or memory cells (cells that have previously participated in an antigen-specific immune response). Those T or B lymphocytes that are active in an immune response are present as large lymphocytes or lymphoblasts (12–15 μm), with relatively more cytoplasm and reduced condensation of nuclear chromatin (**25**, **26**). A separate population of large lymphocytes with granular cytoplasm (large granular lymphocytes or natural killer cells [NK]) are recognized.

Plasma cells are an end stage of differentiation of B lymphocytes and are responsible for the synthesis of Ig. These are oval cells (8–18 μm) having an eccentrically placed, round nucleus with linear

25

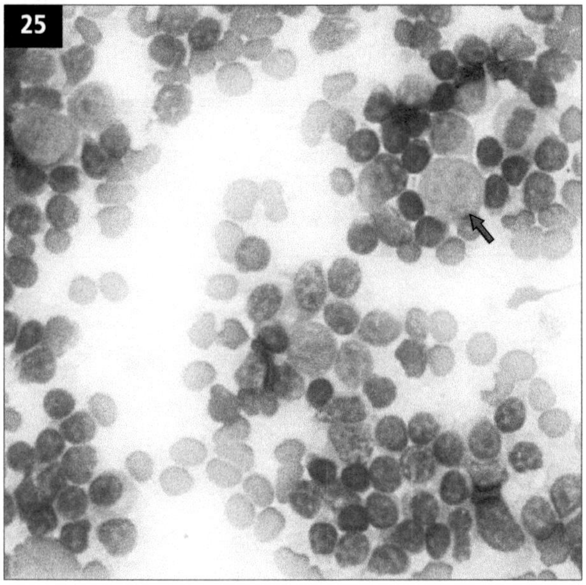

26

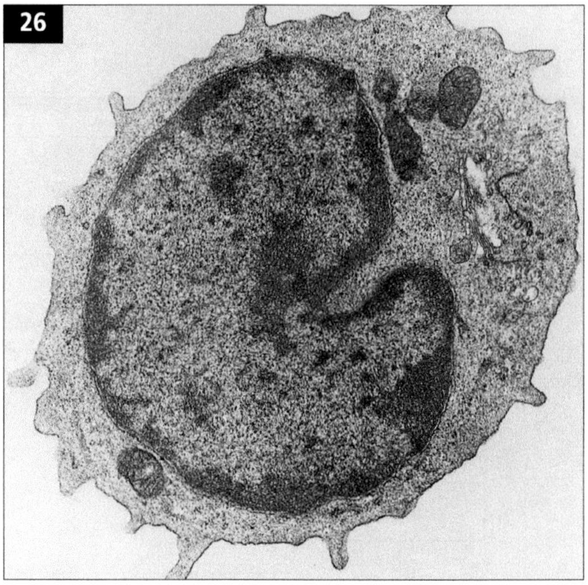

25, 26 Small and large lymphocytes. (**25**) A fine needle aspirate from the lymph node of a dog. The majority of cells are small lymphocytes with a round, basophilic nucleus and a thin rim of pale cytoplasm. A large lymphocyte (lymphoblast) with more cytoplasm and reduced condensation of nuclear chromatin is arrowed. (**26**) Transmission electron micrograph of a canine small lymphocyte. The cell is largely occupied by a rounded nucleus with a small indentation or cleft. The nuclear chromatin is coarsely clumped and there is relatively little cytoplasm and a paucity of organelles.

27

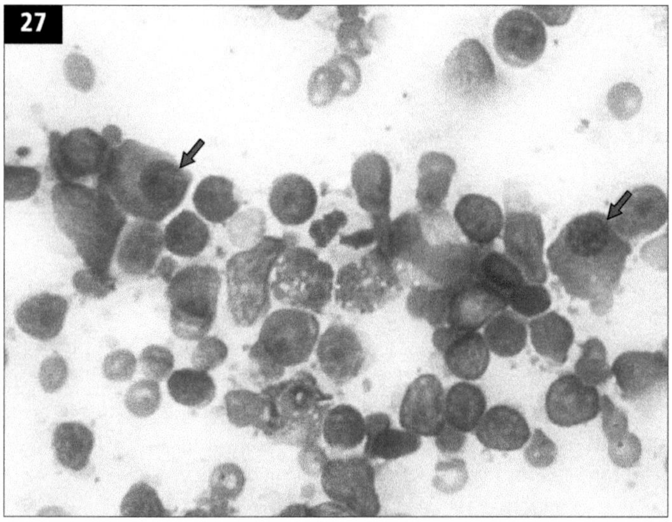

27 Plasma cells. Cytological preparation of a fine needle aspirate from the lymph node of a dog with reactive lymphadenopathy. Two plasma cells (arrowed) are present in addition to several eosinophils. The plasma cells are oval, with an eccentrically placed nucleus with clumped chromatin and a perinuclear 'Golgi zone'.

condensation of chromatin akin to the hands of a clock face. Plasma cells have an abundance of cytoplasmic organelles for protein synthesis, sometimes visible as a perinuclear 'Golgi zone' by light microscopy (27–29).

T and B lymphocytes cannot be distinguished cytologically, but they have different anatomical location (see later), function and expression of surface molecules (phenotype). B lymphocytes and plasma cells are involved in Ig production (humoral immunity), whereas T cells undertake regulatory and cytotoxic functions (cell-mediated immunity [CMI]) and NK cells are cytotoxic (30). T lymphocytes are characterized by expression of

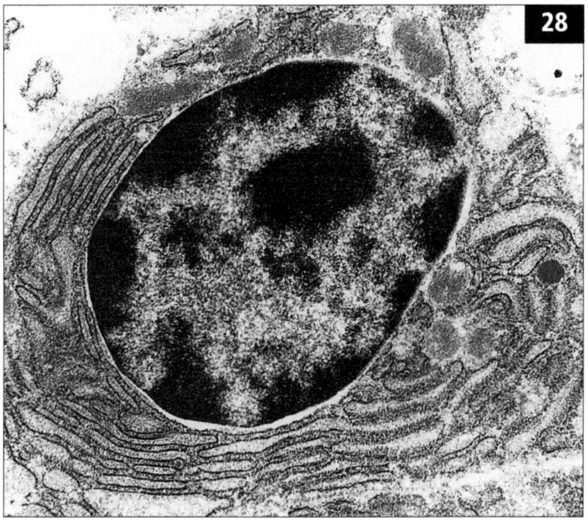

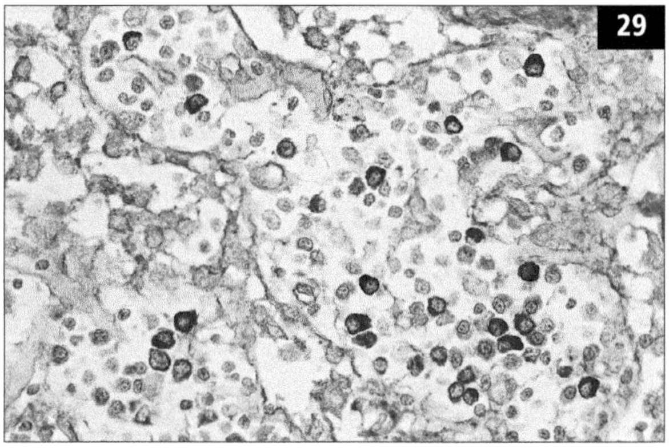

28, 29 Plasma cells. (**28**) Ultrastructure of a feline plasma cell. There is a round nucleus with condensed chromatin and an abundance of cytoplasm enriched with rough endoplasmic reticulum involved in the synthesis of immunoglobulin. (**29**) Section of canine lymph node medullary cord labelled using the immunoperoxidase technique for IgG. The deposition of dark brown chromagen indicates concentration of IgG within the cytoplasm of plasma cells.

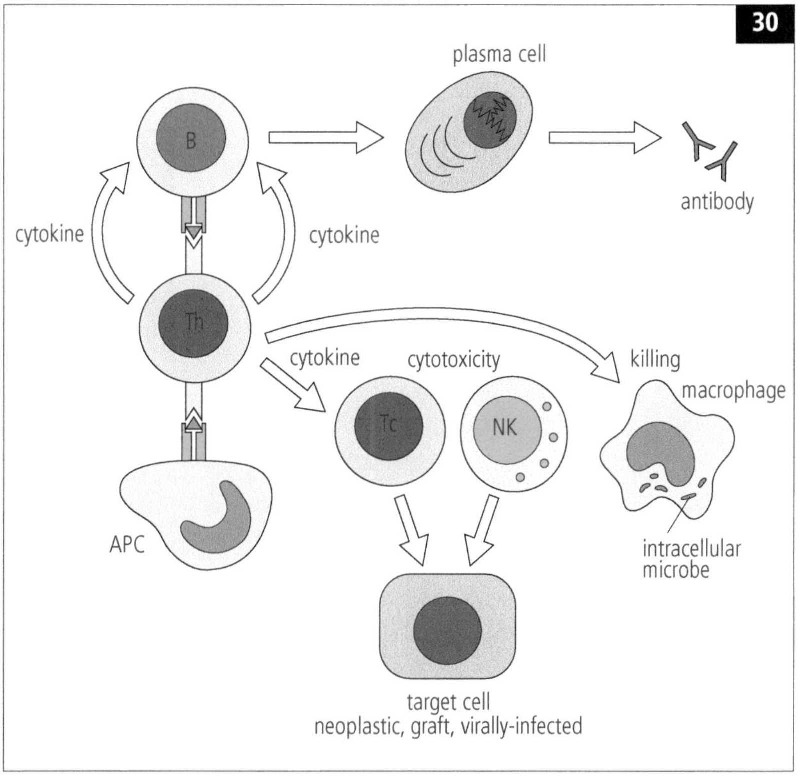

30 Functions of lymphocytes. B lymphocytes transform into plasma cells that produce antibodies, while T helper (Th) cells are stimulated by APCs and B cells to produce cytokines, which regulate immune responses. Macrophages are activated to kill intracellular microorganisms. T cytotoxic (Tc) cells and large granular lymphocytes such as NK cells recognize and kill target cells.

the T cell receptor (TCR) and B lymphocytes have surface membrane immunoglobulin (SmIg) (**31**). A large number of other lymphocyte surface molecules have been identified and some have restricted expression by either T or B lymphocytes. Many of these surface molecules are defined by a 'cluster of differentiation number' (CD number); for example, CD3 is expressed by T lymphocytes and CD79 by B cells.

Antigen presenting cells

Antigen presenting cells (APCs) are crucial to the initiation and perpetuation of immune responses. The classical APCs are macrophages and dendritic

31 amended

31

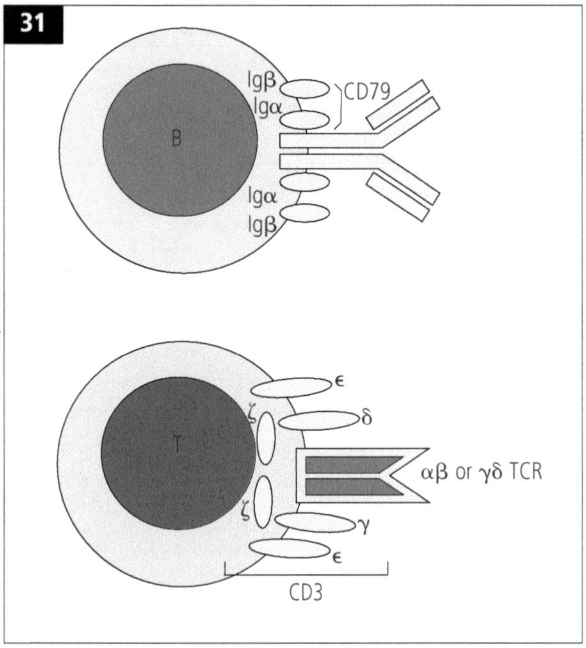

31 Lymphocyte surface molecules. The antigen receptors of T and B cells are derived from a common ancestor and belong to the 'immunoglobulin superfamily'. The B cell Ig receptor consists of two identical heavy and light chains with associated secondary components (CD79). Circulating antibodies are similar, except that they lack the transmembrane and intracytoplasmic regions. The T cell receptor has an antigen-binding portion consisting of α and β (or δ and γ) chains that are associated with a series of other transmembrane molecules (CD3). Each lymphocyte has large numbers of identical receptors in addition to numerous other surface molecules.

32

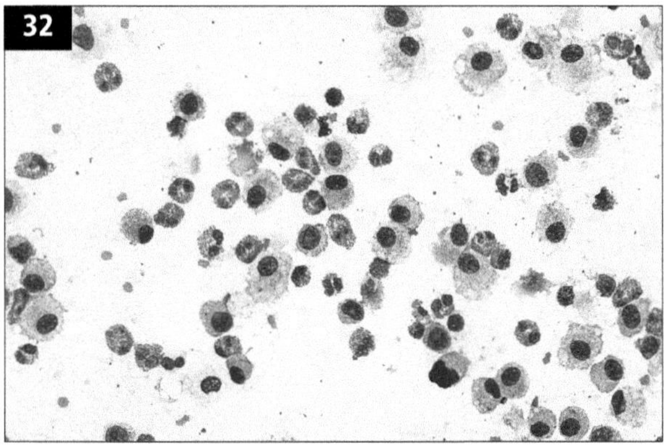

33

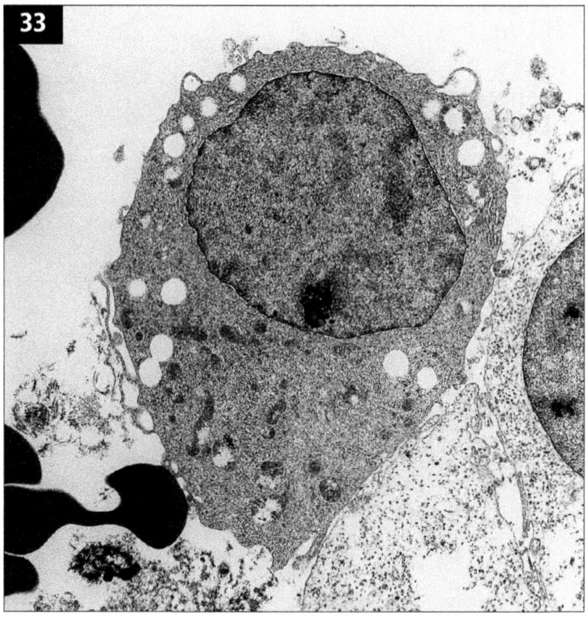

32, 33 Macrophages. (**32**) Cytological preparation of bronchiolar alveolar lavage fluid from a cat, containing numerous macrophages with abundant, sometimes vacuolated, cytoplasm and an oval nucleus. (**33**) Ultrastructure of a canine macrophage. There is a relatively large amount of cytoplasm, with numerous organelles and cytoplasmic vacuoles.

cells (often collectively referred to as 'histiocytes'), which derive from a common $CD34^+$ bone marrow precursor; however, B lymphocytes are also able to function in this manner and other 'non-professional' APCs (e.g. epithelial and endothelial cells) may be recruited in certain circumstances. Blood monocytes differentiate to tissue macrophages (15–30 μm), which, when activated, have abundant, often vacuolated cytoplasm and a bean-shaped nucleus (32–37). Macrophages are most effective at phagocytosis of particulate antigen or pathogens.

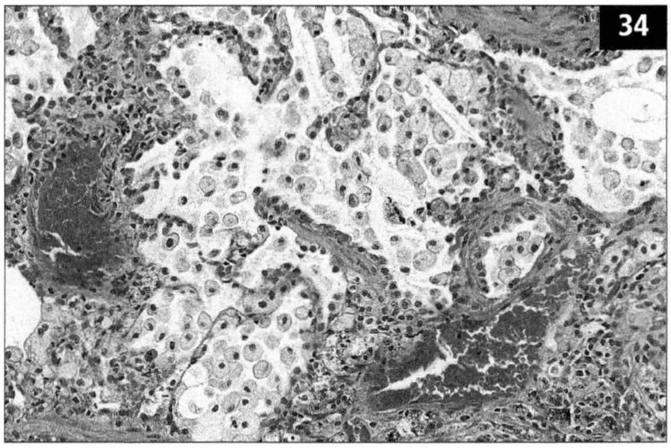
34

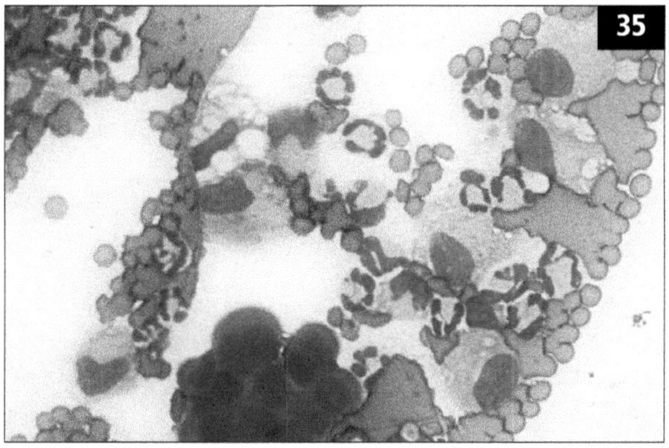
35

34, 35 Macrophages. (**34**) Section of lung from a dog. Large numbers of alveolar macrophages with abundant foamy cytoplasm are seen within the alveolar spaces. (**35**) Abdominal fluid from a cat with feline infectious peritonitis. There are numerous large macrophages with abundant, finely vacuolated cytoplasm, together with neutrophils and a cluster of darkly staining mesothelial cells.

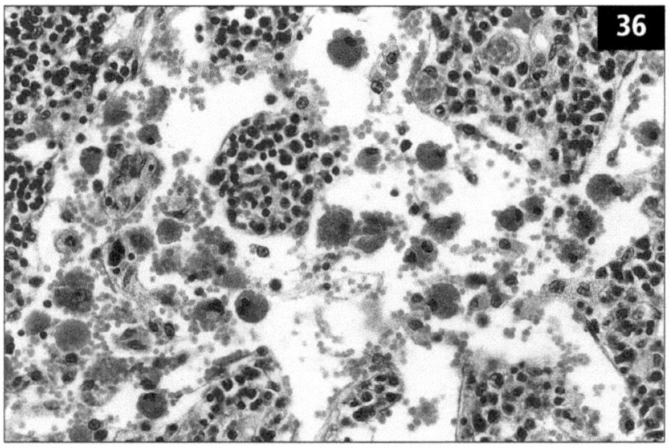
36

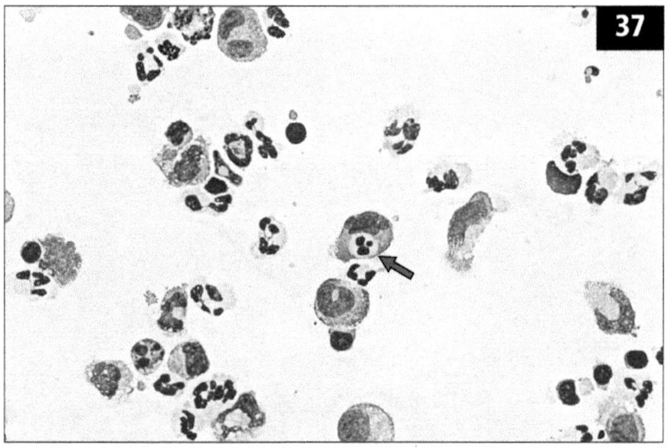
37

36, 37 Macrophage phagocytosis. (**36**) Macrophages within the medullary sinuses of this feline lymph node have phagocytosed numerous erythrocytes following local haemorrhage. (**37**) Macrophages within a sample of abdominal (ascitic) fluid from a cat contain cytoplasmic nuclear debris. These cells have phagocytosed degenerate neutrophils (arrow), which are also present in the preparation.

A family of myeloid dendritic cells is involved in the initial processing and translocation of antigen (**38**). Dendritic cells are generally characterized by the presence of long cytoplasmic projections, giving them a stellate appearance, but occasionally they project large sheets or 'veils' (veiled dendritic cells). Myeloid dendritic cells are widespread in the tissues as Langerhans cells (which localize to the epidermis and express the adhesion molecule E-cadherin in addition to CD1, CD11c and MHC class II) (**39**), dermal dendritic cells or interstitial dendritic cells (which have phenotypic expression of CD1, CD11c, MHC class II and CD90) within viscera. It is suggested that such cells transform morphologically to the veiled type when migrating in afferent lymph to lymph nodes and then become

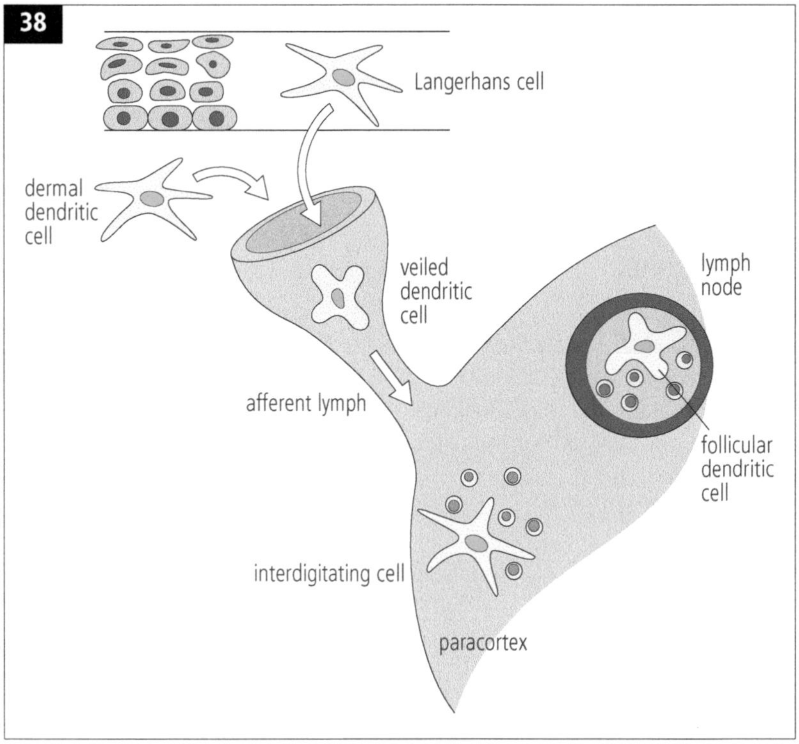

38 The dendritic cell family. Dendritic cells are bone marrow-derived APCs that are found throughout the body and are represented in the skin by the epidermal Langerhans cells. These cells have abundant MHC class II expression and are believed to carry antigens and migrate via the afferent lymphatics (where they appear as 'veiled' cells) into the paracortex of the draining lymph node. Here they interdigitate with T lymphocytes and present antigen to these cells. Presentation to B lymphocytes is by follicular dendritic cells, which are found in the germinal centres of the lymph nodes.

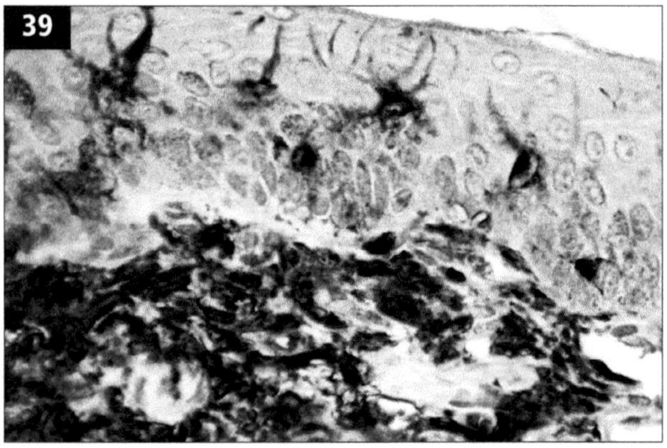

39 Epidermal Langerhans cells. Section of skin from a Japanese Akita dog with uveodermatolgical syndrome labelled by the immunoperoxidase technique for MHC class II. The stellate Langerhans cells are clearly visible within the epidermis and the dermal inflammatory infiltrate includes a population of MHC class II-positive cells. (From Carter J, Crispin SM, Gould DJ *et al.* (2005) An immunohistochemical study of uveodermatologic syndrome in two Japanese Akita dogs. *Veterinary Ophthalmology* **8**:17–24, with permission.) Feline Langerhans cells also express class II in addition to the CD4 molecule.

interdigitating dendritic cells within lymphoid tissue. In some species a distinct lineage of plasmacytoid dendritic cells has been described within lymphoid tissue, but these cells have not yet been recognized in companion animals. The ultrastructure and phenotype of feline dendritic cells has been particularly well defined and feline (but not canine) Langerhans cells contain cytoplasmic Birbeck's granules.

Granulocytes and mast cells

Other white blood cells (WBCs) (neutrophils, eosinophils, basophils and mast cells) have important roles in the immune response.

Neutrophils

Neutrophils (40, 41) may be considered part of the innate immune system and they are the key cells in the early stages of an inflammatory response. Neutrophils are formed within the bone marrow and released to the circulation, where they circulate for a short time (approximately ten hours) before entering tissues. Here, they survive for only a few days before undergoing apoptosis. In response to tissue damage or the presence of infectious agents, neutrophils are rapidly attracted into affected tissue, where they may engulf particulate material by phagocytosis. The process of phagocytosis may be enhanced by the interaction of particle opsonins (Ig and/or complement) with neutrophil membrane receptors, as described in the preceding section on complement. Phagocytosed particles are contained within cytoplasmic compartments (phagosomes), which fuse with cytoplasmic azurophilic and specific granules to form a phagolysosome. Within this compartment, the phagocytosed material is exposed to a range of degradative enzymes (e.g. lysozyme, acid hydrolases, neutral proteases and cationic proteins). Specific granules may also fuse with the cell membrane, resulting in extracellular release of their contents; this causes tissue damage and regional inflammation. Reactive oxygen intermediates generated by oxygen consumption during phagocytosis (the 'respiratory burst') may also damage phagocytosed material and be released to surrounding tissues and contribute to tissue damage. Finally, neutrophils may release arachadonic acid metabolites that may further enhance inflammation.

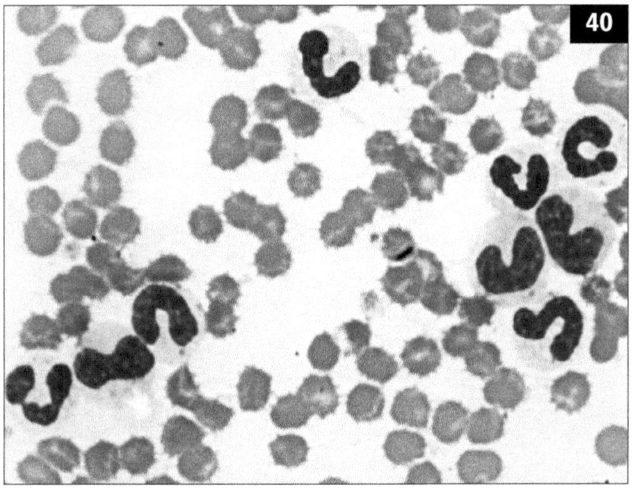

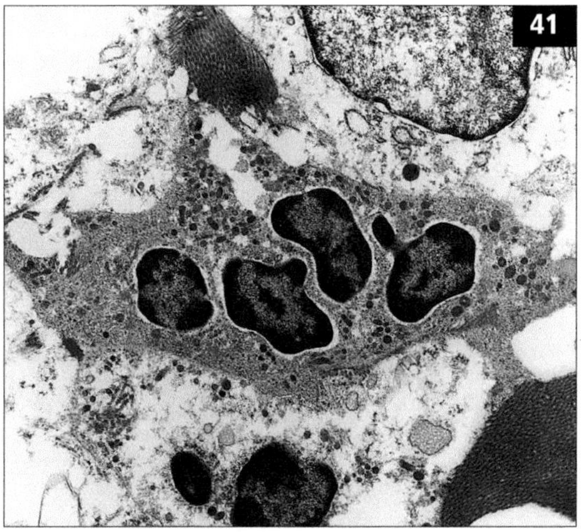

40, 41 Neutrophils. (**40**) Blood smear from a dog with left shift neutrophilia. A range of developmental stages is present, including metamyelocytes, band and segmented neutrophils. (**41**) Transmission electron micrograph of a feline neutrophil. The lobulated nucleus appears in several portions.

Eosinophils

Eosinophils (42, 43) also have a major role in inflammation and are selectively recruited into the sites of particular types of immune response (see Chapter 2, p. 62). The cytoplasmic granules of eosinophils contain a range of enzymes similar to those within neutrophils, but with the addition of other degradative and oxidative proteins (e.g. major basic protein, eosinophil cationic protein, eosinophil peroxidase, eosinophil-derived neurotoxin) and antiinflammatory enzymes (e.g. histaminase, kinase). Circulating eosinophils are relatively fewer in number than neutrophils, but these cells are readily mobilized from bone marrow. Eosinophils have limited ability to phagocytose particles, but they may damage larger targets (e.g. parasites) by extracellular degranulation following interaction between antibody or complement-coated target and eosinophil Fcγ, Fcε or C3b receptors. They are able to contribute to an inflammatory response, but there is debate as to whether these cells may also modulate such responses by counteracting the products released from mast cells.

Mast cells

Mast cells (44, 45) are widespread throughout the connective tissues and are particularly prominent at mucosal surfaces. They function in a similar manner to circulating basophils (but form a distinct lineage to basophils, with a poorly characterized circulating precursor) and the cytoplasmic granules of these cells contain a potent array of inflammatory mediators (described fully in Chapter 2). Studies in the dog and cat suggest that subtypes of mast cell may exist, as is the case for other species. Three canine mast cell subtypes have been defined: those that express tryptase, those that

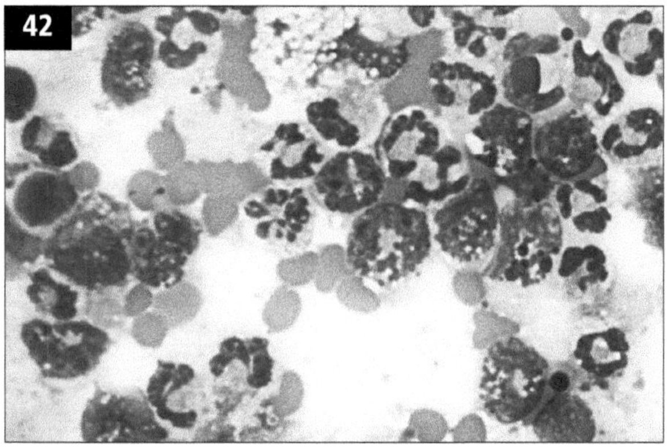

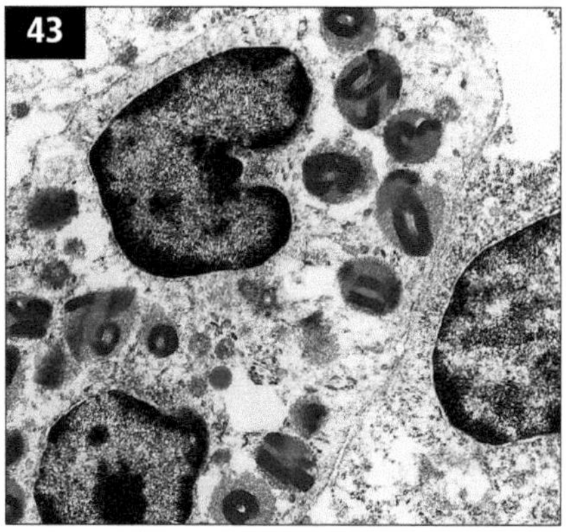

42, 43 Eosinophils. (**42**) Bronchiolar-alveolar lavage fluid from a dog with parasitic respiratory disease. Numerous eosinophils are present in the sample, which also includes neutrophils and vacuolated macrophages. (**43**) Transmission electron micrograph of a feline eosinophil with prominent cytoplasmic granules.

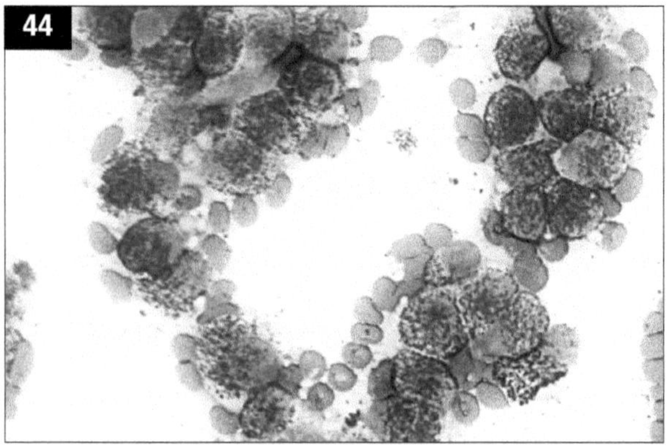

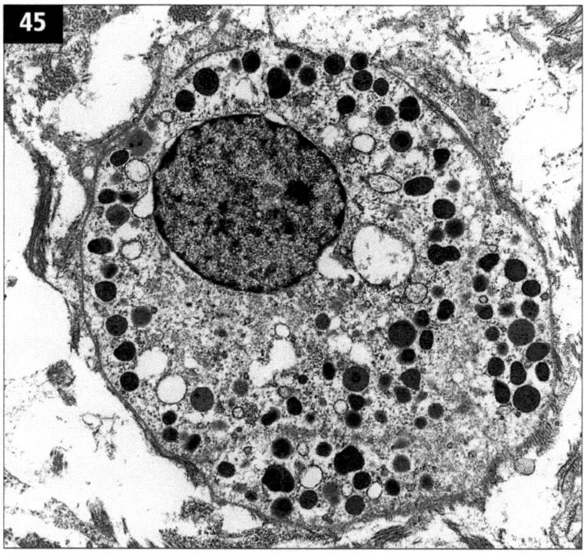

44, 45 Mast cells. (**44**) Fine needle aspirate from a canine cutaneous mast cell tumour. There is prominent granularity of the cytoplasm in this well-differentiated population. (**45**) Transmission electron micrograph of a feline mast cell with prominent cytoplasmic granules.

express chymase, and those that express both of these proteases. A range of stimuli may cause mast cell degranulation. In addition to cross-linking of surface IgE or IgG (see Chapter 2, p. 62) and binding of anaphylotoxins (see Complement), degranulation may be induced by physical stimuli (e.g. cold, trauma), neuropeptides or cytokines. The inflammatory effects of mast cell degranulation include vasodilation, tissue oedema, smooth muscle spasm, leukocyte chemoattraction, mucus secretion, tissue damage and anticoagulation.

TISSUES OF THE IMMUNE SYSTEM

Immune system tissues may be considered as primary (sites of development and maturation of lymphoid cells) or secondary (sites where mature lymphocytes may participate in an immune response). In mammals the primary lymphoid organs are the bone marrow and thymus. All haemopoietic and immunological cells arise from a common bone marrow stem cell (**46, 47**). B lymphocytes undergo development in the bone marrow and intestinal tract, whereas immature T cells are exported to the thymus (**48–50**) for final maturation. Secondary lymphoid tissue may be divided into encapsulated or unencapsulated forms. Encapsulated tissues include the lymph node (**51–55**) and spleen (**56–58**), and unencapsulated tissue is associated with mucosal (Peyer's patch, tonsil) and cutaneous surfaces (**59–66**).

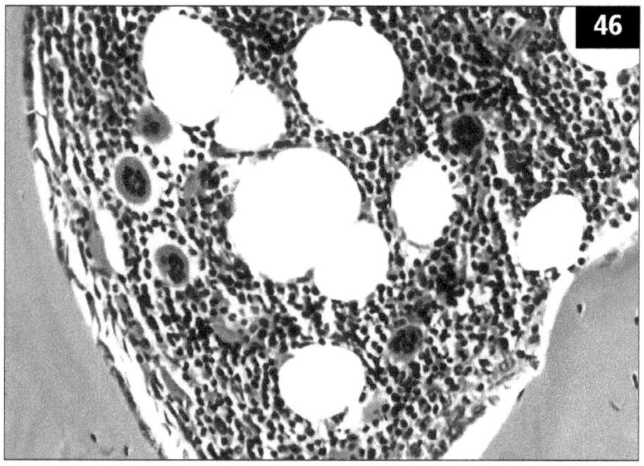

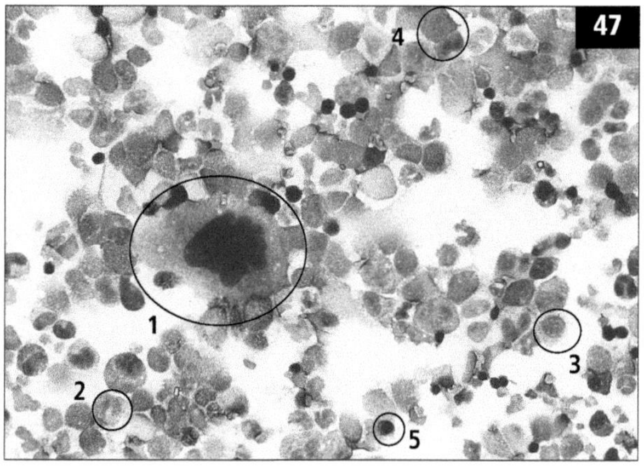

46, 47 Bone marrow. (**46**) Section of normal canine femoral bone marrow. Megakaryocytes are clearly seen. (**47**) Fine needle aspirate of canine bone marrow demonstrating various haemopoietic lineages. Indicated are a megakaryocyte (1), metamyelocyte (2), eosinophil promyelocyte (3), blast cell (4) and metarubricyte (5).

48 Structure of the thymus. The thymus is an encapsulated organ divided into lobules by septa. The cortex contains densely packed, dividing lymphocytes in a network of epithelial cells extending into the medulla. The medulla contains fewer lymphocytes but more APCs (interdigitating dendritic cells and macrophages). Developing lymphocytes are closely associated with epithelia and APCs. The whorled epithelial Hassall's corpuscles may produce cytokines that influence dendritic cell selection of lymphoid populations.

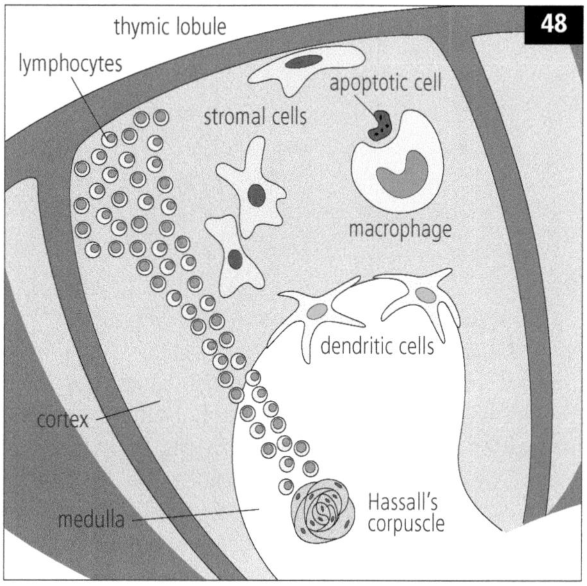

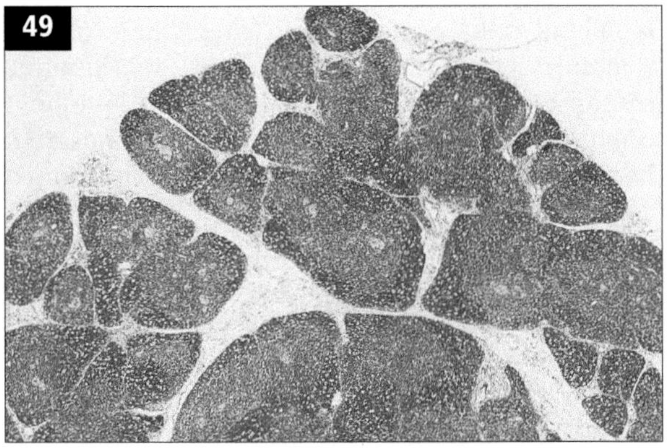

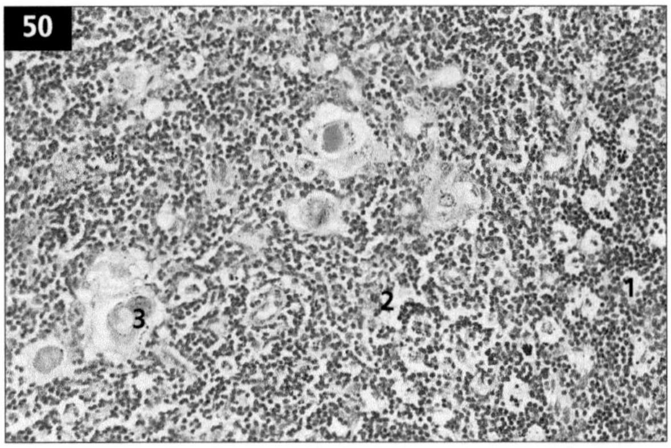

49, 50 Thymus. (**49**) Normal canine thymus. Low power view demonstrates the lobular structure of the tissue. The thymus is encapsulated and each lobule is delineated by a band of connective tissue. (**50**) High power view of a thymic lobule. The lymphocytes within the cortex (1) are more densely packed than in the medulla (2). Apoptotic thymocytes are removed by phagocytic cells, seen as a clear space within the cortex. The position of Hassall's corpuscles (3) is indicated.

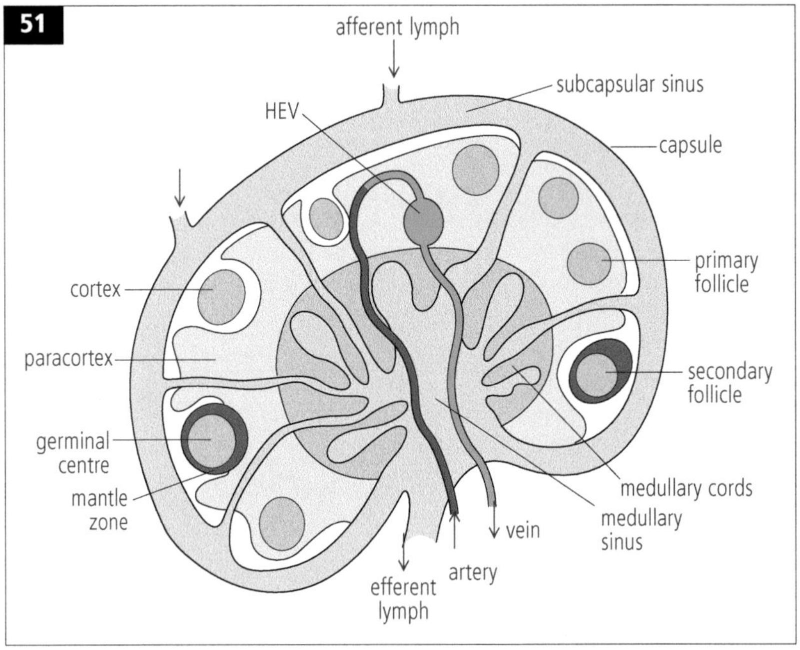

51 Structure of the lymph node. The lymph node has a connective tissue capsule with an underlying subcapsular sinus. Lymphocytes, APCs and antigens from nearby tissue or adjacent lymph nodes drain into the sinus via the afferent lymphatics. The cortex contains aggregates of B lymphocytes (primary follicles) which, when stimulated, become secondary follicles with a site of active proliferation (germinal centre) surrounded by a mantle zone. The paracortex contains mainly T lymphocytes, and APCs are found throughout. There is an arterial and venous blood supply; lymphocytes may also enter the node from the bloodstream via specialized high endothelial venules (HEVs) in the paracortex. The medulla contains T and B cells, as well as numerous plasma cells within the medullary cords. Lymphocytes leave the lymph node via efferent lymphatics.

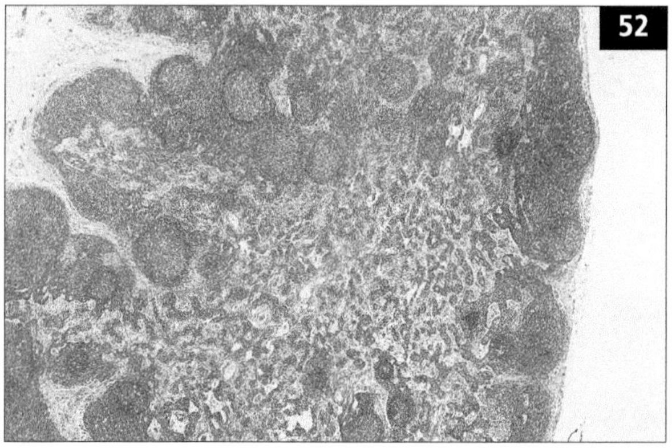

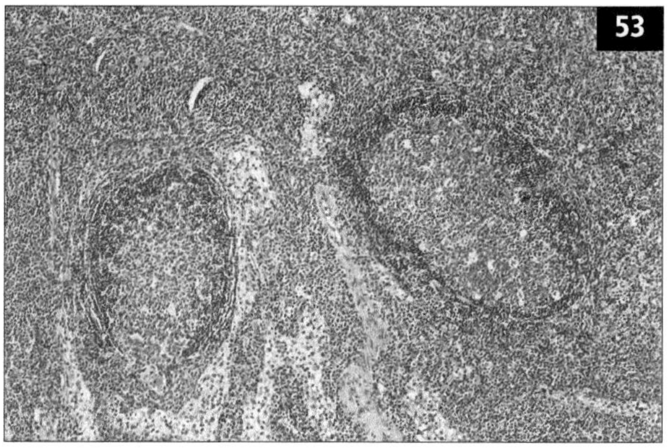

52, 53 Lymph node. (**52**) Cross-section of canine lymph node. The cortex contains prominent lymphoid follicles (B cells) and surrounding paracortex (T cells). The medullary sinuses are crossed by medullary cords of mixed lymphoid cells, particularly plasma cells. (**53**) Secondary follicles within the cortex of a canine lymph node. The actively proliferating blast cells within the germinal centre are surrounded by a mantle zone of small lymphocytes.

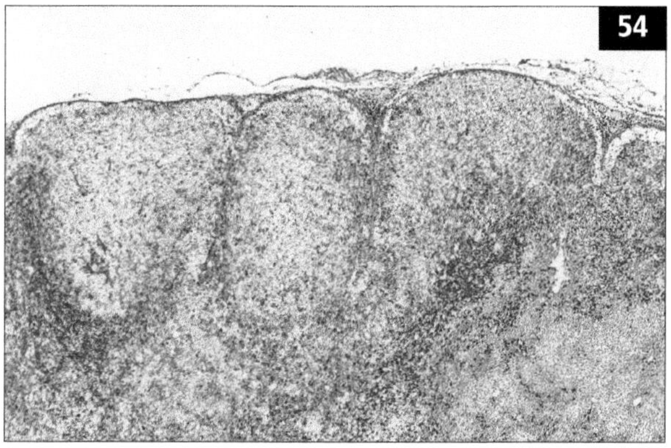

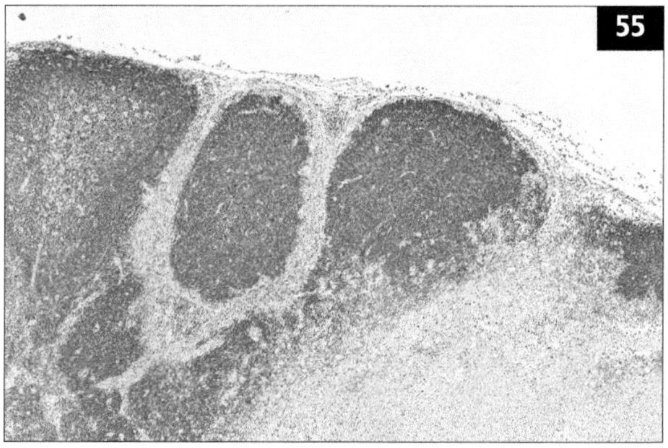

54, 55 T and B cell areas of the lymph node. Serial sections of feline lymph node labelled by the avidin-biotin immunoperoxidase technique using antiserum against T lymphocytes (anti-CD3) (**54**) and B lymphocytes (anti-CD79) (**55**). The localization of B cells to cortical follicles, and T cells to the intervening paracortex, can be seen clearly.

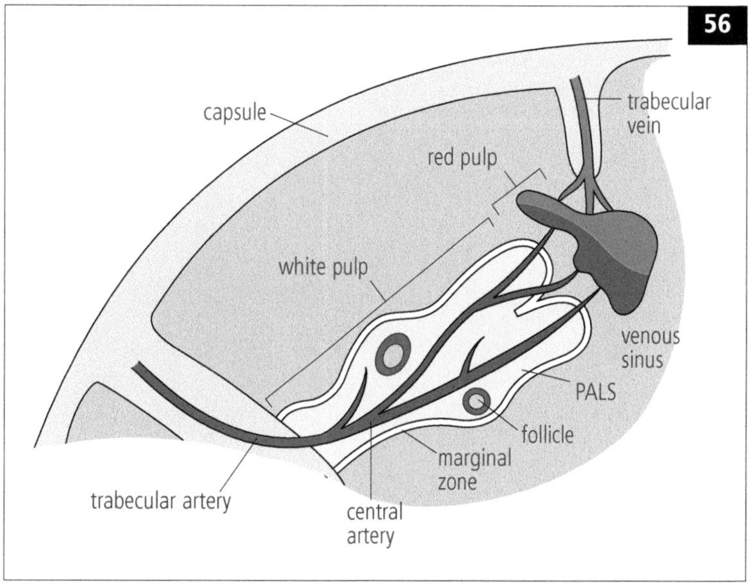

56 Structure of the spleen. The splenic white pulp consists of the periarteriolar lymphoid sheaths (PALS) (T cell area), which may contain lymphoid follicles (B cell area). The white pulp is surrounded by a narrow marginal zone that contains a mixture of macrophages and other APCs, B cells and NK cells. The red pulp contains venous sinuses separated by splenic cords. Blood enters the splenic tissue via the trabecular arteries, which branch into the central arteries. These latter may end in the white pulp or marginal zones. Some arterial branches terminate in the red pulp, where blood drains into the venous circulation. The dog has a sinusal spleen with well-developed vascular sinuses lined by endothelial cells, whereas the cat spleen is considered non-sinusal, having poorly developed sinuses. The spleen has no afferent lymphatic input.

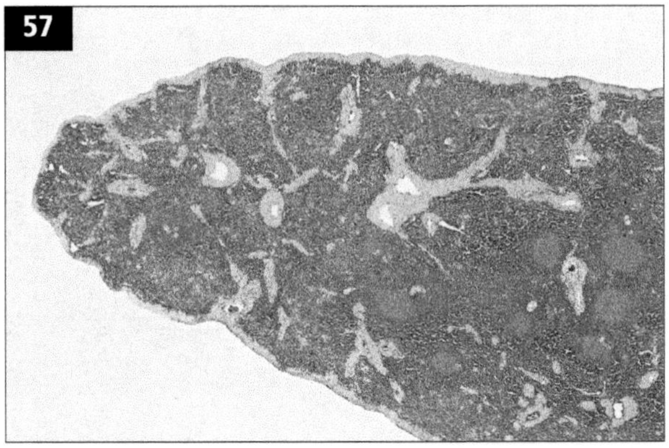

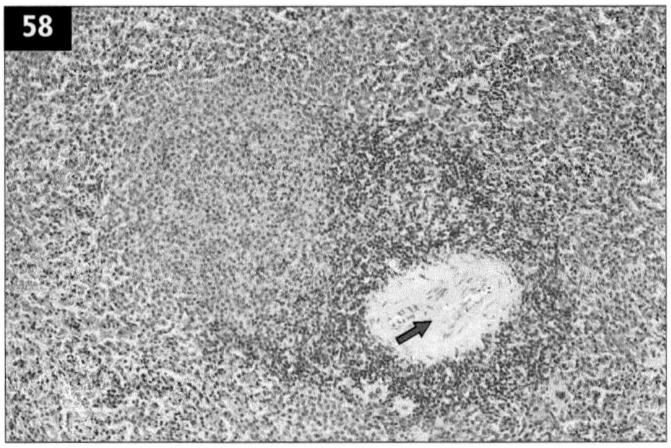

57, 58 The spleen. (**57**) Low power view of the canine spleen. The connective tissue capsule and trabeculae are prominent and foci of white pulp are scattered throughout the predominant red pulp. (**58**) Splenic white pulp. The periarteriolar lymphoid sheath of T lymphocytes (arteriole arrowed) is associated with a peripheral nodular aggregate of proliferating blast cells that are likely B lymphocytes.

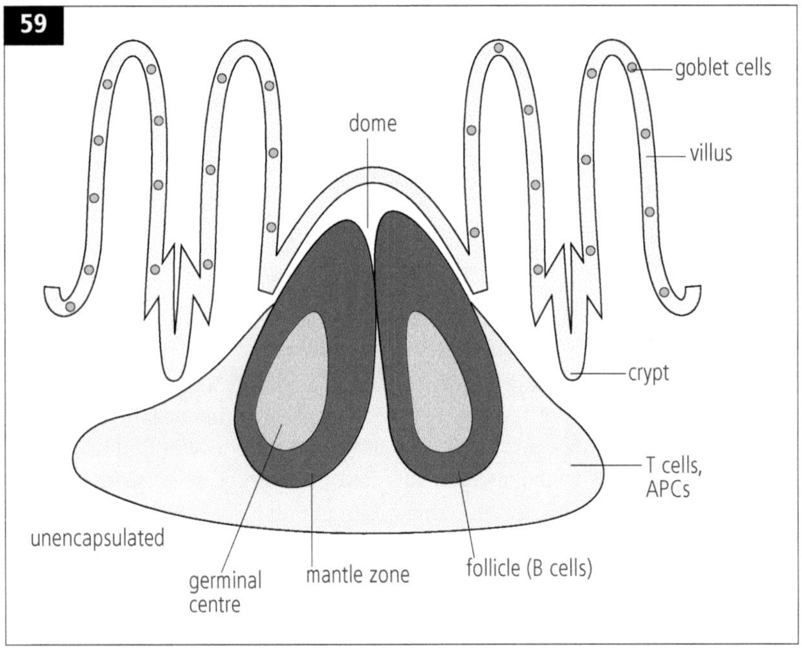

59 Structure of the Peyer's patch. Peyer's patches are found along the length of the small intestine and are an example of unencapsulated, mucosa-associated lymphoid tissue. The overlying villus structure may be distorted by prominent follicular aggregates of B lymphocytes, with surrounding populations of T cells and APCs. The lymphoid aggregates may form a dome-shaped area that abuts the overlying enterocytes. The dome epithelium contains specialized antigen-capturing cells (M cells), and there are fewer goblet cells. These M (microfold) cells absorb and transfer (and possibly process) luminal antigen to underlying immunological populations.

text removed

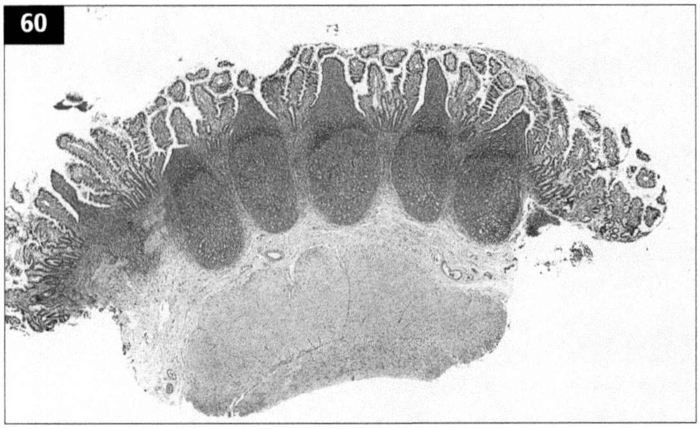

60 Peyer's patches. Low power view of a Peyer's patch in the small intestine of a dog. The region is unencapsulated and consists of a series of prominent secondary follicles with intervening lymphoid tissue, extending into the superficial lamina propria as 'dome' areas.

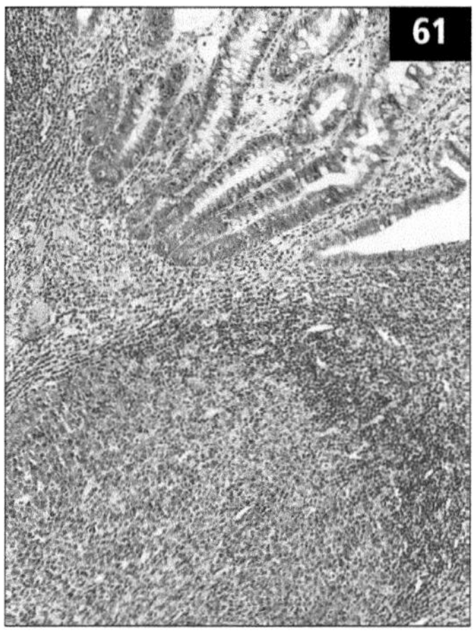

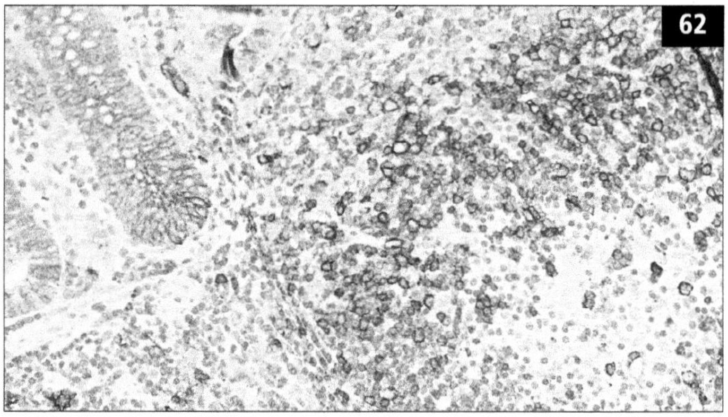

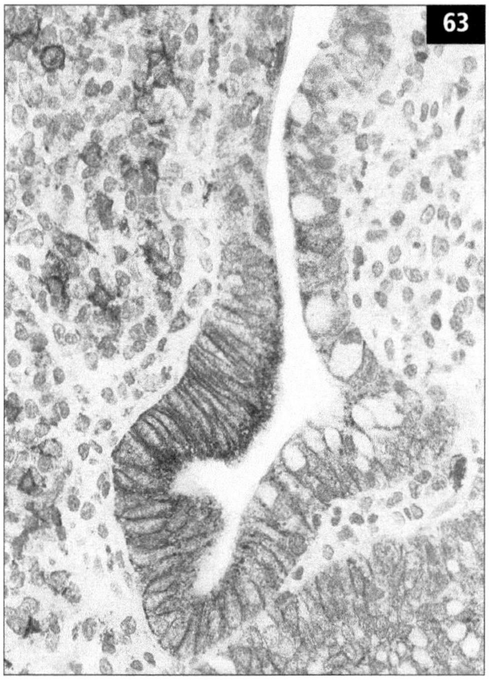

61–63 Peyer's patches (**61**)The Peyer's patch follicle has a germinal centre of proliferating blast cells and a mantle zone of small lymphocytes. A mixture of cell types (predominantly T cells) will be found in the intervening areas. (**62, 63**) Section of canine small intestine including Peyer's patch labelled for MHC class II. There is expression of class II by cells forming the follicular mantle and by adjacent crypt enterocytes.

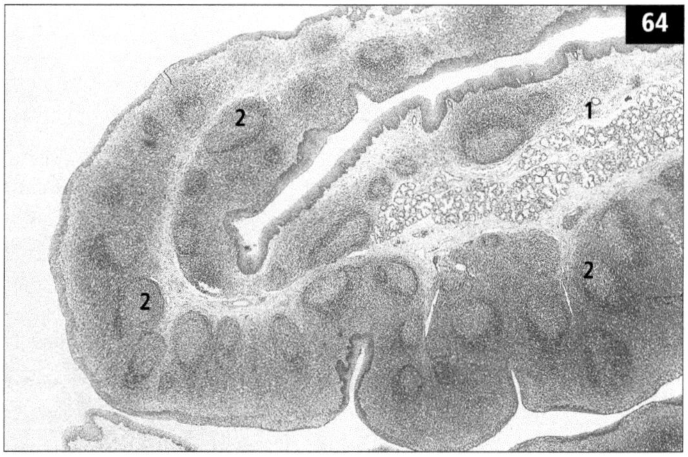

64 Canine tonsil. Section of tonsil from a dog. The overlying squamous epithelium is folded to form a tonsilar fossula. Salivary tissue (1) and active lymphoid follicles (2) are indicated.

65 Canine gastric lymphoid follicle. Gastric lymphoid aggregates are located within the mucosa of the stomach of the cat and dog. These follicles have distinct T and B cell areas.

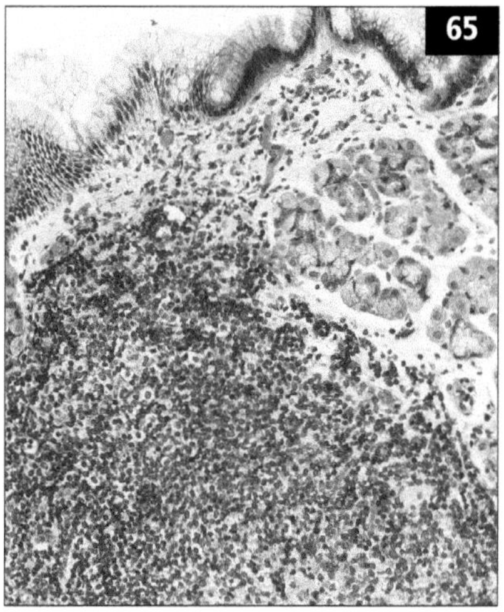

66

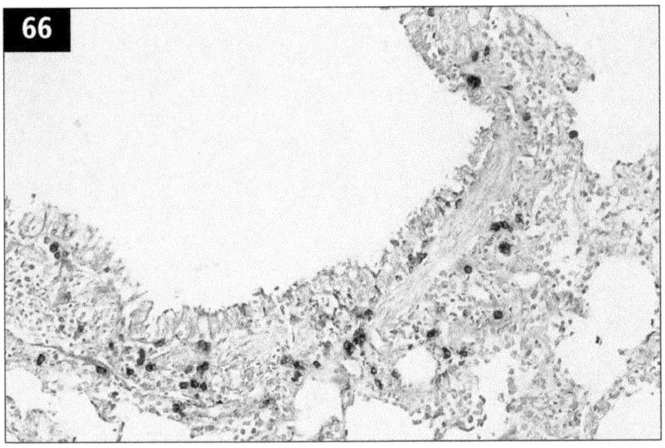

66 Bronchial-associated lymphoid tissue. Section of lung from a dog labelled by the immunoperoxidase technique for canine IgA. Plasma cells with cytoplasmic IgA are seen in close apposition to the bronchial mucosa. The dog appears to lack the well-developed and organized BALT that is found in other species.

67

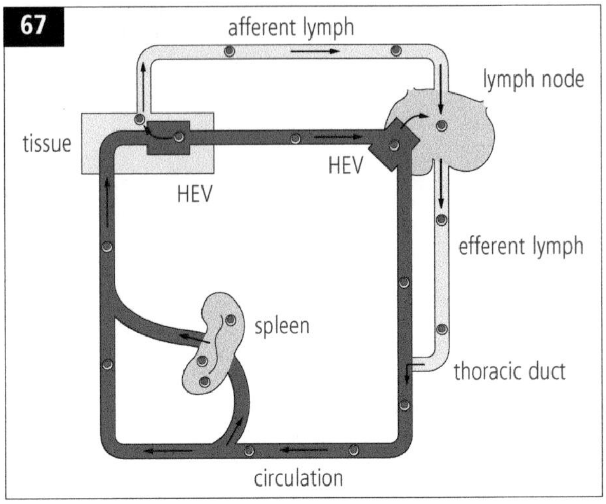

67 Lymphocyte recirculation pathways. The lymphocytes of the immune system have wide access to body tissues by the ability to migrate in blood and lymphatic vessels. Lymphocytes enter the lymph node from the tissues via the afferent lymph or from the circulation via the specialized endothelial cells of post-capillary venules (HEVs). They leave the lymph node by the efferent vessels and pass through other lymph nodes, finally entering the thoracic duct, which drains into the circulation. Lymphocytes may then leave the circulation at HEVs within inflamed tissue, or they may pass into the white pulp of the spleen and from there to the red pulp sinuses and back to the circulation.

LYMPHOCYTE RECIRCULATION

Lymphocytes actively recirculate in great numbers throughout the body via blood and lymphatic vessels (67), enabling all sites of the body to be patrolled (immune surveillance). Such recirculation is necessary, as all lymphocytes have a unique pre-programmed specificity for antigen, which may only be encountered at particular anatomical locations. Initial contact with antigen is most likely to occur within regional lymphoid tissue draining the source of antigen. Following antigen recognition, stimulated lymphocytes are clonally expanded to create large numbers of antigen-specific cells, which must migrate back to the site of antigen deposition to effect the local immune response. Recirculation must have specificity to enable the clonally expanded cells to identify the particular sites of inflammation or infection where they encountered antigen, and to enter the tissues at these points. This is achieved by the presence of modified vascular endothelium (high endothelial venules [HEVs]) at such sites (and within some normal lymphoid tissues), which causes local turbulence and margination of WBCs within the vascular flow. A complex array of adhesion molecules on the HEVs and their ligands on the lymphocyte surface enables binding and local diapedesis only of those populations that have direct relevance (specificity) for the inflammatory process within the tissue (68–70). Several families of leukocyte adhesion molecules are recognized (selectins, mucin-like vascular addressins, integrins, some members of the Ig superfamily), and these mediate the egress of leukocytes from vessels. In addition to the adhesion molecules, migration of leukocytes into tissue is mediated by the family of chemoattractant low molecular weight proteins, collectively known as chemokines. These molecules establish chemotactic gradients within tissue to direct leukocyte recruitment in a similar fashion to the complement proteins described above. Over 50 chemokine molecules are now recognized and they mainly fall into one of two subfamilies, defined

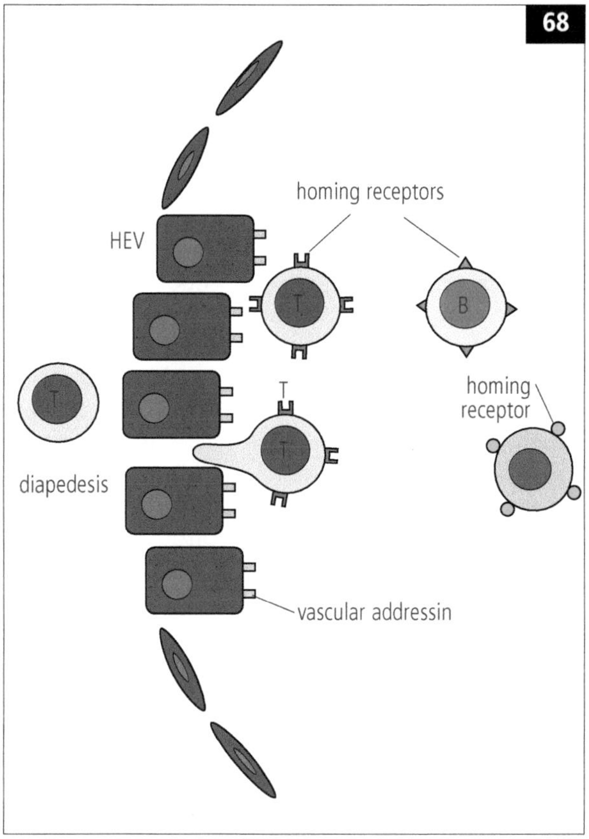

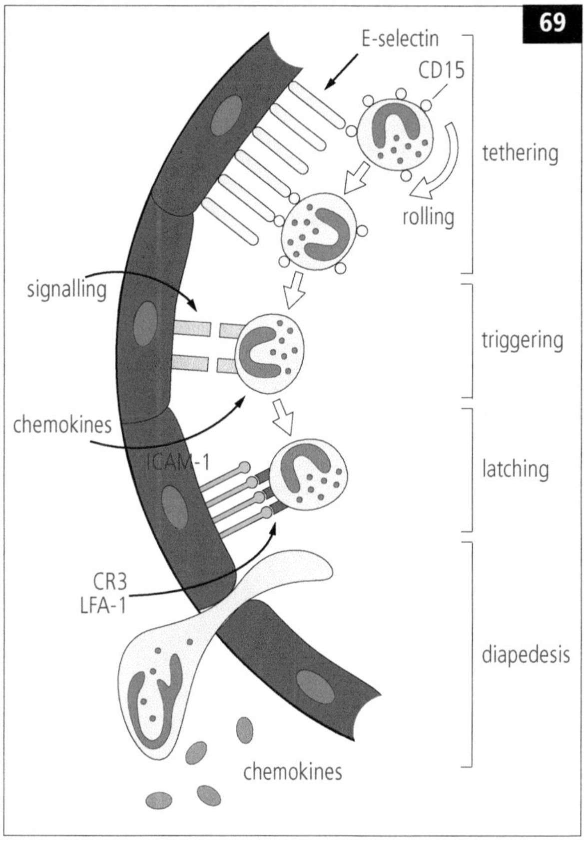

68–69 Leukocyte–endothelial interactions. (**68**) The modified HEVs are found within some normal lymphoid tissues and at sites of tissue inflammation. Low shear forces within the venule permit leukocyte adhesion to endothelium and subsequent diapedesis between endothelial cells into the tissue. HEVs express a range of site-specific adhesion molecules (collectively referred to as 'vascular addressins'), which interact with specific ligands on the surface of particular leukocytes (collectively known as 'homing receptors'). Not all leukocytes express homing receptors that will allow extravasation at a particular site. (**69**) The process of leukocyte adhesion involves a series of stages. During tethering the leukocyte is slowed down by molecular interactions (e.g. E-selectin and CD15) and rolls along the endothelial surface, making and breaking contact as this binding is insufficient to counteract the shearing force of blood flow. The second stage involves signalling events mediated by surface molecules or chemokines (e.g. IL-8) that upregulate and trigger conformational changes in leukocyte integrins that bind to endothelial ICAM-1. The leukocyte is now firmly attached, and further molecular interactions mediate diapedesis across the endothelium.

70 Leukocyte–endothelial interactions. The migration of neutrophils from bloodstream to inflamed tissue can be seen in this section of canine skin.

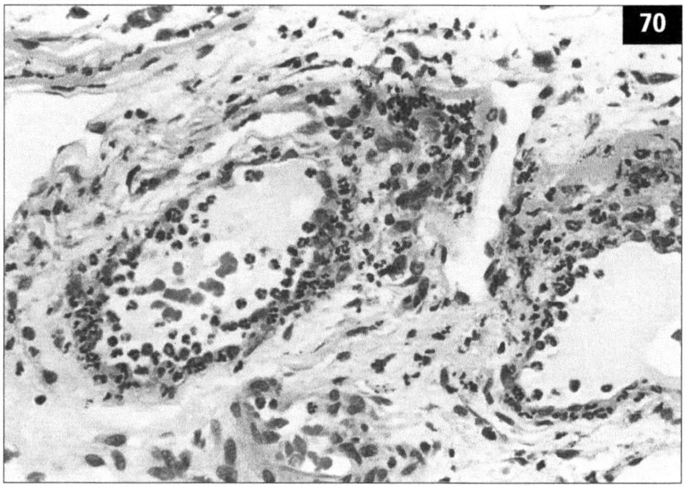

structurally. The CXC chemokines act primarily on neutrophils, whereas CC chemokines act on monocytes, lymphocytes and eosinophils. Chemokines bind to specific chemokine receptors, but several chemokines might share a single receptor type. A number of chemokines and chemokine receptors have now been defined in the dog and cat, primarily at the molecular level (71).

Various levels of lymphocyte recirculation are recognized. For example, the extent of lymphocyte recirculation may vary with the stage of lymphocyte activation (72) and lymphocytes may circulate preferentially between mucosal sites via the common mucosal system (73).

THE MAJOR HISTOCOMPATIBILITY COMPLEX

Histocompatibility antigens are cell-surface molecules that are responsible for the phenomenon of graft rejection (see Chapter 16, p. 408). There are two major classes of such molecules, which differ in structure and distribution (74). Class I histocompatibility antigens are found on all nucleated cells of the body, whereas class II histocompatibility antigens are normally found only on cells of the immune system (B cells, macrophages, dendritic cells) but may be expressed by other cells (e.g. epithelial, endothelial) within inflammatory lesions. Unlike other species, canine and feline T cells constitutively express class II molecules, and puppies develop this expression within the first weeks of life. Within histocompatibility molecules there are areas of variable and constant amino acid sequence, and as the constant domains have homology with the Ig Fc region, these molecules are considered part of the evolutionarily conserved 'immunoglobulin superfamily' that also includes CD4, CD8 and the T cell receptor.

71

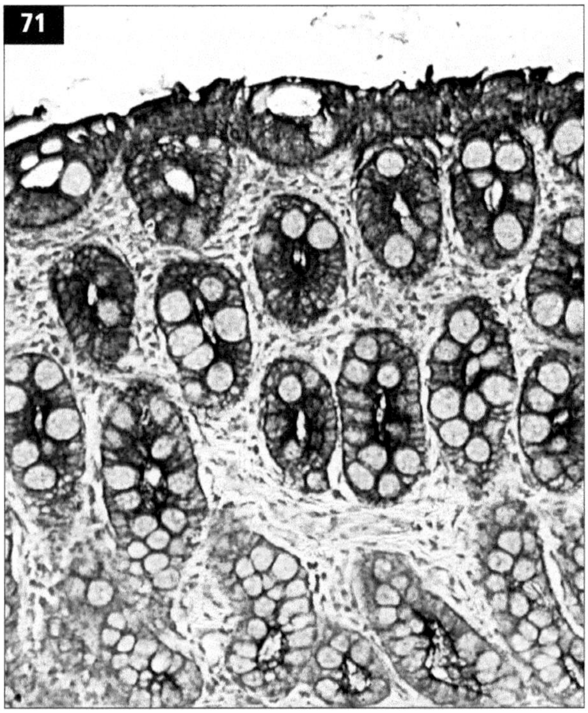

71 Chemokines. Section of feline colon demonstrating expression of mRNA encoding the chemokine receptor CCR3 by *in situ* hybridization. Expression of chemokine receptors by colonic epithelial cells may enable infection by FIV, which utilizes these molecules as co-receptors. (From Caney SMA, Day MJ, Gruffydd Jones TJ *et al.* (2002) Expression of chemokine receptors in the feline reproductive tract and large intestine. *Journal of Comparative Pathology* **126**:289–302, with permission.)

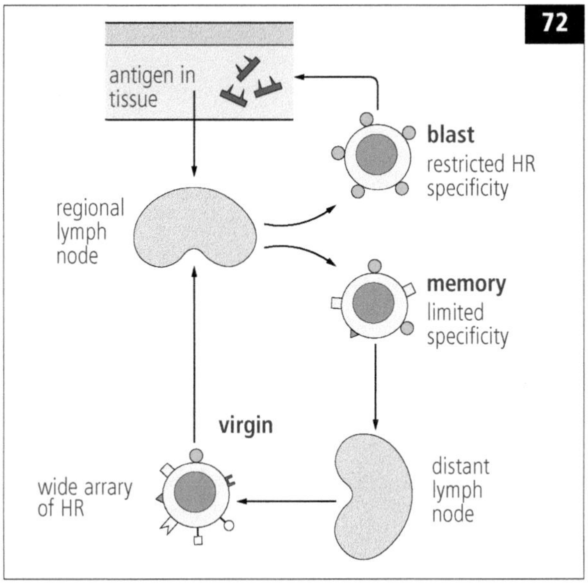

72 Homing receptor expression by activated lymphocytes. Virgin lymphocytes must have access to regional lymphoid tissue draining wide areas of the body in order to make contact with the antigen they are pre-programmed to recognize. For this reason, virgin lymphocytes may express a range of different homing receptor molecules. Following activation, the clonally expanded antigen-specific effector cells enter the recirculation pathway to reach the tissue within which the antigen is located. These effector cells express a restricted array of homing receptors. Immunological memory is generated as part of the immune response, and memory lymphocytes may selectively display homing receptor molecules, enabling them to have access to areas of the body where they are likely to re-encounter antigen.

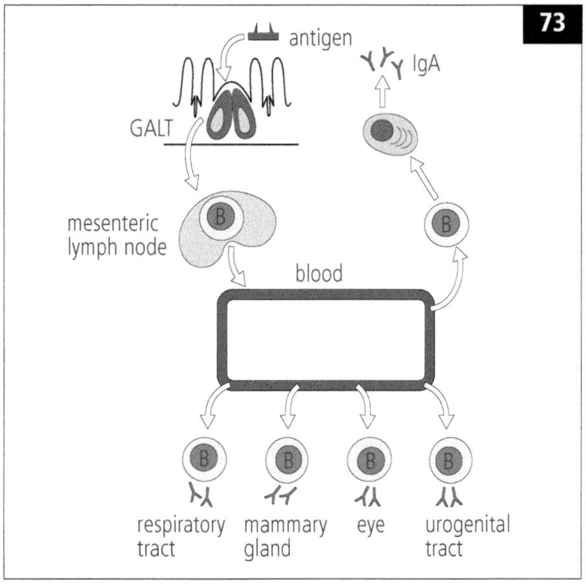

73 The common mucosal system. Lymphocytes activated by antigen in the context of one of the mucosal surfaces of the body may recirculate to other mucosae in addition to the surface of antigen exposure. This 'common mucosal system' may arise through vascular adhesion molecules shared by mucosal sites and allows differentiation of antigen-specific B lymphocytes at more than one mucosal surface. In domestic species this is of great importance because it enables the production of IgA antibodies specific for enteric or respiratory pathogens within the mammary gland and the passive transfer of such antibodies to neonates.

74 Structure of histocompatibility antigens. Class I histocompatibility antigens consist of a transmembrane α chain with three external domains, and the associated β_2 microglobulin. There is conserved sequence in the α_3 domain that has homology with the constant region of the Ig molecule (part of the 'immunoglobulin superfamily'), and the α_1 and α_2 domains have variable sequence. Class II histocompatibility molecules consist of two transmembrane chains (α and β), each of which has two external domains with sequence conservation (α_2 and β_2) or variability (α_1 and β_1). Class I molecules are found on the surface of all nucleated cells of the body and class II molecules on cells of the immune system.

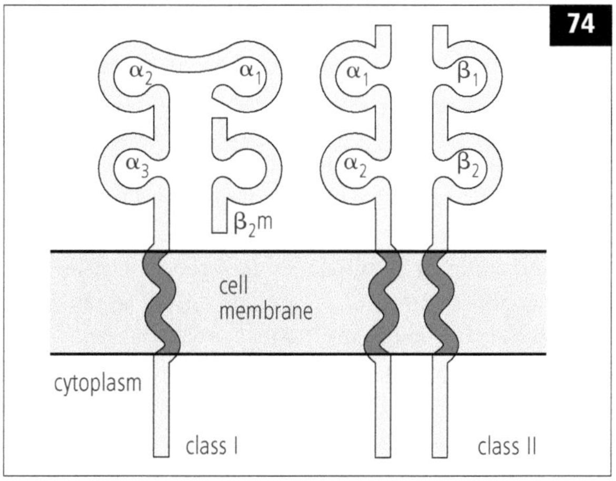

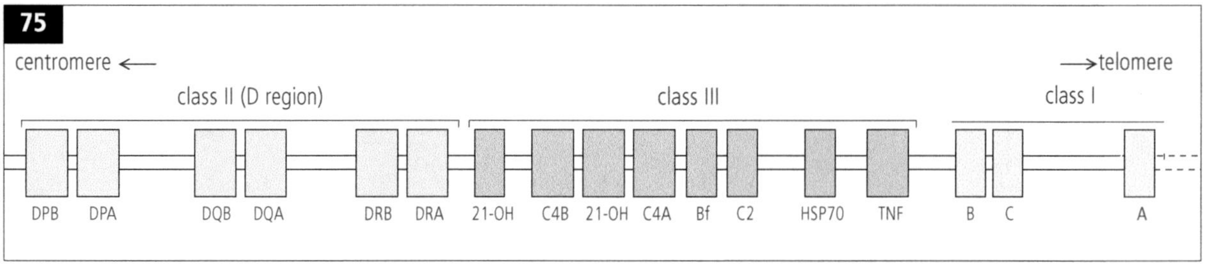

75 The major histocompatibility complex. Genes that encode the class I and II histocompatibility molecules are clustered together at a specific chromosomal location. The gene cluster is known as the 'major histocompatibility complex' (MHC). The human MHC has been mapped and consists of a series of class I genes (A, B and C) and class II genes encoding α and β chains (D region genes). Between these loci are a series of 'class III' genes, which encode a variety of molecules including some complement proteins (C2, C4 and factor B), the enzyme 21-hydroxylase, heat shock protein 70 and the cytokine tumour necrosis factor. The genes encoding the TAP-1 and TAP-2 transporter molecules and some proteasome subunits are located in the class II region. The canine and feline MHCs have similar arrangement, but during evolution (55 million years ago) there was a chromosomal break in these species, which separated an area of the MHC within the chromosome (cat) or to a different chromosome (dog).

gene names made italic

The genes encoding histocompatibility antigens are clustered in a specific chromosomal region known as the major histocompatibility complex (MHC) (**75**). The MHCs of man (human leukocyte antigen [HLA]) and mouse (H2) have been best characterized. In man there are three major class I loci (A, B and C) and a series of class II (D) genes. Sandwiched between these are loci encoding unrelated complement molecules, cytokines and others. The dog leukocyte antigen (DLA) system (canine MHC) and feline leukocyte antigen (FLA) system (feline MHC) are similar but have not been completely mapped. To date, the DLA system has been shown to comprise four major class I genes (*DLA I-12*, *DLA I-64*, *DLA I-79* and *DLA I-88*) and class II genes including *DLA-DRB1*, *DLA-DQA1* and *DLA-DQB1*. Two 'pseudogenes' are recognized as *DLA-DQB2* and *DLA-DRB2*. The DLA system is predominantly found on chromosome 12 with a separate section on chromosome 35. FLA genes have also been characterized. There are at least two classical class I loci and several class II genes (encoding α and β chains), and the FLA system is situated in two separate areas of chromosome B2. A major difference between FLA and canine or human MHC gene clusters is the absence of DQ genes and in dogs and cats there is only vestigial presence of DP genes. This more restricted feline MHC repertoire may have consequences for the range of immune responses that may be made by the cat. The histocompatibility genes are generally markedly polymorphic, with numerous different allelic forms at most loci. The genes are co-dominantly expressed, so products from each are found on the cell membrane (**76**). Histocompatibility antigens are inherited by the laws of mendelian genetics. The maternal and paternal sets of genes (a haplotype) are generally inherited as a block without genetic recombination (**77**). Studies of the DLA system have revealed differences between breeds in the range of DLA alleles and haplotypes expressed. A greater diversity of alleles is found in older breeds (e.g. GSD), whereas some breeds have restricted diversity or unique alleles. The degree of polymorphism in DLA class II genes is currently in the order of 31 *DLA-DQA1* alleles, 90 *DLA-DQB1* alleles and 144 *DLA-DRB1* alleles.

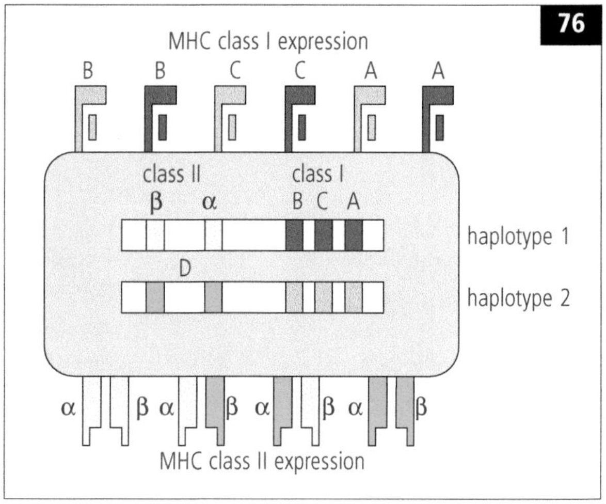

76 Expression of MHC products. MHC genes are co-dominant, such that the product of each is expressed on the cell surface. For each of the six class I loci (three maternal and three paternal) there is expression of a class I molecule on the cell surface. For each class II α and β gene there are α and β chains on the cell surface but, as in the example shown, these can associate to form four different molecules. In reality, expression of class II is more complex, as there are other D region genes not depicted on the diagram. Approximately 2×10^6 class I and class II molecules are found on the surface of a B lymphocyte. T lymphocytes in the cat and dog constitutively express only a single subtype of class II and may express only a single class I gene product.

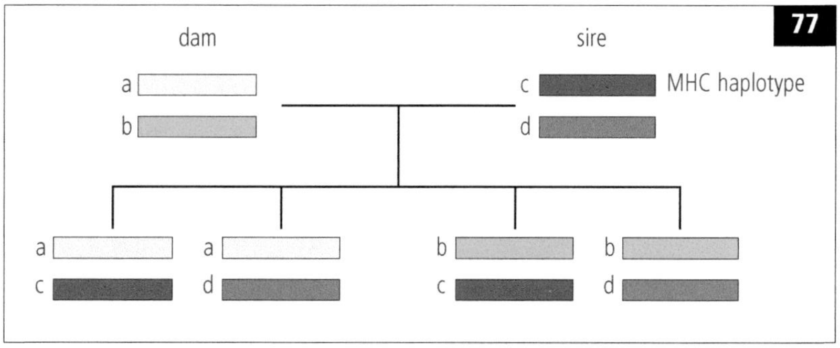

77 Inheritance of histocompatibility antigens. Each individual has two sets of MHC genes, one half ('haplotype') inherited from the sire and one from the dam. The MHC is generally inherited *en bloc* by the laws of simple mendelian genetics. In theory there is a one in four chance of two offspring sharing identical MHC.

CYTOKINES

Cytokines are a group of soluble mediators of the immune and inflammatory response. They are released by one cell and generally have an effect on either the same cell (autocrine) or a nearby cell (paracrine). Alternatively, some cytokines may circulate within the bloodstream and have (endocrine) effects distant from the site of production. Individual cytokines can be synthesized by, and act on, many different cells, and one cell can produce many different cytokines. Cytokines are low molecular weight proteins; are produced locally and transiently; are potent at picomolar concentrations; bind to a specific receptor, which initiates intracellular signalling pathways; and often work in a network involving multiple cells.

A number of structural cytokine families exist (interleukins, interferons, cytotoxins and growth factors) and they have diverse roles in:

- Haemopoiesis and development.
- Activation of T and B lymphocytes, NK cells and ancillary WBCs.
- Leukocyte chemotaxis.
- Clonal expansion of T and B lymphocytes.
- Regulation (or suppression) of T and B lymphocytes.
- Cytotoxicity.
- Inflammation.

78

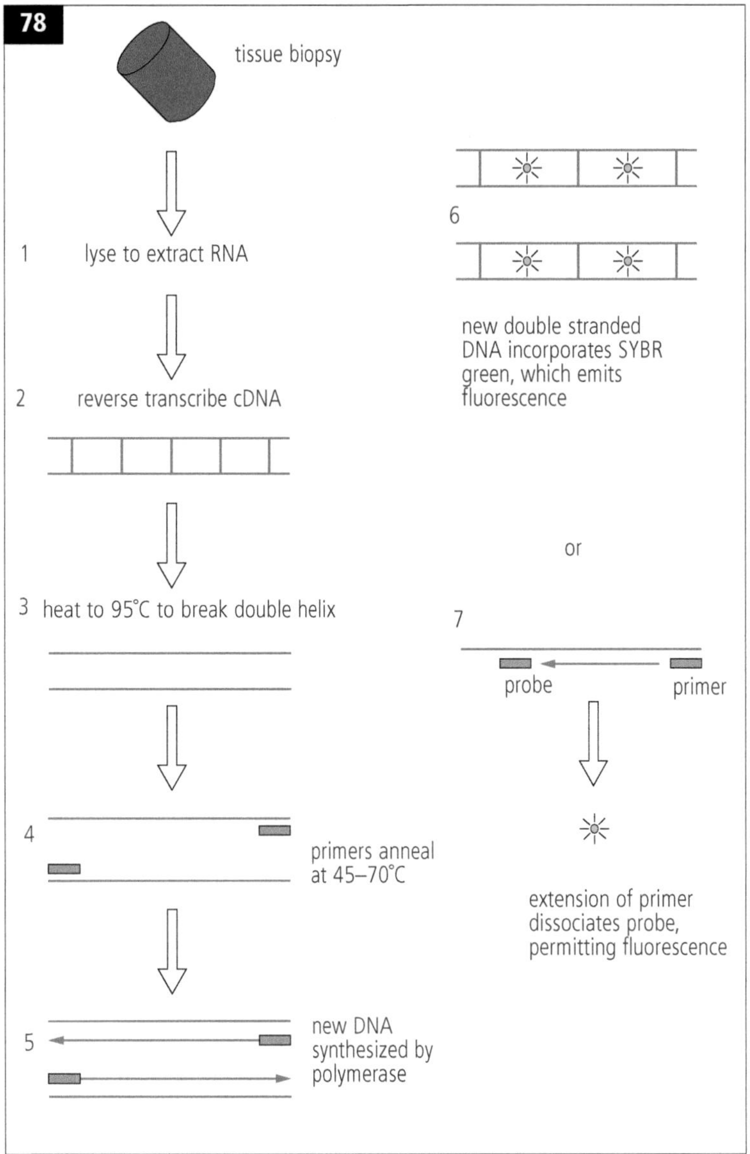

79

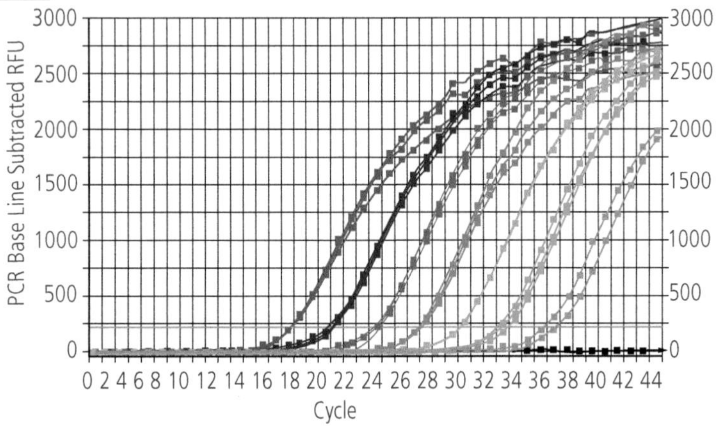

78, 79 Real-time reverse transcriptase polymerase chain reaction. (**78**) Real-time RT-PCR provides a means by which gene transcription within a tissue can be quantified. In this way the activity of genes encoding many inflammatory mediators can be assessed when reagents able to detect the proteins encoded by the genes are not available. In this process, RNA is first extracted from a tissue sample (1) and then reverse transcribed to cDNA (2). In a thermal cycler, the double-stranded DNA is heated to 95°C to denature the double helix (3). When the reaction is cooled to 45–70°C, small complementary sequences (primers) at each end of the gene sequence of interest are able to anneal to the appropriate nucleotides within the single stranded DNA (4), following which a heat stable DNA polymerase adds bases complementary to those in the DNA strands to synthesize new double-stranded DNA (5). This cycle of heat and cooling is subsequently repeated up to 40 times, leading to an exponential increase in the amount of target gene. In the highly sensitive real-time method, the production of DNA is measured at each cycle (in 'real-time') using a fluorescence read out. Fluorescence is emitted (and measured) each time double-stranded DNA is produced in the reaction. This may be achieved via the use of an 'intercalating dye' (e.g. SYBR green), which only binds double-stranded DNA to emit fluorescence (6), or via the use of labelled reporter oligonucleotide 'probes' that emit fluorescence when they are dislodged from the template DNA by the process of extension mediated by the DNA polymerase (7). The point at which the fluorescence value crosses a threshold detection value (the Ct value) is related to the amount of target DNA in the sample. (**79**) In the graph from an experiment detecting mRNA within tissue samples, the samples on the left, which cross the threshold (the orange line parallel to the x axis) with lower cycle number, have more copies of the target DNA than samples on the right, which require many more cycles of amplification to cross the threshold.

The recent application of molecular technology has enabled the characterization of most of the major canine and feline cytokines. Messenger RNA encoding cytokines can be quantified within tissue samples or cultured leukocytes by real-time reverse transcriptase polymerase chain reaction (RT–PCR) and numerous studies have now applied this technology (**78, 79**). The relative amount of mRNA transcripts provides an indication of gene activity and likely correlates with translation into cytokine protein. More recently, monoclonal antibodies that permit quantification of canine and feline cytokine proteins have become available. These commercial test kits enable measurement of key cytokines including IFNγ, TNFα, IL-1β, IL-4 and IL-10 in serum or cell culture supernatants. A novel, bead-based, multiplex kit for detection of canine cytokines, using a very small sample volume, is also available.

T LYMPHOCYTES

The T cell receptor

T lymphocytes are characterized by expression of the antigen-specific T cell receptor (TCR)-CD3 complex and they fall into two non-overlapping subsets defined by mutually exclusive expression of the CD4 or CD8 molecules. The majority of TCRs comprise transmembrane α and β chains (**31**). Each of these two chains consists of a number of distinct regions. The conserved (constant, C) regions of either the α or β chains are nearest the cell surface and have sequence homology with the Ig Fc region, as discussed for MHC molecules. The opposite end of each chain (furthest from the cell membrane) has variable amino acid sequence (akin to the Ig Fab region), and this variable (V) region is largely responsible for the unique antigen-restriction of the T cell. The C and V regions of the α chain are separated by a joining (J) region. The C and V regions of the β chain are linked by both a J and diversity (D) region.

At the molecular level, there are relatively large numbers of V, J and D region genes, but only a single Cα or two Cβ genes. Each Cβ gene is associated with a complete set of D and J genes, a phenomenon that likely arose by evolutionary duplication of this genetic region. In the formation of a single unique TCR α chain, one each of the V and D genes are selected and brought into apposition by the process of DNA rearrangement. The Cα region is subsequently attached by RNA splicing following transcription. A similar process occurs for the TCR β chain, although there is rearrangement of V, D and J genes before combination with a Cβ region. The mechanisms by which these genetic rearrangements arise parallel those used to create the Ig heavy and light chains, and they are explained more fully in the following section on B lymphocytes and in (**85**).

The possible number of combinations of these genes is a major mechanism by which the immune system generates a vast number of unique TCRs (the 'germline repertoire'). The germline repertoire can be further increased by the pairing of α and β chains of the TCR and by the process of 'junctional diversity', whereby the V, D and J segments combine at the level of different nucleotides. Once a T cell has formed a specific TCR, the genes encoding the molecules do not undergo somatic mutation (single nucleotide substitutions).

It has long been assumed that selection of a single TCR from the germline repertoire confers a unique antigen specificity on that T cell expressing the receptor. However, it is now known that there are insufficient T cells in the body to permit each one a unique specificity and that T cells likely cross-react with numerous different peptides bearing appropriate contact residues (see below).

image amended

80

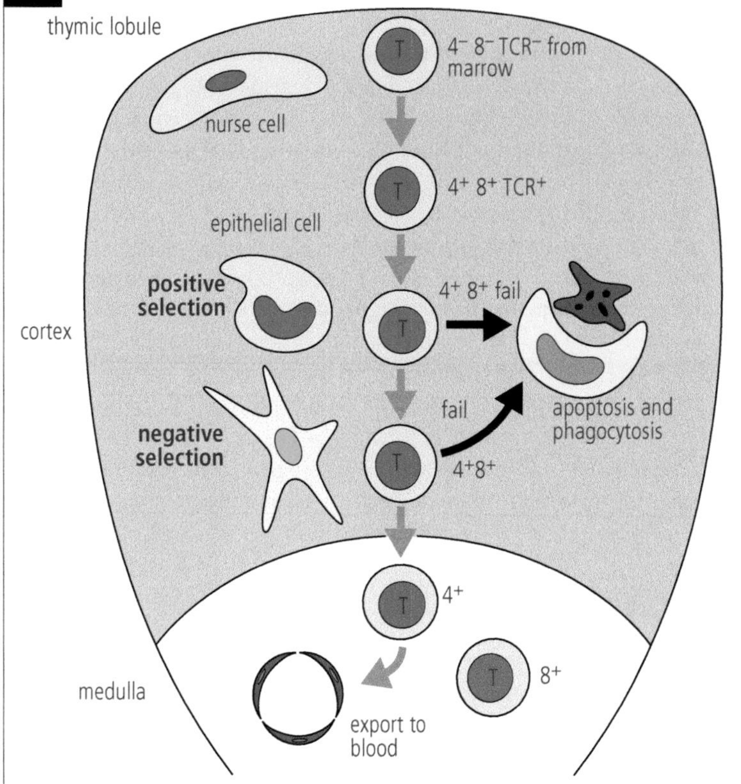

80 Intrathymic T cell development. Immature T cells enter the thymus from the bone marrow and proliferate in the subcapsular region to give rise to cells that enter the differentiation pathway. Subcapsular cells are often associated with epithelial cells (thymic nurse cells), but the role of these cells is unknown. In the thymic cortex the T cells acquire the TCR in addition to both of the CD4 and CD8 molecules before migrating deeper into the cortex and coming into contact with cortical epithelial cells. Self-MHC molecules are expressed on these epithelial cells and these interact with the thymocyte TCRs. Those cells with TCRs able to recognize self-MHC are 'positively selected' for further development, whereas those that cannot mediate this interaction die by apoptosis and are phagocytosed by macrophages. At the corticomedullary junction the developing thymocytes come into contact with dendritic cells presenting self-antigens in the context of MHC. T cells carrying a TCR that can recognize these self-antigens with high affinity die by apoptosis ('clonal deletion') in the process known as 'negative selection'. Finally, medullary thymocytes retain expression of either CD4 or CD8 and leave the thymus via vessels near the corticomedullary junction.

81

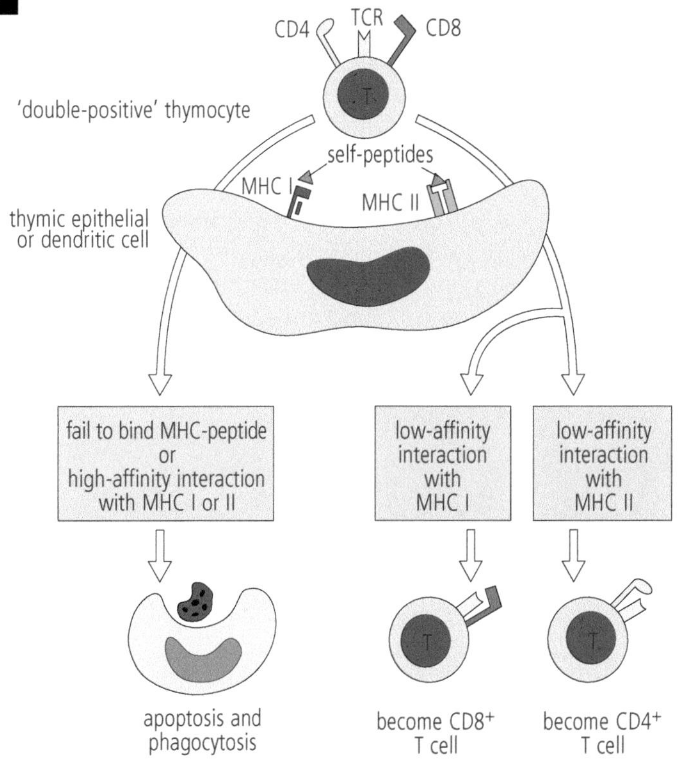

81 T cell differentiation in the thymus. Immature T cells expressing both CD4 and CD8 interact with thymic epithelial or dendritic cells expressing MHC class I and class II molecules containing antigenic peptides derived from self-antigens. Cells that cannot recognize self-MHC are deleted, as are thymocytes that form high affinity interactions with self-peptides expressed on class I or II molecules. Those cells with low affinity for MHC are positively selected. Thymocytes demonstrating a low affinity interaction with class I will become $CD8^+$ T lymphocytes, and those with low affinity for class II will become $CD4^+$ T cells.

82 CD4+ T lymphocyte subsets. There are two major subsets of CD4+ T lymphocytes that are characterized by a distinct pattern of cytokine production. Activation of Th1 cells results in cell-mediated immune effects such as macrophage activation by IFNγ. Th2 cells mediate the humoral effects of antibody synthesis (IgE and IgG subclass) and regulation of mast cell and eosinophil differentiation and mobility. Th2 cells produce IL-10, which can render Th1 cells unable to respond to antigen (anergic), as there is interference with production of APC co-stimulatory signals. The Th2 cytokines IL-4 and IL-13 also negatively influence Th1 cells. Th1 cells directly inhibit the function of Th2 cells via IFNγ production.

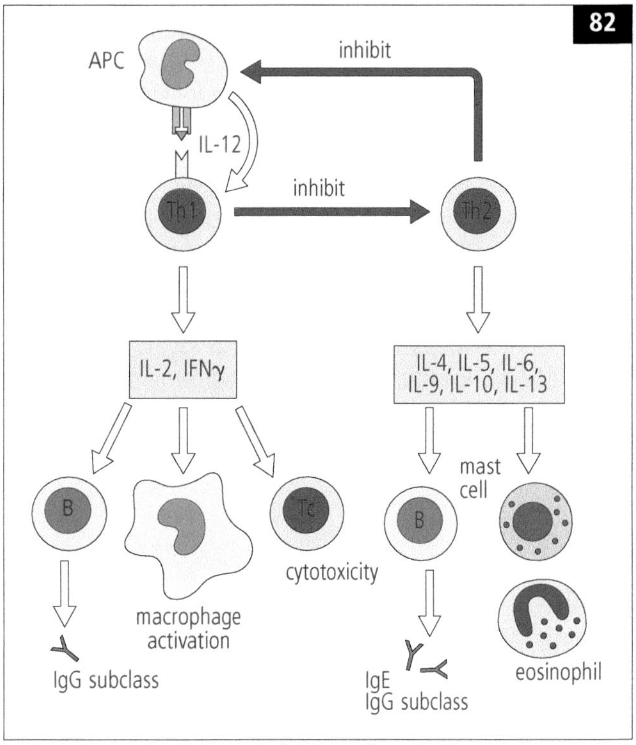

T cell development

Immature bone marrow-derived T cells are exported to the thymus in the bloodstream, where they undergo a sequence of maturation events (**80, 81**). The vast majority of T cells that enter the thymus do not 'pass the tests' of positive and negative selection and die by apoptosis (programmed cell death). T cells released by the thymus are able to participate in productive immune responses against foreign antigens, but a small proportion of T cells with TCRs having low affinity for self-antigens escape clonal deletion and can potentially mediate self-reactivity (autoimmunity).

Subsets of CD4+ T lymphocytes

The subpopulation of T cells that expresses the CD4 molecule (T helper [Th] cells) can be further subdivided into the major Th1 and Th2 subsets (**82**), defined by the profile of cytokines that they produce and the immunological effects they orchestrate. Th1 cells:

- Produce predominantly IL-2 and IFNγ.
- Undertake intracellular signalling from surface cytokine receptors via the use of signal transducers and activators of transcription (STAT) 4.
- Initiate cell-mediated immunity and cytotoxicity.
- Have limited effect on antibody production, but enhance production of a specific IgG subclass (IgG2a in mice).
- Antagonize the action of Th2 cells (via IFNγ).

Th2 cells:

- Produce IL-4, IL-5, IL-9, IL-10, IL-13, IL-25, IL-31 and IL-33.
- Undertake intracellular signalling from surface cytokine receptors via the use of STAT6.
- Mediate humoral immunity, particularly the synthesis of IgE and a subclass of IgG (IgG1 in mice).
- Antagonize the action of Th1 cells (via IL-4, IL-10 and IL-13).

The two populations have a common precursor (Th0) that is able to produce IL-2, IL-4 and IFNγ (**83**); differentiation into a Th1 or Th2 cell may depend upon:

- The nature of the APC and the co-stimulatory molecules expressed by the APC.
- The type and dose of antigen and the nature of the PAMP-PRR interaction (see below) that occurs on the surface of the APC.
- The route of exposure to antigen (local tissue factors). For example, the presence of IL-12 and IL-18 locally may direct development of a Th1 response, whereas the presence of glucocorticoid, IL-4 or IL-6 may select for Th2 activity.
- The stage of the immune response.

Th1 and Th2 cells may be selectively recruited into inflamed tissue via expression of specific adhesion molecules and their response to particular chemokines. Similar functional subsets are recognized among $CD8^+$ T lymphocytes, and these cells may act in parallel with their $CD4^+$ counterparts to mediate a type 1 (Th1) or type 2 (Th2) response. Most immune responses use a balance of both type 1 and type 2 elements, but some antigens may induce a polarized response (e.g. nematodes or aeroallergens preferentially induce type 2, viruses or intracellular protozoa induce type 1).

Many recent studies have shown that dogs and cats are likely to have these functional T cell subsets directing immune responses. However, in companion animals (as in humans) the polarization

83

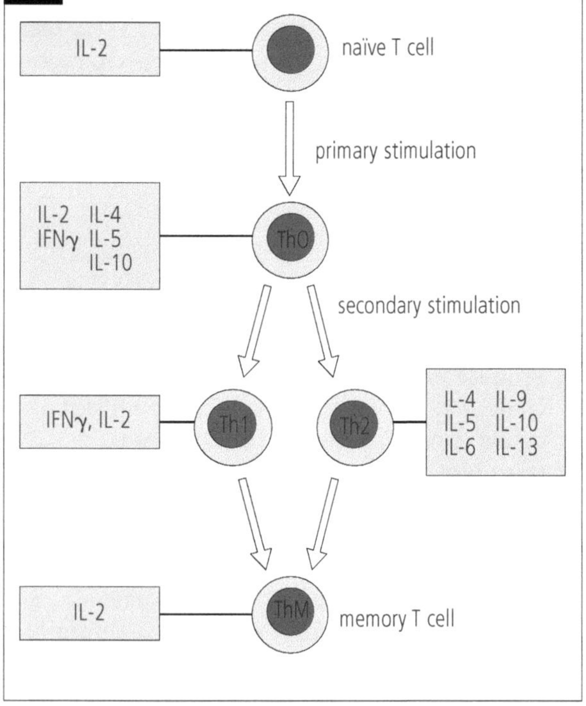

83 Differentiation of $CD4^+$ T cells. $CD4^+$ Th cells may be divided into different subsets by the profile of cytokines produced. The major effector populations are the Th1 and Th2 cells, which likely arise from a common precursor (Th0) able to express a combination of cytokines. Differentiation of these precursors towards Th1 or Th2 cells is likely to depend on a number of factors related to the nature of the antigen, type of APC and route of antigen exposure. Although such cells are likely to exist in the dog and cat, they have been poorly characterized to date.

84

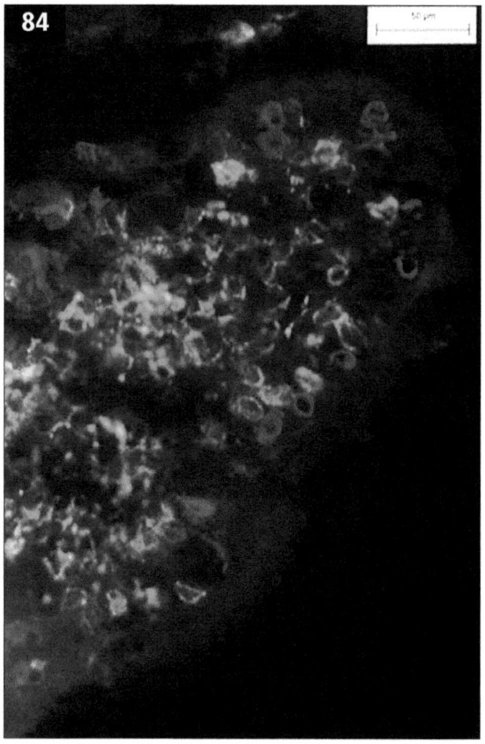

84 γδ T cells. Section of canine intestinal villus stained by dual colour immunofluorescence. T cells expressing the αβ TCR fluoresce green, while γδ TCR^+ T cells show red fluorescence. Note that the γδ T cells are localized to the epithelial lining of the villus, consistent with their putative role as 'front line' immunological cells important in any encounter with bacterial pathogens. (From German AJ, Hall EJ, Moore PF *et al.* (1999) Analysis of the distribution of lymphocytes expressing the αβ and γδ T cell receptors and expression of mucosal addressin cell adhesion molecule-1 in the canine intestine. *Journal of Comparative Pathology* **201:**249–263, with permission.)

of these responses is not as distinct as in experimental rodent models. Exceptions to this are the type 1 immune response that mediates resistance of dogs to *Leishmania* infection and the type 2 responses that occur in the early stages of allergic disease in both dogs and cats.

Other CD4+ T cell subsets are those involved in immunoregulation (see below) and the Th17, Th9 and T follicular helper (TFh) cells. Th17 cells preferentially produce IL-17 and IL-22 in response to APC production of IL-6, IL-23 and TGFβ, the use of STAT3 in signal transduction and have a functional role in the immune response to particular parasites and bacteria. Th17 cells may also have a pathogenic role, as they are increased in number in some autoimmune responses, and IL-17 expression is increased in neoplasia. Th9 cells (key cytokine IL-9) are also involved in inflammatory responses and TFh cells (IL-21) in humoral immunity.

γδ T lymphocytes

T cells expressing a TCR consisting of γ and δ chains (with CD3) are less common than αβ T cells, are found predominantly at body surfaces (e.g. skin and mucosae) and are thought to be important in the 'first line' immune response to bacterial pathogens, as they are activated in response to a range of bacteria (*Mycobacterium* spp., *Listeria* spp., *Salmonella* spp., *Escherichia coli*) and conserved heat shock proteins. These cells are poorly characterized, but they arise in the thymus, where the γδ receptor may be an evolutionarily older form of TCR. γδ T cells generally do not express CD4 or CD8 and are therefore not MHC-restricted, but they may produce either Th1 or Th2 cytokines and thus act with αβ Th cells to participate in type 1 or type 2 responses. Canine γδ T cells have been identified and are reported to comprise up to one third of T cells within the spleen (84).

B LYMPHOCYTES

The B lymphocyte antigen receptor

B lymphocytes are characterized by expression of SmIg (31). Each B cell carries Ig of a unique specificity, which is the same specificity as the antibody eventually produced by the plasma cell derived from that lineage. In man and rodents, Ig diversity is achieved in similar fashion to that of the TCR, where light chains comprise V, J and C regions and heavy chains are formed from the combination of V, D, J and C regions. The genes encoding the κ, λ and heavy chains of Ig are located on three separate chromosomes. In the case of the heavy chains, there are a large number of V region genes, with fewer D and J region loci, and constant region genes corresponding to each Ig class (Cμ, Cδ, Cγ, Cε and Cα) and subclass. The genes encoding the κ and λ light chains differ in number. For λ light chains there are fewer V region loci but several Cλ genes, whereas for the κ chain there are a large number of V region genes and a single Cκ locus.

text removed

The formation of an Ig molecule requires DNA rearrangement such that the genes encoding the V, D and J regions are associated, and the C region is subsequently associated by RNA splicing during transcription (85). The means of DNA recombination in the formation of Ig and TCRs likely involves looping out and deletion of introns, mediated by 'recombinase' enzymes that are either regulated or encoded by recombination activating genes (*RAG1*, *RAG2*), together with DNA repair enzymes. The possible permutations and combinations of the Ig genes creates a vast diversity in antibody specificity. This can be further increased by variable boundary recombination between V-J and V-D-J segments ('junctional alternatives') and by single nucleotide substitutions ('point mutations') in the process of 'somatic mutation'.

made italic

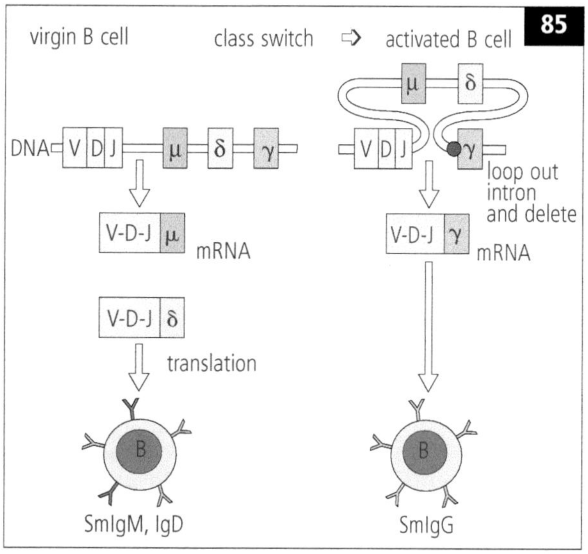

85 The Ig class switch. Virgin B cells concurrently express SmIgM and SmIgD. The VDJ region of the heavy chain is created by DNA rearrangements and either the μ or the δ C region is added by differential RNA splicing. After activation, the Ig class switch involves a second DNA rearrangement whereby the μ and δ genes are looped out and an alternative C gene is moved up to exchange at the switch region (red).

86

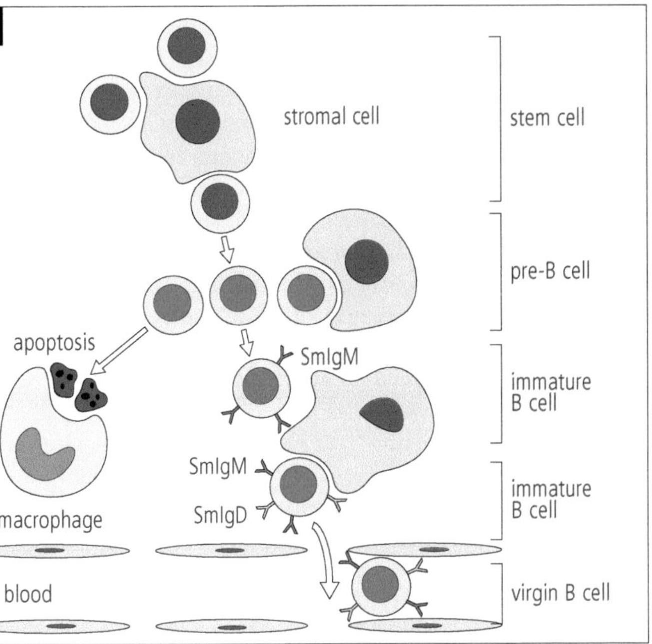

86 B cell development. Bone marrow stem cells mature into pre-B cells (cytoplasmic μ chain), most of which die and are engulfed by macrophages. Immature B cells then express SmIgM and finally a combination of SmIgM and SmIgD before being released to the circulation as virgin B cells. During development the B cell precursors interact with stromal cells via surface adhesion molecules, and stromal cell-derived IL-7 is required for maturation.

The principle of 'allelic exclusion' means that each B cell produces only a single heavy and light chain, as gene rearrangement on one chromosome inhibits that of the corresponding loci on the other chromosome. The formation of SmIg in animals (including presumptively the dog and cat) occurs by the process of 'gene conversion'. Animals have a restricted V, D and J gene repertoire and V region diversity is achieved by incorporation of DNA segments from up-region pseudogenes into the V region DNA.

B cell differentiation

B cell maturation in rodents largely occurs in the bone marrow following development from the stem cell (**86**), but in man and animals this process occurs in the intestine, particularly in the ileal Peyer's patch that is of maximum size in neonates and progressively involutes with age. The earliest B cell (pre-B cell) is characterized by the presence of cytoplasmic μ chains, as only heavy chain gene rearrangements have occurred at this stage. The majority of developing B cells die by apoptosis and are then phagocytosed by macrophages. B cell development likely involves some form of selection via interaction with stromal cells, with clonal deletion of autoreactive cells. Following light chain gene rearrangement, the next developmental stage is characterized by the expression of SmIgM. All immature B cells initially express IgM, even if they will eventually express Ig of another class. Finally, B cells are released to the periphery as virgin B lymphocytes, which are characterized by the concomitant expression of SmIgM and SmIgD.

ANTIGEN PRESENTATION

The first stage in the initiation of an immune response is conversion of antigen into a 'user friendly' form for T lymphocytes. This involves antigen uptake, processing and presentation by the APC. The initial encounter between antigen and APC as part of the innate immune response determines the nature of the subsequent adaptive response. Many foreign antigens (particularly pathogenic organisms) carry on their surface a relatively restricted array of unique molecules known collectively as pathogen-associated molecular patterns (PAMPs). These interact with a series of receptor molecules expressed on the surface of APCs, collectively termed the pattern recognition receptors (PRRs). PRRs are also sometimes referred to as Toll-like receptors (TLRs), after the homologous molecule 'Toll' that was first defined in *Drosophila*. TLR gene expression has been demonstrated in canine and feline lymphoid tissue and some TLRs have been cloned and sequenced in these species. One PRR may recognize several different PAMPs (**87**, **88**). Engagement of a PRR leads to translocation of signals to the cell (**89**), with upregulation of genes encoding specific cytokines and co-stimulatory molecules that are expressed on the surface of the APC. The array of these co-stimulatory factors

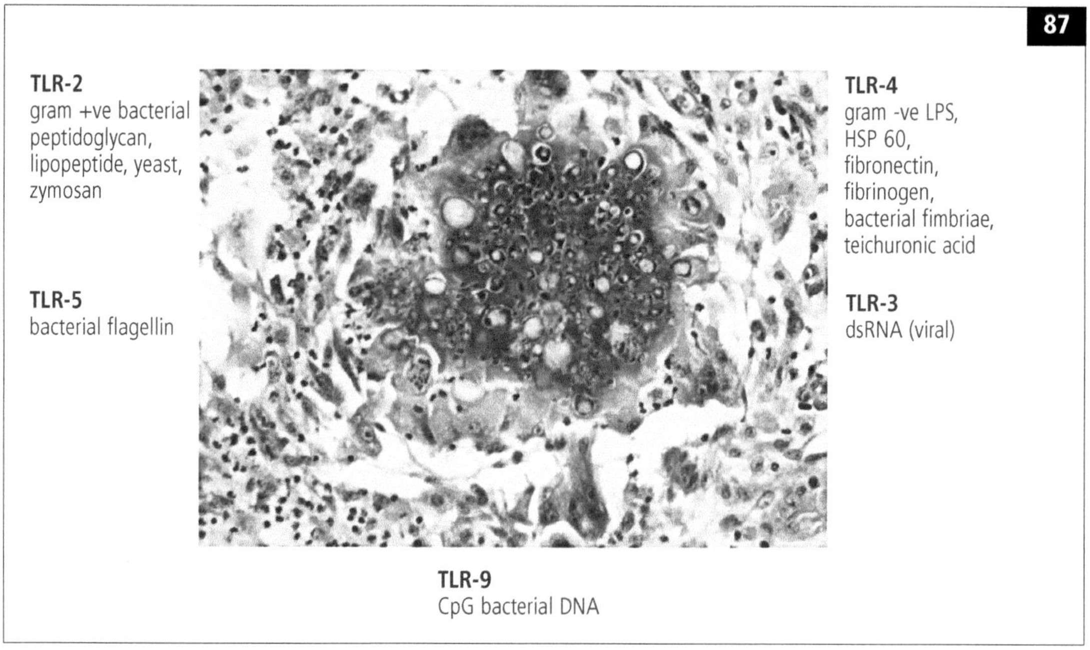

87 Pattern recognition receptors. A range of pattern recognition receptors (PRRs; also known as Toll-like receptors [TLRs]) has been defined. PRRs are found on the surface of APCs. They interact with a number of highly conserved and structurally stable molecules (sugars, proteins, lipids and nucleic acids) that are termed pathogen-associated molecular patterns (PAMPs). PAMPS are often microbial in origin. The central image shows a granulomatous inflammatory reaction around fungal elements in a skin biopsy from a cat with mycotic dermatitis. It is likely that such cells express PRRs for interaction with antigen derived from the organism.

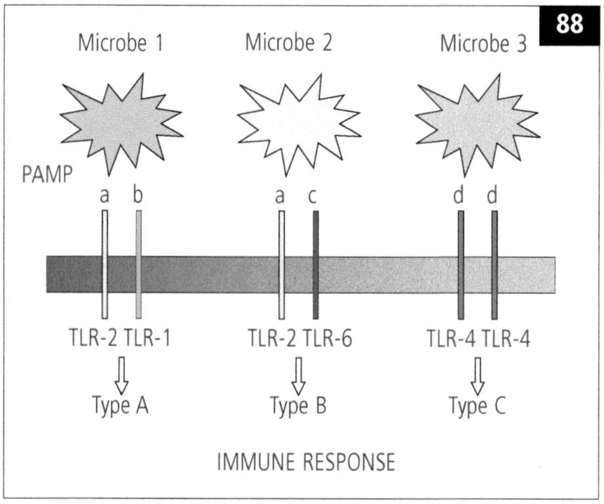

88 Engagement of PRRs. Different microbes may express different combinations of PAMPs and may therefore engage different PRRs on the surface of APCs. The type and combination of PRR ligated determines the nature of signalling to the APC, which in turn directs the form of the immune response that will be made to that microbe.

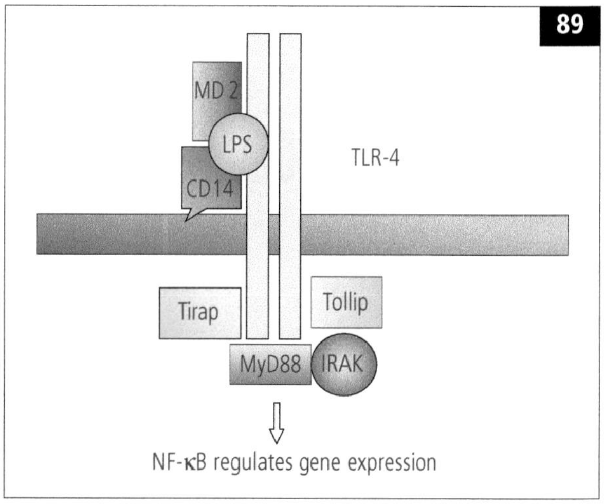

89 Intracellular signalling through PRRs. Binding of PAMPs by PRRs leads to induction of a complex intracellular signalling pathway, the net effect of which is to activate nuclear factor B mediated regulation of gene expression in the APC. The nature of the genes activated determines how the APC will direct the ensuing adaptive immune response. The diagram shows the interaction of bacterial lipopolysaccharide (LPS) with TLR-4.

induced by the PAMP-PRR interaction determines the nature of the subsequent T cell response to the initiating antigen (e.g. type 1 or type 2) (90). Other families of PRRs are intracellular and include:

- NOD-like receptors that specifically detect a range of bacterial antigens and activate signalling pathways for cytokine production. The best characterized of this family are the molecules NOD1 and NOD2.
- RIG-like receptors that specifically interact with viral antigens, activating pathways that lead to the production of a range of anti-viral proteins.

In similar fashion, molecules released by damaged or dying host cells (damage-associated molecular patterns; DAMP) interact with the same range of PRRs, thereby alerting the immune system to tissue damage ('danger signals').

Following recognition, the antigen must be taken into the cytoplasm of the APC (e.g. by phagocytosis for the prototypic APC, the macrophage), where it localizes within a cytoplasmic compartment (e.g. the endosome). It is within this compartment that 'antigen processing' occurs. Crude antigen is converted to constituent peptide fragments, which are subsequently re-expressed on the surface of the APC, nestled within a groove formed by the variable domains of either class I or class II histocompatibility molecules (antigen presentation). A single MHC molecule may bind many different peptides, but each must have specific anchor residues that fit into specific pockets of the antigen binding groove. There are two major intracellular antigen processing pathways: exogenous antigens (e.g. bacteria) are dealt with by the endosomal pathway and re-expressed on class II molecules (**91, 92**); whereas endogenous (cytoplasmic) antigens (e.g.

90

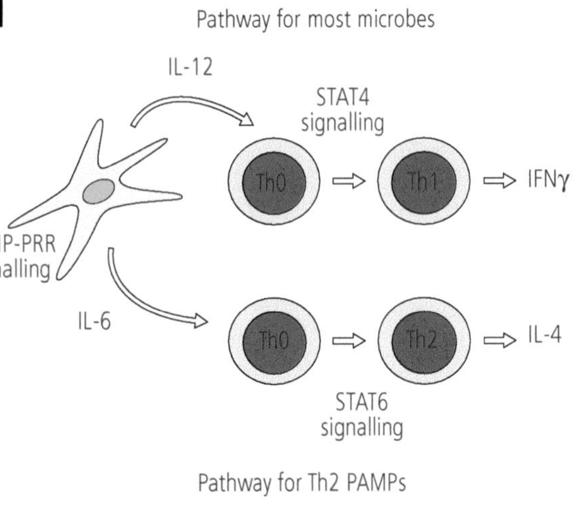

90 Outcome of PRR signalling. Different microbial antigens activate specific Th1 or Th2 immune responses dependent on the nature of the PAMP-PRR interaction. Recognition of the majority of microbial antigens results in production of IL-12 by the APC and activation of the Th0 cell via the STAT4 signalling pathway. The effect of this stimulation is development of a Th1 immune response. By contrast, some infectious agents (e.g. *Bordetella* spp., nematode parasites) induce IL-6 production by the APC and stimulation of the Th0 cell through the STAT6 signalling pathway. These interactions result in production of a Th2 immune response.

91

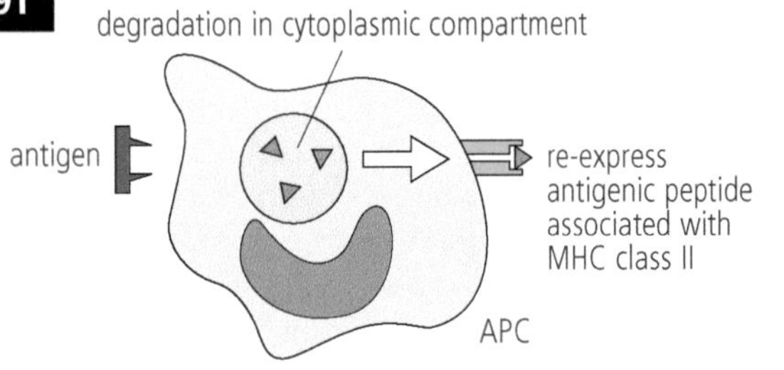

92

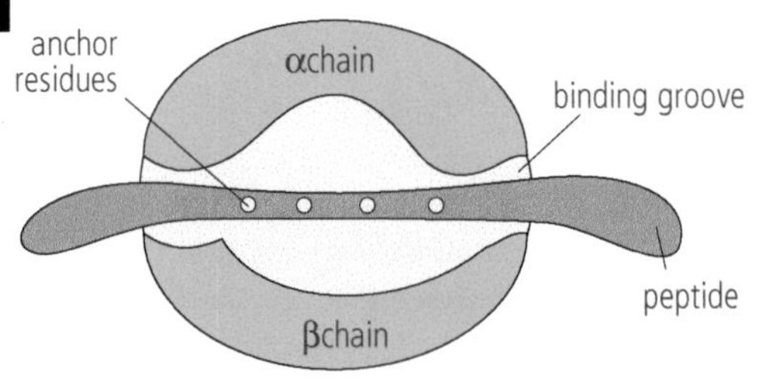

91, 92 Processing of exogenous antigen. (**91**) Exogenous antigens are internalized by APCs and broken down by proteolytic enzymes within the cytoplasmic endosomal compartment. Antigenic peptide fragments associate with class II MHC molecules within specialized cytoplasmic compartments, and the combination of MHC and peptide is re-expressed on the cell surface. (**92**) MHC class II-associated peptides may be longer than the binding groove (12–25 amino acids) and anchor via the insertion of specific residues into pockets in the groove (viewed from above).

viral) are passed through the endoplasmic reticulum and Golgi apparatus and re-expressed on class I molecules (**93–95**). The pathways are not mutually exclusive as exogenous antigen may enter the endogenous pathway ('cross-presentation'). Multiple different peptides (often with limited sequence homology) may compete for binding to any one MHC molecule, suggesting that much of the specificity of antigen recognition lies with the TCR. The peptide–MHC interaction is mediated only by some amino acids within the peptide, and others likely interact with the TCR.

A third antigen processing pathway involves the presentation of lipid antigen (e.g. derived from organisms such as *Mycobacterium*) by a class of antigen presenting molecules known as the CD1 family. CD1 molecules are likely evolutionarily related to MHC, but diverged at an early stage of mammalian development. The CD1 molecule is a transmembrane glycoprotein with three extracellular domains that associates with β2 microglobulin but has limited homology to MHC class I. There is a family of genes that encodes a number of non-polymorphic forms of CD1 that

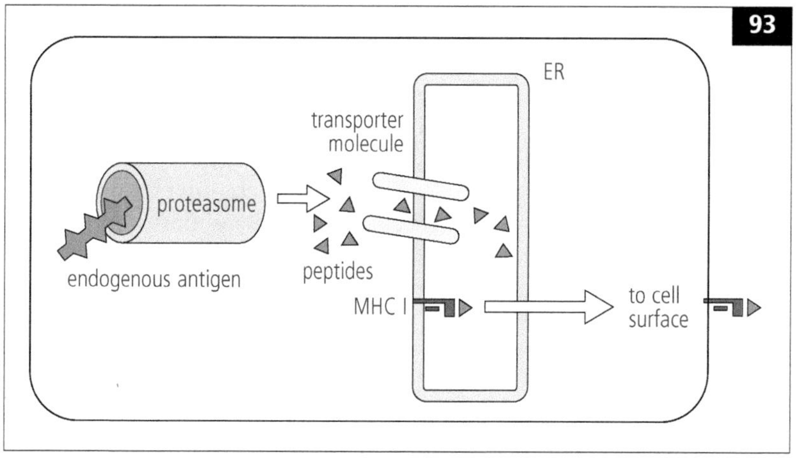

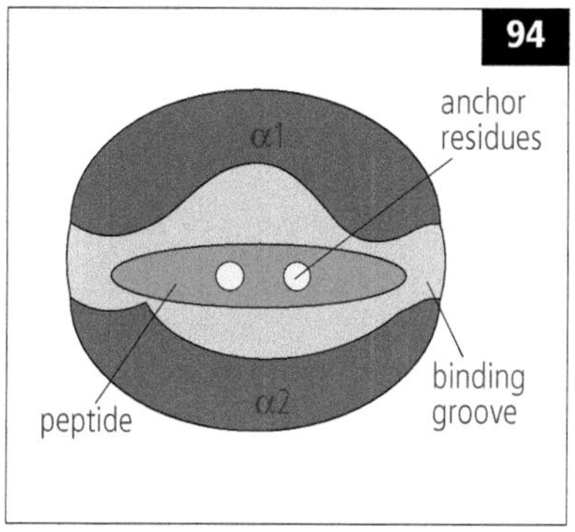

93, 94 Processing of endogenous antigen. (**93**) Endogenous cytoplasmic antigens are processed by proteasomes, then peptides are transported by 'transporter molecules' into the endoplasmic reticulum. Antigenic peptides associate with class I MHC molecules and are then transported to the cell surface. (**94**) Class I-associated peptides (8–9 amino acids long) are contained within the peptide binding groove and anchor residues insert into pockets within the groove (viewed from above).

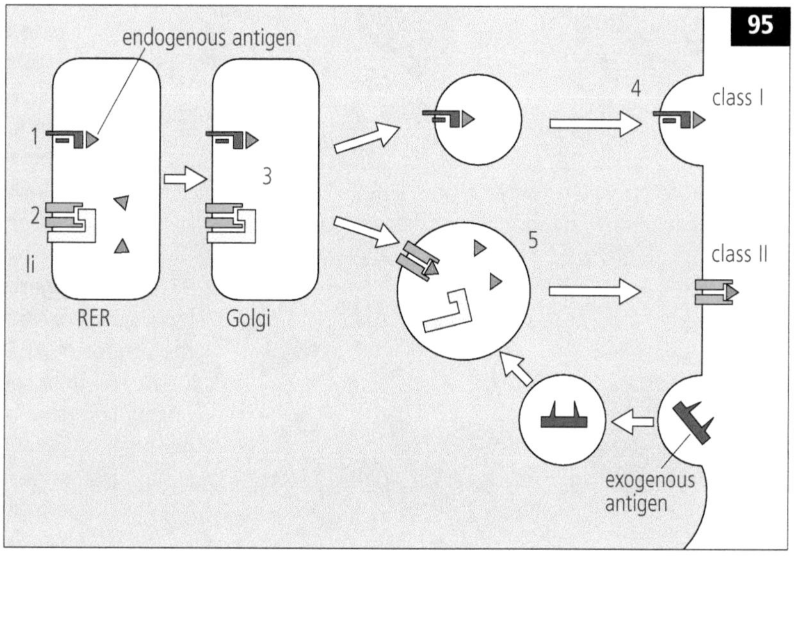

95 Antigen processing pathways. Endogenous peptide fragments associate with class I within the endoplasmic reticulum (1) but are prevented from associating with class II as the peptide-binding site is occupied by the invariant chain (Ii), which contains sequences that permit the class II molecule to exit the rough endoplasmic reticulum (RER) (2). After passage through the Golgi apparatus (3), class I molecules loaded with antigen pass directly to the cell surface (4). Class II molecules are transferred to endosomal compartments where the acidic and enzyme-rich environment results in displacement of the invariant chain and association with peptides derived from exogenous antigens (5).

may have a variable cellular distribution. The association of lipid antigen with CD1 is likely to occur within the environment of the endosome, with subsequent translocation of the antigen-loaded molecule to the surface of the APC.

Antigen presentation by dendritic cells (**96**) differs from that of macrophages in several respects. Dendritic cells constitutively express high levels of MHC class II (it must be induced on macrophages) and may take up antigen by phagocytosis or by sampling extracellular material via large pinocytic vesicles (macropinocytosis). It is now recognized that both immature and mature forms of dendritic cell exist. Immature dendritic cells may be found normally throughout the body, where they sample autoantigens and allergens that are presented to T cells to maintain a default tolerance response. However, in situations where there is infection or inflammation, dendritic cells become fully mature and are able to induce active immune protection. Dendritic cells are considered to be the most potent APCs and are thus more important in initiating primary immune responses in immunologically naïve individuals. B lymphocytes can also present antigen (**96**), but such presentation is unlikely to be significant in the initial stages of an immune response.

T LYMPHOCYTE ACTIVATION

Activation of antigen-specific T lymphocytes occurs following recognition of the combination of processed antigen and histocompatibility molecule by the TCR (**97**). This recognition event is termed 'signal 1' for T cell activation. T cell activation also requires co-stimulatory signals delivered by the interaction of other surface molecules and their ligands on the two cells (signal 2), and the release of a cytokine (e.g. IL-1, IL-12, IL-18) by the APC, which binds to its specific receptor on the T cell (signal 3) (**98**). The clustering of co-stimulatory molecules in the vicinity of the TCR-MHC interaction forms points of close association between the T cell and APC known as the 'immunological synapse'. These interactions trigger complex intracellular signalling pathways within the T lymphocyte, leading to specific gene expression that results in:

- Transformation to a blast cell.

96

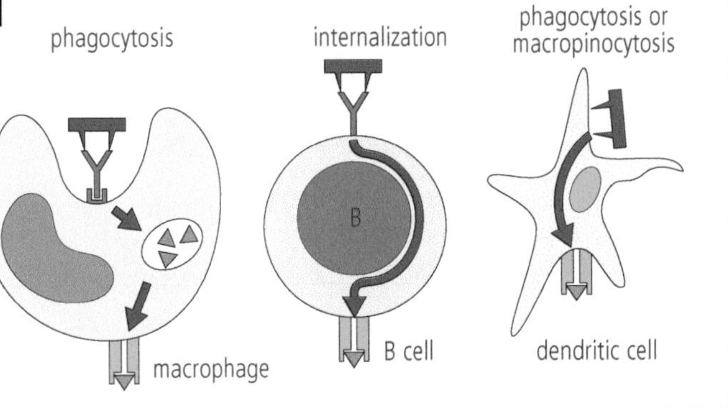

96 Antigen presenting cells. The major classes of APCs presenting antigen to Th cells are the macrophages, B lymphocytes and dendritic cells. Macrophages phagocytose antigen either non-specifically or following opsonization, and peptide fragments are generated in cytoplasmic compartments before re-expression on surface MHC class II molecules. B cells may also internalize antigen following capture with surface immunoglobulin molecules. The B cell is also able to generate peptide fragments of antigen that are re-expressed on surface class II molecules. Dendritic cells are known to constitutively express MHC class II and take up antigen by phagocytosis or macropinocytosis.

97

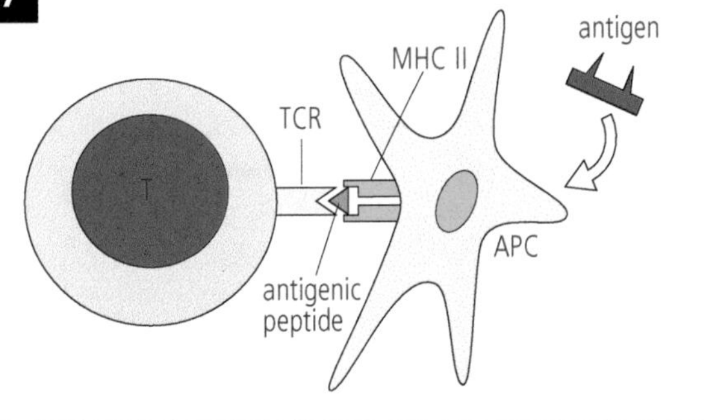

97 T cell antigen recognition. T cells recognize antigens by binding specifically to antigenic peptides presented on the surface of APC by class I or class II MHC molecules. The T cells use their specific receptors (TCRs) to recognize the unique combination of MHC molecule and antigenic peptide.

- Secretion of cytokines (e.g. IL-2) and expression of high affinity cytokine receptors (IL-2R), enabling these cytokines to act in an 'autocrine' fashion to maintain activation.
- Rapid division to form large numbers of identical T cells ('clonal proliferation').
- Differentiation of the cloned cells to an effector or memory function (99, 100).

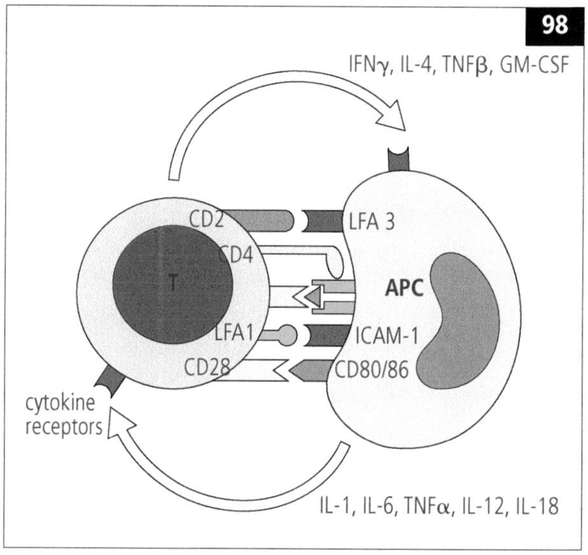

98 Co-stimulatory signals for T cell activation. The interaction between TCRs and the MHC-peptide complex is insufficient to activate a T lymphocyte. Additional molecular interactions between surface molecules on the APC and T cell are required, in addition to the action of soluble factors (cytokines) released by one cell and binding to specific cytokine receptors on the other. One such molecular interaction involves CD28 and CD80/86.

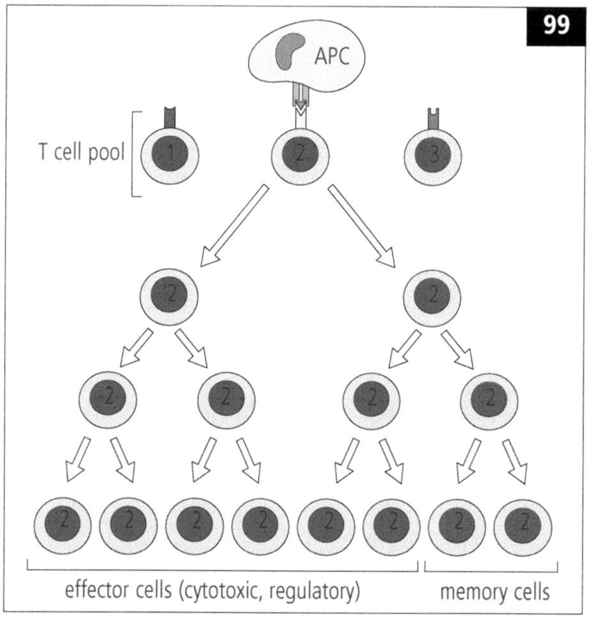

99 Clonal selection of T lymphocytes. T lymphocytes are programmed to recognize antigenic peptide in the context of a self-MHC molecule through the TCR. When appropriate antigen-specific T cells are selected from the circulating pool, they are increased in number (clonal proliferation) and mature into effector and memory T cells (clonal differentiation). All daughter cells share the same TCR.

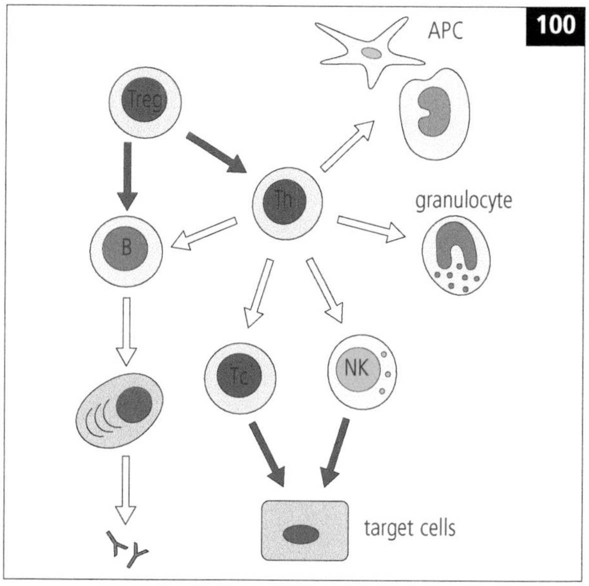

100 T lymphocyte functions. T lymphocytes have three major roles in generation and regulation of the immune response. Activated helper T cells provide co-stimulatory signals to B lymphocytes for the production of antibody, and, through cytokine production, can enhance or suppress the actions of a range of other effector cells including NK cells, macrophages and granulocytes. Cytokines derived from other cell types may also influence the activity of these populations. Some T lymphocytes are directly cytotoxic (Tc cells) and others (Treg) may regulate (suppress) the action of lymphoid cells.

B LYMPHOCYTE ACTIVATION

Recognition of antigen by B lymphocytes differs from T cells in that B cell SmIg recognizes a conformational epitope of an antigen that is not necessarily associated with the surface of an APC. A small group of antigens is able directly to activate B cells in the absence of T cell 'help' (T-independent antigens). These are generally molecules with simple repeating units (e.g. bacterial polysaccharide) that are able to cross-link the B cell receptors (SmIg). The majority of antigens, however, can only activate B cells in the presence of T cell help (T-dependent antigens).

Activation of B cells again requires a combination of signals. Signal 1 for a B cell is antigen recognition, which occurs through the B cell receptor. The co-stimulatory signals for B lymphocytes are T cell derived cytokines (e.g. IL-4), in addition to interactions between surface molecules on the B and T cells including recognition of antigenic peptides presented by MHC class II (**101**). Activated B cells migrate into the germinal centres of secondary lymphoid tissue, where they transform to lymphoblasts, rapidly divide (clonal proliferation), undergo somatic mutation of V region genes and are directed by the action of specific cytokines to undertake a second rearrangement of Ig genes known as the 'immunoglobulin class switch'. In this instance there is replacement of the μ and δ genes by a further heavy chain gene downstream of these loci.

101

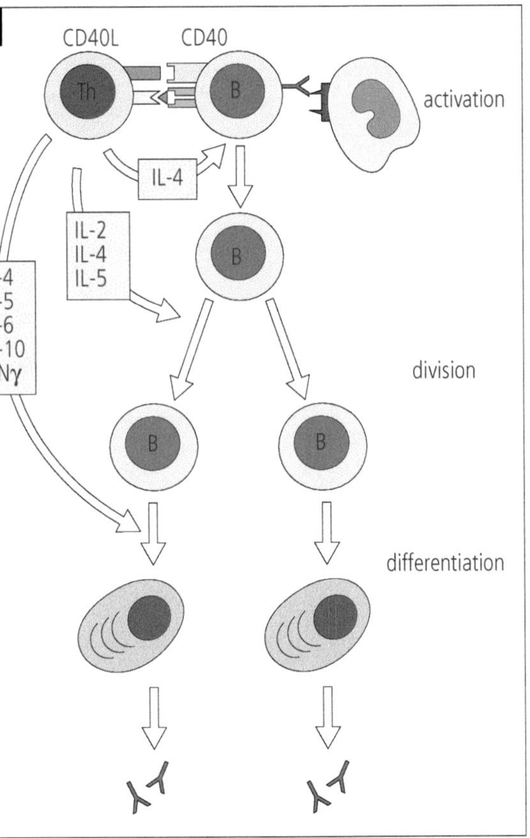

101 B lymphocyte activation. B cell activation requires recognition of a conformational determinant of antigen (possibly on the surface of an APC) with co-stimulatory signals provided by Th cells in the form of interactions between molecules on the surface of the B and T cells (including TCR recognition of processed peptide) and released cytokines (e.g. IL-4). Cytokines are also involved in B cell division and the differentiation of B cells into plasma cells for antibody production.

102

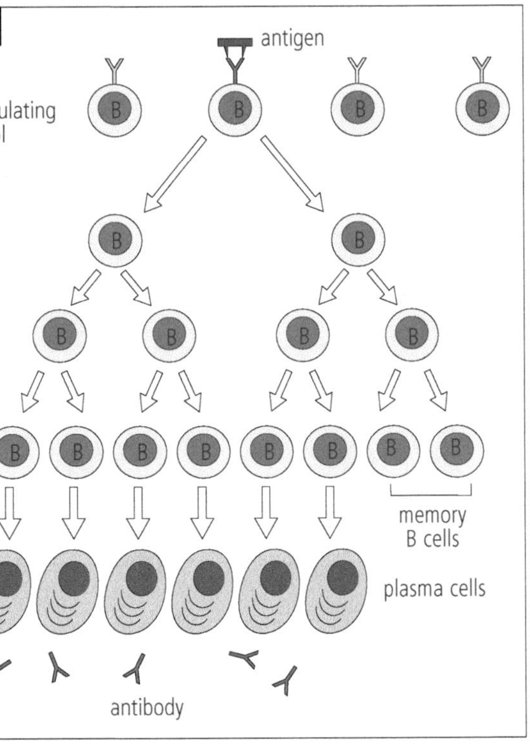

102 Clonal selection of B cells. B cells are programmed to make antibody of a single specificity. In an immune response, antigen-specific B cells are selected from the circulating pool, expanded in number (clonal proliferation) and differentiate into plasma cells that secrete antibody and memory B cells (clonal differentiation). The specificity of B cell SmIg is identical in all daughter cells and for the secreted antibody.

The μ and δ genes are likely looped out and deleted and the B cell becomes committed to production (and surface membrane expression) of Ig of a single class (e.g. IgG) (**85**). These B lymphocytes then migrate to the periphery of the germinal centre, where they re-encounter antigen on dendritic cells. The majority of B cells have mutated receptors that interact with low affinity; therefore, the cells undergo apoptosis, but those cells with appropriate receptors leave the germinal centre to differentiate into memory B cells or plasma cells that secrete antibody (**102**).

CYTOTOXICITY

Cytotoxicity is mediated by phagocytes, antibody and complement, $CD8^+$ T cells and NK cells (**103**).

The cytotoxic destruction of a target cell (e.g. neoplastic or virally infected cell) by a cytotoxic T cell or NK cell proceeds through a series of stages.

Recognition

The cytotoxic cell must recognize the target cell in an MHC-restricted or non-MHC-restricted fashion. The former involves target cell expression of peptide by surface MHC class I for $CD8^+$ T cells. NK cells mediate recognition through the NK receptor, but these lymphocytes also have surface FcR and can mediate cytotoxicity following the interaction of target cell-bound Ig with the FcR (antibody-dependent cell-mediated cytotoxicity [ADCC]) (**103**). A range of other molecular interactions between the target and cytotoxic cells is likely to be important (**104**).

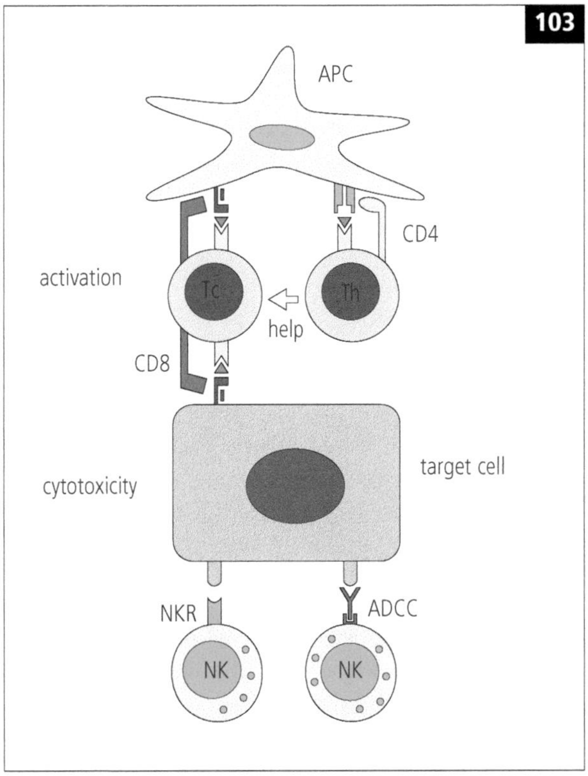

103 Target cell recognition by cytotoxic lymphocytes. A range of lymphocytes can mediate cytotoxic destruction of a target cell and these may be distinguished by the recognition events that precede cytotoxicity. $CD8^+$ T cells recognize antigen expressed on class I histocompatibility antigens, whereas NK cells have a unique NK receptor that permits non-MHC restricted recognition. NK cells also have surface FcRs, allowing recognition of antibody coated target cells. Initial activation of the $CD8^+$ T cell by professional APCs may require help from $CD4^+$ T cells.

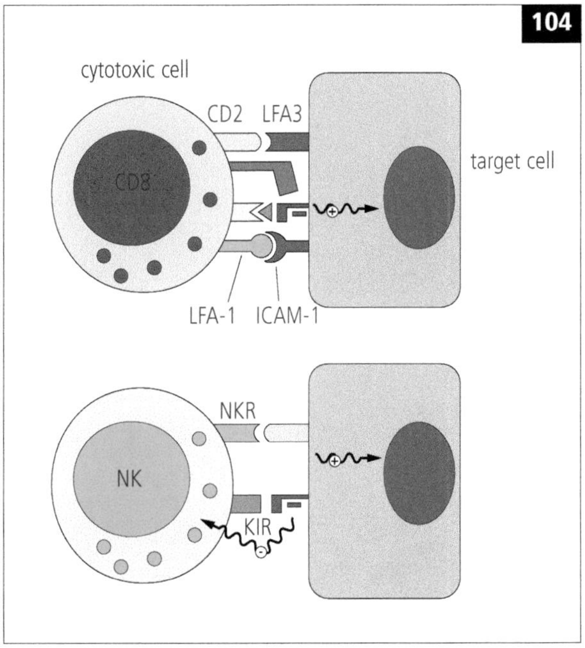

104 Molecular interactions between Tc and target cells. The interaction between $CD8^+$ cytotoxic and target cells may involve numerous molecular interactions in addition to the antigen-specific recognition mediated by the TCR. One such interaction is the binding of CD8 to MHC class I. The NK cell recognizes surface carbohydrate via the NK receptor. NK cells can be inhibited by the interaction of class I with the killer-cell inhibitory receptor (KIR).

Adhesion

Following recognition, the target and cytotoxic cells have close cytoplasmic apposition, with the formation of tight junctions to contain the cytotoxic process and prevent 'innocent bystander' cytolysis of nearby cells. The cytoplasmic granules of the cytotoxic cell migrate towards the target cell surface.

Cytolysis

The final stage of cytotoxicity involves destruction of the target cell. This largely occurs following induction of apoptosis within the target cell, which may be initiated by the different mechanisms summarized in **105**. Cytotoxic lymphocytes are 'multi-hit' cells and may detach from the target cell and subsequently kill other targets.

IMMUNOREGULATION

Like all biological systems, the immune system must be able to regulate its own activity. Failure to do so may result in the undesirable consequence of damage to self-tissue. This does not refer, in this context, to positive immunoregulation (such as the effects of IL-2 in initiating an immune response), but to regulatory mechanisms that limit the immune response by 'suppressing' activity of antigen-specific lymphocytes. Immunoregulation remains a poorly understood area of immunology, and there are numerous mechanisms that likely work in combination to 'down-regulate' an immune response.

105

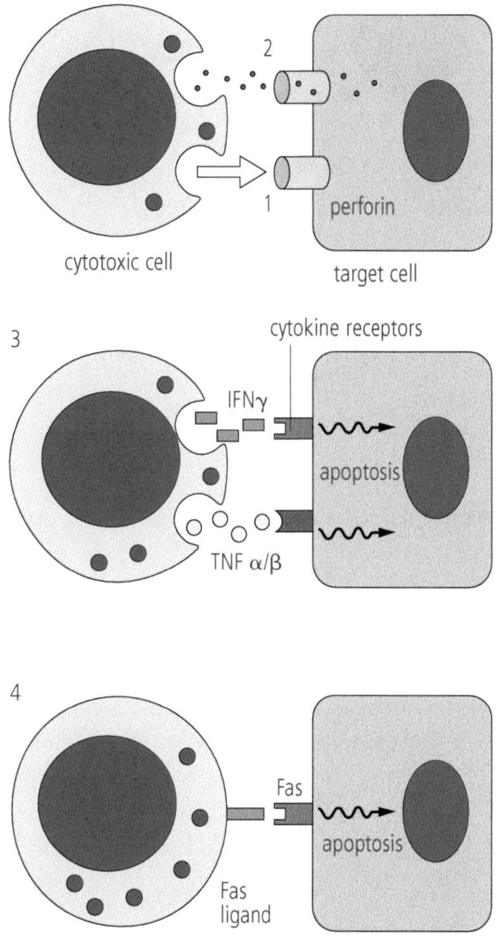

105 Mechanisms of cell-mediated cytotoxicity. Killing of a target cell by a cytotoxic lymphocyte may involve a number of different mechanisms. Following recognition and adhesion, the cytotoxic cell degranulates and releases pore forming molecules (perforin) and enzymes into the area adjacent to the target cell membrane. Perforin is polymerized and inserts into the target cell as a transmembrane channel akin to the MAC of the complement pathways (1). Although osmotic imbalance may occur, other enzymes and toxic substances (fragmentins) may enter the target cell via these channels and mediate target cell apoptosis (programmed cell death) (2). Cytokines released from the cytotoxic cell may bind to receptors on the target cell membrane and trigger cell death (3). Finally, target cell apoptosis may occur independently of perforin and be mediated by direct interaction between Fas ligand (on the lymphocyte surface) and the Fas molecule on the target cell (4).

Antigen removal

In an effective immune response, antigen is destroyed and less is available to perpetuate the function of activated lymphocytes.

Regulation by antibody

Antibody binds antigen, thereby blocking the availability of antigenic epitopes to SmIg on B lymphocytes. Immune complexes of antigen and antibody may bind to FcR on B lymphocytes and cross-link SmIg, thereby inhibiting B cell activation (**106**). Alternatively, immune complexes may be taken up by phagocytic cells that release suppressive substances (e.g. prostaglandin E_2).

Regulation by hormones

There are complex regulatory interactions between the immune and endocrine systems and the brain referred to as the 'neuroendocrine immunological loop'. For example, endogenously released glucocorticoid can suppress the immune system (**107**) and hormones derived from non-endocrine tissue may have local autocrine or paracrine effects on immune or inflammatory cells.

Cell-mediated regulation

It is well recognized that subpopulations of lymphocytes are able to regulate the activity of others, and such 'suppressor cells' can be

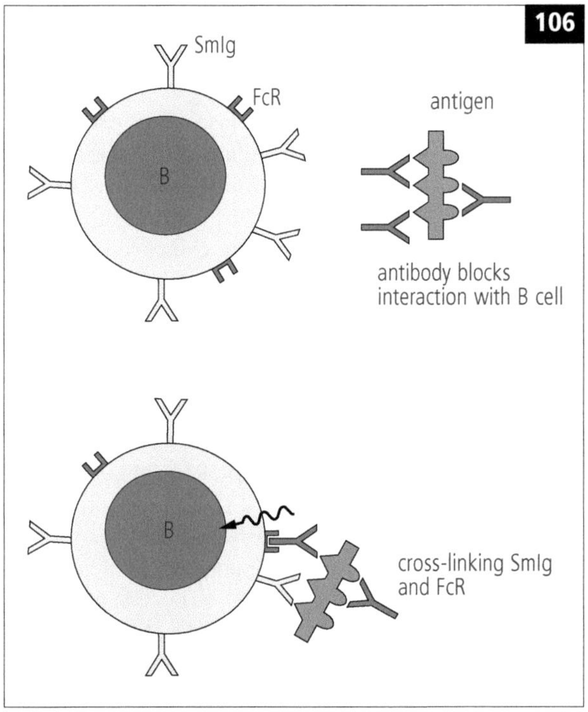

106 Antibody-mediated suppression of the immune response. Antibody may coat antigen and block the interaction between an epitope and B cell SmIg, preventing B cell activation. Alternatively, immune complexes of antigen and antibody bind to B cell FcRs and cross-link the B cell SmIg. This allows B cell priming but prevents antibody synthesis. This effect is not epitope specific.

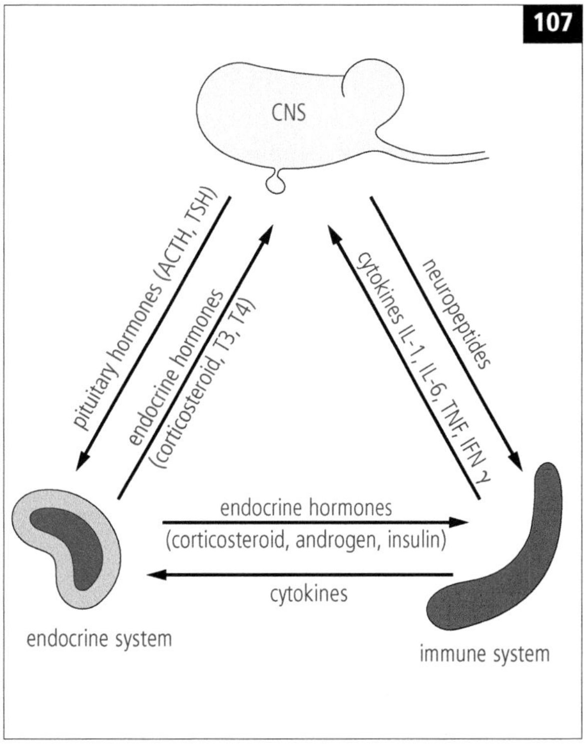

107 The neuroendocrine immunological loop. These three body systems are able to cross-regulate each other. For example, immune cytokines (IL-1, IL-6, TNF) may re-set body temperature (pyrexia) via the hypothalamus, endogenous glucocorticoid may be immunosuppressive, and neuropeptides may be immunoregulatory.

demonstrated in many experimental models of immunological disease (**108**). Both CD8⁺ and CD4⁺ T cells can have suppressor function, although it is now generally accepted that CD4⁺ T cells are dominant in this regard. Suppression is generally antigen-specific and likely involves the suppressor cell using a TCR specific for the antigen driving the immune response (but perhaps different 'suppressor epitopes' on the antigen). However, antigen-activated suppressor cells may in some circumstances inhibit the activity of other unrelated lymphocytes in their immediate vicinity ('bystander suppression'). Understanding of the mechanisms of suppression has been one of the growth areas of immunology in recent years. Initially, much emphasis was placed on the ability of antigen-specific Th1 and Th2 cells to 'cross-regulate' each other by production of inhibitory cytokines (termed 'immune deviation'), but although this undoubtedly occurs, it may not be a significant means of immunoregulation. At least three other specific regulatory populations have been described. Th3 cells are characterized by the preferential production of the cytokine TGFβ and are important in the maintenance of oral tolerance. CD4⁺ T cells that express the molecule CD25 (the IL-2 receptor) are normally found in the body and are thought to act as 'natural suppressors' of deleterious immune responses. These lymphocytes (generally known as Treg cells) are thought to function by directly contacting the cell that they intend to suppress, and they are also characterized by IL-10 production and expression of a range of other molecules (e.g. CTLA-4, some PPRs) and genes (*GITR* and *Foxp3*). CD4⁺CD25⁺ T regulatory cells have been identified in cats in an experimental study of FIV infection, and Foxp3⁺ regulatory cells are recognized in the dog.

In experimental systems, a further population of CD4⁺ T cells that preferentially express IL-10 (Tr1 cells) are recognized, and these are termed 'induced suppressors'. Induced suppressors do not require direct contact with their target cell, but influence the target through the secreted IL-10. Finally, the TCR of a suppressor cell may recognize epitopes (idiotypes) derived from the antigen-specific receptor (TCR or SmIg) of cells that are effectors in an immune response. Such idiotype-specific cells may suppress those lymphocytes bearing receptor molecules containing the idiotypic region.

It is now recognized that there is a fine balance between the effector and suppressor functions of T lymphocytes. Although regulatory cells are essential to control an overzealous or unnecessary immune response, their function would clearly be undesirable in the effector phase of a productive immune response. Down-regulation of Treg activity might be achieved through limiting the provision of key cytokines (e.g. IL-2) or by engaging specific surface receptor molecules. Treg cells are known to express PRRs, and microbial engagement of these molecules inhibits their suppressive function.

108

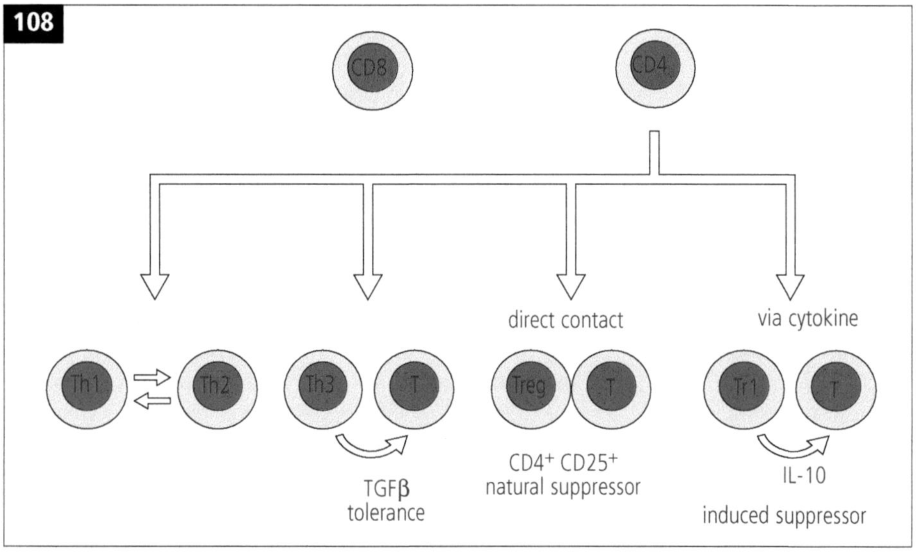

108 Types of regulatory T cell. Regulatory activity of T cells resides primarily with the CD4⁺ subpopulation, although CD8⁺ T cells can also be suppressive. Models of CD4⁺ T cell regulation include (1) cross-regulation by mutually antagonistic Th1 and Th2 cells; (2) the action of TGFβ secreting Th3 cells that are likely of importance in mediating mucosal antigen tolerance; (3) the presence of CD4⁺CD25⁺ 'natural suppressor' (Treg) cells that mediate suppression by direct contact with their target; and (4) the action of IL-10 producing 'induced suppressor' (Tr1) cells that inhibit the function of target cells via release of this cytokine.

Lymphocyte apoptosis

Elimination of antigen-specific lymphocytes by apoptosis (following occupation of Fas or tumour necrosis factor [TNF] receptors) may also be a means of switching off an immune response. Apoptosis may also occur when lymphocytes are no longer stimulated at the conclusion of an immune response. A further means of down-regulating an immune response involves the nature of the interaction between T cell surface molecules and ligands expressed by the APC. As shown in **98**, activation of a naïve T cell involves the interaction of the T cell CD28 molecule with CD80 or CD86 expressed by the APC, with subsequent transduction of a co-stimulatory signal to the T cell. Following activation, the T cell expresses the molecule CTLA-4 that can also bind CD80/86, but with much greater affinity. Co-stimulation via the interaction of CTLA-4 and CD80/86 causes an inhibitory signal to be delivered to the T cell and shuts down the proliferative phase of the immune response.

IMMUNOLOGICAL MEMORY

Following an immune response, the immune system retains specific memory of the antigen so that subsequent antigen exposure results in a more effective 'secondary' immune response. Immunological memory is mediated by long-lived memory T and B cells, which are more sensitive to antigen and may express surface molecules that differ from virgin cells. For example, naïve T cells express a form of the leukocyte common antigen (CD45) known as CD45RA, which is a high molecular weight isoform that incorporates three variable exons, A, B and C. Memory and effector T cells express CD45RO, a low molecular weight isoform in which none of these three exons is included. The CD45RO is more closely associated with the TCR and may allow more efficient signal transduction on encounter with antigenic peptide. Memory T cells also have increased levels of the surface adhesion molecules L-selectin and CD44.

Memory cells are likely to undergo continual low level division following periodic stimulation by antigen that may be:

- Sequestered in a reservoir in lymphoid tissue (associated with dendritic cells).
- Periodically reintroduced to the body (booster vaccinations).
- Derived from an environmental antigen with common epitopes ('cross-reactive' antigen).

The effectiveness of immunological memory is best demonstrated by following the kinetics of antibody production after primary and secondary exposure to antigen (**109**).

109 B lymphocyte memory. Secondary antigenic challenge results in activation of memory B cells. The characteristics of the secondary antibody response are a shorter lag phase, a higher antibody titre, which persists for longer, and a dominance of IgG over IgM, with synthesis of antibody of greater affinity ('affinity maturation').

109

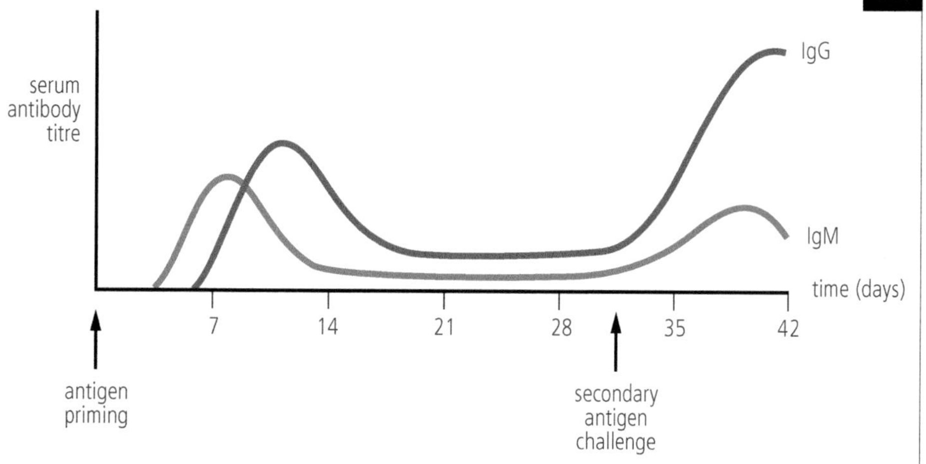

IMMUNOLOGICAL TOLERANCE

In contrast to the normal functioning of the immune system, exposure to antigen may on occasion fail to induce an active immune response, a situation termed 'immunological tolerance'. Tolerance has been recognized in several different contexts:

- **Neonatal tolerance** occurs when an animal is exposed to foreign antigen either *in utero* or within the immediate post-natal period. Such exposure appears to persuade the developing immune system that the antigen is part of 'self' and therefore should be ignored immunologically. The concept of neonatal tolerance was first proposed with the observation that transplants performed between genetically dissimilar dizygotic bovine twins were not rejected, presumptively due to exposure *in utero* to antigens expressed by cells of the twin and the development of tolerance to these antigens. Experimentally, tolerance can be induced in this way by deliberate exposure of neonates to foreign antigen, and transgenic mice are tolerant to the product of the inserted gene.
- Tolerance can also be induced experimentally in adult animals. **Adult tolerance** occurs following delivery of antigen by specific dosage regimes. 'High zone' adult tolerance results from exposure to a single very high concentration of antigen, whereas 'low zone' tolerance occurs following repeated exposure to small doses of antigen. Adult tolerance is readily induced in rodent experimental systems, and allergen-specific immunotherapy for allergic disease (see Chapter 5, p. 133) may be considered a form of adult tolerance.
- Another manifestation of this phenomenon is **oral tolerance**, whereby experimental delivery of antigen across the intestinal mucosa leads to a failure to respond to the same antigen when subsequently injected parenterally. In addition to being an interesting experimental procedure, the induction of oral tolerance likely has physiological relevance in preventing the gut immune system from responding to dietary antigens and epitopes derived from the gut microflora. Indeed, failure of oral tolerance is likely to underlie diseases such as dietary hypersensitivity and inflammatory bowel disease (see Chapter 7, p. 212. The tolerance response can also be induced by delivery of antigen across other mucosal barriers (e.g. intranasal tolerance), and these mechanisms have been exploited in the development of novel immunotherapies (see Chapter 16, p. 403).
- Finally, **self tolerance** relates to failure of the normal immune system to respond to self-tissue antigens, producing an autoimmune response that may lead to autoimmune disease (see Chapter 3, p. 78). Low levels of self-immune reactivity do occur naturally (i.e. for the removal of senescent cells), but these must be tightly controlled to prevent deleterious side-effects.

Understanding the tolerance response has been a major research theme in immunology. There are likely numerous mechanisms by which this immunological 'paralysis' arises. Although there is some evidence that exposure to antigen in a tolerizing protocol might induce apoptosis (and therefore deletion from the repertoire) of the responding T cells, it is considered more likely that the antigen-specific T cells persist in the body but are regulated by the range of mechanisms discussed above, in particular involving 'anergy' (failure of an APC to deliver the full range of co-stimulatory signals for T cell activation) or the action of regulatory T cells (see also Chapter 3, p.78).

AGE-RELATED CHANGES IN THE IMMUNE SYSTEM

A number of studies have now investigated the development of the immune system in neonatal companion animals and the alterations in immune parameters that occur with increasing age (immunosenescence). These changes are broadly in line with those described for man, and some examples are cited below.

The number and proportions of feline blood lymphocytes alters in the 90-day period after birth. The absolute lymphocyte count rises, as do the numbers of T and B lymphocytes, but the proportion of $CD4^+$ and $CD8^+$ T cells changes from a relatively high CD4:CD8 ratio at birth (4.4) to a lower value at 90 days of age (2.9). These data are derived from animals housed in an experimental facility. The thymus of these kittens was of maximal size at days 23 and 46 of monitoring, and there was a similar change in the proportion of T cell subsets over time, with a relative increase in $CD8^+$ cells. The numbers of double negative or double positive (CD4 and CD8) cells remained stable at all time points. Thymic involution begins at around

6–8 months of age in the kitten, and in puppies there is progressive decline in thymus weight to 23 months of age. The lymph nodes of kittens in this study also showed expansion of the CD8 population (with reduced CD4:CD8) over time, together with an increase in the number of IgG^+ lymphocytes.

Very similar data are reported for Beagle puppies from birth to 90 days of age. An initial high CD4:CD8 ratio decreases as the proportion of $CD8^+$ cells increases, achieving almost adult levels by day 90. Over the same time period, the number of $CD21^+$ B cells decreases from the newborn level. The ability of blood lymphocytes to respond to stimulation by mitogens (see Chapter 12, p. 298) gradually increases to near adult level by day 90. There are also breed influences on these parameters. In a comparative study of Beagles, GSDs, Dalmatians and Dachshunds, significant differences were found; for example, Beagles had the highest total lymphocyte counts, whereas GSDs had the lowest.

In aged dogs, immunosenesence is characterized by similar changes to those occurring in geriatric humans. These include reduction in the number of circulating B cells and T cells; an increase in the proportion of blood $CD8^+$ cells and reduction in $CD4^+$ cells (with reduced CD4:CD8 ratio from 3.0 to 1.8); an increase in the relative proportion of memory to naïve T cells; reduced capacity of blood lymphocytes to respond to non-specific stimulation by mitogens; and reduced intradermal delayed-type hypersensitivity reactions (see Chapter 2, p. 69). In contrast, there is elevation in serum IgG and IgA concentration with age, with increased concentration of salivary IgA and no impairment in serological responsiveness to vaccination or exposure to a novel antigen. Innate immune function also appears relatively age-resistant, with no impairment in neutrophil phagocytosis or NK cell activity in older dogs. Canine immunosenescence is an active area of research, as pet food manufacturers attempt to formulate diets that slow this range of changes in geriatric animals. Of interest is a study that reports reversal of these trends by lifetime caloric restriction in experimentally housed Labrador Retriever dogs. A molecular basis for the observation that canine body size is inversely related to life span has been described. A unique haplotype of 20 individual single nucleotide polymorphisms is found in the gene encoding the insulin-like growth factor-1 (IGF1) in small breed dogs.

Feline immunosenescence follows the same trends as described for the dog. The blood CD4:CD8 ratio drops from 1.75 to 1.35 and the total numbers of lymphocytes and all subsets ($CD4^+$, $CD8^+$ T cells, B cells and NK cells) reduces. There is evidence for reduced proliferative response to mitogen stimulation of blood lymphocytes and intradermal delayed type hypersensitivity response. Concentrations of serum IgA and IgM are elevated in older cats, but there is no change in function of the complement pathway or in the concentration of acute phase proteins.

FURTHER READING

Bao Y, Guo Y, Xiao S *et al.* (2010) Molecular characterization of the VH repertoire in *Canis familiaris*. *Veterinary Immunology and Immunopathology* **137**:64-75.

Blount DG, Pritchard DI, Heaton PR (2005) Age-related alterations to immune parameters in Labrador Retriever dogs. *Veterinary Immunology and Immunopathology* **108**:399–407.

Burgener IA, Jungi TW (2008) Antibodies specific for human or murine Toll-like receptors detect canine leukocytes by flow cytometry. *Veterinary Immunology and Immunopathology* **124**:184-191.

Campbell DJ, Rawlings JM, Koelsch S *et al.* (2004) Age-related differences in parameters of feline immune status. *Veterinary Immunology and Immunopathology* **100**:73–80.

6 ref removed 8 (red) to replace

Day MJ (2007) Immune system development in the dog and cat. *Journal of Comparative Pathology* **137**:S10–S15.

Day MJ (2007) Immunoglobulin G subclass distribution in canine leishmaniosis: a review and analysis of pitfalls in interpretation. *Veterinary Parasitology* **147**:2–8.

Day MJ (2010) Ageing, immunosenescence and inflammageing in the dog and cat. *Journal of Comparative Pathology* **142**:S60-S69.

Faldyna M, Leva L, Knotigova P *et al.* (2001) Lymphocyte subsets in peripheral blood of dogs: a flow cytometric study. *Veterinary Immunology and Immunopathology* **82**:23–37.

Greeley EH, Spitznagel E, Lawler DF *et al.* (2006) Modulation of canine immunosenescence by lifelong caloric restriction. *Veterinary Immunology and Immunopathology* **111**:287–299.

Harley R, Gruffydd-Jones TJ, Day MJ (2003) Characterisation of immune cell populations in oral mucosal tissue of healthy adult cats. *Journal of Comparative Pathology* **128**:146–155.

HogenEsch H, Thompson S, Dunham A *et al.* (2004) Effect of age on immune parameters and the immune response of dogs to vaccines: a cross-sectional study. *Veterinary Immunology and Immunopathology* **97**:77–85.

Horiuchi Y, Nakajima Y, Nariai Y *et al.* (2007) Th1/Th2 balance in canine peripheral blood lymphocytes: a flow cytometric study. *Veterinary Immunology and Immunopathology* **118**:179–185.

Ignacio G, Nordone S, Howard KE *et al.* (2005) Toll-like receptor expression in feline lymphoid tissues. *Veterinary Immunology and Immunopathology* **106**:229–237.

Kennedy LJ, Barnes A, Happ GM *et al.* (2002) Extensive interbreed, but minimal intrabreed, variation of DLA class II alleles and haplotypes in dogs. *Tissue Antigens* **59**:194–204.

Kjelgaard-Hansen M, Luntang-Jensen M, Willesen J *et al.* (2007) Measurement of serum interleukin-10 in the dog. *Veterinary Journal* **173**:361–365.

Matiasovic J, Andrysikova R, Karasova D *et al.* (2009) The structure and functional analysis of canine T-cell receptor beta region. *Veterinary Immunology and Immunopathology* **132**:282-287.

Peeters D, Day MJ, Farnir F *et al.* (2005) Distribution of leucocyte subsets in the canine respiratory tract. *Journal of Comparative Pathology* **132**:261–272.

Peeters D, Peters IR, Farnir F *et al.* (2005) Real-time RT–PCR quantification of mRNA encoding cytokines and chemokines in histologically normal canine nasal, bronchial and pulmonary tissue. *Veterinary Immunology and Immunopathology* **104**:195–204.

Peters IR, Calvert EL, Hall EJ *et al.* (2004) Measurement of immunoglobulin concentrations in the faeces of healthy dogs. *Clinical and Laboratory Diagnostic Investigation* **11**:841–848.

Peters IR, Helps CR, Calvert EL *et al.* (2004) Identification of four allelic variants of the dog IGHA gene. *Immunogenetics* **56**:254–260.

Peters IR, Helps CR, Calvert EL *et al.* (2005) Cytokine mRNA quantification in histologically normal canine duodenal mucosa by real-time RT–PCR. *Veterinary Immunology and Immunopathology* **103**:101–111.

Pinheiro D, Singh Y, Grant CR *et al.* (2010) Phenotypic and functional characterization of a $CD4^+$ $CD25^{high}$ $FOXP3^{high}$ regulatory T-cell population in the dog. *Immunology* **132**:111-122.

Sutter NB, Ostrander EA (2004) Dog star rising: the canine genetic system. *Nature Reviews Genetics* **5**:900–910.

Sutter NB, Bustamante CD, Chase K *et al.* (2007) A single IGF1 allele is a major determinant of small size in dogs. *Science* **316**:112–115.

Valli JL, Williamson A, Sharif S *et al.* (2010) *In vitro* cytokine responses of peripheral blood mononuclear cells from healthy dogs to distemper virus, *Malassezia* and *Toxocara*. *Veterinary Immunology and Immunopathology* **134**:218-229.

Waly N, Gruffydd-Jones TJ, Stokes CR *et al.* (2001) The distribution of leucocyte subsets in the small intestine of normal cats. *Journal of Comparative Pathology* **124**:172–182.

Wood BA, O'Halloran KP, Vande Woude S (2011) Development and validation of a multiplex microsphere-based assay for detection of domestic cat (*Felis catus*) cytokines. *Clinical and Vaccine Immunology* **18**:387-392.

Yuhki N, Beck T, Stephens R *et al.* (2007) Comparative genomic structure of human, dog, and cat MHC: *HLA, DLA,* and *FLA*. *Journal of Heredity* **98**:390-399.

2 IMMUNOPATHOLOGICAL MECHANISMS

Michael J. Day

INTRODUCTION

The adaptive immune system has evolved in order to combat the multitude of potential pathogens that may penetrate host defences and initiate disease. The immune system responds to individual pathogens by selecting from its repertoire those mechanisms that are most likely to eliminate the organism. At either end of the spectrum lie cell-mediated immunity (CMI) and humoral immunity, but in many infections aspects of both processes are incorporated into the immune response.

The same immunological effector mechanisms that make up the protective immune response may sometimes be utilized inappropriately and cause pathological change. For example, in some infections the disease process is extended beyond that caused by the pathogen by the development of immune-mediated sequelae such as immune-complex deposition. Alternatively, some pathological immune responses are not driven by pathogens, but by innocuous foreign substances (causing allergic disease) or by self-antigens (causing autoimmunity).

The immunological mechanisms involved in these different types of immune response may conveniently be classified as one of four 'hypersensitivity reactions' (type I–type IV). The use of the word 'hypersensitivity' implies that the mechanisms are allergic responses that develop in individuals sensitized over time to allergens, but as this is not always the case, it may be more appropriate to consider 'immunopathological mechanisms' of types I–IV that may be utilized appropriately (in protective immunity) or inappropriately (in allergy or autoimmunity). These mechanisms are not mutually exclusive and it is possible for more than one to be involved in any one immune response.

The original classification of hypersensitivity has been modified to take into account non-classical mechanisms such as the interaction of antibody with cell surface receptor molecules. Other forms of immunopathology are not readily incorporated into the classification; for example, disease that may be induced following lymphocyte activation by microbial 'superantigens' or that involving amyloid deposition. This chapter examines immunopathological mechanisms (*Table 1*) that underlie protective and pathological immune responses.

Table 1: Summary of immunopathological mechanisms. The four major immunopathological mechanisms (types I–IV hypersensitivity) may be utilized appropriately in the protective immune response or inappropriately to cause hypersensitivity (allergic) or autoimmune diseases. Types I–III involve antibody (IgE or IgG) mediated effects, whereas type IV is initiated by antigen-specific T lymphocytes. Some classes of microbes produce 'superantigens' that can also mediate immunopathology by non-specifically activating clones of T and B lymphocytes.

Type	Major immune reactants	Antigen	Effector mechanisms	Examples
Type I (immediate)	IgE mast cells Th2 cells	Soluble antigen	IgE coated mast cell degranulation and inflammation	Response to intestinal nematodes, atopic dermatitis
Type II (cytotoxic)	IgG IgM	Cell-associated antigen	Complement fixation, FcR and C3bR binding to phagocytic or NK cells	FIA, AIHA

Continues on page 62

Table 1: Summary of immunopathological mechanisms. (*Continued*)

Type	Major immune reactants	Antigen	Effector mechanisms	Examples
		Cell surface receptors	Agonist or antagonist of receptor function	Myasthenia gravis
Type III (immune complex)	IgG	Soluble antigen	Immune complex formation, complement fixation, phagocytic cells	Leishmaniosis, SLE
Type IV (delayed)	T cells	Soluble or cell-associated antigen	Th1 cells, cytotoxic lymphocytes,macrophage activation, IFNγ production	Obligate intracellular parasites, rheumatoid arthritis, contact dermatitis
Microbial superantigens	T and B cells	Superantigen	Non-classical activation of T and B cells	Bacterial or viral infection, autoimmunity

TYPE I HYPERSENSITIVITY

Type I hypersensitivity (**110**) is utilized protectively in the immune response to agents that establish at mucosal sites (e.g. intestinal nematodes) and pathologically in response to environmental allergens (e.g. house dust mite) that cross the skin, respiratory or gastrointestinal tracts in allergic diseases such as asthma or atopic dermatitis.

The first phase of this process involves sensitization to the causative antigen (or allergen); this may occur over a long period of time. Factors such as the nature and dose of antigen, the site of exposure and the available APCs result in a Th2-dominated response. Expression of Th2 cytokines orchestrates production of antigen-specific IgE that binds initially to high affinity Fcε receptors on the surface of local mast cells and may then 'spill over' into the bloodstream to coat circulating basophils and tissue mast cells at other sites. The individual is then said to be 'sensitized'. IgE may remain attached to the mast cell surface for many months (**111**).

On subsequent local exposure to multivalent antigen, the IgE recognizes appropriate epitopes. There is cross-linking of Fcε receptors, which triggers an intracellular calcium influx, elevation of cAMP and activation of intracellular signalling pathways. The combined effect of these three events leads to rapid mast cell degranulation. Mast cell degranulation may also be mediated by allergen cross-linking IgG molecules bound to mast cell membrane FcγRIII, the binding of the biologically active complement fragments C3a and C5a to their specific receptors, or the action of a variety of drugs or lectins that bind non-specifically to carbohydrate residues on the FcεR. Mast cell degranulation may also occur following the effect of physical stimuli (e.g. cold, trauma), neuropeptides or cytokines.

Mast cell granules contain a potent combination of preformed inflammatory mediators including histamine, heparin, serotonin, kininogenase, tryptase, chymase, exoglycosidases, eosinophil and neutrophil chemotactic factors, and platelet activating factor. Additionally, there are a series of synthesized mediators, the most important of which are derived from the precursor molecule arachidonic acid, which in turn is a cleavage product of membrane phospholipids. Arachidonic acid is modified by two distinct pathways to give rise to prostaglandins, thromboxanes (cyclooxygenase pathway) and leukotrienes (lipoxygenase pathway). Mast cells are also a potent source of proinflammatory and immunoregulatory cytokines including IL-1, IL-3, IL-4, IL-5, IL-6, IL-8, IL-9, IL-13, TNFα, TGFβ and GM-CSF.

The release of this range of molecules in turn mediates local vasodilation, tissue oedema and

110a, b Type I hypersensitivity mechanism. (**a**) During the sensitization phase, allergen enters via cutaneous or mucosal surfaces and is processed by local APCs. There is preferential activation of antigen-specific Th2 cells. These provide help for B cell differentiation to IgE secreting plasma cells, while inhibiting activation of the antigen-specific Th1 population. This may occur in an immunological background deficient in Tregs, which permits expansion of allergen-specific Th2 cells. IgE antibodies occupy the Fcγ receptor on the surface of mast cells. (**b**) When a sensitized animal re-encounters allergen, there is cross-linking of IgE with an influx of intracellular calcium and triggering of degranulation. The potent inflammatory mediators released by mast cells cause vasodilation and oedema, eosinophil chemotaxis, bronchoconstriction and pruritus. Mast cell derived cytokines contribute to inflammation and enhance local IgE production.

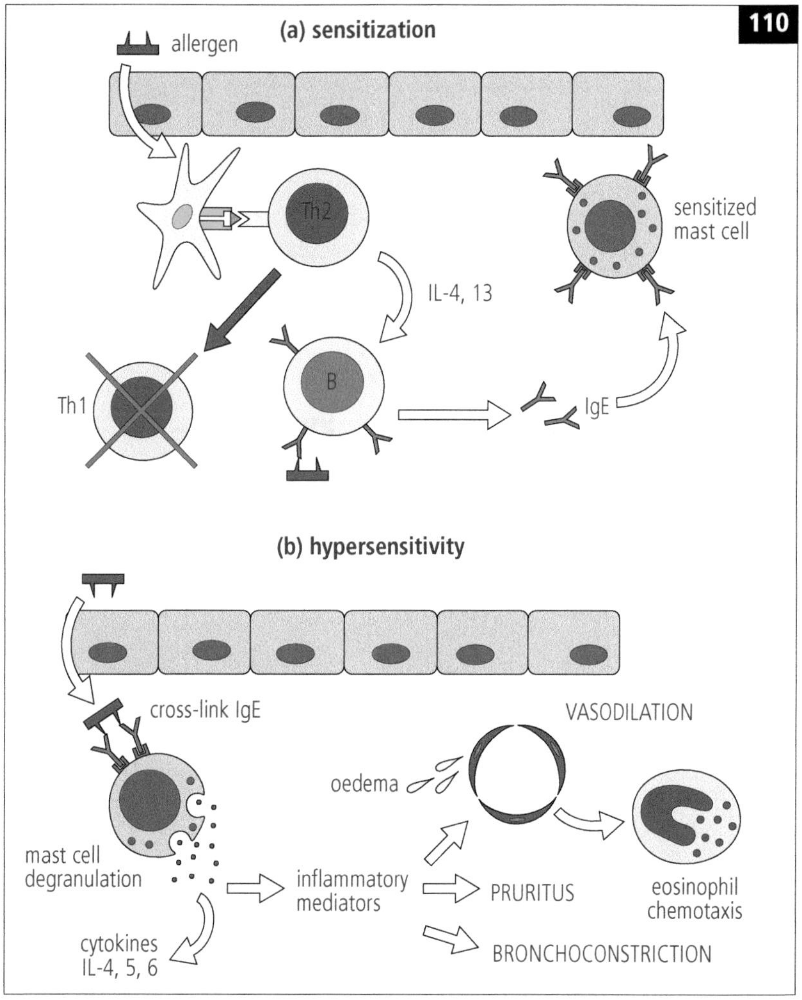

111 Mast cells in cutaneous type I hypersensitivity. Skin biopsy, stained with toluidine blue, from a dog with cutaneous hypersensitivity. Mast cells have purple cytoplasmic granules and are prominent within the superficial dermis. These cells are coated by allergen-specific IgE and will degranulate upon contact with multivalent allergen.

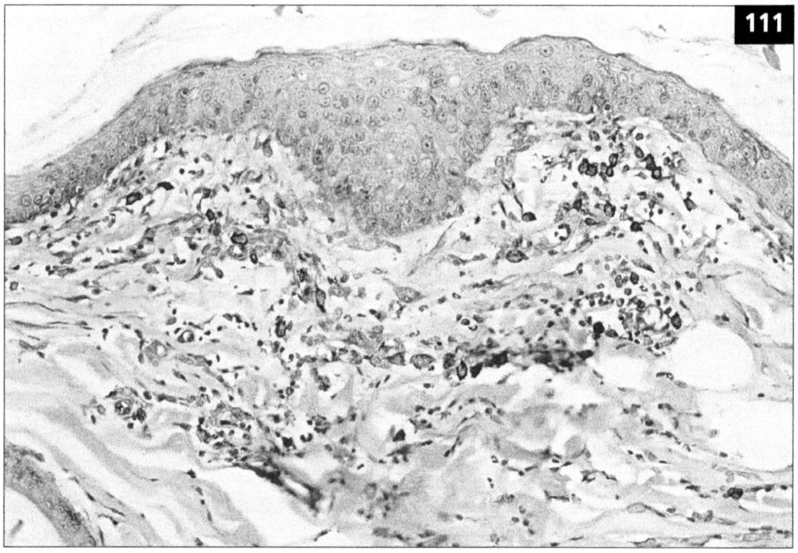

extravasation of serum proteins and inflammatory cells (particularly eosinophils) (**112–115**). In the bronchus, mast cell degranulation causes smooth muscle contraction (bronchoconstriction) and in the skin, neurological reactions stimulate pruritus. The vasoactive effect of mast cell degranulation is rapid and the process is described as 'immediate hypersensitivity'. An influx of eosinophils, macrophages and T cells occurs some 6–12 hours later and is known as the 'late phase response'. This egress of cells may be regulated by the expression of particular vascular adhesion molecules (e.g. VCAM-1) induced by Th2-derived cytokines, and by chemotactic factors including the chemokines eotaxin, eotaxin-2, eotaxin-3, RANTES and MCP-2, -3 and -4.

Although the effects of mast cell degranulation are usually localized (skin, respiratory tract), it is possible for systemically administered antigen (e.g. drugs) to activate connective tissue mast cells

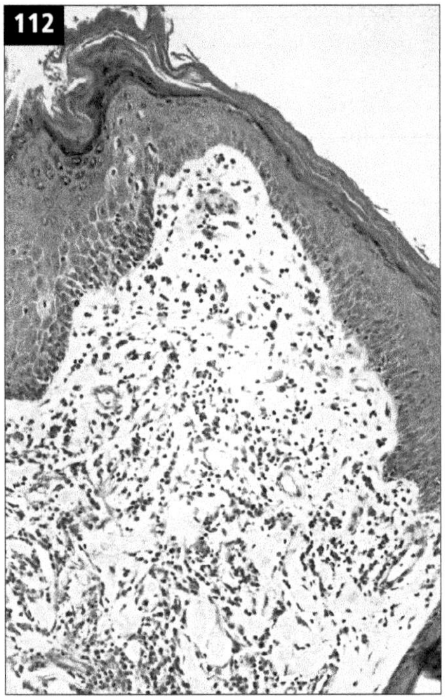

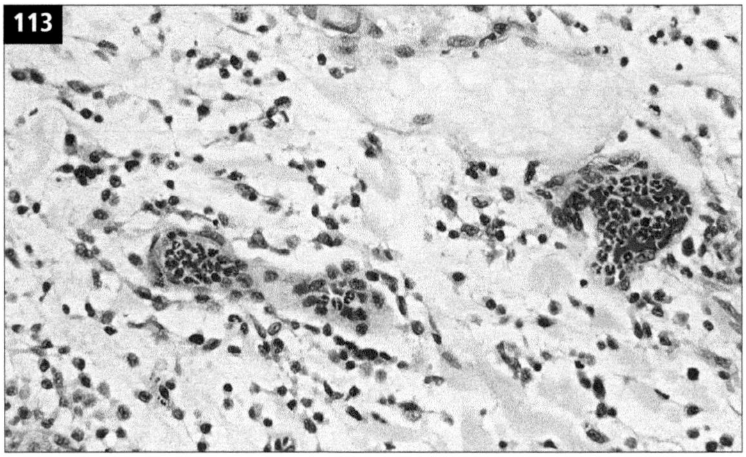

112, 113 Eosinophil chemotaxis in cutaneous type I hypersensitivity. Skin biopsies from dogs with cutaneous hypersensitivity. The effects of mast cell degranulation are clearly seen. (**112**) There is dilation of superficial dermal blood vessels with local dermal oedema and an influx of inflammatory cells (superficial perivascular dermatitis). (**113**) The blood vessels contain numerous eosinophils, which are attracted into the oedematous superficial dermis.

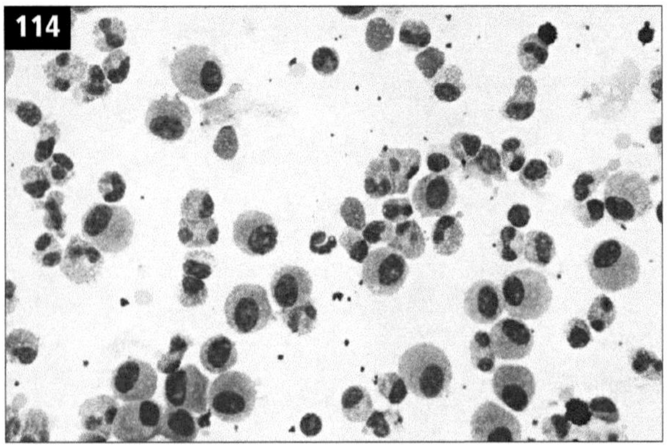

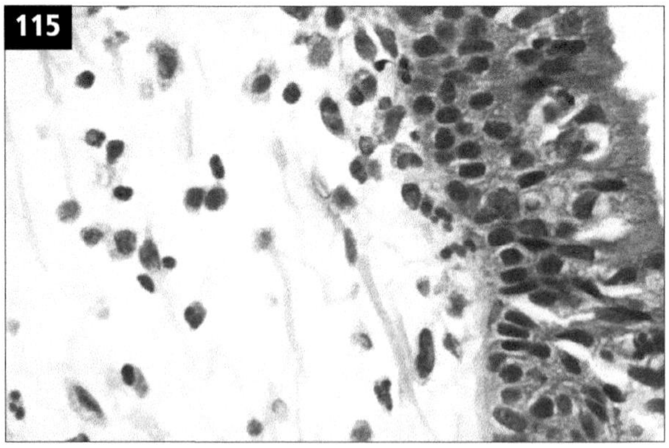

114, 115 Type I hypersensitivity mechanism in small animal airway disease. (**114**) Bronchiolar-alveolar lavage fluid from a four-year-old DSH cat with dyspnoea. There is a mixed inflammatory population of macrophages and eosinophils, suggesting that hypersensitivity (or parasitic disease) may be a component of the respiratory pathology. (**115**) Bronchial biopsy from a 12-year-old Poodle with chronic coughing and rales. The mucosa is oedematous and the presence of an infiltrate of mast cells and eosinophils suggests a hypersensitivity component to the disease.

throughout the body, causing anaphylactic shock due to generalized vasodilation (and reduced blood pressure) and localized oedema. The clinical presentation of anaphylaxis varies in dogs and cats, as the target 'shock organs' differ. In the dog, hepatic veins are affected, producing collapse, sometimes preceded by vomiting and diarrhoea. In cats both the respiratory (coughing, dyspnoea) and gastrointestinal (vomiting and diarrhoea) tracts are affected.

The same type I mechanism may be used in protective immune responses, for example to intestinal nematode parasites (e.g. *Toxocara canis*), where eosinophils are thought to have an effector role in damaging the outer surface of the parasite (**116, 117**).

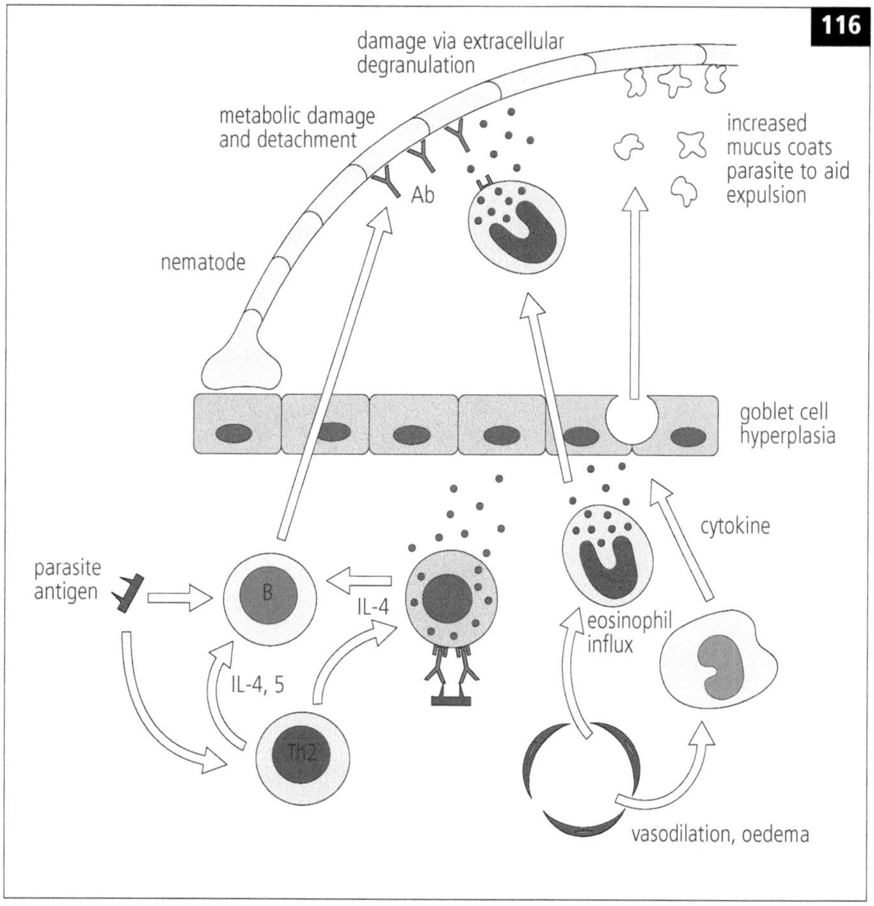

116, 117 The immune response to intestinal nematodes involves type I hypersensitivity. (**116**) Parasite antigens preferentially activate Th2 lymphocytes, which direct B cell differentiation to IgE secreting plasma cells. Parasite-specific IgE coats mucosal mast cells, which degranulate following cross-linking of surface IgE by multivalent parasite antigen. Parasite damage results from the combined effects of antibody (IgE, IgG and IgA), which may cause direct damage or interfere with parasite metabolism, and the toxic contents of mast cell and eosinophil granules. Mast cell degranulation results in local intestinal inflammation and eosinophil chemotaxis, and eosinophils may be localized to the parasite surface by antibody in an ADCC-like fashion. Macrophage-derived cytokines (TNF and IL-1) cause goblet cell hyperplasia, with increased mucus production, which coats the damaged parasite and aids in expulsion. (**117**) Duodenal biopsy from a dog showing a cross-sectioned nematode parasite in the intestinal lumen adjacent to a villus.

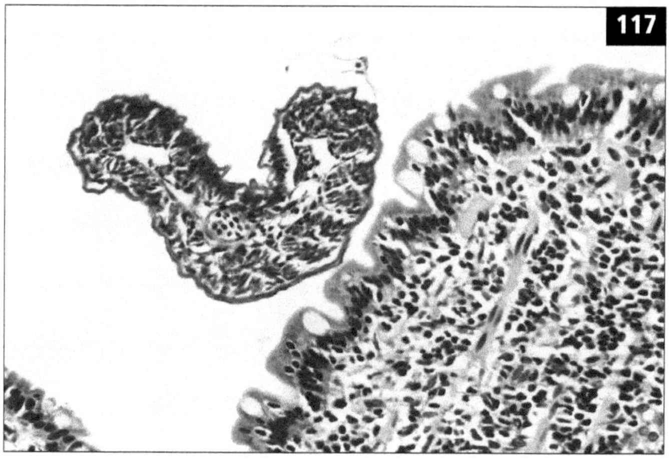

TYPE II HYPERSENSITIVITY

Type II ('cytotoxic') hypersensitivity involves destruction of a target cell following binding of IgG (or IgM) antibody to molecules on the cell surface (**118**). The classical example of such a target cell is the erythrocyte, and molecules involved may be normal self-antigens (e.g. erythrocyte membrane glycophorin in autoimmune haemolytic anaemia, blood group antigen in transfusion reaction), infectious agents (e.g. *Mycoplasma haemofelis* in feline infectious anaemia [FIA]) (**119**) or non-biological antigens (e.g. penicillin in drug-induced anaemia).

In organ-specific autoimmune disease, tissue-specific IgG autoantibodies are produced that may initiate pathology via a type II mechanism. For example, in the autoimmune skin disease pemphigus foliaceus (see Chapter 5, p. 150), autoantibodies contribute to disruption of keratinocyte adhesion, leading to vesicle formation. In other autoimmune diseases, tissue-specific autoantibodies may be present but are non-functional and regarded as an 'epiphenomenon'. These autoantibodies are often specific for intracellular molecules and are formed following cell-mediated tissue destruction and exposure of these epitopes.

118

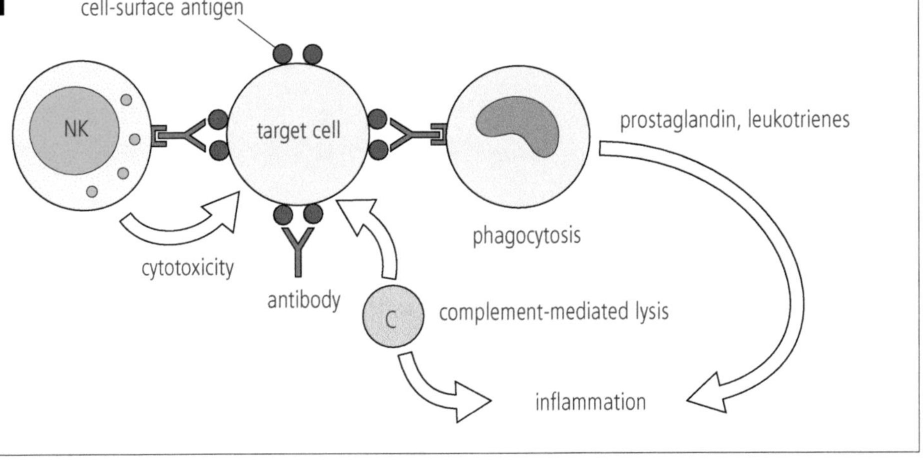

118 Type II hypersensitivity mechanism. Type II hypersensitivity involves cytotoxic destruction of a target cell coated by antibodies (usually IgG) specific for cellular antigens or molecules (drugs, infectious agents) that have been adsorbed onto the cell surface. A range of cytotoxic mechanisms may be employed including complement fixation via the classical pathway, phagocytosis of the opsonized target by macrophages or cytotoxicity mediated by NK cells via ADCC.

119

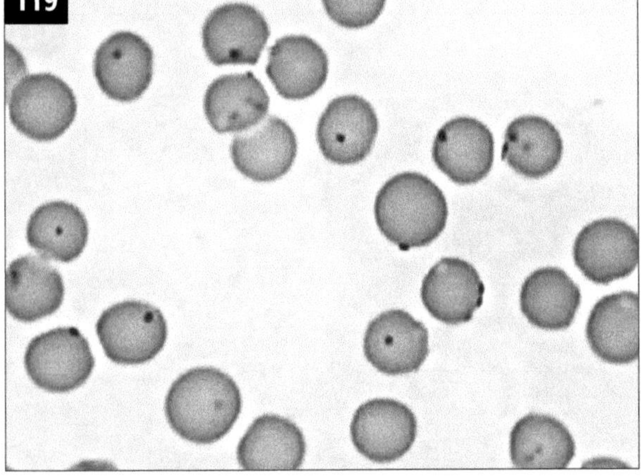

119 Type II hypersensitivity in feline infectious anaemia. Blood smear from a cat with RBCs parasitized by the epicellular organism *Mycoplasma haemofelis*. Such erythrocytes are cleared by macrophages in a type II (antibody-dependent) fashion. The antibody may be directed towards the organism or to erythrocyte antigens exposed or modified following association of the parasite with the erythrocyte plasmalemma. (Photograph courtesy S. Tasker.)

Antibody–receptor interactions

The agonist or antagonist interaction of IgG antibody with cell-surface receptor molecules is also considered a form of type II immunopathology, although the effects are not necessarily dependent upon cytotoxicity. The agonist action of antibody is typified by Grave's disease of man in which antibodies directed against the thyroid stimulating hormone receptor on thyroid follicular epithelium cause uncontrolled thyroid activation with clinical hyperthyroidism. The antagonist effect of antibody to acetylcholine receptors (AChRs) at the neuromuscular junction, together with antibody-mediated cytotoxic destruction of these receptors, is the mechanism underlying myasthenia gravis (see Chapter 6, p. 193).

TYPE III HYPERSENSITIVITY

The third type of hypersensitivity involves formation or deposition of immune complexes of soluble antigen and antibody (generally IgG) within tissue, with subsequent complement fixation and localized inflammation. Immune complex formation occurs in most immune responses, but the complexes are generally removed by phagocytes after complement fixation. Excessive immune complex formation occurs in many infectious diseases (e.g. feline infectious peritonitis [FIP]) and some autoimmune diseases (e.g. systemic lupus erythematosus [SLE]).

Two types of immune complex may form depending upon the relative amounts of antigen and antibody available. Where there is an excess of antibody in a sensitized individual, immune complex may remain localized within tissue at the site of antigen exposure (Arthus reaction) (**120**).

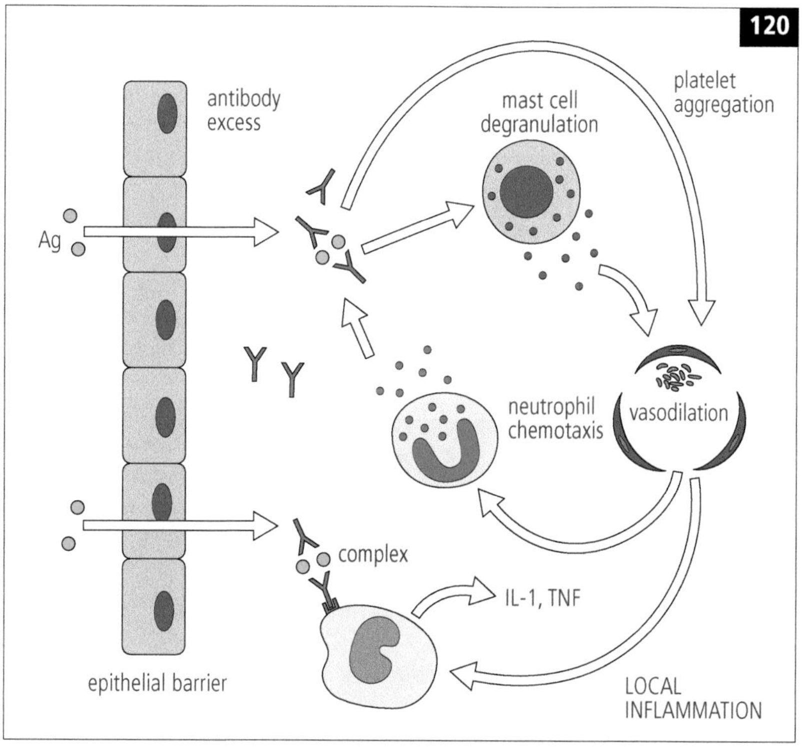

120 Type III hypersensitivity mechanism. Antibody excess (the Arthus reaction). In sensitized individuals with high levels of circulating antibody (antibody excess), immune complexes form locally at the site of antigen exposure (e.g. skin or lungs). Complement activation results in mast cell degranulation, platelet activation with release of vasoactive substances, and chemotactic attraction and activation of WBCs (particularly neutrophils). Phagocytosis of immune complex by macrophages is associated with the release of pro-inflammatory cytokines.

121

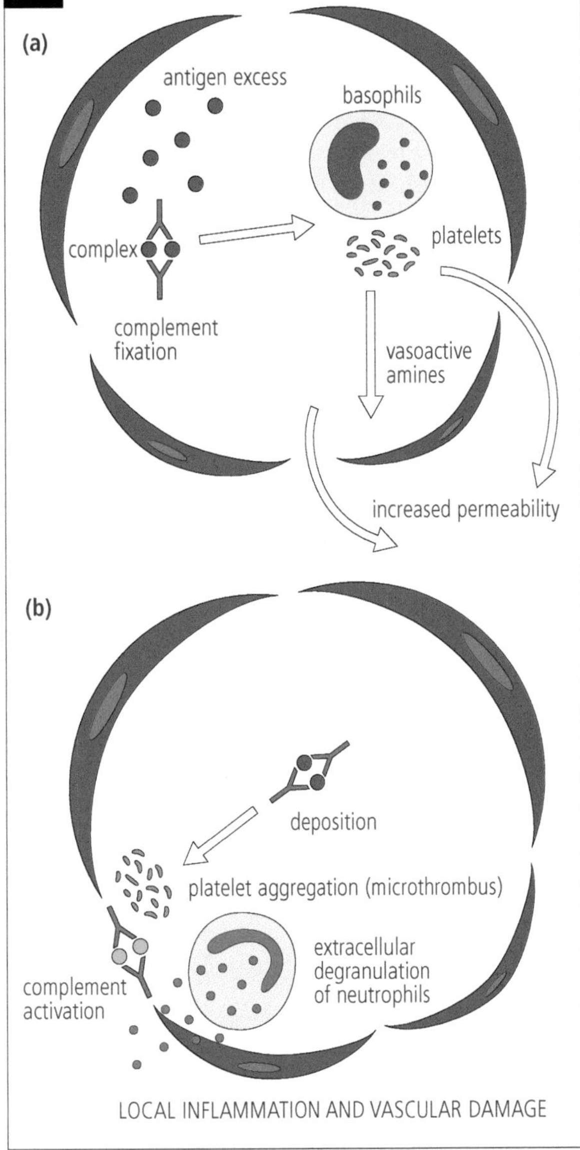

Alternatively, with an excess of circulating antigen, soluble immune complexes may form within the circulation (121) and become deposited in capillary beds, especially those of the kidney, joints, eye or skin (122). The deposition of such immune complexes is dependent upon:

- The size of the complex. Large complexes will be phagocytosed and removed and small complexes will be unable to induce a type III response. The size of the complex also partially determines the site of deposition; for example, in the glomerulus, only small complexes can pass the glomerular basement membrane.
- The nature of the antigen, including the chemical composition (degree of glycosylation) and charge.
- The class, subclass and glycosylation of the Ig involved.
- Increased vascular permeability with exposure of basement membrane enables immune complexes to lodge within vessel walls.
- High blood pressure and turbulent flow pushes immune complexes to the vascular periphery.

121a, b Type III hypersensitivity. Antigen excess (circulating immune complexes). (a) In sensitized individuals exposed to high levels of circulating antigen, immune complexes form within the bloodstream, fix complement and cause release of vasoactive amines from basophils and platelets. **(b)** In areas of increased vascular permeability with altered vascular flow, complexes deposit within the vessel wall, resulting in localized platelet aggregation (microthrombus formation) and inflammation mediated by extracellular degranulation of neutrophils that are unable to phagocytose the immune complexes.

122

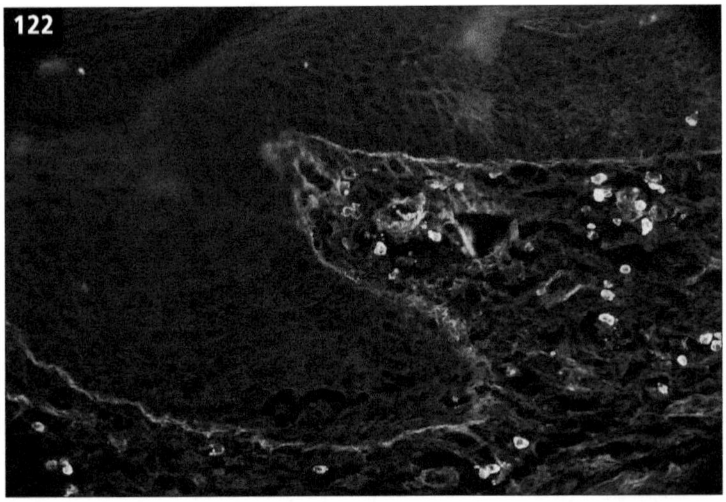

122 Immune complex deposition at the epidermal BMZ. Skin biopsy from a dog with cutaneous lupus erythematosus labelled by the indirect immunofluorescence method for canine IgG. There is strong, irregular labelling of the BMZ consistent with deposition of immune complexes at this site. Plasma cells within the dermis are labelled for cytoplasmic IgG. Parallel labelling using antibody specific for complement C3 may demonstrate complement fixation by the immune complexes.

TYPE IV HYPERSENSITIVITY

This immunopathological mechanism involves antigen-sensitized Th1 and CD8 lymphocytes, cytokines and macrophages rather than IgE or IgG antibodies. The activation and effector function of sensitized lymphoid cells requires between 24 and 72 hours, and type IV hypersensitivity is often referred to as 'delayed-type hypersensitivity' (DTH). Two forms of DTH reaction may be considered. The first is triggered by soluble antigen (or hapten-carrier complexes) and involves Th1 recognition of antigen presented by macrophages or dendritic cells with release of cytokines such as IFNγ. The second mechanism involves cytotoxic destruction of target cells following recognition of cell-associated antigen by Th1 or CD8 lymphocytes. In either instance, after activation of previously sensitized Th1 cells, there is transformation of local vascular endothelium (mediated by IFNγ), with expression of adhesion molecules and recruitment of further macrophages, neutrophils and T lymphocytes to the site of antigen exposure (**123–125**).

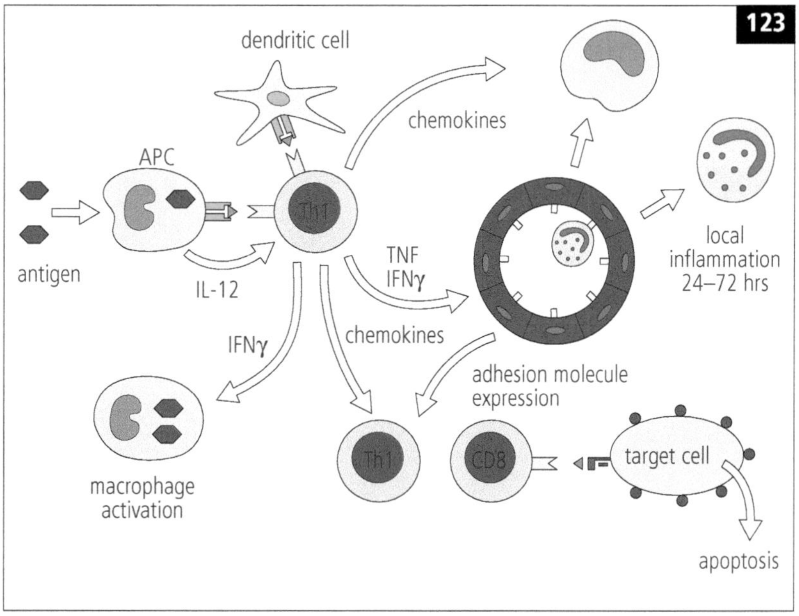

123, 124,125 Type IV hypersensitivity mechanism. Type IV immunopathology involves activation of sensitized Th1 lymphocytes by antigen, with T cell-derived cytokines causing expression of specific adhesion molecules by local vascular endothelium. Cytokines and chemokines released by activated T cells permit local recruitment of further T cells, macrophages and neutrophils. The effector functions of recruited T cells are in macrophage activation or cytotoxic destruction of target cells. The local inflammatory response takes 24–72 hours to become apparent, and this process is sometimes called 'delayed type hypersensitivity' (**124**) A rat was sensitized by immunization with a synthetic peptide in adjuvant by subcutaneous injection. Four weeks later the rat was challenged by intradermal injection of peptide into the skin overlying the ear. Marked increase in ear thickness was evident 24 hours after challenge and histological examination revealed an extensive infiltrate of mononuclear cells. (**125**) A section from the contralateral ear injected with an irrelevant peptide as a control indicates the specificity of the type IV response.

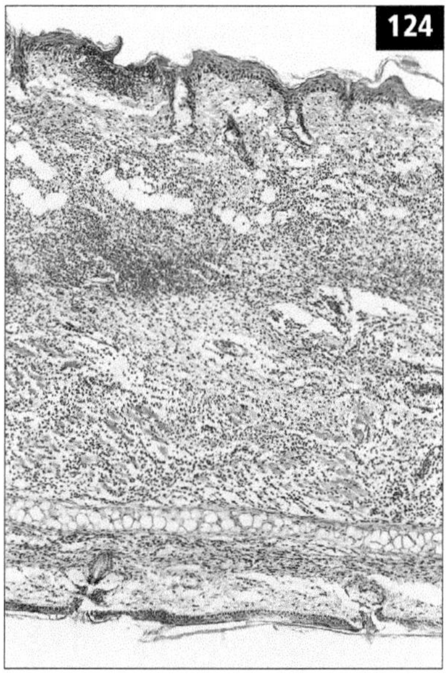

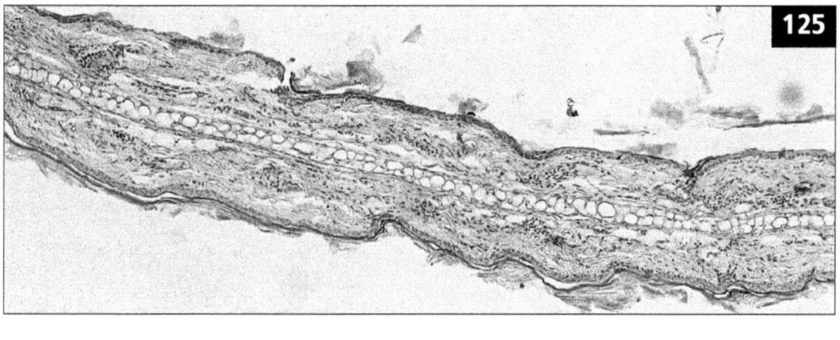

Type IV hypersensitivity is also of importance in the protective immune response to obligate intracellular microbes that target macrophages and induce granulomatous lesions (**126, 127**). Persistence of the pathogen (chronic antigenic stimulus) can result in formation of multinucleate giant cells (**128**) and tissue granulomas.

An effective immune response to intracellular protozoan parasites of the genus *Leishmania* is dominated by the regulatory effects of Th1 lymphocytes (**129–132**). Leishmaniosis occurs in dogs in those parts of the world where appropriate sandfly vectors are found. The amastigote stage of the organism divides within macrophages and these cells require activation signals (e.g. IFNγ) from *Leishmania*-specific Th1 cells to eliminate organisms and resolve disease. Although parasite-specific antibody is produced, individuals that make a dominant antibody response (Th2 regulation) have progressive, non-healing disease. In contrast, dogs that have a dominant cell-mediated response, with production of IL-2, TNF and IFNγ, are able to resolve infection. These clinically significant polarized immune responses are an example of the phenomenon of 'immune deviation'.

Studies have also attempted to define the balance of Th1/Th2 activity in cats infected experimentally with agents that would be predicted to induce either response preferentially, but the data are not clear-cut. Cats infected with the intracellular bacterium *Listeria* made strong DTH responses and little antibody, whereas infection with the extracellular organism *Serratia* gave the reverse profile of effects. However, when cytokine mRNA expression in

126

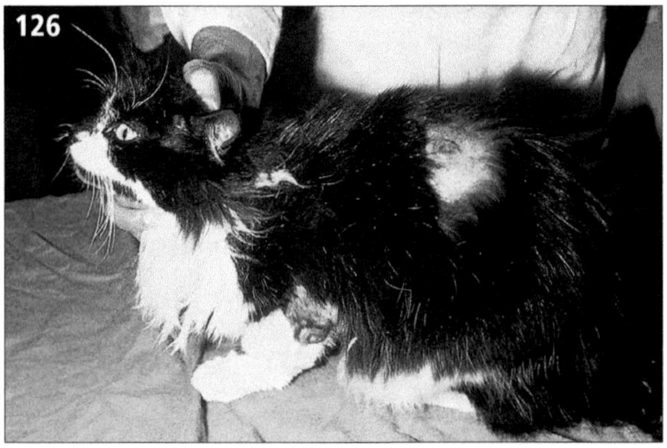

127

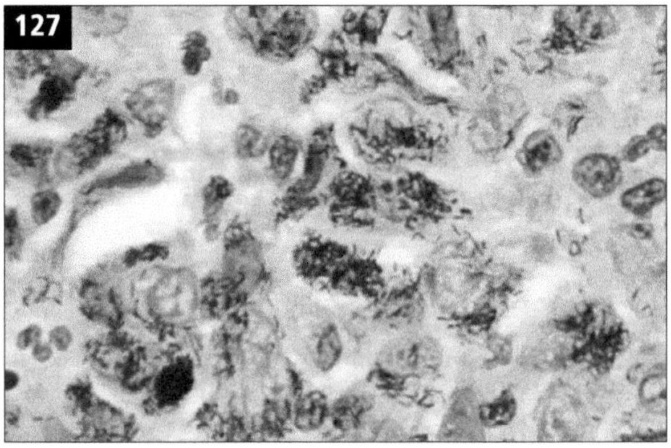

126, 127 Feline leprosy. The immune response of the cat to cutaneous infection with *Mycobacterium* involves type IV immunopathology. (**126**) A cat with 'feline leprosy' has multiple well-circumscribed, alopecic and ulcerated cutaneous nodules. (From Gunn-Moore D, Shaw SE (1997) Mycobacterial disease in the cat. *In Practice* **19**:493-501, with permission.) (**127**) A biopsy from such a lesion reveals a diffuse granulomatous dermatitis, and Ziehl-Neelsen staining demonstrates numerous acid fast bacteria within the cytoplasm of many macrophages. Elimination of these intracellular bacteria requires macrophage activation by T cell-derived IFNγ.

128

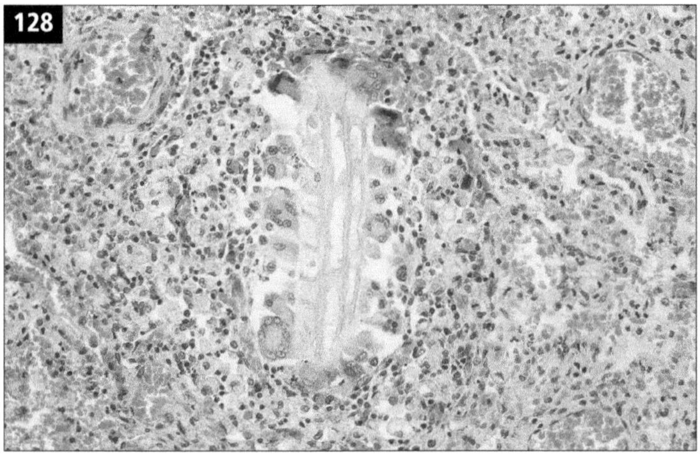

128 Multinucleate giant cells. Persistence of antigen in chronic granulomatous disease results in high levels of TNF production by activated macrophages that may fuse to produce multinucleate giant cells. In this section of lung from a dog with long-standing aspiration pneumonia, the presence of a large fragment of plant material has induced a localized giant cell reaction.

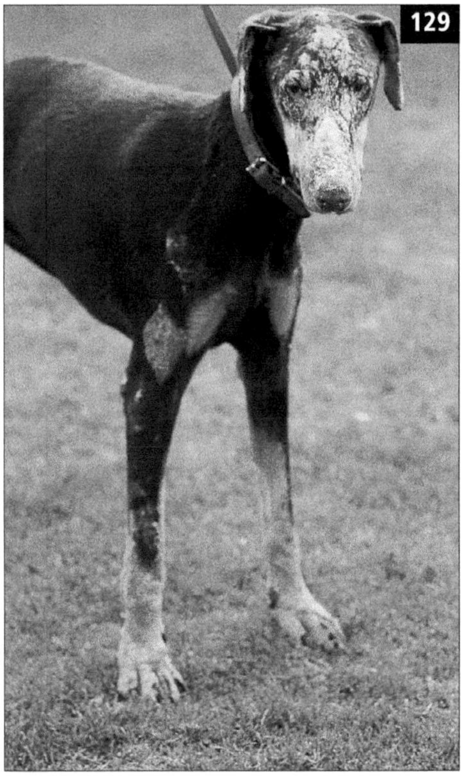

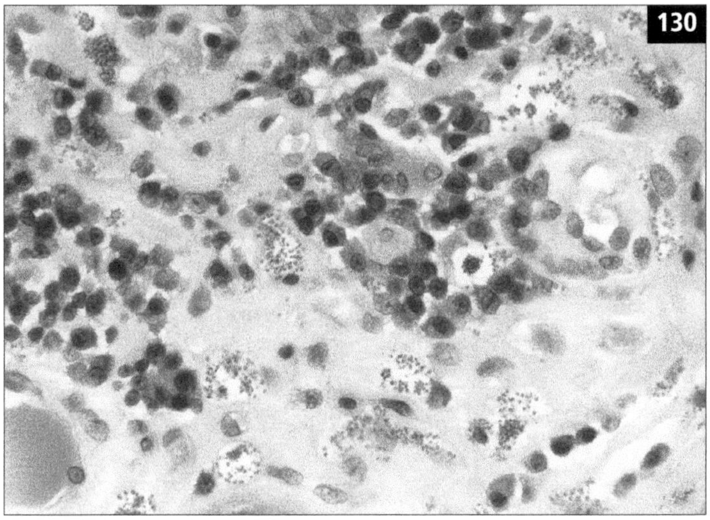

129, 130 Canine leishmaniosis. Type IV hypersensitivity is crucial to the resolution of lesions induced by *Leishmania*. (**117**) Cutaneous leishmaniosis in a dog, with extensive areas of crusting and alopecia. (Photograph courtesy S.E. Shaw) (**118**) Biopsy from the skin of a dog with leishmaniosis demonstrates amastigote forms of the parasite within the cytoplasm of dermal macrophages.

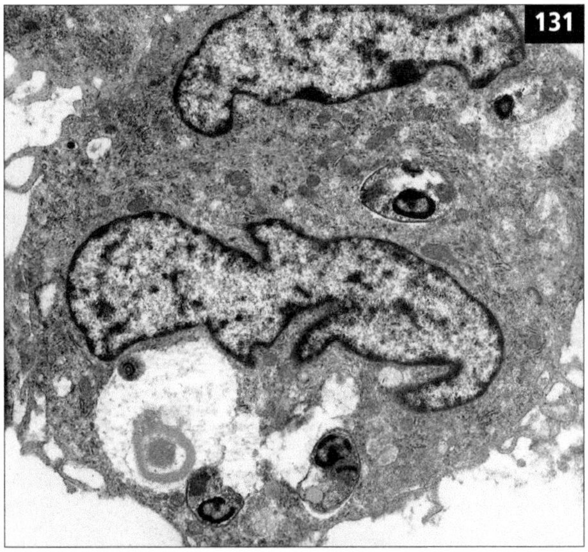

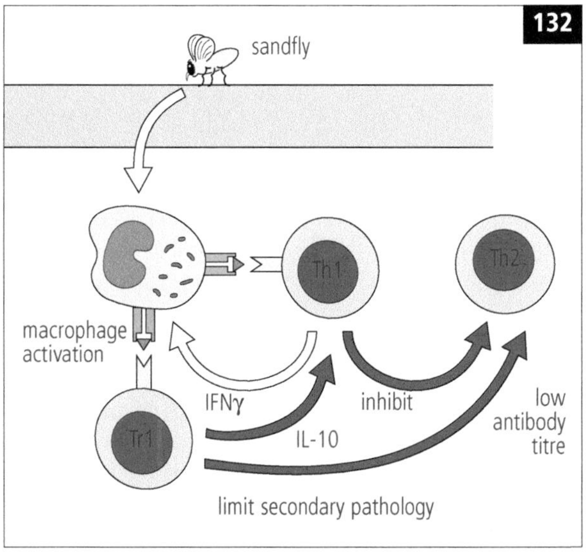

131, 132 Canine leishmaniosis. The *Leishmania* protozoan is an obligate intracellular organism and it resides within the macrophage cytoplasm. (**131**) Transmission electron micrograph of an infected macrophage demonstrating amastigotes. (**132**) An effective immune response to the parasite necessitates stimulation of Th1 lymphocytes, with production of IFNγ to activate parasitized macrophages. By contrast, dogs that have a dominant Th2-driven antibody response are not able to resolve the infection. Dogs mounting an appropriate Th1 response may also show activation of IL-10 producing Treg cells, which serve to limit secondary immune-mediated tissue pathology, but may also permit persistence of the infection.

82 CD4+ T lymphocyte subsets. There are two major subsets of CD4+ T lymphocytes that are characterized by a distinct pattern of cytokine production. Activation of Th1 cells results in cell-mediated immune effects such as macrophage activation by IFNγ. Th2 cells mediate the humoral effects of antibody synthesis (IgE and IgG subclass) and regulation of mast cell and eosinophil differentiation and mobility. Th2 cells produce IL-10, which can render Th1 cells unable to respond to antigen (anergic), as there is interference with production of APC co-stimulatory signals. The Th2 cytokines IL-4 and IL-13 also negatively influence Th1 cells. Th1 cells directly inhibit the function of Th2 cells via IFNγ production.

82

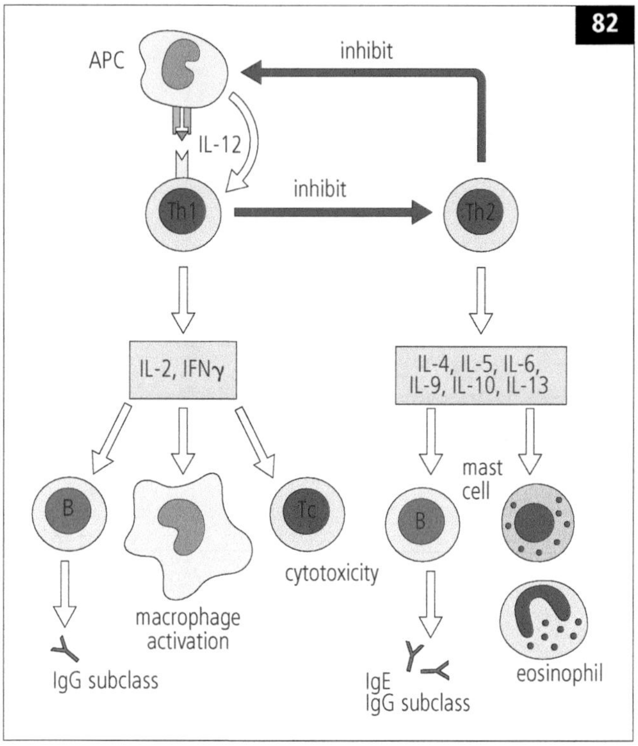

T cell development

Immature bone marrow-derived T cells are exported to the thymus in the bloodstream, where they undergo a sequence of maturation events (80, 81). The vast majority of T cells that enter the thymus do not 'pass the tests' of positive and negative selection and die by apoptosis (programmed cell death). T cells released by the thymus are able to participate in productive immune responses against foreign antigens, but a small proportion of T cells with TCRs having low affinity for self-antigens escape clonal deletion and can potentially mediate self-reactivity (autoimmunity).

Subsets of CD4+ T lymphocytes

The subpopulation of T cells that expresses the CD4 molecule (T helper [Th] cells) can be further subdivided into the major Th1 and Th2 subsets (82), defined by the profile of cytokines that they produce and the immunological effects they orchestrate. Th1 cells:

- Produce predominantly IL-2 and IFNγ.
- Undertake intracellular signalling from surface cytokine receptors via the use of signal transducers and activators of transcription (STAT) 4.
- Initiate cell-mediated immunity and cytotoxicity.
- Have limited effect on antibody production, but enhance production of a specific IgG subclass (IgG2a in mice).
- Antagonize the action of Th2 cells (via IFNγ).

Th2 cells:

- Produce IL-4, IL-5, IL-9, IL-10, IL-13, IL-25, IL-31 and IL-33.
- Undertake intracellular signalling from surface cytokine receptors via the use of STAT6.
- Mediate humoral immunity, particularly the synthesis of IgE and a subclass of IgG (IgG1 in mice).
- Antagonize the action of Th1 cells (via IL-4, IL-10 and IL-13).

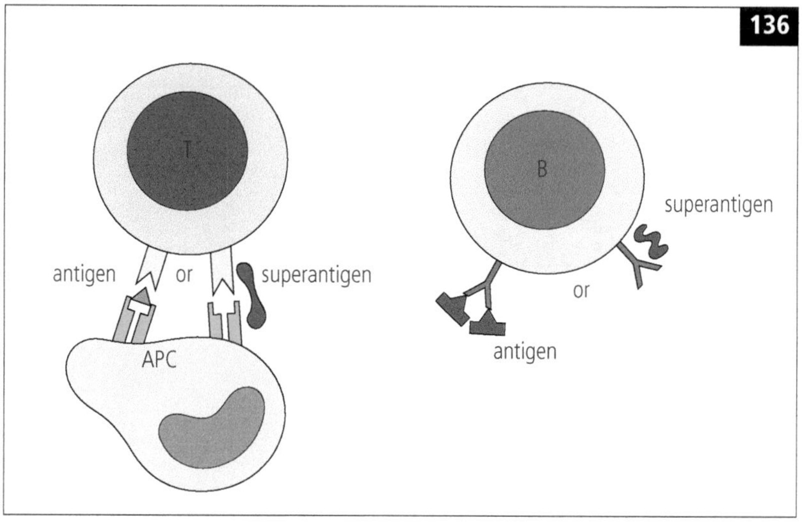

136 Superantigens. Microbially derived superantigens activate multiple clones of T and B lymphocytes by non-antigen specific binding to SmIg (B cell) or binding between the MHC class II molecule and particular types of Vβ chain of the T cell receptor. The activated lymphocytes may mediate inappropriate tissue immunopathology.

SUPERANTIGENS

The immunological effects of the so-called 'superantigens' may contribute to many disease states. Superantigens are generally microbially derived molecules (e.g. staphylococcal enterotoxin B). They may activate non-specifically numerous clones of T and B lymphocytes (including autoreactive cells) by mechanisms that do not involve occupation of the antigen-specific TCR or SmIg and lead to uncontrolled release of cytokines, with subsequent systemic shock (**136**). Superantigens have affinity for specific Vβ types utilized by the TCR molecule and they may be soluble (bacterial) or membrane-bound (viral).

AMYLOIDOSIS

Amyloidosis refers to a diverse group of diseases characterized by extracellular deposition of fibrils formed by polymerization of protein subunits. Development of amyloidosis requires a sustained supply of an amyloid fibril precursor protein, which can fold into an abnormal conformation that facilitates its incorporation into fibrillar aggregates. The fibrillar precursors are produced in abnormal abundance and/or have abnormal primary structure. Despite the heterogeneity of precursor proteins, the structure and biochemical properties of all amyloid fibrils are remarkably similar. Little is known about the factors that govern the anatomical distribution of the deposits, their clinical effects and why certain forms of amyloid are deposited in some patients but not others.

Amyloidosis is classified by the distribution of the deposits (i.e. systemic or localized) and by the nature of the protein involved. Localized syndromes usually affect one organ and are uncommon in animals. Examples include:

- Pancreatic islet cell amyloid in cats (see Chapter 9, p. 248).
- Amyloid protein in the cerebral vessels of aged dogs that is related to β protein in humans with Alzheimer's disease. Similar extracellular accumulation of β amyloid plaque has been documented within the cortex of aged cats.
- Apolipoprotein A-1 in the pulmonary vasculature of dogs.

Reactive (secondary) amyloidosis is a systemic syndrome characterized by tissue deposition of amyloid-associated protein (AA amyloid), an amino-terminal fragment of the acute phase reactant serum amyloid-associated protein (SAA). SAA is one of several acute phase reactants synthesized by the liver in response to cytokines (e.g. IL-1, IL-6, TNFα) released from macrophages after tissue injury. It is assumed that SAA has a role in the response to tissue injury, and the

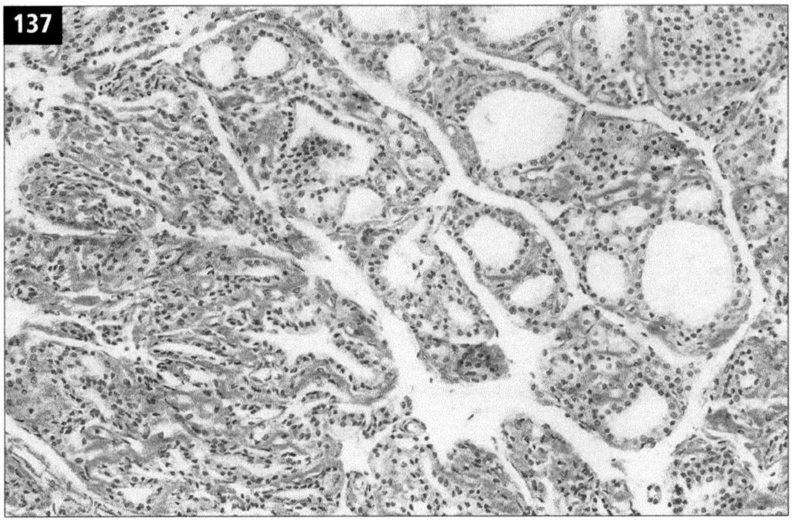

137 Amyloidosis. Section of thyroid stained by Congo red from a five-year-old female DSH cat with systemic amyloidosis. The kidneys, liver, spleen and adrenal corticies were also involved. The AA amyloid in Siamese cats is distinct from that in the Abyssinian breed, as there is a two-amino acid substitution in the amino acid sequence.

plasma concentration of SAA increases before amyloid deposits are observed in the tissues. Not all patients with chronic inflammatory disease develop amyloidosis, so other factors (e.g. genetic) are likely to be involved in the pathogenesis.

Systemic amyloidosis is usually a progressive and fatal disease; however, control of underlying conditions can improve clinical outcome and there are anecdotal reports of histological regression of amyloid in such patients. Reactive amyloidosis occurs in many chronic inflammatory or neoplastic diseases of dogs and cats; however, many dogs with reactive amyloidosis have no discernible underlying disease. AA amyloidosis usually presents with proteinuria, renal dysfunction, or both. Clinical involvement of the liver, spleen and, sometimes, the gut may occur at a later stage. Familial amyloidosis is documented in Abyssinian and Siamese cats (**137**) and Shar Pei dogs (see Chapter 6, p. 185).

Ig-associated (primary) amyloidosis is characterized by tissue deposition of aminoterminal fragments of amyloid (Ig) light chain protein (AL amyloid); however, it is rare in animals (see Chapter 13, p. 339).

Amyloidosis is confirmed by demonstrating tissue amyloid deposition by Congo red staining. This imparts birefringence to the material under polarized light. Pretreatment of sections with potassium permanganate may abolish positive staining of AA amyloid, but not AL or islet cell amyloid. Immunohistochemistry can identify fibril type, although it may not be definitive in identifying AL amyloid.

FURTHER READING

Francis AH, Martin LG, Haldorson GJ *et al.* (2007) Adverse reactions suggestive of type III hypersensitivity in six healthy dogs given human albumin. *Journal of the American Veterinary Medical Association* 230:873–879.

Gunn-Moore DA, McVee J, Bradshaw JM *et al.* (2006) Ageing changes in cat brains demonstrated by β-amyloid and AT8-immunoreactive phosphorylated tau deposits. *Journal of Feline Medicine and Surgery* 8:234–242.

Robinson A, Sparkes AH, Day MJ (2002) Local cell recruitment and cytokine production following intradermal injection with *Microsporum canis* antigen in cats. *Advances in Veterinary Dermatology* 4:100–108.

Trichieri G (2007) Interleukin-10 production by effector T cells: Th1 cells show self control. *Journal of Experimental Medicine* 204:239–243.

3 THE BASIS OF IMMUNE-MEDIATED DISEASE

Michael J. Day

THE SPECTRUM AND INTERRELATIONSHIP OF IMMUNE-MEDIATED DISEASES

Immune-mediated disease arises following primary dysfunction of the immune system in the absence of a recognized underlying disease state. In contrast, immune-mediated pathology occurs commonly as part of the pathogenesis of many chronic inflammatory, infectious or neoplastic diseases, but the immunological dysfunction is readily identified as secondary to the underlying disorder. For example, immune complex formation is a feature of some primary immune-mediated (autoimmune) diseases such as SLE, but it also occurs in infectious (e.g. FeLV, canine leishmaniosis) or neoplastic (e.g. canine mammary tumours) disease.

Primary immune-mediated disease is the focus of this book; however, such conditions are relatively uncommon in small animal medicine, whereas secondary immune-mediated phenomena are not. In a referral hospital survey conducted over a ten-year period, primary immune-mediated disease (excluding cutaneous hypersensitivity) accounted for 2% of total case accessions.

Immune-mediated diseases may be grouped as:

- Hypersensitivity (allergic) diseases.
- Autoimmune diseases.
- Immune system neoplasia.
- Immunodeficiency diseases.

Primary immune-mediated diseases have a multifactorial aetiopathogenesis, involving interaction of an optimal combination of predisposing factors, permitting imbalance in normal immune system homeostasis and clinical expression of immune-mediated disease. The nature of the imbalance determines the type of immunological abnormality expressed, but immune-mediated disease should be considered as a continuum in which a particular set of predisposing factors may initiate concurrent clinical expression of more than one immunological abnormality (**138**). Alternatively, the presence of one immunological abnormality may alter the immune system to allow subsequent expression of a second immune-mediated disease. For example, canine IgA deficiency may occur concurrently with autoimmunity or hypersensitivity, thymoma in dogs and cats is often associated with myasthenia

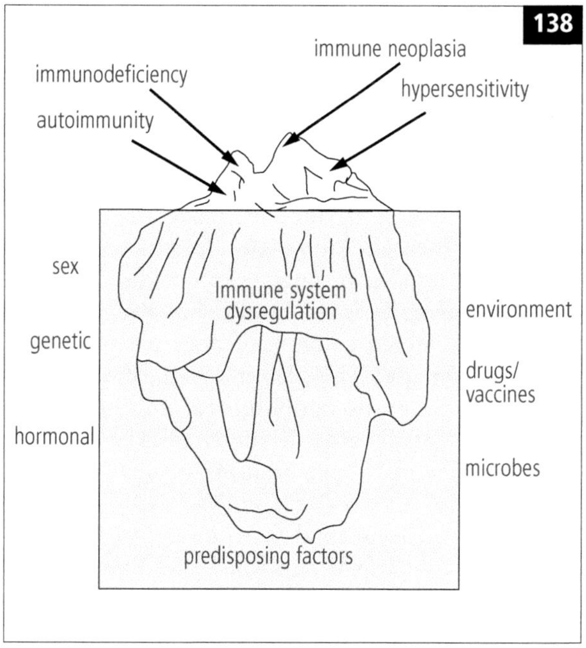

138 The basis of immune-mediated disease. Immune-mediated disease may best be considered using the 'iceberg model'. There are four broad categories of immune-mediated disease: hypersensitivity, autoimmune disease, primary immunodeficiency and immune-system neoplasia. These are all manifestations of an imbalance in normal immune system homeostasis, which occurs following exposure of an individual to a particular set of predisposing and trigger factors. The iceberg floats in a sea of predisposing factors, which interact with the 'body' of the iceberg hidden below the waterline. Disturbed immune system homeostasis may become expressed clinically (i.e. above the waterline) as immune-mediated disease. Because the four categories of immunological disease are linked by the underlying immune system, one or more peaks of the iceberg may present above the waterline at any one time. For example, a dog may have concurrent lymphoma and autoimmune haemolytic anaemia, suggesting that in that animal the immune disturbance is clinically manifest as two different abnormalities.

gravis or megaoesophagus, and lymphoma may be diagnosed concurrently with autoimmune haematological disease in both species.

In general terms there are a number of factors that predispose animals to immune-mediated diseases. Such conditions often occur with greatest frequency in animals of particular age and gender. Autoimmunity and idiopathic immune system neoplasia occur in middle-aged to older animals, immunodeficiency is generally recognized before 12 months of age, and atopic dermatitis is usually first recognized in dogs under three years of age. Hormonal influences are recognized in man and rodent models of immune-mediated disease, but such factors are more difficult to define in the cat and dog, which likely reflects the effect of neutering in these species.

The occurrence of immune-mediated disease is heavily influenced by genetic factors. Particular breeds and families of dogs are more susceptible to immunological disorders, and it has been possible to establish inbred colonies of dogs with immune-mediated disease. The identification of the genes that determine susceptibility to immunological disease is a major area of contemporary research, but limited studies have been performed in the cat and dog.

Finally, environmental factors (e.g. exposure to pollutants, microbial antigens [by infection or vaccination], or preceding drug therapy) are documented susceptibility factors in human immunological diseases, and these are becoming recognized in studies of the equivalent disorders in dogs and cats.

IMMUNOLOGICAL MECHANISMS UNDERLYING ALLERGIC DISEASE

The major allergic diseases of the cat and dog are those affecting the skin, although dietary hypersensitivity and 'asthma' are recorded in both species. The common underlying pathogenesis involves type I hypersensitivity, but other mechanisms may act concurrently in disorders such as flea allergy dermatitis (FAD) or dietary hypersensitivity. Less commonly, pathology caused by type IV hypersensitivity underlies disease (e.g. contact dermatitis). A number of factors predispose to type I hypersensitivity, and the hypothesis of 'allergic breakthrough' suggests that clinical disease requires a particular level of immunological activity, which may be dependent upon the interaction of such predisposing factors.

Genetic factors

Diseases such as canine atopic dermatitis are recognised in particular breeds or families, and it is likely that specific genes underlie this susceptibility. Some of these genes may lie within the MHC, but non-MHC susceptibility loci are recognized in man, including the genes encoding Th2 cytokines (IL-3, IL-4, IL-5, IL-9 and IL-13) that are clustered on a specific chromosome. People with type I hypersensitivity disease may have a hereditary predisposition to high serum IgE levels, but this is not recognized in the dog.

Immunoregulatory imbalance

Type I hypersensitivity disorders were initially considered to be a form of polarized immune response in which exposure to allergen preferentially activated Th2 over Th1 lymphocytes. It is now recognized in both people and companion animals that such diseases may in their chronic stages involve an equally significant Th1

139

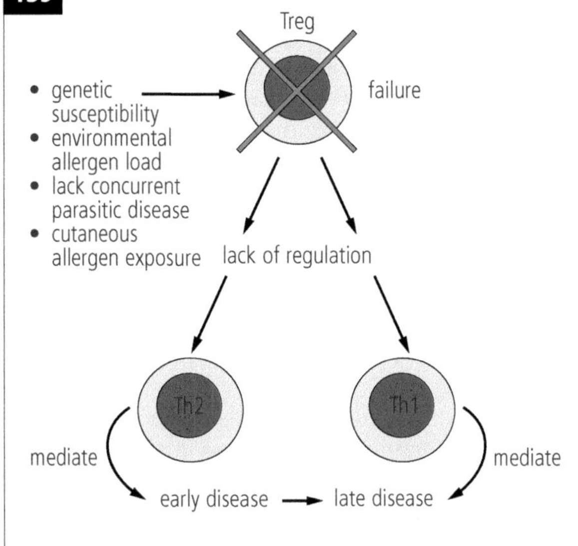

139 Immunoregulatory imbalance underlies allergic disease. In type I hypersensitivity (allergic) disease such as canine atopic dermatitis, a combination of predisposing factors may be required in order to disturb the balance of immunoregulation. The fundamental immunological abnormality might be failure of IL-10 producing regulatory T cells, which in turn allows over-activity of allergen-specific Th2 cells in the initial phases of the hypersensitivity response, followed by activity of allergen-specific Th1 cells in the later stages of chronic disease.

response. There is mounting evidence that the fundamental immune defect in allergic disease is lack of function of regulatory cells, which permits inappropriate activity of both allergen-specific Th1 and Th2 effector cells (**139**).

Environmental factors

The most important environmental factor is exposure to causative allergen during the sensitization and hypersensitivity phases of disease. Particular environments favour the presence of large numbers of fleas, dust mites or pollen grains, and thus increase the level of exposure. Some studies have shown that vaccination enhances production of pollen-specific or food allergen-specific IgE in the dog, although it has been difficult to directly associate this with clinical allergic disease or an increased prevalence of atopic dermatitis. This situation is said to mimic the proposed effects of childhood viral infection on development of allergic disease in man. There is a recognized association between human allergic disease and environmental pollutants (e.g. diesel exhaust) that affect mucosal permeability and enhance penetration of allergens in addition to altering immunoregulation to enhance IgE production. Dogs and cats also inhale pollutants (**140**), but the potential for these to enhance susceptibility to allergic disease has not been examined.

Perhaps the greatest discussion of environmental influences on the development of human allergic (and autoimmune) diseases has related to the 'hygiene hypothesis'. There is now little doubt that the incidence of both allergy and autoimmunity has risen dramatically since the 1960s in western populations. The hygiene hypothesis suggests that this is directly related to the more 'sanitized' lifestyle that we lead, with small family size, high standards of environmental and personal cleanliness, ingestion of processed foods and the active use of vaccination. Numerous epidemiological studies have shown that in places (e.g. farms) where there is greater exposure to microbial infection (particularly in childhood) there is reduced development of immune-mediated disease, and that deliberate re-exposure to infectious agents (e.g. the ingestion of probiotic bacteria by pregnant women) might reverse this trend (**141**).

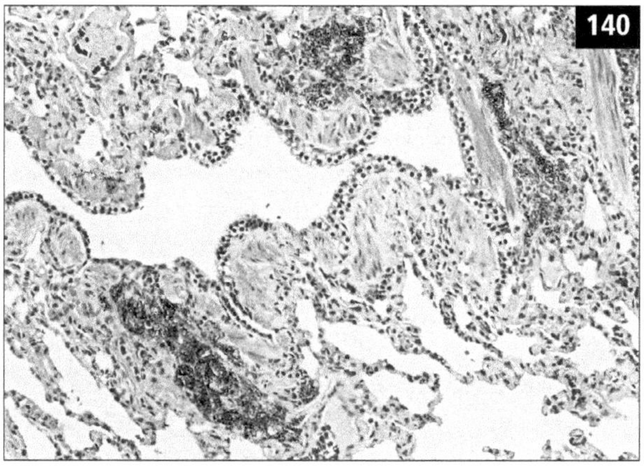

140 Environmental pollutants may predispose to immune-mediated disease. The expression of human respiratory diseases with a type I hypersensitivity mechanism may be enhanced by inhalation of a range of environmental pollutants that may weaken the mucosal barrier and directly modify normal mucosal immunoregulation. Such effects have been poorly characterized in small animals, but as these species share an environment with man it might be predicted that similar factors may have a role in development of such diseases in the cat and dog. Shown is a section of lung from a dog in which there is a peribronchiolar aggregation of macrophages containing carbon and birefringent crystalline material that is determined to consist of an array of exogenously derived elements by electron microprobe analysis.

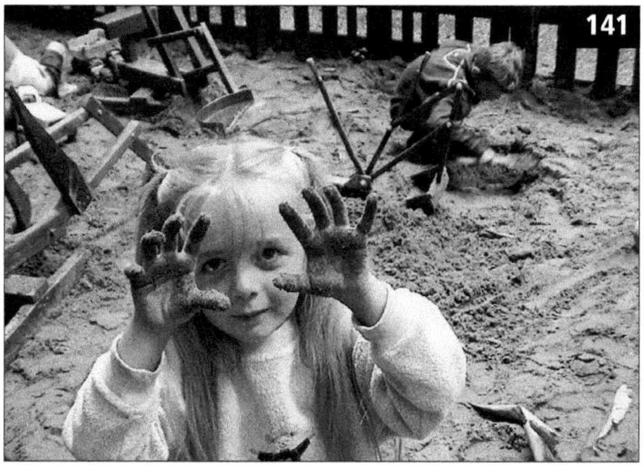

141 The hygiene hypothesis. Reduced exposure to microbial antigens as part of the more sanitized western lifestyle may underlie an increasing incidence of human allergic and autoimmune diseases. Here the author's children demonstrate the principle that exposure to dirt is fundamentally beneficial to the immune system!

Immunologically, the hygiene hypothesis, as first proposed, suggested that these observations were related to an imbalance in Th1 versus Th2 immunity in susceptible individuals. Interesting studies of human cord blood lymphocytes suggested that all human babies are born with a Th2-dominated immune system, which likely relates to the immune imbalance that occurs in the pregnant mother in order to maintain the pregnancy. In infancy the immune system normally 'resets' to a Th1-dominance, with exposure to microbial antigens, but in an ultra hygienic environment this may not be possible and such children may go on to develop allergy. More recently, the explanation has altered to suggest that exposure to infectious agents in fact drives the expansion of regulatory T cells, which in turn control both allergen-reactive and autoreactive clones. Lack of expansion of regulatory cells would thus underlie the development of allergy. It is arguable whether similar background changes have altered the incidence of allergy in companion animals, and such epidemiological data are lacking in veterinary medicine. It is interesting to speculate, however, about the effects on some companion animals of living a largely indoor life in a human environment.

Neurological factors

The pruritus that occurs in type I hypersensitivity requires interaction of the immune system with the autonomic and central nervous systems. The autonomic nervous system of some individuals may be imbalanced and hyperresponsive to mast cell-derived inflammatory mediators. Conversely, a neuropeptide derived from cutaneous nerves (substance P) can degranulate mast cells.

Co-existing type I hypersensitivity

If the immune system of an individual is primed to make a type I hypersensitivity response, immune responses to other antigens may be influenced by the presence of activated Th2 lymphocytes. Dogs with atopic dermatitis are susceptible to the development of FAD and they may have concurrent respiratory or conjunctival allergic disease. Dogs with intestinal parasitism may have serum IgE specific for aero-allergens, but they do not necessarily develop atopic disease. There are, again, human parallels for this observation in that the prevalence of allergic (and autoimmune) diseases is lower in geographical areas where the population may have greater carriage of intestinal nematode parasites. The current hypothesis that explains this finding is that intestinal parasitism induces a strong T regulatory response, and it is these regulatory cells that control the emergence of allergic or autoimmune pathologies. To progress this concept, recent human clinical studies have examined the effect of deliberately establishing nematode infection in the gut of patients with allergic (e.g. hay fever) or immune-mediated (e.g. Crohn's disease) diseases. These preliminary studies show striking protective effects in some individuals, which may be related to induction of regulatory cells. It has been suggested that the increased hygiene of the past century has removed a 'natural' exposure of people in western civilization to intestinal parasites, and that this might explain the rising prevalence of allergic and autoimmune diseases in these populations. It is interesting to speculate that actively seeking to remove parasite burdens from companion animals (for the benefit of the pets as well as their owners) over the same time frame might underlie the increasing occurrence of immune-mediated disease in pets as well as in man.

IMMUNOLOGICAL MECHANISMS UNDERLYING AUTOIMMUNE DISEASE

The relative uncommonness of autoimmunity is a reflection of the effectiveness of self-tolerance, whereby the immune system is generally incapable of mounting a pathological response to self-tissue. Both T and B lymphocytes must be tolerant of self, although tolerance of Th cells might be sufficient to prevent activation of autoreactive B cells. Self-tolerance likely arises through a combination of effects. There is negative selection of potentially autoreactive T and B cells during maturation (see Chapter 1, p. 43). However, the fact that autoimmunity does arise means that T and B cell clonal deletion is not absolute and self-reactive lymphocytes must escape to the 'periphery'. In normal individuals, such cells must be kept in check by the mechanisms described below (**142**):

- Autoreactive T cells may recognize self-antigen presented by MHC in the extrathymic environment and undergo 'peripheral deletion' by apoptosis following Fas-Fas ligand interaction. Peripheral deletion of B cells may also occur.
- Autoreactive T cells may be specific for peptides derived from self-molecules that are normally hidden (e.g. intracellular domains of membrane proteins) from the immune system ('cryptic'

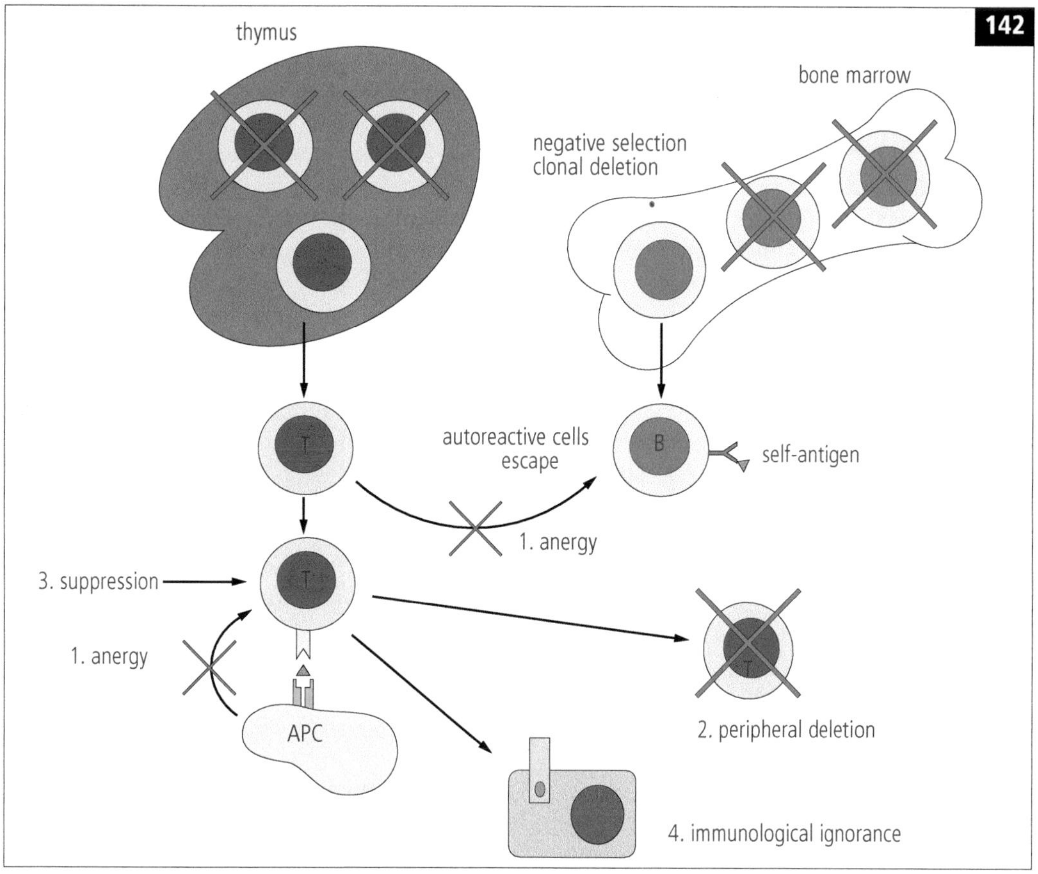

142 Failure of self-tolerance underlies autoimmune disease. Autoreactive T and B lymphocytes must exist to mediate autoimmune disease, but in clinically normal individuals their function must be strictly controlled. Autoreactive clones may be deleted during lymphocyte maturation in the thymus or bone marrow. Alternatively, autoreactive cells that escape negative selection may be regulated in the periphery by (1) recognizing self-antigen but not receiving costimulation (anergy); (2) recognizing self-antigen and undergoing apoptosis (peripheral deletion); (3) active suppression; or (4) failure to recognize hidden (cryptic) self-antigen that is not normally processed and presented to the immune system (immunological ignorance).

epitopes) or for peptides that have low affinity for MHC and are not presented by routine antigen processing ('immunological ignorance'). Altered antigen processing and presentation (perhaps following infection) may permit presentation of cryptic epitopes, with subsequent 'epitope spreading' to involve other determinants within the same molecule and to related molecules during maturation of the autoimmune response.

- Autoreactive T and B cells may be rendered 'anergic' in the periphery. Such cells may recognize autoantigen but not receive co-stimulatory molecular interactions or cytokines allowing activation.
- Autoreactive T cells may be actively suppressed, most likely by a phenotypically distinct population of regulatory T cells (e.g. $CD4^+CD25^+$ 'natural' suppressor cells) that maintains a homeostatic balance with autoreactive T cells.

Autoimmune disease occurs when these regulatory factors fail and permit activation of autoreactive T and B cells. The factors involved in 'breaking tolerance' are likely to be multiple, and an optimum combination may be required for expression of disease.

Age

Autoimmunity generally arises in middle-aged to older animals, which may reflect increased risk of immunoregulatory failure with increasing age.

Hormonal background

There are documented hormonal influences on expression of autoimmune disease in people (i.e. females are predisposed) and laboratory rodents. Limited evidence suggests that female dogs are predisposed to some forms of autoimmunity and oestrus or whelping are known triggers for development of autoimmune haemolytic anaemia (AIHA). Some lymphocytes express oestrogen receptors and oestrogen is able to regulate IFNγ gene expression in these cells. Interactions of the neuroendocrine immunological loop may also be of significance. The hormones of pregnancy induce spontaneous remission from autoimmunity in people with rheumatoid arthritis (RA), but this effect has not been studied in the dog.

Genetic background

There is strong genetic influence on the development of autoimmune disease. Autoimmunity is frequently recognized in particular breeds of dog and is often familial. Autoimmunity is more prevalent in geographically isolated areas where inbreeding occurs, and colonies of dogs with various autoimmune diseases have been established by selective inbreeding (**143**). One study of inherited canine autoimmune disease has involved the Old English Sheepdog, where reports from the USA, the UK and Australia have demonstrated susceptibility to a range of autoimmune diseases (AIHA, AITP, lymphocytic thyroiditis), and common ancestry has been identified in affected dogs. Familial autoimmunity is poorly documented in the cat.

A variety of genetic associations with autoimmune disease are described. The strongest are with loci, which encode molecules that are intrinsically involved in the initiation of autoimmunity. For example, there are associations between autoimmune disease and specific allotypic variants of molecules of the MHC (see below). Particular autoantibody allotypes and T cell receptor Vβ, and Vα genes are more frequently utilized in some experimental autoimmune responses. IgA deficiency is associated with autoimmunity in man and dogs, likely due to increased susceptibility to infectious agents that cross compromised mucosal barriers (**144**). Susceptibility to autoimmune disease does not entirely rely on genetic factors, as human monozygotic twins that share susceptibility alleles do not invariably develop autoimmune disease; therefore, other predisposing factors must be important.

Altered immunoregulation

Altered immunoregulation may result from perturbation of the immune system by unrelated disease (e.g. lymphoma, infection) or from the use of chemotherapy. Autoimmunity may arise following inappropriate presentation of cryptic self-epitopes by APCs as a sequela to infection (**145**). There is increasing evidence that failure of regulatory cell function or altered balance between Th1 and Th2 cells underlies many autoimmune diseases.

143

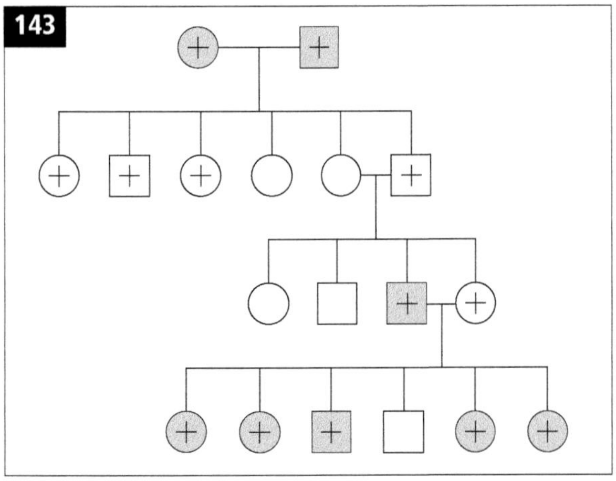

143 Familial autoimmunity in the dog. Pedigree showing four generations of dogs with clinical signs of systemic lupus erythematosus (shaded boxes or circles) with or without serum ANA (+ indicates ANA positive). Five of the eight dogs with clinical signs share the major histocompatibility phenotype DLA A7, B13, C4*2. (Data from Teichner M, Krumbacher K, Doxiadis I *et al.* [1990] Systemic lupus erythematosus in dogs: association to the major histocompatibility complex class I antigen DLA-A7. *Clinical Immunology and Immunopathology*, **55**:255–262.)

144 Association of IgA deficiency and autoimmune disease. Dogs with IgA deficiency have weakened immunological defences against microbial infection at mucosal surfaces. The increased exposure to microorganisms may be related to the development of autoimmune disease by mechanisms involving factors such as cross-reactivity between microbial and self-epitopes.

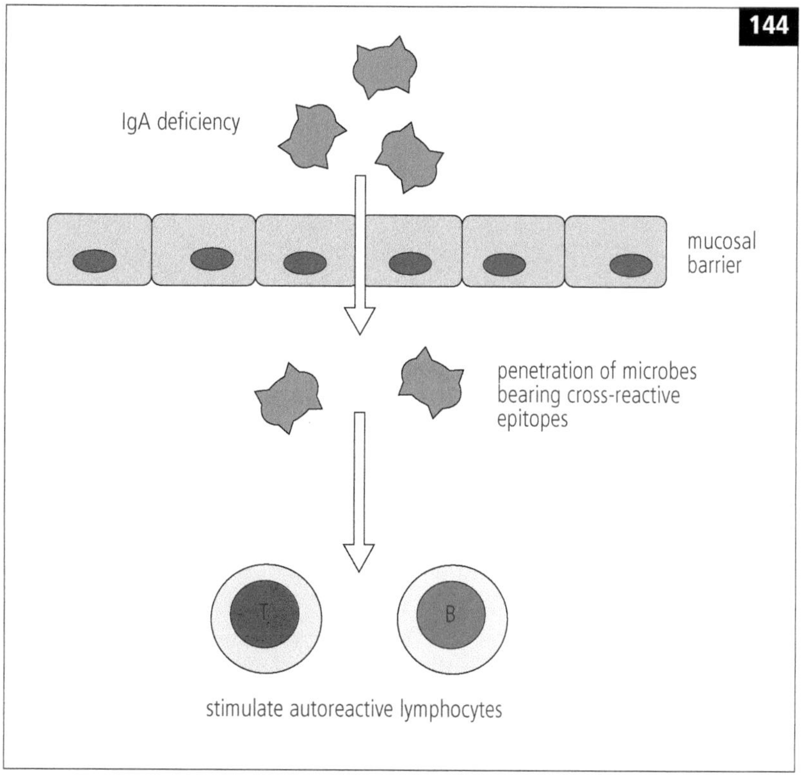

145a, b Loss of immunological ignorance may trigger autoimmunity. (a) In normal individuals, autoreactive B cells do not receive T cell help (anergy) as the appropriate Th cells are deleted, suppressed, anergic or not exposed to suitably processed cryptic epitopes of autoantigens (ignorant).
(b) Immunological ignorance can be reversed if there is an alteration in the way in which self-antigen is processed, thus permitting the expression of cryptic epitopes. Such alteration in antigen processing may be a result of changed cytokine milieu following infection.

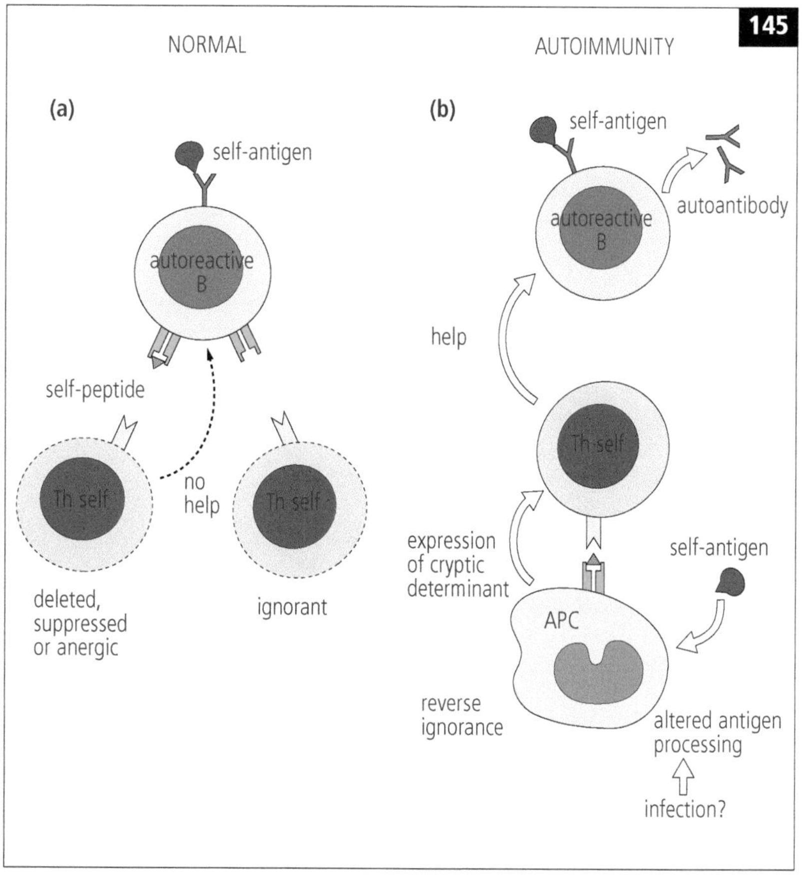

Environmental factors

Environmental factors are increasingly recognized to be important in the development of autoimmune disease, particularly exposure to microbial antigens following infection or vaccination.

Important differentials for autoimmune disease in the dog and cat are the vector-borne infections, including ehrlichiosis, rickettsiosis, borreliosis, leishmaniosis, babesiosis, bartonellosis and haemoplasmosis. These diseases may clinically mimic autoimmunity and induce laboratory abnormalities compatible with autoimmune disease. The reason for this relates to the intrinsic relationship between these pathogens, their vectors and the host immune system. The pathogen and vector may work together to subvert the normally protective Th1 host immune response and allow establishment of infection. For example, the saliva of ticks and sandflies contains potent immunomodulatory substances that preferentially drive a non-protective Th2 immune response within the dermal microenvironment (the site of infection). Activation of Th2-driven humoral immunity may also account for the secondary immune-mediated processes that characterize such infections. These include hypergammaglobulinaemia, immune complex formation and tissue deposition, and triggering of autoantibody responses (**146**).

A good example of this phenomenon is canine leishmaniosis. There is excellent experimental evidence that immunomodulators within sandfly saliva can induce a Th2 immune response. Genetically susceptible dogs (see Chapter 2, p. 70) develop symptomatic infection, the clinical manifestations of which are primarily immune-mediated and may include polyarthritis, glomerulonephritis (**147**), vasculitis (**148, 149**), anaemia, thrombocytopenia (**150**) and serum hypergammaglobulinaemia (**151**). In non-endemic areas it would be relatively easy to mistake this multisystemic clinical presentation for SLE (see Chapter 14, p. 356).

146

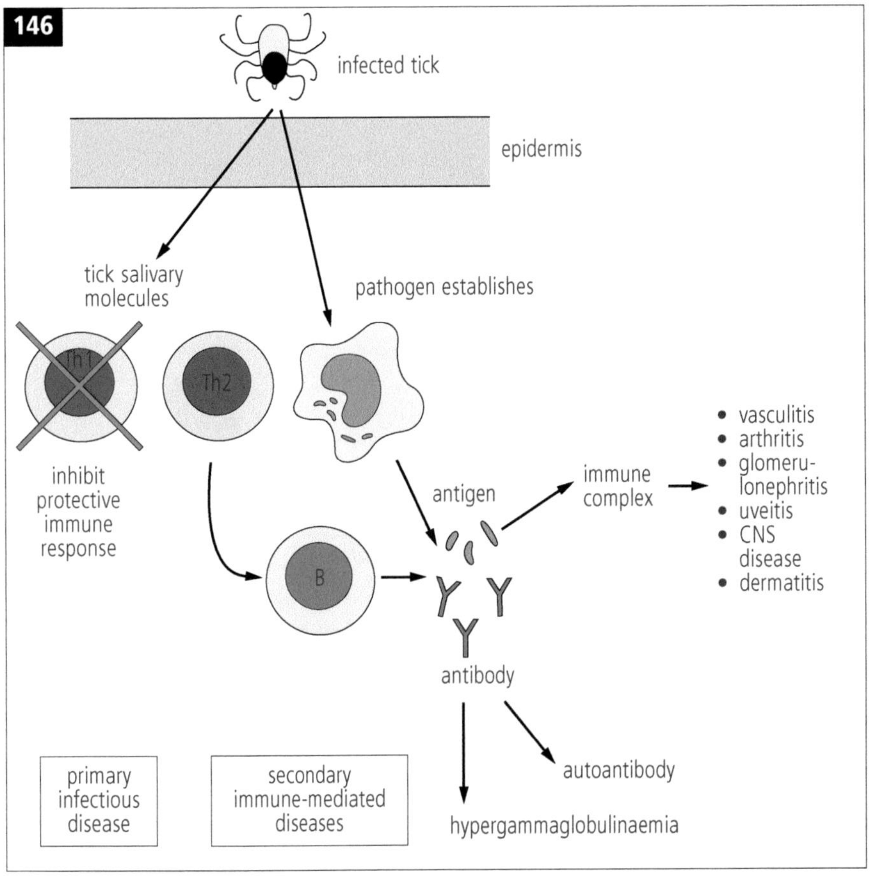

146 Immune-mediated sequelae to arthropod-borne infection. The propensity for animals with arthropod-transmitted infection to develop immune-mediated tissue damage relates to the intrinsic interaction between pathogen, vector and the host immune system. As pathogens are transmitted to the dermal microenvironment through the bite of a haemophagous arthropod (tick, mosquito, fly or flea), salivary molecules modulate the local immune response by altering the Th1-Th2 balance to create a non-protective Th2 environment in which the infection can establish. The expansion of humoral immunity subsequently leads to the development of the antibody and immune-complex mediated clinical manifestations of disease.

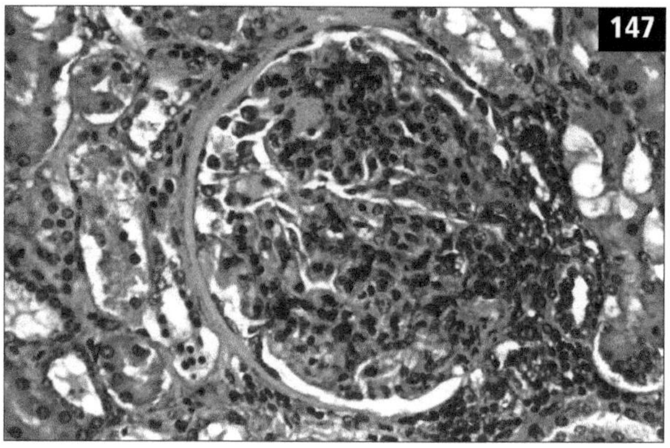

147 Glomerulonephritis in canine leishmaniosis. Section of kidney from a Greyhound dog with leishmaniosis imported into the UK from an area endemic for the disease. The dog had elevated serum BUN and creatinine, hypoalbuminaemia and proteinuria, in addition to cutaneous and ocular disease. There is a pronounced periglomerular and glomerular inflammatory response.

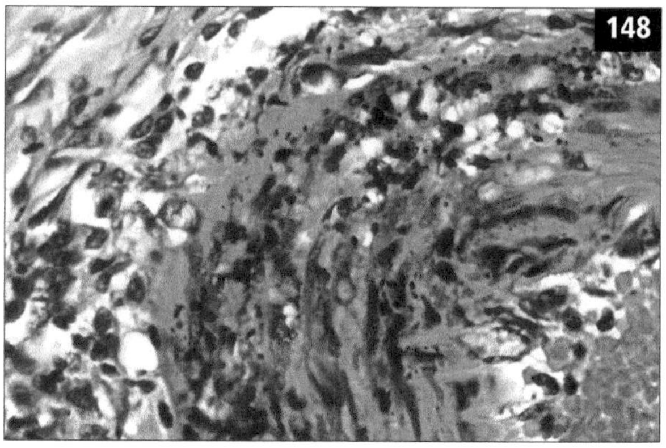

148 Vasculitis in canine leishmaniosis. Section of arterial wall from the dog described in **147**. There are inflammatory cells and nuclear debris within the vessel wall, together with a perivascular inflammatory infiltrate and evidence of fibrin deposition.

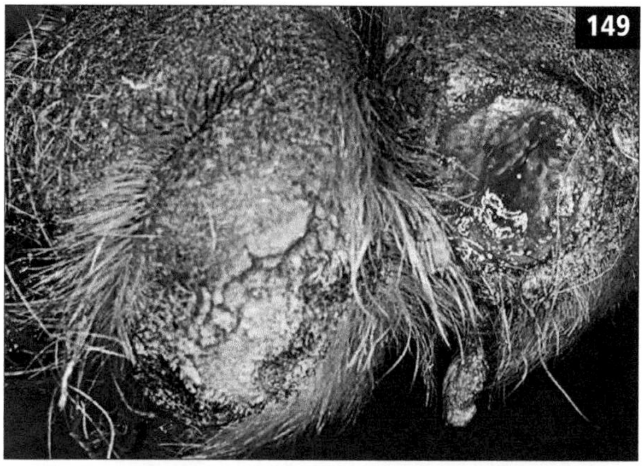

149 Vasculitis in canine leishmaniosis. Focal ulceration in the centre of a footpad in a dog with leishmaniosis. This location and the appearance of this lesion is consistent with vasculitis, but may also involve local granulomatous dermal inflammation. (From Shaw SE, Day MJ [2005] *Arthropod-Borne Infectious Diseases of the Dog and Cat*. Manson Publishing, London, with permission.)

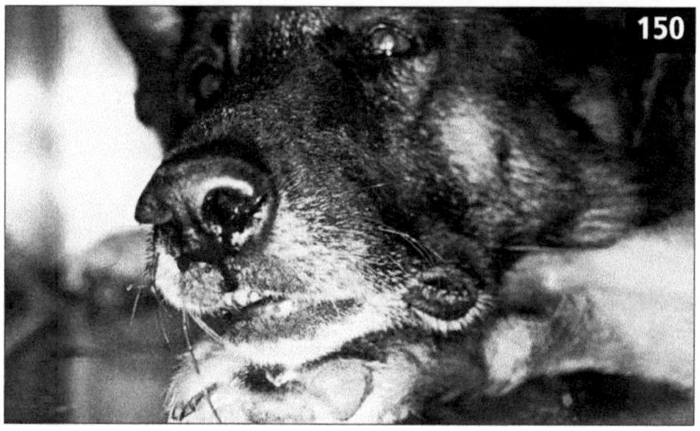

150 Thrombocytopenia in canine leishmaniosis. Epistaxis in this dog with leishmaniosis may relate in part to the induction of anti-platelet antibodies as a secondary immune-mediated sequela to infection. (From Shaw SE, Day MJ [2005] *Arthropod-Borne Infectious Diseases of the Dog and Cat*. Manson Publishing, London, with permission.)

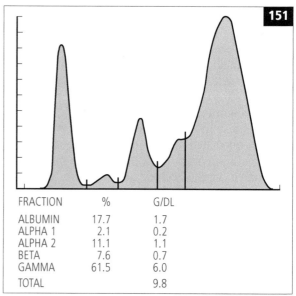

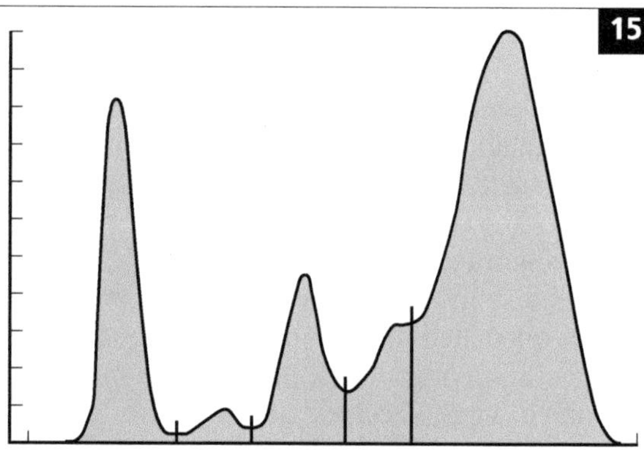

FRACTION	%	G/DL
ALBUMIN	17.7	1.7
ALPHA 1	2.1	0.2
ALPHA 2	11.1	1.1
BETA	7.6	0.7
GAMMA	61.5	6.0
TOTAL		9.8

151 Hypergammaglobulinaemia in leishmaniosis. Serum protein electrophoretic trace from a dog with leishmaniosis showing polyclonal gammopathy.

At least part of the pathogenesis of the anaemia and thrombocytopenia that occurs in dogs with babesiosis relates to the development of anti-erythrocyte and anti-platelet antibody. There is evidence from studies of dogs infected with small *Babesia* that the erythrocyte-bound antibody may have specificity for membrane autoantigens rather than microbial epitopes expressed on the surface of the target cells. A similar hypothesis is proposed for the red cell-associated antibodies that appear in cats with haemoplasmosis.

In endemic areas, practitioners are attuned to the diagnosis of these infections and would rarely consider autoimmune disease without first ruling out underlying infection. However, in non-endemic areas this distinction may not be readily made. There is at present great concern over the growing geographical distribution of arthropod-transmitted infections. This relates to a range of factors including climate change, extension of the geographical range of vector arthropods and the increasing mobility of companion animals brought about by legislation such as the European Pet Passport Scheme. There are well-documented examples of such change; for example, the establishment of canine babesiosis in traditionally non-endemic European countries (Belgium, Germany and Switzerland) and the spread of canine small *Babesia* and *Leishmania* within North America. Characteristically, such infections may be very difficult to diagnose, but the advent of PCR-based detection methods have enhanced the ability to detect these pathogens. Practitioners in traditionally non-endemic areas should be aware of these changes, as animals presenting with clinical signs once considered to be compatible with primary idiopathic autoimmunity might actually be harbouring infection.

A second possible environmental trigger for immune-mediated disease in companion animals is administration of vaccines, in particular multivalent attenuated viral vaccines or vaccines containing adjuvant. Although not common occurrences when considered in light of the number of vaccines administered to dogs and cats (*Table* 2), there is mounting evidence that in individual animals vaccination might act as a trigger for immune-mediated disease. Such instances are mostly recorded in dogs, where there are suggested associations between vaccination and the onset of diseases such as polyneuritis, pemphigus, cutaneous vasculitis (**152–155**), polyarthritis, IMHA and IMTP. In most studies, an association is defined as disease onset occurring within a four-week period after vaccination. Similar linkage between vaccination and a spectrum of immune-mediated disease is proposed in man.

Despite these proposed associations, there is little understanding of the mechanisms that might underlie this phenomenon. A series of recent experimental studies have shown that both IgG and IgE responses are made to extraneous bovine proteins incorporated into canine vaccines (bovine serum is utilized in cell culture for propagating virus) and that true autoantibody responses to the homologous canine molecules may also be triggered. For example, antithyroglobulin antibody develops in vaccinated dogs, although there is no suggestion that this leads to clinical hypothyroidism. Similarly, vaccinated cats have

Table 2: Incidence of vaccine-associated autoimmunity in dogs and cats. Vaccination may trigger a range of immune-mediated adverse reactions in dogs and cats, but these are rare complications. The figures in this Table come from an analysis of the UK Suspected Adverse Reactions Surveillance Scheme database between 1995 and 1999. The figures refer to incidence per 10,000 vaccines sold (and presumptively administered) in the UK during that period of time. Reactions with a possible autoimmune/immune-mediated mechanism are less common than type 1 hypersensitivity reactions or local injection site reactions. (Data from Gaskell RM, Gettingby G, Graham SJ *et al.* (2002) *Veterinary Products Committee (VPC) Working Group on Feline and Canine Vaccination: Final Report to the VPC.* DEFRA Publications, London.)

	Dog	**Cat**
Anaphylaxis	0.026	0.018
Injection site reaction	0.012	0.099
IMHA	0.001	0
IMTP	0.002	0.001
Blue eye	0.002	0
Polyarthropathy	0.006	0.044

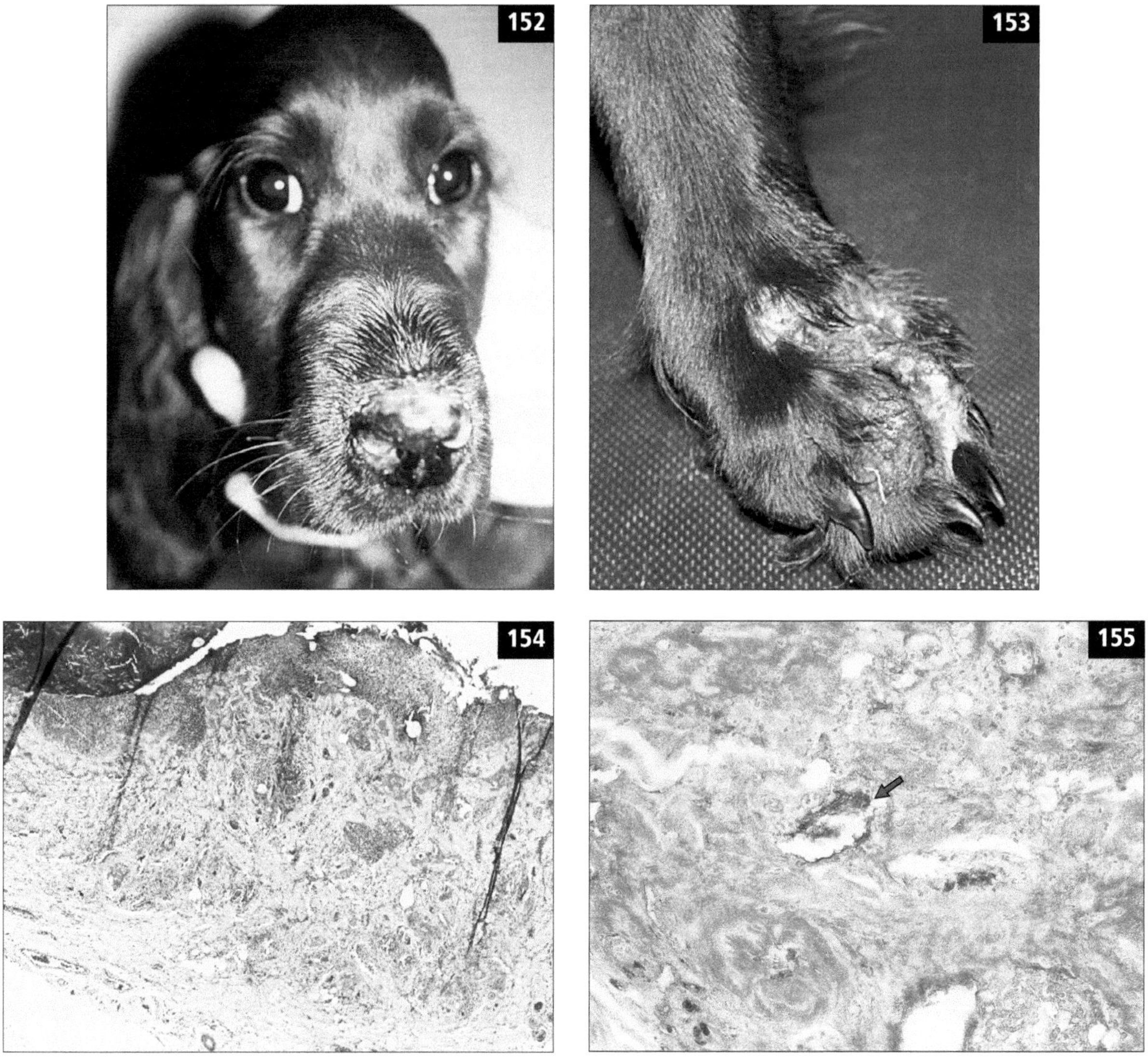

152–155 Vaccine-associated vasculitis. This young Irish Setter dog developed focal areas of alopecia and depigmentation in peripheral sites including the nasal planum (**152**) and feet (**153**). A biopsy from an affected site demonstrates a localized zone of ischaemic necrosis secondary to vasculitis and thrombosis affecting deep dermal vessels (**154**). Immunoglobulin was demonstrated in the walls of affected vessels (arrowed), consistent with an immune complex vasculitis (**155**). (Photographs **152** and **153** courtesy O.A. Garden.)

been shown to develop antibody to renal epithelial cells secondary to incorporation of residual Crandall Rees feline kidney epithelial cells (CRFK) used for producing vaccine virus. These seropositive cats do not, however, appear to develop significant renal pathology or clinical renal failure. It is also possible that the microbial component of vaccine stimulates autoimmunity via mechanisms that are discussed below. In this context, both distemper virus antigen and antibody have been found in the joints of dogs with RA, and immune complexes of rabies virus antigen and immunoglobulin have been identified in dermal vessel walls of dogs with rabies virus vaccine-associated alopecia. The well-documented phenomenon of adenovirus-associated canine 'blue eye' is described in Chapter 11 (p. 275). Finally, the potent immunomodulatory effects of vaccine adjuvant (**156**) might also act to trigger autoimmunity in genetically predisposed individuals.

Numerous experimental studies have now been conducted to investigate the potential immunological mechanisms that might underlie the association between infectious agents and autoimmunity. For example:

- The immune response to infectious agents may involve production of IFNγ, which causes expression of MHC class II by tissue cells that would not normally express these molecules (e.g. thyroid follicular epithelial cells). Such cells may express self-antigen within these MHC molecules and become targets for autoreactive T lymphocytes (**157, 158**).

156

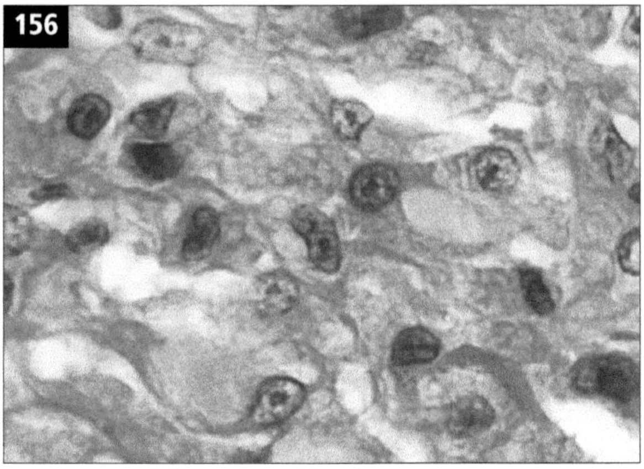

156 Vaccine adjuvant. Section taken from a vaccine injection site in a cat. There is a granulomatous inflammatory response and the blue-grey material within the cytoplasm of some macrophages is alum adjuvant. The inflammatory response induced by adjuvanted vaccines may trigger the subsequent development of neoplasia (i.e. feline vaccine associated fibrosarcoma) or, in theory, trigger other immunological consequences.

157

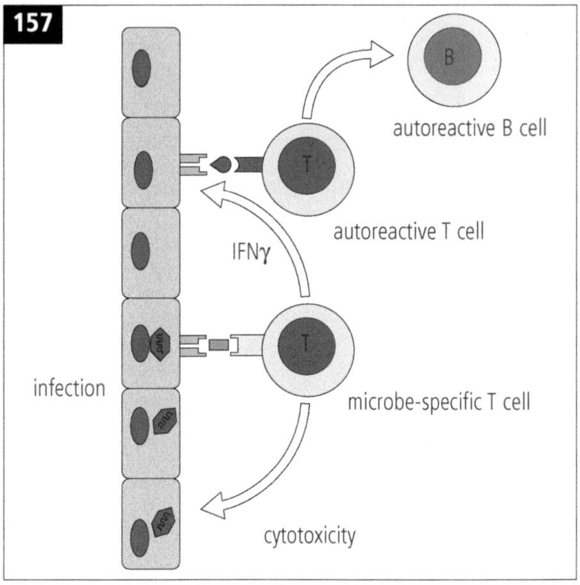

157 Aberrant expression of MHC II by target cells in autoimmunity. The normal immune response to viral infection involves cytotoxicity and local production of IFNγ. One action of this cytokine is to initiate expression of MHC class II molecules by cells that would otherwise not display this molecule. If these MHC II molecules contain appropriate self-peptides, autoreactive T cells may be activated.

158

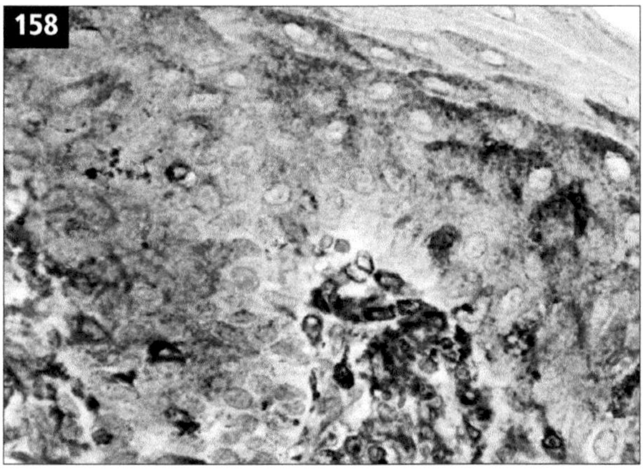

158 Expression of MHC II by keratinocytes in autoimmune skin disease. Skin biopsy from a Japanese Akita dog with uveodermatological syndrome labelled by the immunoperoxidase method for MHC class II. A number of the keratinocytes express cytoplasmic and membrane class II, whereas this molecule is not found within the normal canine epidermis. (From Carter J, Crispin SM, Gould DJ *et al.* [2005] An immunohistochemical study of uveodermatologic syndrome in two Japanese Akita dogs. *Veterinary Ophthalmology* **8**:17–24, with permission.)

- Microbes may induce non-specific polyclonal activation of numerous T and B cell clones, some of which may be autoreactive. Microbial 'superantigens' may act in this fashion. Increased numbers of a subset of B cells ($CD5^+$), which produce low affinity IgM autoantibody and polyspecific anti-microbial antibody, are identified in autoimmune disease.
- Microbial infection of a cell may lead to 'innocent bystander' destruction of that cell when an immune response is directed towards microbial antigens expressed on the cell surface or to a combination of microbial and self-determinants ('modified self').
- Microbial antigens may cross-react with self-antigens by sharing conformational epitopes or linear peptides ('molecular mimicry') (**159**). In this regard, heat shock proteins (HSPs) are of importance in some autoimmune diseases. HSPs are a series of families of proteins with highly

159

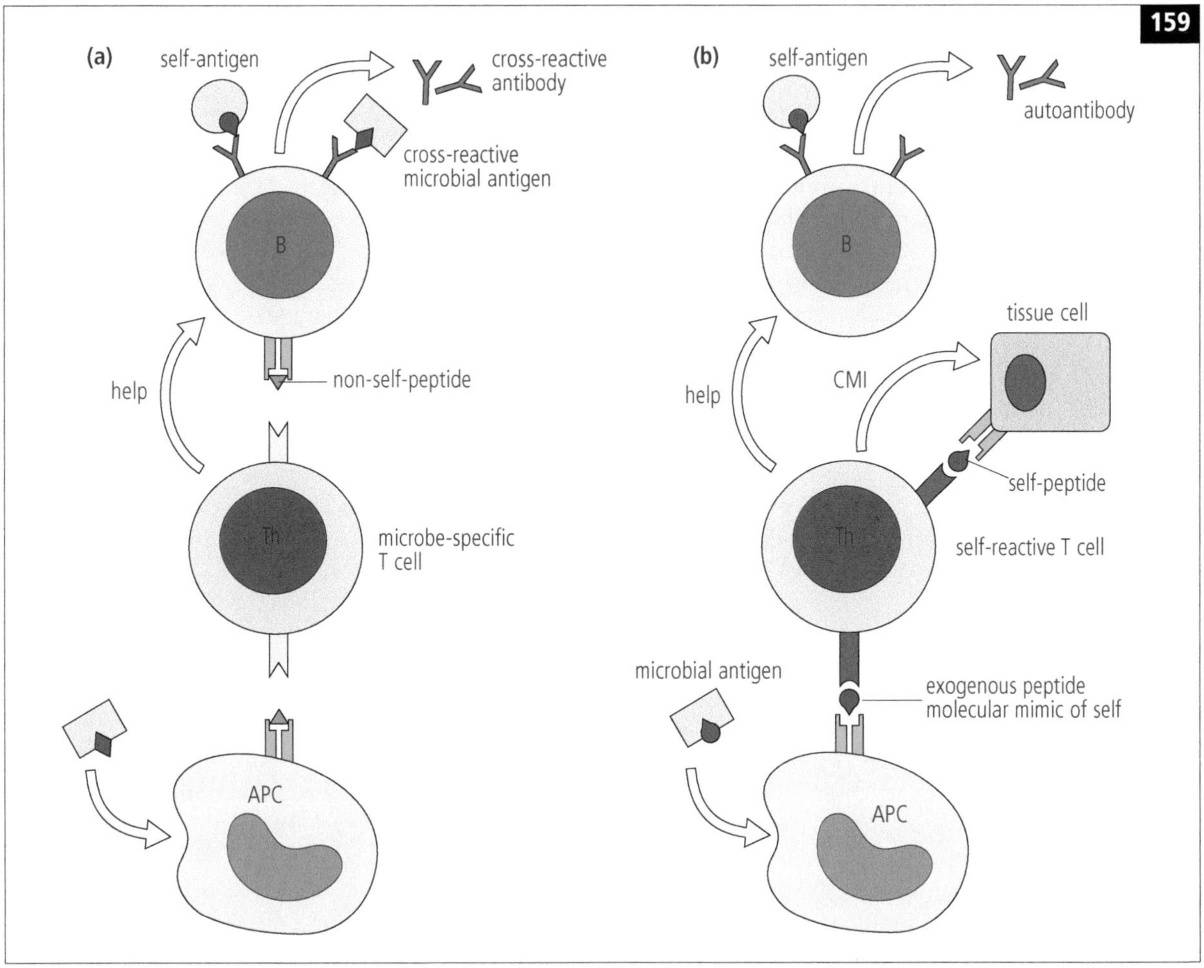

159a, b Microbial infection may break self-tolerance and initiate autoimmunity. (a) A microbe bears a cross-reactive epitope that allows the organism to bind to B cell SmIg and be internalized. The microbe is processed by the B cell and non-self, microbially derived peptides are presented on MHC class II molecules. The subsequent activation of microbe-specific T cells provides a source of help for the cross-reactive B cell, bypassing self-tolerance and allowing production of cross-reactive antibodies. **(b)** A microbe bears a peptide sequence that is shared by a self-antigen (molecular mimicry). During processing of the organism there is presentation of this cross-reactive sequence, which may bind MHC with greater affinity than cryptic self-peptide and allow activation of autoreactive T lymphocytes. These T cells may then provide a source of help for autoreactive B cells, bypassing self-tolerance and allowing production of autoantibodies that do not necessarily cross-react with the initiating organism. Alternatively, the activated T cells may subsequently recognize self-peptide presented by tissue cells (non-professional APC) and cause cell-mediated tissue pathology.

> conserved amino acid sequence between species as diverse as plants and mammals. HSPs are produced by heated or stressed cells, where they have a protective function, but they are also involved in the assembly, translocation and degradation of cytoplasmic proteins. In many autoimmune diseases, HSPs are a target autoantigen, which may reflect surface expression of self-HSP by stressed cells or preceding bacterial infection with release of cross-reactive bacterial HSP.

A final example of an 'environmental' trigger for autoimmunity is administration of drugs. A wide range of drugs may potentially act in this fashion, but the best example is antibiotics. In dogs there is a well-documented association between administration of trimethoprim-sulphonamide and immune-mediated haematological disease (IMHA, thrombocytopenia and neutropenia). Although initially described in the Doberman Pinscher, a wide range of breeds has now been reported to be affected. Administration of carbimazole/methimazole to hyperthyroid cats is also a known trigger for autoimmunity (IMHA, thrombocytopenia and serum antinuclear antibody).

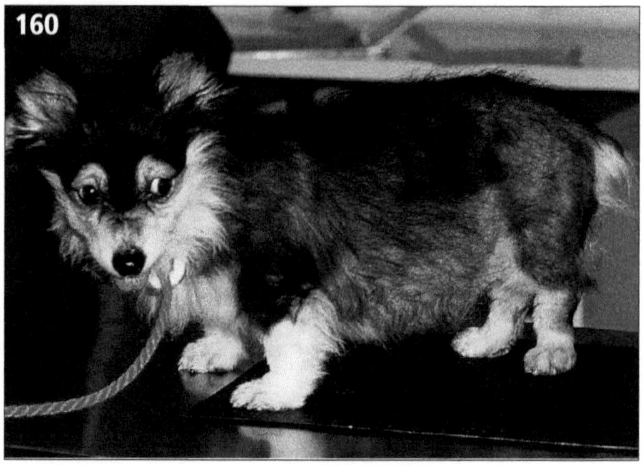

160 Secondary immunodeficiency. Secondary suppression of the immune system may occur in a wide range of diseases. Shown is a dog with hyperadrenocorticism demonstrating the classical features of symmetrical alopecia and abdominal enlargement. The high levels of endogenous glucocorticoid produced by such dogs may cause atrophy of lymphoid tissue and increase susceptibility to secondary infection. (Photograph courtesy S.E. Shaw.)

GENETIC DEFECTS UNDERLYING IMMUNODEFICIENCY DISEASE

There are two situations in which the immune system fails to function adequately and mount a protective immune response when required. The most common involves mature animals, in which an identifiable factor causes suppression of the immune system (acquired immunodeficiency). Such factors include chronic infectious (e.g. FIV), inflammatory or neoplastic disease, drug therapy, malnutrition, toxins or stress (**160**). Alternatively, younger animals may be immunodeficient due to:

- *In utero* infection that targets immunological tissue (e.g. feline infectious enteritis virus).
- Failure to absorb sufficient colostrum.
- Congenital, inherited diseases (primary immunodeficiency) whereby one or multiple components of the immune system are absent or functionally defective.

A number of primary immunodeficiency diseases are recognized in the dog, but such diseases are rare in cats. The precise genetic defects are generally poorly characterized, but they may occur at any stage of immunological maturation, resulting in a spectrum of change from profound immunological unresponsiveness to more subtle deficiencies of a single Ig class or complement component (see Chapter 12, p. 291).

THE INDUCTION OF LYMPHOID NEOPLASIA

The cell types that make up the immune system may all potentially undergo neoplastic transformation. In practice, lymphoid neoplasia in the dog and cat (lymphoma, lymphoid leukaemia) and canine cutaneous histiocytoma (Langerhans cell origin) are relatively common, whereas tumours of other developmental stages or cell types (multiple myeloma, plasmacytoma, histiocytic sarcoma) are less prevalent.

Lymphoma and lymphoid leukaemia in the cat were once almost always attributed to FeLV infection (**161**); however, since the advent of improved diagnostic test methods and vaccination for this retroviral infection, a change in the pattern of feline lymphoid neoplasia has occurred. Feline lymphoma is now recognized in an older cohort of

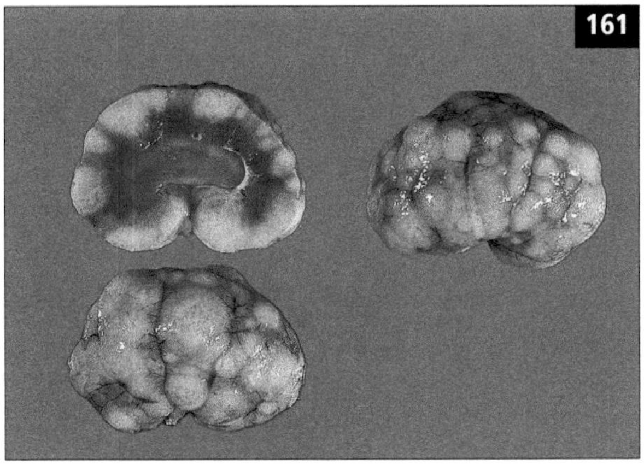

161 Feline lymphoma. Lymphoma in the cat may be caused by infection with FeLV. Shown are the kidneys from a nine-year-old DSH cat with multicentric lymphoma. Much of the cortex is replaced by a series of coalescing cream nodules.

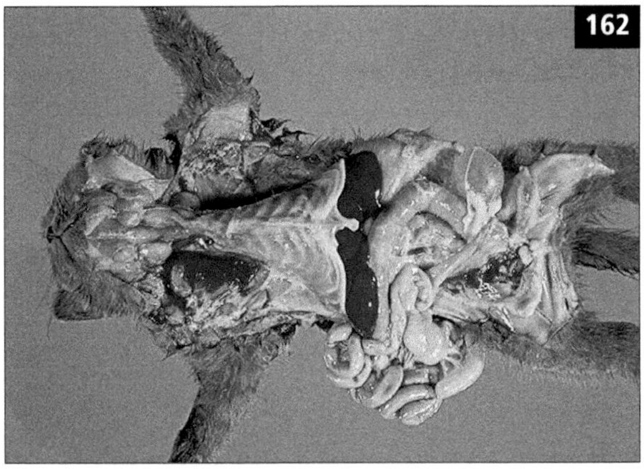

162 Genetic susceptibility to lymphoma. This eight week old, British blue kitten has massive generalized lymphadenopathy. Histologically this is consistent with lymphoma, and immunophenotyping defines these as neoplastic T cells. Over several years, numerous affected kittens were born in this particular cattery in which the animals were consistently FeLV negative by routine serological diagnostic methods. Although this does not exclude a retroviral aetiology for this very early onset disease, a genetic predisposition may also be suggested.

cats that serologically test negative for FeLV. Moreover, the most common anatomical presentation is now alimentary rather than thymic lymphoma. Although this might reflect the emergence of non-retroviral-associated feline lymphoid neoplasia, there is not yet clear information concerning the presence of FeLV provirus within such tumours. In some geographical areas (e.g. Sydney, Australia) the prevalence of FeLV infection has always been low, although feline lymphoma is as common as in other countries. Despite occasional reports over many years, there is still no definitive evidence to suggest that canine lymphoid neoplasia is virally induced.

Lymphoid tumours arise through the concerted action of predisposing, initiating and promoting factors. These include genetic background (e.g. the prevalence of lymphoma in Boxers and familial lymphoma in some canine pedigrees) (**162**), age (middle-aged to older dogs are most often affected) and environmental factors, including exposure to carcinogens. The role of carcinogenic agents in the induction of small animal neoplasia is poorly documented (**163**). Such factors induce transformation in particular lymphocytes, involving

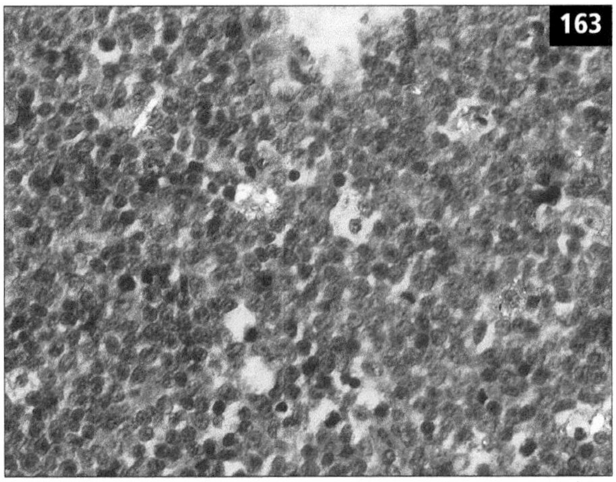

163 Crystalline material in canine lymphoma. The lymph nodes of dogs with multicentric lymphoma sometimes contain large quantities of birefringent crystalline material that comprises a combination of exogenously derived elements. An association has been proposed between the accumulation of such mineral material within lymph nodes and the subsequent development of lymphoid neoplasia or autoimmunity. Shown is a section of canine lymph node in which normal histological structure is largely replaced by a sheet of neoplastic lymphocytes. Amidst these cells are portions of extracellular crystal and similar material within the cytoplasm of macrophages (taken under polarized light).

genetic alterations that result in uncontrolled clonal proliferation of the transformed cells (**164, 165**). Early studies investigated the relationship between chemical exposure and canine lymphoma, and recent epidemiological investigations have suggested a link between feline lymphoma and passive exposure to cigarette smoke.

MAJOR HISTOCOMPATIBILITY COMPLEX AND OTHER GENETIC ASSOCIATIONS WITH IMMUNE-MEDIATED DISEASE

Individual humans that express particular allotypes of MHC-encoded molecules have a greater relative risk for development of a range of immune-

164

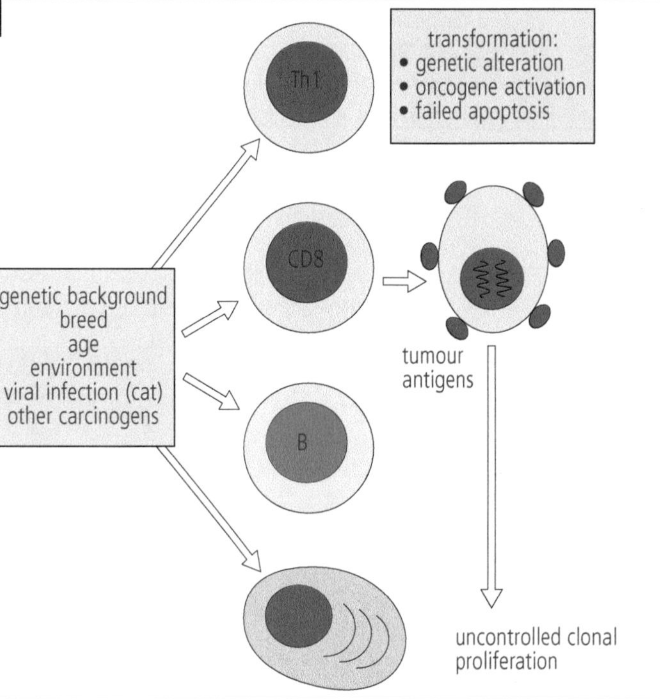

164 The basis of lymphoid neoplasia. The expression of lymphoid neoplasia is likely to involve the interaction of a series of susceptibility, initiating and promoting factors. The best defined of these is FeLV infection in the cat. These factors will cause transformation of a particular lineage of lymphoid cell. Inappropriate oncogene activation or failure of programmed cell death (apoptosis) results in uncontrolled proliferation of the transformed cell, and there will be cytological and phenotypic alterations within the tumour population.

165

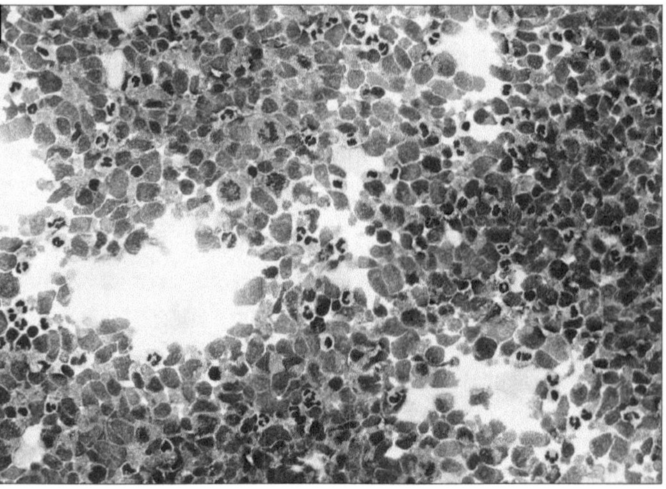

165 Cytological abnormalities in lymphoid neoplasia. Abdominal fluid from a four-year-old crossbred dog with hepatomegaly. There are large numbers of actively mitotic lymphoblastic cells. A needle core biopsy of liver confirmed the presence of lymphoma.

mediated and autoimmune diseases. Similarly, inbred strains of laboratory rodents have a variable susceptibility to spontaneously arising or experimentally induced autoimmune disease that is in part dependent upon their MHC type (**166**). The strongest such 'MHC disease associations' are with particular alleles of MHC class II loci, and the associations are even more significant when combinations of alleles at different loci are considered ('haplotypes'). Allotypic variants of the MHC-encoded complement C4 molecules are also associated with expression of immune-mediated diseases.

These genetic associations are not completely understood, but as MHC molecules are intrinsically involved in the presentation of antigens to T cells, it may be that the sequence of the variable region of specific molecules confers greater ability to present antigen optimally for T cell activation or to alter T cell selection during intrathymic development. An alternative hypothesis is that these associations are not of primary importance, but are simply genetic markers for other 'disease genes' that have a more direct role in the causation of disease or for other MHC-encoded genes involved in generation and transportation of peptides or production of cytokines.

MHC disease associations have been studied in the dog (*Table 3*), but there is little information available for the cat. The original studies were performed in the late 1970s and early 1980s using complex and technically demanding serological and cellular techniques to define the DLA (canine MHC) allotypes. These studies involved relatively

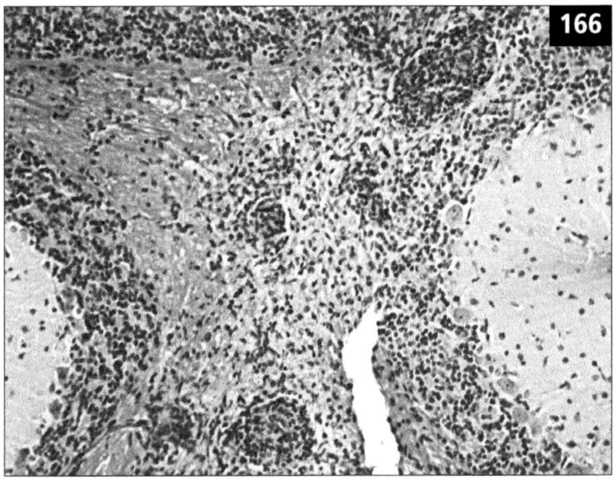

166 MHC type in rodent autoimmune disease. Section of cerebellum from a mouse with experimental autoimmune encephalomyelitis (EAE), a model of human multiple sclerosis. There is a series of perivascular lymphoid cuffs within the white matter, which also shows granulomatous inflammation and demyelination. T lymphocyte-mediated models of autoimmune disease, such as EAE, have variable expression in different inbred strains of laboratory mice. The MHC type of the mouse strain is one factor that determines this susceptibility.

Table 3: MHC disease associations in the dog. A number of studies have examined the association between canine disease states and expression of specific allotypes of canine MHC molecules.

Disease	Study population (n=)	DLA association
AIHA	108	Risk haplotypes include: DRB1*000601, DQA1*005011, DQB1*00701 and DRB1*015, DQA1*00601, DQB1*00301
Immune-mediated polyarthritis	61	DRB1*002 DRB1*009 DRB1*018
Diabetes mellitus	460	Risk haplotypes include: DRB1*009, DQA1*001, DQB1*008 and DRB1*015, DQA1*0061, DQB1*023 and

Continues on page 92

Table 3: MHC-disease associations in the dog. (*Continued*)

Disease	**Study population (n=)**	**DLA association**
		DRB1*002, DQA1*009, DQB1*001 Protective haplotype is: DQA1*004, DQB1*013
Susceptibility to leishmaniosis	109 study dogs typed for DRB1, DQA1 and DQA2 alleles	DRB1*01502 associated with high serum IgG and PCR positivity for infection
Dermatouveitis in Japanese Akitas	26	DQA1*00201 associated with development of disease (relative risk 15.3)
Anal furunculosis	107	DRB 1*00101
Anal sac carcinoma in English Cocker Spaniel	42 cases 75 controls	DQB1*00701
Doberman hepatitis	37 cases 37 controls	DRB1*00601/DQA1*00401/ DQB1*01303 homozygosity [susceptibility] DRB1*01501 [protection]
Pug Dog necrotizing meningoencephalitis	43 cases 147 controls	DRB1*010011/DQA1*00201/ DQB1*01501
Juvenile demodicosis	56 cases [mixed breeds] 60 controls	Microsatellite marker associations
Lymphocytic thyroiditis in Giant Schnauzers	74 cases 30 controls	DRB1*01201/DQA1*00101/ DQB1*00201
Hypoadrenocorticism in Nova Scotia Duck Tolling Retrievers	29 cases 34 controls	DRB1*01502/DQA1*00601/ DQB1*02301

low numbers of animals, but they provided 'proof of principle' that there was DLA linkage to canine immune-mediated disease. These early studies were a spin-off from research into organ and bone marrow transplantation using the canine model, where matching transplants by MHC type was essential.

In the past decade the advent of molecular technology has made it possible to redefine the canine and feline MHC (see Chapter 1, p. 36) and apply high throughput rapid testing to large numbers of samples from animals with well-phenotyped clinical disease. Associations have been found between DLA type and canine anal furunculosis, RA, AIHA, diabetes mellitus and hypothyroidism. These associations are strongest when analysed by comparison of cases versus controls within specific dog breeds. The association with canine RA is particularly intriguing, as the DLA class II molecule that has strong linkage shares structural similarity with the HLA molecule associated with human RA. This in turn suggests that a common antigenic epitope might trigger both the canine and human disease. As proof that the MHC is fundamental to immune responsiveness, associations have also been found with susceptibility to canine leishmaniosis, and current research is investigating whether MHC type (in both dogs and cats) influences the response to routine vaccination. One study has examined feline MHC class II polymorphism in cats with coronavirus (FIP) infection, but has not shown an association between FLA DR allotype and clinical outcome of infection.

The availability of the canine and feline genomes has meant that a range of other genetic markers for immune-mediated disease may be investigated.

Based on human studies, linkage of canine disease to specific 'candidate genes' likely to play a role in disease pathogenesis has been investigated. Such studies often utilize the technique of searching for unique disease-associated single nucleotide polymorphisms (SNPs) within the genes of interest. A range of putative susceptibility genes for human Crohn's disease has been reported (e.g. NOD-2, some cytokine and Toll-like receptor genes), and current research is examining whether similar associations may be found with canine inflammatory enteropathy. Similar studies of SNPs in candidate genes have defined 'risk' and 'protective' genes for the development of canine diabetes mellitus and examined such genetic associations with susceptibility to canine leishmaniosis. More recently, disease-associated SNPs across the entire genome have been identified through genome wide association studies (GWAS). For example, the SLE-like disease of the Nova Scotia Duck Tolling Retriever has been linked to SNPs in a group of genes encoding molecules involved in T-cell activation. In addition to investigation of disease associations at the DNA level, the use of gene microarray or even proteomic or metabolomic screening is now being applied to identify levels of expression of these candidate genes in disease animal blood, tissue or secretions.

FURTHER READING

Agguirre-Hernandez J, Polton G, Kennedy LJ et al. (2010) Association between anal sac gland carcinoma and dog leukocyte antigen-DQB1 in the English Cocker Spaniel. *Tissue Antigens* 76:476–481.

Barnes A, O'Neill T, Kennedy LJ *et al.* (2009) Risk of anal furunculosis in German shepherd dogs is primarily associated with DLA-DRB1 and not TNF-α. *Tissue Antigens* 73:218–224.

Dyggve H, Kennedy LJ, Meri S *et al.* (2010) Association of Doberman hepatitis to canine major histocompatibility complex II. *Tissue Antigens* 77:30–35.

Greer KA, Wong AK, Liu H *et al.* (2010) Necrotizing meningoencephalitis of Pug Dogs associates with dog leukocyte antigen class II and resembles acute variant forms of multiple sclerosis. *Tissue Antigens* 76:110–118.

Hughes AM, Jokinen P, Bannasch DL *et al.* (2010) Association of a dog leukocyte antigen class II haplotype with hypoadrenocorticism in Nova Scotia Duck Tolling Retrievers. *Tissue Antigens* 75:684–690.

It V, Barrientos L, Lopez Gappa J *et al.* (2010) Association of canine juvenile generalized demodicosis with the dog leukocyte antigen system. *Tissue Antigens* 76:67–70.

Kennedy LJ, Barnes A, Ollier WER *et al.* (2006) Association of a common DLA class II haplotype with canine primary immune-mediated haemolytic anaemia. *Tissue Antigens* 68:502–506.

Mellersh C (2008) Give a dog a genome. *Veterinary Journal* 178:46–52.

Ollier WER, Kennedy LJ, Thomson W *et al.* (2001) Dog MHC alleles containing the human RA shared epitope confer susceptibility to canine rheumatoid arthritis. *Immunogenetics* 53:669–673.

Quinnell RJ, Kennedy LJ, Barnes A *et al.* (2003) Susceptibility to visceral leishmaniasis in the domestic dog is associated with MHC class II polymorphism. *Immunogenetics* 55:23–28.

Rook GAW (2008) Review series on helminthes, immune modulation and the hygiene hypothesis: the broader implications of the hygiene hypothesis. *Immunology* 126:3–11.

Shearin AL, Ostrander EA (2010) Leading the way: canine models of genomics and disease. *Disease Models and Mechanisms* 3:27–34.

Wilbe M, Jokinen P, Truve K *et al.* (2010) Genome-wide association mapping identifies multiple loci for a canine SLE-related disease complex. *Nature Genetics* 42:250–254.

Wilbe M, Sundberg K, Hansen IR *et al.* (2010) Increased genetic risk or protection for canine autoimmune lymphocytic thyroiditis in Giant Schnauzers depends on DLE class II genotype. *Tissue Antigens* 75:712–719.

Wood SH, Ollier WE, Nuttall T *et al.* (2010) Despite identifying some shared gene associations with human atopic dermatitis the use of multiple dog breeds from various locations limits detection of gene associations in canine atopic dermatitis. *Veterinary Immunology and Immunopathology* 138:193–197.

4 IMMUNE-MEDIATED HAEMATOLOGICAL DISEASE

Michael J. Day and Andrew J. Mackin

INTRODUCTION

Anaemia or thrombocytopenia due to immune-mediated destruction of red blood cells (RBCs) or platelets, respectively, are among the most commonly diagnosed immunological disorders of cats and dogs. In immune-mediated haemolytic anaemia (IMHA) or immune-mediated thrombocytopenia (IMTP), the underlying pathogenesis involves destruction of RBCs or platelets via a type II (antibody-dependent cytotoxicity) mechanism (**167**). The antibody may attach to the surface of the RBC or platelet by several different means (**168**). In many cases there is a specific underlying cause for this antibody binding, but where a true autoantibody binds to a structural component of the erythrocyte or platelet membrane (self-antigen), in the absence of underlying disease, the haemolysis or thrombocytopenia is autoimmune in nature and the disease is autoimmune haemolytic anaemia (AIHA) or autoimmune thrombocytopenia (AITP; also called idiopathic thrombocytopenia purpura [ITP]). IMHA or IMTP should only be defined as autoimmune in the absence of identified underlying factors. Although AIHA and AITP most commonly occur in isolation, the two conditions may occur together (Evans' syndrome) or as part of the multisystemic autoimmune disease SLE. Recently, it has become clear that dogs may also be affected by immune-mediated neutropenia (IMNP) and that this entity may occur concurrently with either or both IMHA/IMTP.

167

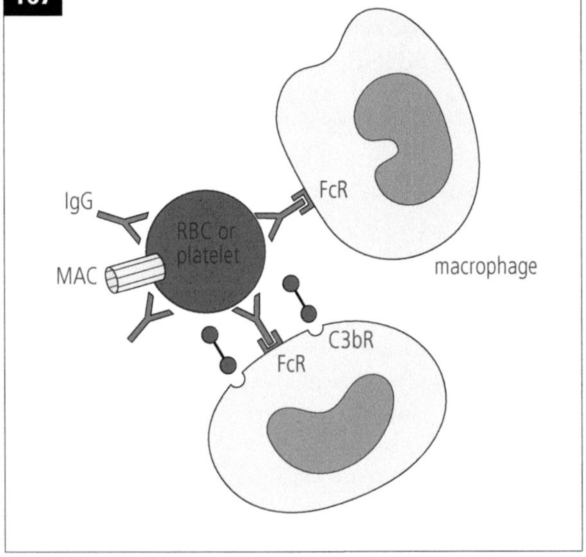

167 IMHA or IMTP. Destruction of RBCs or platelets by the immune system occurs via a type II (antibody-dependent) cytotoxic mechanism. Antibody (IgG or IgM) coated RBCs or platelets may be removed following formation of the MAC of the terminal pathway of complement (intravascular lysis) or following opsonization by IgG and/or complement C3b and phagocytosis by macrophages in sites such as the spleen and liver (extravascular lysis).

IMMUNE-MEDIATED HAEMOLYTIC ANAEMIA IN THE DOG

Immunopathogenesis

IMHA is the most common cause of haemolytic anaemia in the dog. Initiating factors for canine secondary IMHA include:

- Infectious disease, particularly the range of arthropod-borne infections described in Chapter 3 (babesiosis, ehrlichiosis, leishmaniosis, rickettsiosis). *Mycoplasma haemocanis* does not appear to trigger canine IMHA.
- Neoplasia, particularly lymphoma, myeloproliferative disease and haemangiosarcoma. The reasons for these associations remain speculative, but may include disturbed immunoregulation by clonal proliferation of neoplastic T lymphocytes, production of autoantibody by neoplastic B lymphocytes, and erythrocyte damage with exposure of cryptic autoantigens in haemangiosarcoma.
- Vaccination within the preceding four-week period (see Chapters 3 and 17).

- Drug therapy, particularly with trimethoprim-sulphonamide drugs, although cephalosporins also act in this fashion.

Despite the increasing awareness that many dogs with IMHA have disease of a secondary nature, in geographical areas non-endemic for arthropod-borne infectious disease the majority of patients with IMHA are still considered to have primary idiopathic disease (AIHA) when clinical and laboratory investigation fails to reveal an underlying causation.

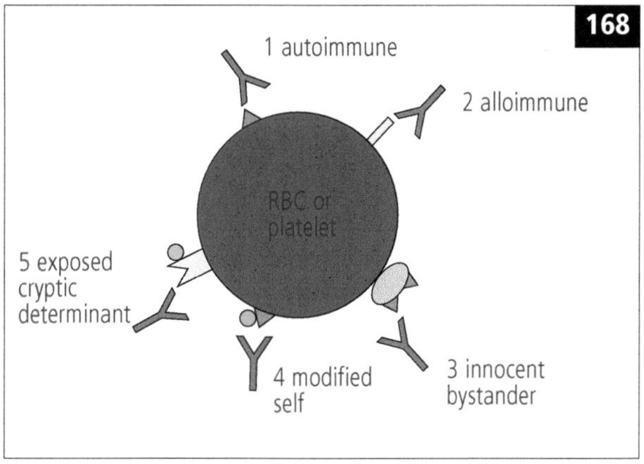

168 Mechanisms of antibody binding in IMHA or IMTP. (1) In primary autoimmune disease an autoantibody binds to a membrane structural determinant. The autoantibody may develop following primary immunological dysregulation or secondary to infection by a microbe that carries a cross-reactive epitope or induces immunological dysregulation (e.g. FeLV). (2) An alloantibody binds to a blood group antigen. Such antibodies may be spontaneously arising, induced by incompatible blood transfusion or passed to neonates in colostrum (neonatal isoerythrolysis). (3) An antibody binds to a foreign epitope carried by an infectious agent (e.g. *Mycoplasma haemofelis*) or drug (e.g. penicillin) that is attached non-specifically to the cell surface ('innocent bystander' destruction). (4) A drug (acting as a hapten) binds to an erythrocyte surface molecule creating a novel epitope ('modified self'), recognized as foreign by the immune system. (5) Binding of a drug or microbe causes exposure of a previously cryptic determinant. In this case the antibody is an autoantibody, but the disease is secondary to the initiating cause. Additionally, immunoglobulin or immune complexes may be absorbed non-specifically on to the surface of the erythrocyte or platelet (not via Fab binding), but will not necessarily mediate cell destruction.

IMHA is most often a disease of middle age, although young dogs (<12 months of age) can uncommonly be affected. There are breed predispositions for the Cocker Spaniel, Old English Sheepdog, English Springer Spaniel and Poodle, and other breeds may have increased susceptibility. A predisposition in the Maltese Terrier is reported in Australia. AIHA within pedigrees has been reported. Many reports suggest a higher prevalence in female dogs, and episodes of IMHA may be precipitated by stressful events such as oestrus or whelping. Seasonal associations have been observed in the northern hemisphere, but these are not consistent, with reported peak incidence in either summer or winter. It has been suggested that such seasonality relates to factors such as exposure to arthropod-borne infectious agents during warmer months or vaccination before travelling with, or kennelling, dogs during vacation periods.

The immunopathogenesis of AIHA involves presentation of erythrocyte membrane self-antigen by MHC molecules and interactions between autoreactive T and B lymphocytes, resulting in synthesis of autoantibody (**169**). Antibody-coated

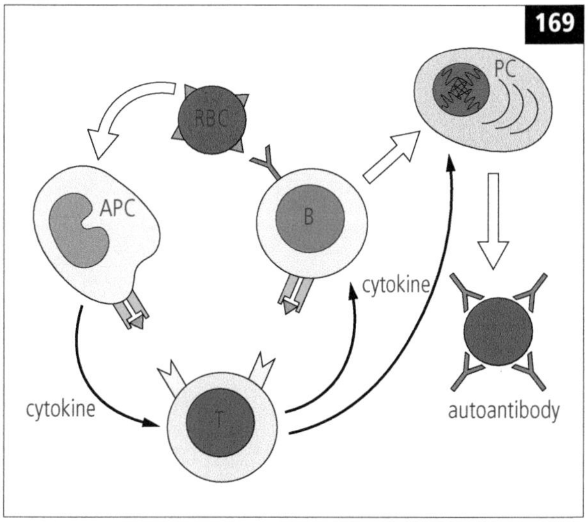

169 Immunological events in the initiation of IMHA. Development of IMHA requires bypass of self-tolerance by presentation of erythrocyte autoantigenic epitopes by APCs, with activation of autoreactive T cells able to provide help for autoreactive B lymphocytes. Clonal proliferation and differentiation of these cells results in the synthesis of autoantibody by plasma cells.

erythrocytes may be removed by extravascular haemolysis in the spleen (**170**) and, to a lesser extent, the liver (**171**) or, less frequently, by intravascular haemolysis following complement fixation by the autoantibody. In some cases the autoantibody is directed against bone marrow erythroid precursors, and a severe form of non-regenerative IMHA occurs. In the literature this form of disease is often subclassified into two entities, which probably form a single spectrum of

170

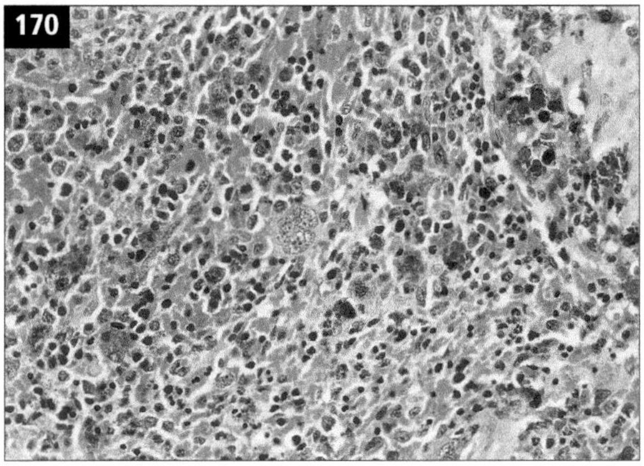

170 Splenic extravascular haemolysis and extramedullary haemopoiesis. Section of spleen from a dog with IMHA. There are prominent stores of haemosiderin (golden-brown pigment) within phagocytic cells, consistent with excessive erythrocyte breakdown. Additionally, haemopoietic precursors are present within the red pulp. This is indicative of extramedullary haemopoiesis as part of a regenerative response to the chronic anaemia.

171

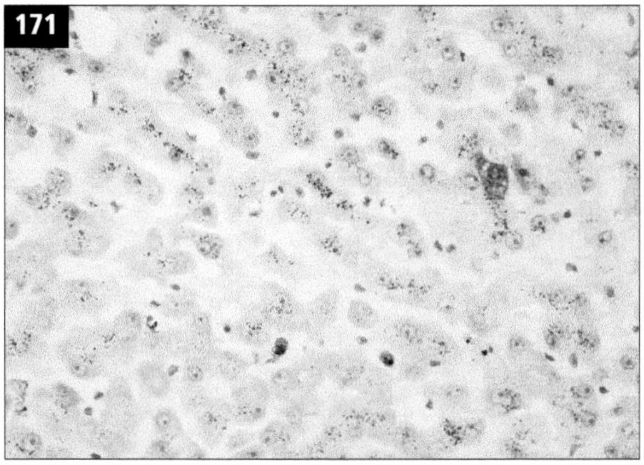

171 Hepatic extravascular haemolysis. Section of liver from a cat with immune-mediated haemolysis. Sinusoidal Kupffer cells contain prominent aggregates of haemosiderin that stains positive for iron by Perls' Prussian blue. Hepatocytes also contain a scattering of cytoplasmic haemosiderin.

172

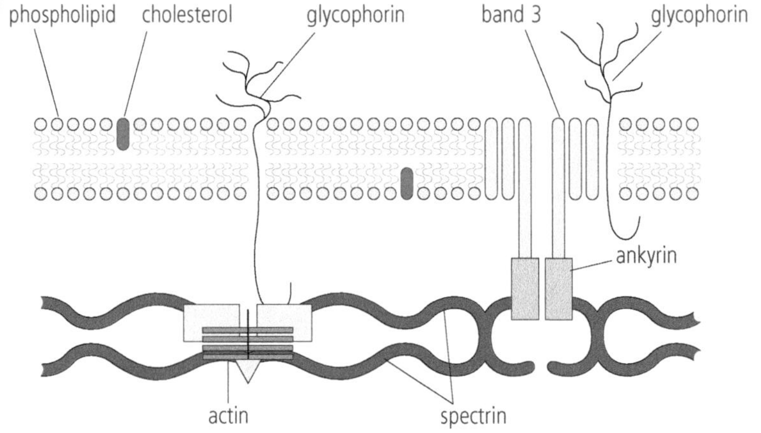

172 Erythrocyte autoantigens in canine IMHA. The specificity of autoantibodies in canine IMHA has been demonstrated by eluting antibodies from patient erythrocytes and using them to immunoprecipitate autoantigens from normal canine RBCs. The major autoantigenic molecules are depicted in this diagrammatic representation of the RBC membrane. These include the family of erythrocyte membrane glycoproteins termed 'glycophorins' and the components of the erythrocyte anion exchange channel (band 3). Autoantibodies specific for the cytoskeletal molecule spectrin are recognized in dogs with IMHA as well as in normal dogs, and these may be involved with clearance of senescent RBCs. The heterogeneity of these autoantibody responses suggests that the underlying aetiology of IMHA may vary in individual dogs.

disease. Acquired pure red cell aplasia (PRCA) involves immune-mediated destruction of marrow erythroid precursors such that these are markedly reduced in number and function. In contrast, non-regenerative IMHA (NRIMHA) is also thought to involve immune-mediated interference with marrow erythropoiesis, but the marrow has evidence of erythropoietic activity. It is likely that NRIMHA progresses to acquired PRCA; in this chapter the name PRCA will be used to describe both entities. Dogs with PRCA may not necessarily have antibody bound to circulating RBCs, but serum IgG from such cases can inhibit erythropoiesis *in vitro*.

In recent years, understanding of the immunological basis of canine AIHA has been extended by identification of the following features:

- Autoantibody of the IgG (all four subclasses, but IgG1 and IgG4 may predominate), IgM and IgA classes may be identified on the erythrocyte surface, although the significance of relatively low levels of IgA is questionable.
- These autoantibodies have been eluted from the RBC surface and their specificity determined (172).
- *In vitro* phagocytosis of opsonized erythrocytes is greater by monocytes derived from dogs with AIHA compared with monocytes from normal dogs.
- Autoreactive T cells (specific for RBC membrane proteins and glycophorin peptides) are found in the blood of some normal dogs; however, they are readily identified in the blood of dogs with AIHA or normal relatives of affected dogs.
- Elevation of serum pro- and anti-inflammatory cytokine concentrations, with elevation in IL-18 and MCP-1 associated with poor prognosis.

Clinical signs

The clinical presentation of IMHA may be acute, subacute or chronic. The majority of affected dogs have extravascular destruction of RBCs and a relatively protracted (days to weeks) history. In these dogs, clinical signs may reflect the anaemia itself (pale mucous membranes, weakness, lethargy, exercise intolerance, tachypnoea, tachycardia and anorexia) (173–175) or the underlying destruction of RBCs (hepatosplenomegaly, lymphadenopathy

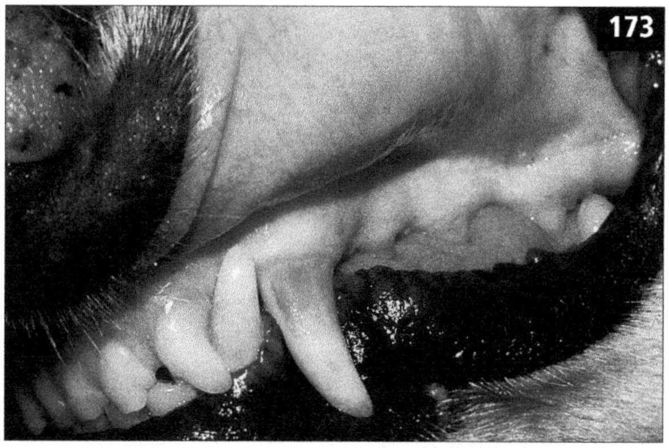
173

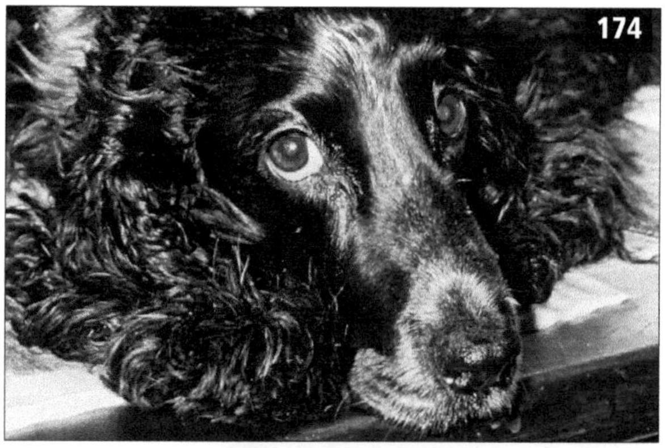
174

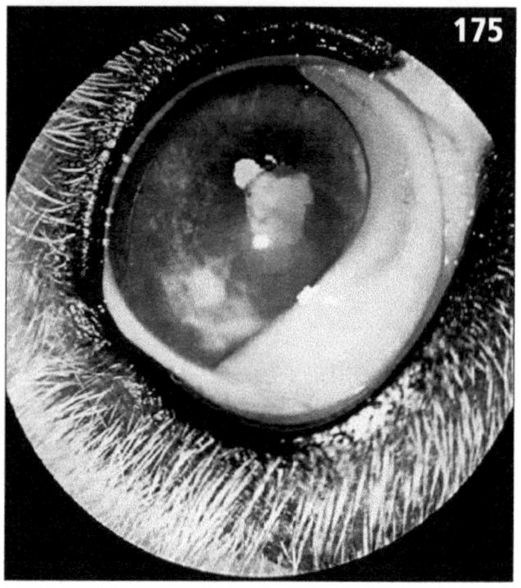
175

173–175 Clinical presentation of canine IMHA. (**173**) Pale mucous membranes in a dog with severe anaemia due to chronic IMHA. (**174**) Cocker Spaniel dog with acute onset IMHA. The dog is depressed and lethargic and there is pallor and mild icterus of the conjunctival mucous membranes. (**175**) Pallor of the ocular mucous membranes in a dog with IMHA.

and pyrexia). In those uncommon patients with PRCA, anaemia may take months to develop, since the loss of circulating RBCs is due to normal ageing rather than accelerated destruction. Since chronic anaemia is remarkably well tolerated, dogs with PRCA or chronic extravascular haemolysis often show minimal clinical signs. Dogs with chronic IMHA may have transient episodes of jaundice associated with flare-ups of subacute or acute intravascular haemolysis.

Patients with acute or subacute intravascular haemolysis have a rapid onset (one to two days) of severe anaemia and jaundice, often with associated vomiting and pyrexia. Dogs with intravascular haemolysis may also have haemoglobinaemia and haemoglobinuria. Liver enzymes (alanine aminotransferase and alkaline phosphatase) are often elevated in patients with severe, acute haemolytic anaemia, likely as a result of hepatic hypoxia. Dogs with acute severe anaemia have little time in which to develop adaptive responses and are therefore often extremely weak and depressed. Acute or subacute RBC destruction, especially that due to intravascular haemolysis, is far less common than chronic haemolytic anaemia.

Some dogs with IMHA develop disseminated intravascular coagulation (DIC) or thromboembolism (particularly within the pulmonary artery) (**176–178**). Dogs with pulmonary thromboembolism develop moderate to severe dyspnoea of acute onset that is unrelated to the magnitude of their anaemia. Thoracic radiography may be normal or it may show either areas of pulmonary hypovascularity or an alveolar or interstitial pattern with a slight pleural effusion.

Diagnosis

Diagnosis of IMHA should proceed through the stages of clinical examination, haematological investigation and definitive immunodiagnostic procedures (**179**). A clinical suspicion of AIHA should be investigated by ruling out possible underlying causes. Some precipitating causes of IMHA (e.g. neoplasia, particularly lymphoma) can be difficult to identify and may only be revealed by extensive investigations including thoracic and

176

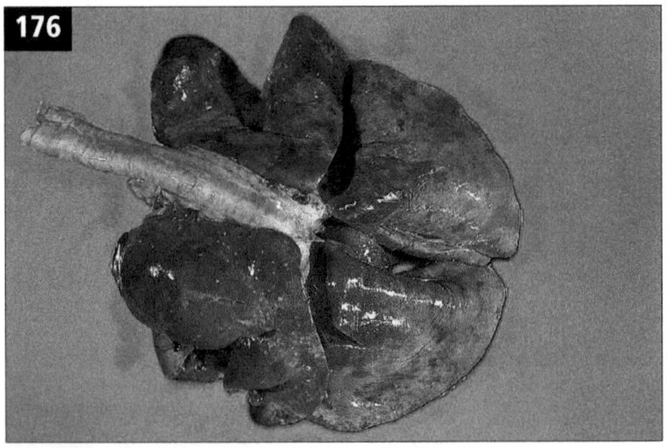

177

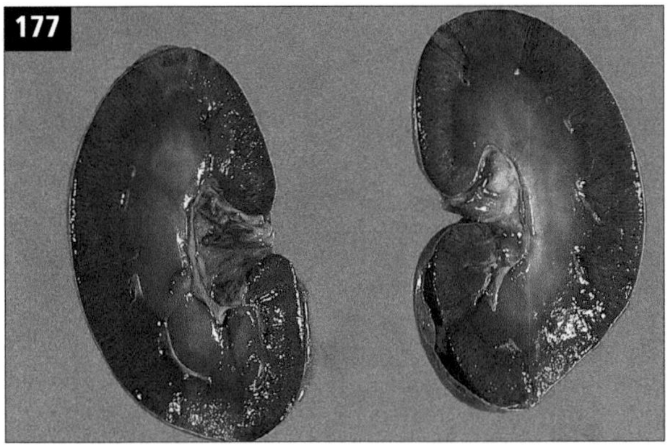

178

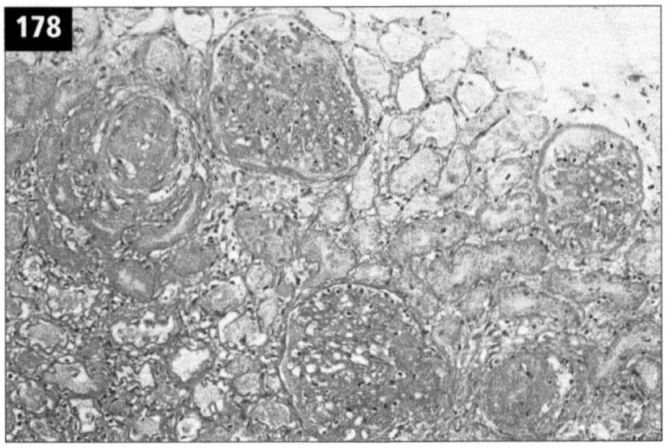

176–178 Thromboembolism in canine IMHA. (**176**) Lungs from an eight-year-old Golden Retriever with IMHA. The dog developed dyspnoea during an episode of relapse of disease. There are areas of discoloration and consolidation within all the lobes. Microscopic examination reveals areas of necrosis, with thrombus formation in major vessels. (**177**) Sagitally sectioned kidney from the same dog demonstrating a wedge-shaped region of corticomedullary infarction. (**178**) There is thrombus formation within the blood vessels supplying the affected area of kidney. (This section, stained by Martius scarlet blue, demonstrates fibrin within the thrombus.)

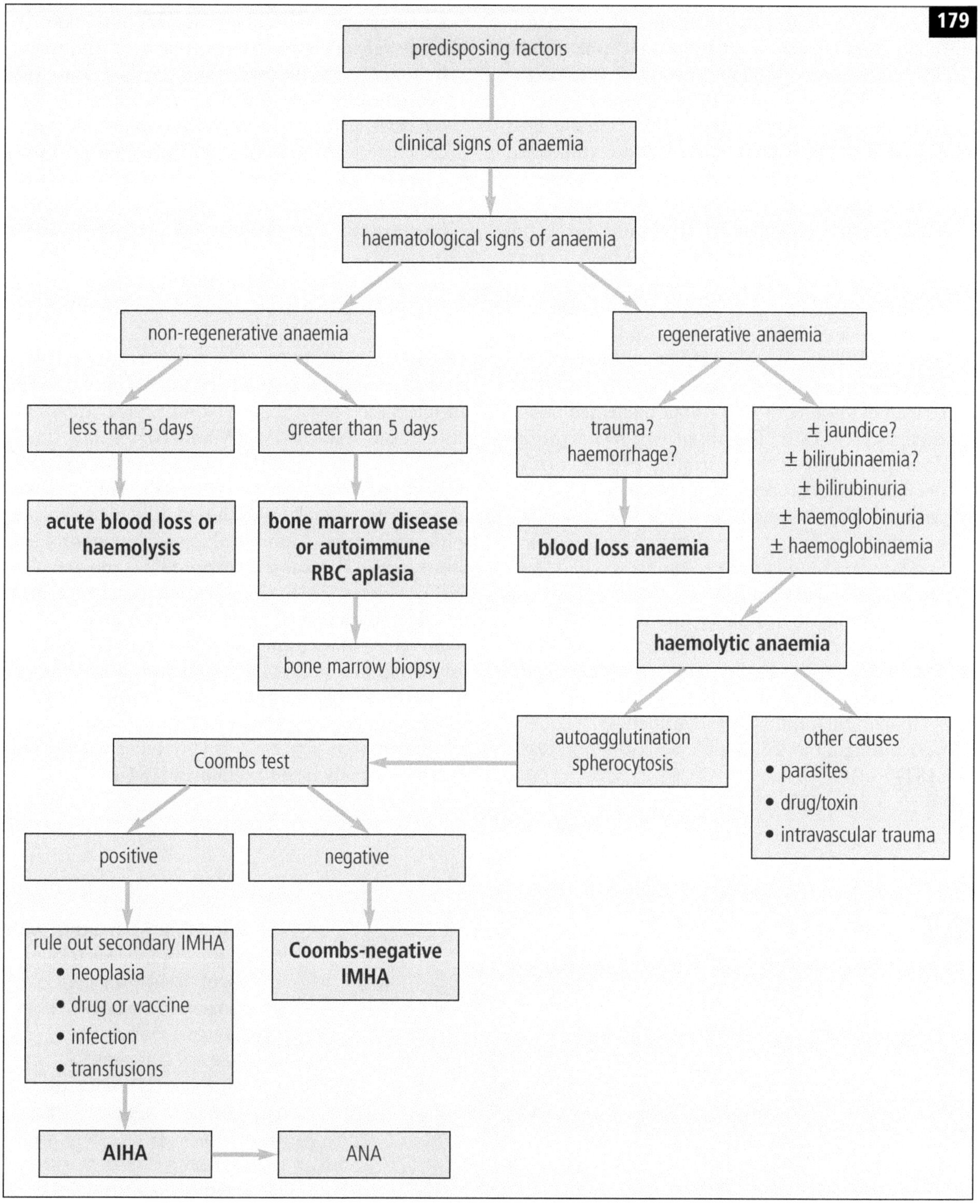

179 Diagnostic flow chart for canine IMHA. Diagnosis of IMHA in the dog should proceed through the stages of clinical examination, haematological assessment and specific immunodiagnostic tests. A dog with clinical signs of anaemia and haematological data consistent with haemolysis and erythroid regeneration, with features such as spherocytosis or agglutination, is a candidate for a Coombs test. A positive Coombs test may be consistent with primary IMHA (AIHA) in the absence of any underlying cause. A proportion of dogs with AIHA will also be positive for ANA.

abdominal radiography, abdominal ultrasonography, bone marrow analysis and fine needle aspiration cytology of lymph nodes. Such testing is probably 'diagnostic overkill' in patients with a signalment highly suggestive of AIHA (middle-aged dogs of a susceptible breed), but it is recommended in those dogs that do not fit the typical autoimmune profile (e.g. geriatric dogs).

The primary diagnostic test should be a full haematological examination, which may demonstrate:

- Anaemia (PCV <0.35 l/l [<35%]) that ranges from mild to marked (PCV <0.1 l/l [<10%]).
- Erythroid regeneration as indicated by the presence of anisocytosis, polychromasia and reticulocytosis, with or without nucleated erythrocytes (**180**). The absence of regeneration does not eliminate the possibility of PRCA or of peracute IMHA (present for less than 3–5 days) with insufficient time to permit a bone marrow response.
- Spherocytosis indicative of immune-mediated damage to circulating RBCs.
- Autoagglutination of blood grossly in the collection tube or microscopically on the blood smear. Autoagglutination may not become apparent until the blood is cooled to 4°C. Autoagglutination is best identified by performing an in-saline slide agglutination test (**181–183**).
- Leukocytosis, particularly neutrophilia, that likely reflects bone marrow regeneration, tissue hypoxia (particularly hepatic) or the release of cytokines by activated phagocytic cells. In contrast, persistent neutropenia might indicate concurrent IMNP.
- The platelet count should be normal unless the dog has concurrent IMTP or DIC. A range of haemostatic abnormalities may be present (refer below).
- Elevation of serum acute phase proteins (e.g. C-reactive protein) occurs in IMHA

The definitive diagnostic test is the demonstration of erythrocyte-bound antibody by the Coombs or direct antiglobulin test. The Coombs test does not distinguish between IMHA and AIHA, but simply detects erythrocyte surface Ig and/or complement deposition. A Coombs test is generally only indicated in anaemic animals and should not be performed without first undertaking haematological assessment. The sample required is anticoagulant (EDTA) blood, which should be submitted as soon as possible, although the erythrocyte-bound Igs are relatively robust and samples remain positive following several days transit by post. It is preferable to perform the Coombs test before initiating immunosuppressive therapy, although this is not absolutely necessary as it usually takes some weeks for the antibody titre to diminish (**184**).

180

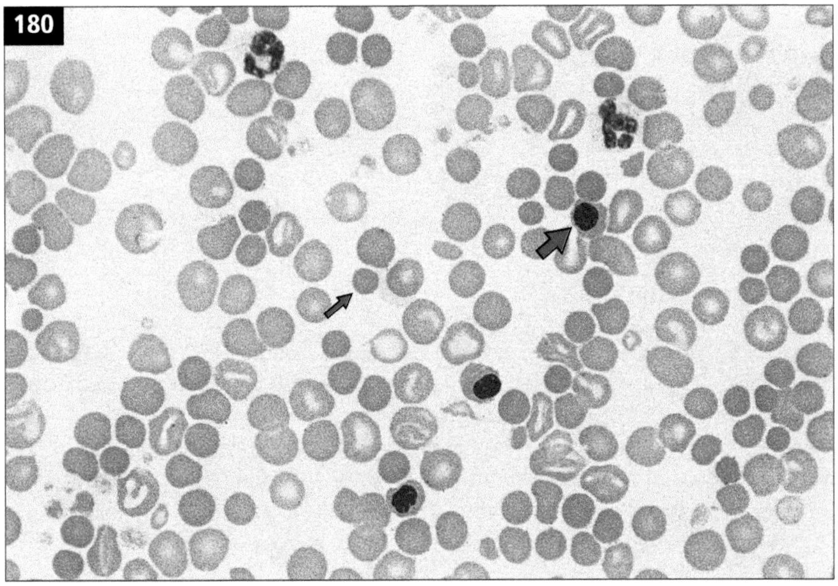

180 Blood film from a dog with IMHA. The major haematological features of IMHA are shown in this blood smear. The anisocytosis and polychromasia likely reflects immature red cells, and regeneration is also suggested by the presence of nucleated RBCs (large arrow). Spherocytes (small arrow) are also consistent with immune-mediated haemolysis. (From Day MJ [1998] Mechanisms of immune-mediated diseases in small animals. *In Practice* **20**:75–86, with permission.)

181

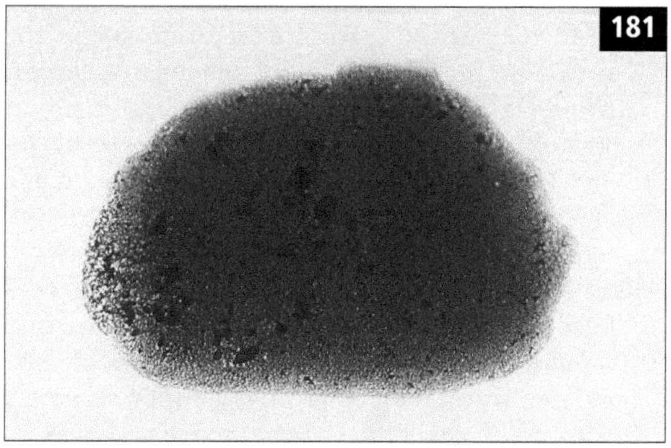

182

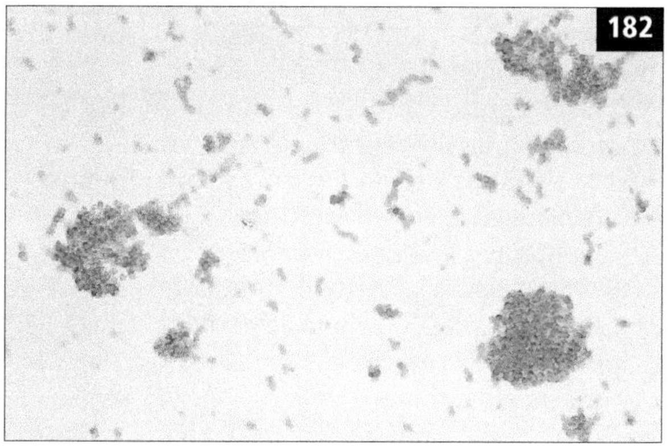

183

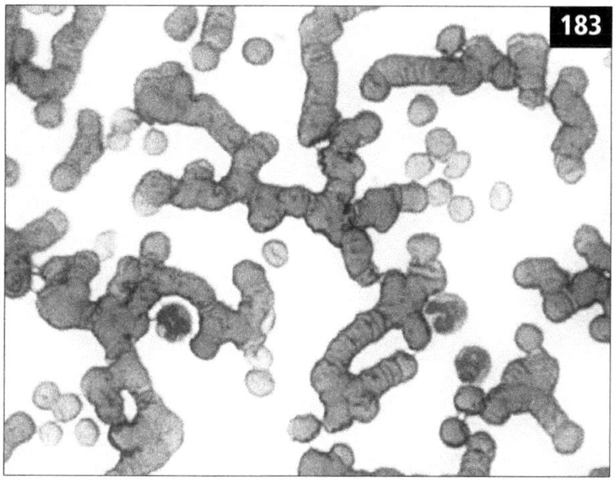

181–183 The in-saline slide agglutination test in canine IMHA. (**181**) One drop of anticoagulated blood from a dog with IMHA is mixed with one drop of saline on a microscope slide and examined against a white background over a period of 1–2 minutes for gross agglutination. (**182**) Gross agglutination can be confirmed by placing a coverslip over the blood/saline mix and examining microscopically. (**183**) Rouleaux (a normal, non-immunological phenomenon) will also appear grossly as speckles in undiluted whole blood, but will usually be dispersed by the 1:1 addition of saline. A positive slide agglutination is strongly suggestive of IMHA and usually indicates the presence of severe disease; however, a negative result does not rule out IMHA. Many relatively stable dogs with chronic IMHA will have a negative slide agglutination; however, the test is still an extremely useful, simple and rapid in-practice test, particularly in critically-ill patients presenting with acute anaemia.

184

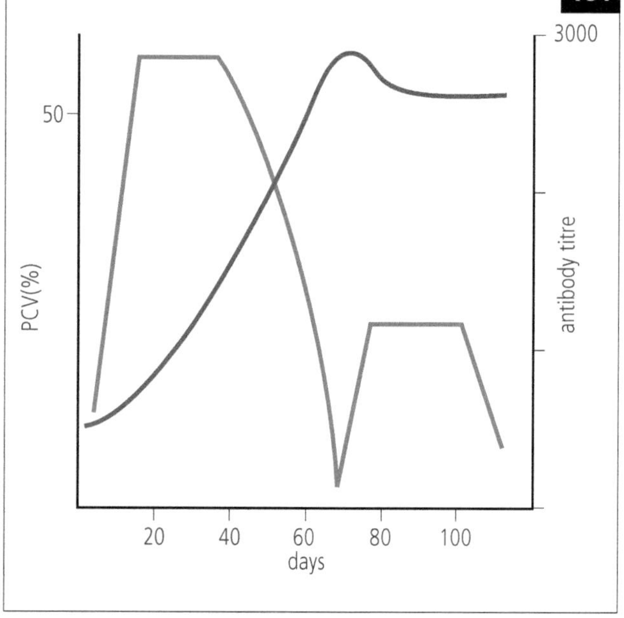

184 Serial monitoring of PCV and autoantibody titre following initiation of treatment for IMHA in a dog. Data from a three-year-old Lurcher with IMHA demonstrating a rapid rise in PCV after initiation of immunosuppressive therapy (red line) but persistence of autoantibody, as shown by a positive Coombs test, for over 100 days after initiation of treatment and clinical recovery (blue line). (Data from Day MJ [1996] Serial monitoring of clinical, haematological and immunological parameters in canine autoimmune haemolytic anaemia. *Journal of Small Animal Practice* **37**:523.)

The Coombs test (**185, 186**) provides information concerning:

- The class of erythrocyte-bound antibody (IgG is more commonly reported than IgM).
- The antibody titre (a low titred reaction more often suggests secondary IMHA).
- The optimal *in vitro* temperature reactivity of the antibody. The test will usually be positive at both 4°C and 37°C, but the antibodies may be preferentially reactive (as indicated by a higher titre) at either temperature.
- Whether the antibody has fixed complement. The presence of C3 alone is considered indicative of secondary IMHA or deposition of immune complexes in chronic disease.

Although a Coombs test confirms IMHA, interpretation of the results may be difficult. In some studies there appears to be no correlation between the titre and pattern of reactivity in the Coombs test and the severity of anaemia or clinical outcome, while other studies have reported an association between the presence of erythrocyte-bound IgM and complement with severe, acute IMHA involving intravascular haemolysis. Generally, when a full Coombs test is performed, false-negative results are uncommon, but instances of false-negative results have been described and may relate to technical as well as *in vivo* factors. The Coombs test may be positive in approximately 30% of dogs with PRCA. Bone marrow should be examined (cytologically or histopathologically) in cases of PRCA (**187, 188**), but methods to identify antibody bound to marrow erythroid precursors have been poorly defined.

It is generally accepted that gross autoagglutination of a blood sample and a strong in-saline slide agglutination test are diagnostic of IMHA and

185

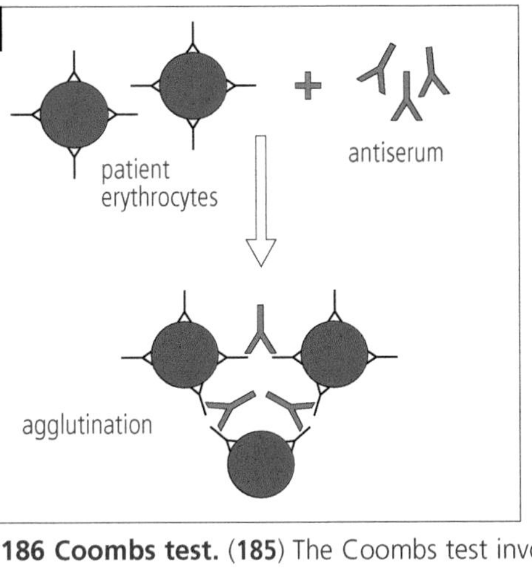

186

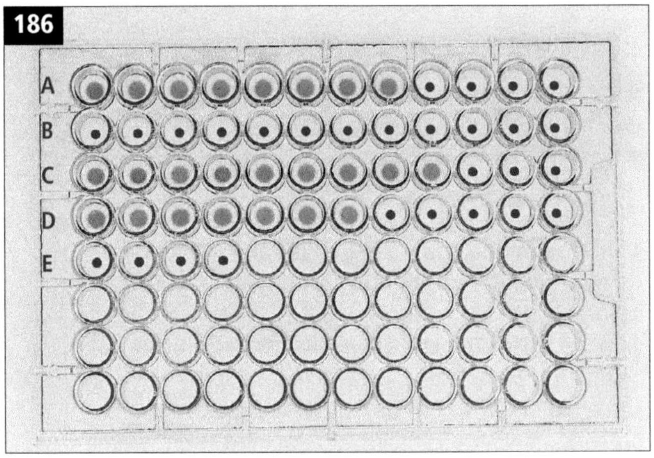

185, 186 Coombs test. (**185**) The Coombs test involves incubation of a suspension of RBCs from the patient (washed several times in buffered saline to remove serum protein, WBCs and RBC debris) with serial dilutions of a polyvalent antiglobulin (Coombs reagent) that is specific for IgG, IgM and complement C3. Additionally, parallel tests are performed using antisera specific for either IgG, IgM or C3. These reagents should be specific for the dog and preabsorbed with pooled normal canine RBCs. The test is performed in duplicate at both 4°C and 37°C (sometimes also at room temperature). RBCs with surface membrane antibody or complement will be agglutinated by the appropriate antisera and the titre of reaction is determined. (**186**) A Coombs test performed in a microtitre system and incubated at 4°C. The antisera are serially diluted across the rows (from 1/5): row A contains polyvalent Coombs reagent; row B anti-dog IgG; row C anti-dog IgM; row D anti-dog C3; and row E a saline control. The test is positive for polyvalent canine Coombs reagent (titre 640), anti-dog IgM (titre 1280) and anti-dog C3 (titre 320), indicating the presence of a cold-reactive IgM autoantibody that has fixed complement. (From Davidson M, Else R, Lumsden J [1998] *Manual of Small Animal Clinical Pathology*. BSAVA, Gloucester, with permission.)

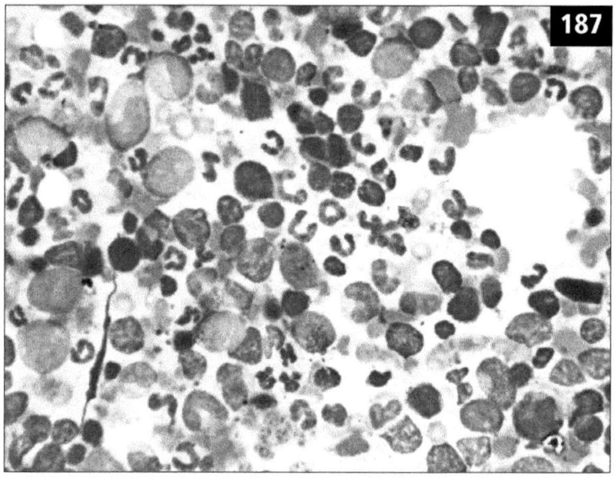

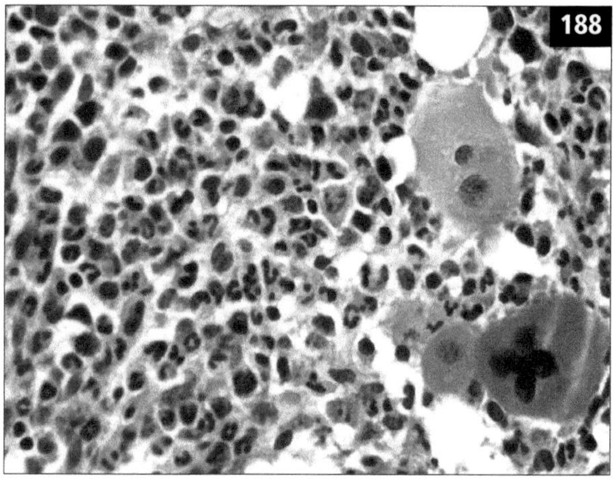

187, 188 Pure red cell aplasia. Examination of bone marrow is indicated in cases with PRCA. These samples are from an 11-year-old Whippet that had Coombs-positive IMHA 18 months previously. The dog has now represented with a non-regenerative anaemia that is Coombs negative. (**187**) In this cytological preparation the majority of cells are myeloid, consistent with destruction of erythroid precursors. (**188**) Similarly, a bone marrow core biopsy reveals adequate leukocyte and platelet precursors but an absence of erythropoiesis.

preclude the necessity, or ability, to perform a Coombs test. While this may sometimes be so, in such instances it is often still possible to undertake a Coombs test after washing the RBCs or by performing all stages of the procedure at 37°C. The indirect Coombs test (testing for serum antibody that can bind to a suspension of normal erythrocytes) is not considered useful in the diagnosis of AIHA in dogs and cats, as most antibody is thought to be erythrocyte bound rather than circulating, but such antibodies can be detected by enzyme-linked immunosorbent assay (ELISA).

The Coombs test remains the test of choice in the diagnosis of IMHA. Relatively crude methods involving papain treatment of patient erythrocytes and reincubation with patient serum are non-specific, and the more complex and lengthy ELISA-based modification of the direct antiglobulin test is a valuable research tool; however, it is not practical for routine diagnosis. Recently, the technique of flow cytometry (see Chapter 12, p. 279) has been applied for the detection of erythrocyte-bound antibodies in dogs with IMHA. This method, which utilizes detecting antibodies with a fluorescent label, has excellent sensitivity and acceptable specificity when compared with the 'gold standard' Coombs test. As flow cytometers remain very expensive pieces of apparatus, this test is unlikely to become widely available in the immediate future. Although not yet widely tested, gel-based tests have been developed for the diagnosis of canine and feline IMHA. In this procedure the antiglobulin reagent is be held within a gel matrix in a tube and patient erythrocytes are loaded into a reservoir above the matrix. During centrifugation the erythrocytes migrate through the gel, but antibody-coated cells will agglutinate when in contact with antiserum and be trapped at the top of the matrix. Non-agglutinated erythrocytes pass to the base of the tube. Alternatively, the antiglobulin–patient red cell interaction can be performed within the reservoir before centrifugation through a neutral gel (which does not contain antiglobulin).

Adjunct immunodiagnostic testing is rarely necessary for canine AIHA, although determination of serum antinuclear antibody (ANA) (see Chapter 6, p. 179) may be useful. Some dogs with primary AIHA may be ANA positive but not have SLE, which by definition requires at least a second clinical manifestation of autoimmunity. Dogs with vaccine-associated IMHA are generally ANA negative, and this criterion may be a useful means of distinguishing these possibilities.

Treatment

A range of therapeutic approaches can be considered in canine IMHA. The most important of these is management of any primary underlying disease (**189**), but specific modalities designed to target the immune-mediated process include:

- In most instances the primary treatment involves immunosuppressive doses of oral glucocorticoid (e.g. prednisolone 2–4 mg/kg q24h then gradually tapered over a period of weeks to months to alternate day maintenance therapy of 0.5–1 mg/kg) with or without the use of an initial injectable glucocorticoid. The major effects of glucocorticoid in IMHA are in blocking the interaction of the phagocyte Fc receptor with erythrocyte-bound Ig and decreasing the binding of Ig and complement to RBC (within hours), and any effect on antibody production via suppression of T cell function will be considerably delayed. In dogs with chronic, stable AIHA, glucocorticoids alone should be tried for a minimum period of four weeks before including other drugs in the regime.

text removedin Danazol bullet point

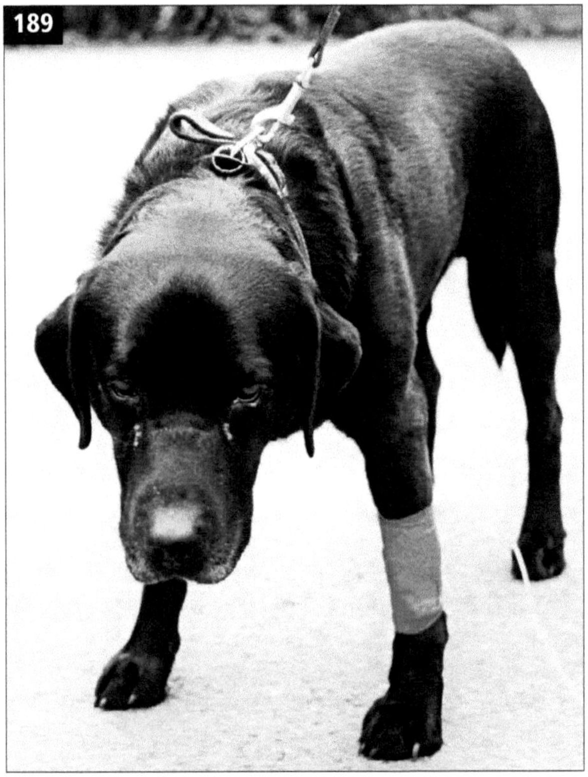

- In patients with refractory or severe anaemia (particularly those with haemoglobinaemia, haemoglobinuria, jaundice or positive slide agglutination) cytotoxic drugs such as azathioprine (2 mg/kg p/o q24h daily then slowly tapered to 1–2 mg/kg on alternate days) should be included in the regime, and will eventually enable a reduced dose of glucocorticoid to be used. Since there is a delay (of approximately ten days) before azathioprine becomes effective, it is advisable to commence combination therapy as soon as possible in those patients with severe disease. Until recently, cyclophosphamide was also widely used as an adjunct to glucocorticoid therapy; however, recent clinical studies have shown that there is no benefit with use of this drug, and in some patients the outcome may actually be worsened with cyclophosphamide combination therapy.
- Danazol (synthetic androgen; 5 mg/kg p/o q12h) may also block the FcR-Ig interaction and reduce long-term production of autoantibody, but recent reviews have suggested that danazol has minimal beneficial effect in terms of survival of IMHA patients.
- Ciclosporin (microemulsion formulation at 5 mg/kg p/o q24h) has been used to treat refractory AIHA, generally in combination with oral prednisolone. Success is reported in individual cases; however, recent reviews have suggested that while this combination therapy is safe, there is minimal benefit (in terms of survival) above the use of glucocorticoid alone. Although ciclosporin has now been licensed for use in the dog, the current legal indication is for atopic dermatitis only and its use remains a relatively expensive treatment modality.

189 Treatment of canine IMHA. The fundamental approach to treatment of IMHA is management of underlying disease. This dog has *Babesia canis canis* infection and requires specific anti-protozoal medication. Although the haemolytic anaemia of babesiosis may in part be immune-mediated (and affected dogs may be Coombs positive) the use of adjunct glucocorticoids in the management of the disease is controversial. (From Shaw SE, Day MJ (2005) *Arthropod-Borne Infectious Diseases of the Dog and Cat.* Manson Publishing, London, with permission.)

- Two further immunomodulatory agents currently being evaluated in the management of canine IMHA are mycophenolate mofetil (an azathioprine-like drug) and liposome-encapsulated clodronate (which is phagotyosed by macrophages leading to apoptosis of these cells)
- Supportive therapy (fluids or blood transfusion) may be required in life-threatening anaemia. Because patients with IMHA have normal blood volume, fluid therapy should not be too aggressive. Transfusion of dogs with IMHA is controversial, since the provision of extra RBCs may 'fuel the fire' of haemolysis. However, transfusion should never be withheld in patients with life-threatening disease (severe clinical signs or PCV <0.1 l/l [<10%]). Transfusion may 'buy time' until drug therapy becomes effective (typically in 3–7 days). When available, the use of packed RBCs is preferable to whole blood, since patients with AIHA do not need plasma. Cross-matching should be performed, but may be of little diagnostic value in animals with positive slide agglutination that typically cross-match positive with blood from all donors. Multiple transfusions at short intervals (as frequently as every 24 hours) may be required in dogs with very acute IMHA. Transfusion is particularly useful in dogs with PRCA since, in the absence of peripheral RBC destruction, the beneficial effects of transfusion may last for several months. In an emergency, polymerized bovine haemoglobin as a blood substitute can be used to provide temporary support, although it has recently been suggested that use of this product may also contribute to poor clinical outcome.
- Approaches such as plasmapheresis (see Chapter 14, p. 361) and high-dose human gamma globulin therapy (0.5–1.5 g/kg i/v given over 4 hours) have been reported. Plasmapheresis will only remove circulating autoantibody and not erythrocyte-bound autoantibody, and it is rarely available. Transfusion with human gammaglobulin is simple and may be life saving in dogs with acute, life-threatening anaemia. Gammaglobulin therapy is reported to saturate macrophage Fc receptors non-specifically. It may also provide Igs that bind to and inactivate circulating anti-RBC antibody or bind to and down-regulate the function of T and B lymphocytes. Dogs appear to tolerate human Ig remarkably well, and anaphylactic reactions have not been reported, although it has been suggested that the treatment may have a prothrombotic effect. Gammaglobulin therapy is, however, very expensive.
- Splenectomy as a means of removing a major site of erythrocyte destruction and antibody production is controversial in the treatment of IMHA. Few published studies indicate that this is a useful procedure, but individual cases appear to benefit. One recent abstract has suggested that early splenectomy (within 48 hours of diagnosis), in addition to medical therapy, is associated with increased survival, but at this time splenectomy should be considered a last resort in patients with life-threatening refractory anaemia.

Prognosis and monitoring

Poor prognostic factors for canine IMHA include very low PCV, poorly regenerative anaemia at presentation, autoagglutination, haemoglobinaemia, haemoglobinuria and hyperbilirubinaemia. Therefore, dogs with acute intravascular haemolytic anaemia or PRCA have a guarded prognosis. Pulmonary thromboembolism has a higher incidence where there is hyperbilirubinaemia, a negative Coombs test or the presence of an indwelling catheter. The mechanism for development of these thrombi is poorly defined, but early reports suggested that this may be associated with the presence of a circulating 'lupus-type anticoagulant' (see Chapter 14, p. 360). Evidence of such antibodies was found in only two of 20 dogs with primary IMHA, although these animals frequently had evidence of altered haemostasis (increased activated partial thromboplastin time, one-stage prothrombin time and fibrinogen concentration, and decreased antithrombin activity). Moreover, platelets from dogs with IMHA appear to circulate in an activated state, as evidenced by marked elevation of P-selectin expression. In contrast, autoantibody to endothelial cells was not identified as a factor contributing to thromboembolism in canine IMHA. Since the most common signs of clinically significant pulmonary thromboembolism are either sudden death or severe unrelenting dyspnoea, and since pre-existing thrombi are extremely difficult to dissolve, prevention of thromboembolism is preferable to treatment. Prophylactic treatment with heparin or ultra-low-dose aspirin, particularly in dogs with acute severe AIHA, has been used. A number of prophylactic regimes using various doses and routes of administration of heparin/aspirin are described.

Dogs with chronic, IgG-mediated IMHA often recover with appropriate therapy; however, there is a high incidence of relapse months to years later and many animals succumb during these subsequent episodes. Additionally, dogs that recover from AIHA may go on to develop other manifestations of autoimmunity (AITP, SLE, immune-mediated skin disease), often years after the initial episode. Several recent studies have examined the long-term survival of dogs with IMHA and have presented Kaplan-Meier survival graphs. In many of these reviews up to 50% of affected animals (with presumptively severe disease) die during the initial period of hospitalization. There is a steady decline in survival thereafter (most due to relapsing IMHA), although in the largest case series, approximately 25% of affected dogs were alive up to ten years after initial diagnosis.

Since relapse is common, long-term monitoring of patients with IMHA is important. After initiation of treatment, the PCV often climbs rapidly, but erythrocyte-bound autoantibody may persist, sometimes for many months. It is not necessary to wait until dogs are Coombs negative to taper immunosuppressive therapy. Regular haematological assessment (every 2–4 weeks) to monitor response to therapy and to detect drug-induced myelosuppression is of value during initial treatment. Since both azathioprine and danazol can cause idiosyncratic hepatotoxicity, liver enzymes should be closely monitored in patients receiving these drugs (although some elevation in alanine aminotransferase, and particularly alkaline phosphatase, is to be expected in dogs receiving concurrent steroids). The long-term aim is to reduce and gradually withdraw immunosuppressive therapy, but in many cases this is not possible and a low maintenance dose is given for long periods. In dogs requiring ongoing steroid therapy, concurrent use of an immunosuppressive agent (e.g. azathioprine) is recommended in order to minimize chronic glucocorticoid side-effects. Long-term administration of azathioprine typically causes a low-grade, non-regenerative anaemia (PCV approximately 0.3 l/l [30%]), which is clinically insignificant and should not be mistaken for disease relapse.

Dogs with secondary IMHA, in which the underlying disease has not been identified and eliminated, are unlikely to respond completely or persistently to immunosuppressive therapy. A meticulous search for underlying disease is therefore recommended in those dogs that respond inadequately to appropriate therapy. Potential initiators of IMHA identified from the patient's history (e.g. drugs, vaccines) should be avoided in the future if possible.

PRCA is reported to have a poor prognosis. Since it can take months for a severely affected marrow to recover erythropoietic activity and replenish circulating RBCs, an apparently poor response to therapy may be due to an inadequate duration of treatment. Treatment with prednisolone with or without concurrent azathioprine (following an initial transfusion if anaemia is severe) for a minimum of 2–3 months is recommended before concluding that PRCA is refractory to therapy.

IMMUNE-MEDIATED HAEMOLYTIC ANAEMIA IN THE CAT

AIHA is infrequently documented in the cat, whereas secondary IMHA is considered to be the most common cause of haemolytic anaemia in this species. Cats with suspected IMHA should therefore be screened for underlying diseases, particularly FeLV and FIA (with clinical anaemia being most frequently related to infection by *Mycoplasma haemofelis*). Coombs-positive anaemia is sometimes reported in cats with FIP or FIV infection, neoplastic disease (especially lymphoma and leukaemia), inflammatory disease (e.g. aural haematoma, pancreatitis, chronic abscessation) or immune-mediated disease (e.g. chronic interstitial nephritis, polyarthritis, inflammatory bowel disease, amyloidosis). The anaemia of FeLV infection is often more complex than simply involving haemolysis, as the virus may induce a range of effects including suppression of haematopoiesis. PRCA has recently been documented in young cats with severe non-regenerative anaemia that tested negative for FeLV and FIV. The disease was responsive to aggressive, long-term immunosuppression and some cats were Coombs positive, suggesting an immune-mediated pathogenesis. Vaccination has not been incriminated as a causative factor for feline IMHA, although recognized side-effects of treatment with carbimazole/methimazole for hyperthyroidism include the induction of IMHA, IMTP and serum antinuclear antibody.

Clinical signs of IMHA in the cat include pallor, lethargy, anorexia, tachycardia and tachypnoea, vomiting, icterus, pyrexia, lymphadenopathy and hepatosplenomegaly (**190–192**). Extravascular haemolysis predominates, so haemoglobinaemia and haemoglobinuria are uncommon. The characteristic haematological feature is a moderate to severe regenerative anaemia, although thrombocytopenia and leukocytosis are sometimes reported. Cat erythrocytes are relatively small, so spherocytes are rarely recognized. Feline haemoplasma (FIA, *Mycoplasma*) should be ruled out by PCR testing. Evaluation of a blood smear for the presence of these organisms (**119**) is a highly inaccurate diagnostic procedure, and excellent sensitivity and specificity may be obtained with a real-time PCR test designed to detect the three feline haemoplasma species that are now recognized. Autoagglutination is common in cats with IMHA, but it must be distinguished from rouleaux (a frequent finding in normal cats) by performing a slide agglutination test using one drop of blood to two drops of saline (in the cat, greater dilution of blood with saline is required to disperse rouleaux).

There is a misconception in the literature that the Coombs test is invalid in cats. This concept is based entirely on one early study, which suggested that 40% of apparently normal cats had a low titred, cold-reactive IgM haemagglutinin. However, the study involved only 20 cats and employed an anti-IgM reagent that was inadequately diluted and so reported positive titres that would now be considered insignificant. A recent re-evaluation of

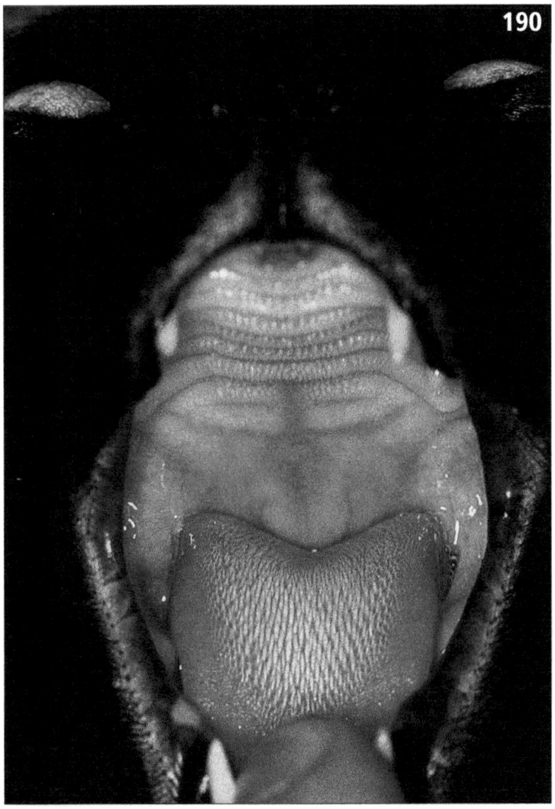

190

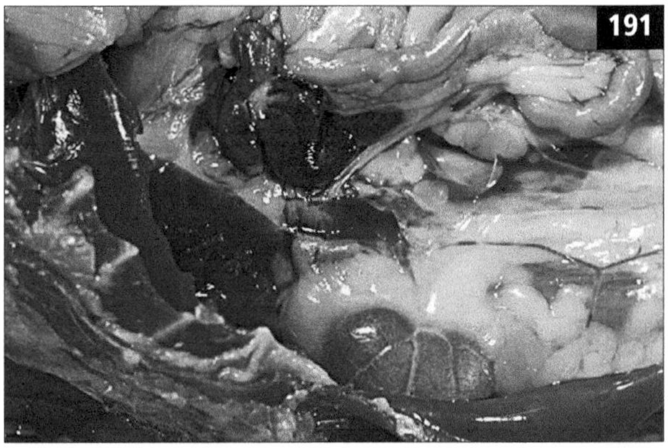

191

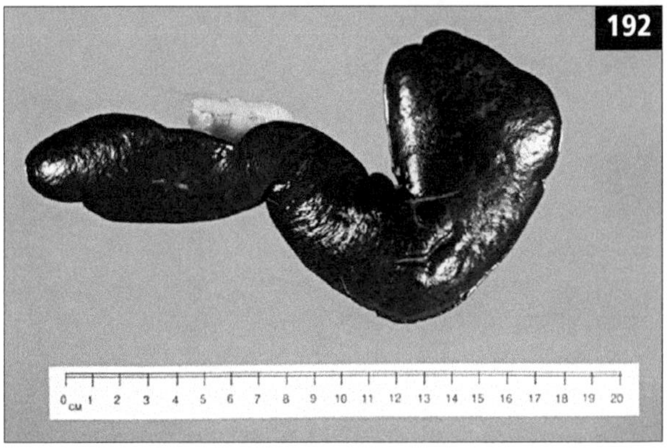

192

190–192 Clinical presentation of IMHA in the cat. (**190**) Generalized jaundice, which is most obvious on careful examination of the oral mucous membranes, in a cat with subacute haemolytic anaemia due to *Mycoplasma haemofelis* infection. (**191**) Marked carcase icterus and splenomegaly (**192**) in a cat that died with Coombs-positive haemolytic anaemia. In this case the IMHA was secondary to underlying lymphoid neoplasia, which also affected a littermate.

the feline Coombs test has demonstrated that this diagnostic procedure has equal utility to the canine test. However, as for the dog, the Coombs test does not distinguish between primary AIHA and secondary IMHA. Cats with FIA will often show autoagglutination of blood and a cold-reactive IgM antibody on Coombs testing. In experimental infection studies, these immunological abnormalities are closely associated with the peaks of cyclical infection and the presence of clinically significant anaemia.

There are few published data on the clinical outcome of cats with IMHA, but one recent report describes a 68% Kaplan-Meier one year survival rate in cats with primary idiopathic IMHA. Treatment with immunosuppressive doses of glucocorticoid (prednisolone 4–8 mg/kg daily) is reported. Cats tolerate high doses of glucocorticoid remarkably well; however, they often tolerate other immunosuppressive agents poorly, so the use of prolonged courses of steroids at high doses in cats with severe or refractory anaemia is often preferable to the use of more powerful immunosuppressive drugs. On the rare occasions where immunosuppressive agents are indicated, concurrent azathioprine can be administered at a starting dose of 0.3 mg/kg daily. Azathioprine does not come in a tablet size suitable for cats and, since overdosage can cause profound myelosuppression, the drug must be carefully formulated into a suspension suitable for oral dosing. Recent studies have shown that cats have lower levels of thiopurine methyltransferase (an enzyme required for the conversion of the active form of azathioprine to inactive metabolites) than either dogs or humans, supporting the concept that this agent should be used with caution in the cat. The other therapeutic modalities used to treat dogs with IMHA have not been evaluated in cats with haemolytic anaemia.

Since most cases of IMHA in the cat are secondary, an underlying disease should always be searched for and eliminated if possible. The most common secondary cause is feline haemoplasma infection and, following PCR diagnosis, appropriate antimicrobial therapy (e.g. doxycycline) should be administered. Cats with severe FIA may be given concurrent glucocorticoids in order to treat the immune-mediated component of the disease. Cats with IMHA secondary to FeLV should still be given steroids, although their long-term prognosis is guarded.

IMMUNE-MEDIATED THROMBOCYTOPENIA IN THE DOG

Pathogenesis

Thrombocytopenia is not uncommon in the dog and, in many cases, elimination of other causes leads to a presumptive diagnosis of IMTP. The reported prevalence of IMTP is probably underestimated due to the lack of readily available definitive diagnostic tests. Canine IMTP can be induced by drugs (e.g. trimethoprim/sulphonamide) or may be associated with vaccination or neoplasia (particularly lymphoma and haemangiosarcoma). A range of infections has been associated with IMTP and/or the presence of platelet-specific antibodies in the dog, including canine distemper virus infection, monocytic ehrlichiosis (**193, 194**), anaplasmosis, babesiosis, leishmaniosis (**150**), rickettsiosis, dirofilariasis (**195**) and angiostrongylosis (**196**). An association between IMTP and inflammatory bowel disease has recently been demonstrated. In the absence of such underlying causes the disease is likely to be AITP. Breed predispositions are suggested for the Poodle, Old English Sheepdog and Cocker Spaniel, and suspected familial AITP is documented. AITP is reported to occur more frequently in female dogs, and it may be initiated by stressful events such as kennelling, oestrus, parturition or surgery.

The pathogenesis of AITP involves removal of antibody-coated platelets in excess of replacement by bone marrow platelet production (thrombopoiesis). The spleen is the primary site of platelet removal and is also likely the major site of autoantibody synthesis. Autoantibody can sometimes also be directed against megakaryocytes, and antibody-mediated inhibition of platelet function has also been reported. IgG antibodies are most frequently documented, and these have been eluted from platelets and shown to be specific for various components of the platelet membrane such as glycoproteins (GP) IIb and/or IIIa.

Clinical signs

Dogs with IMTP generally present with acute onset disease. The thrombocytopenia predisposes to spontaneous haemorrhages, most commonly:

- Petechiae and ecchymoses of the skin (**197, 198**) and the oral, conjunctival, preputial or vaginal mucous membranes.
- Melaena, haematemesis, haematuria or epistaxis.

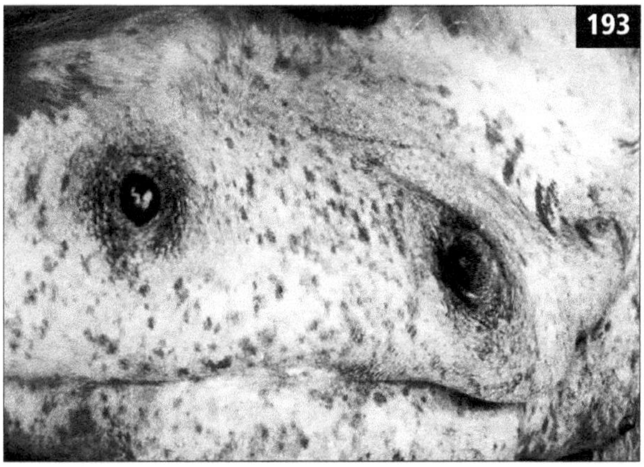

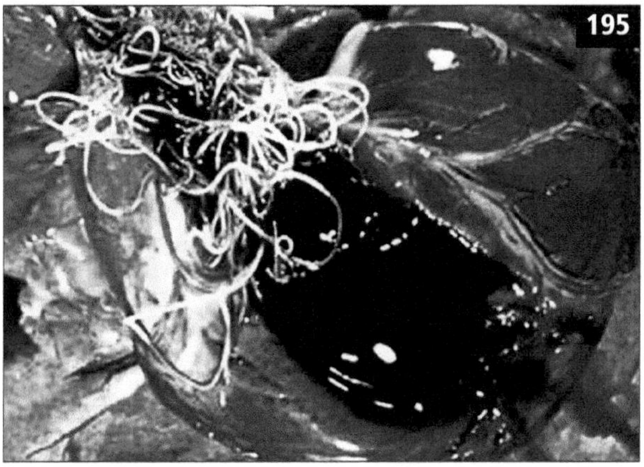

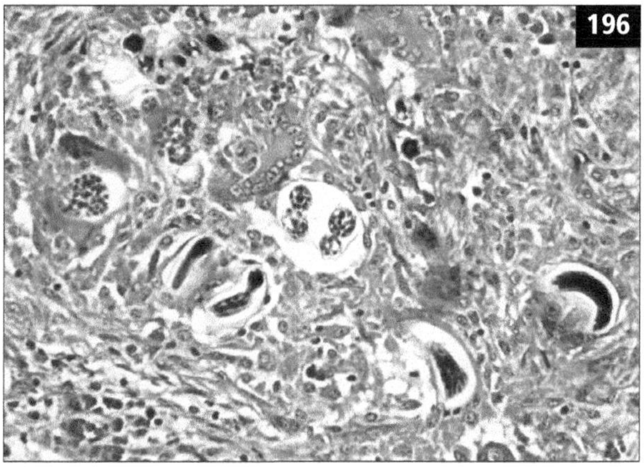

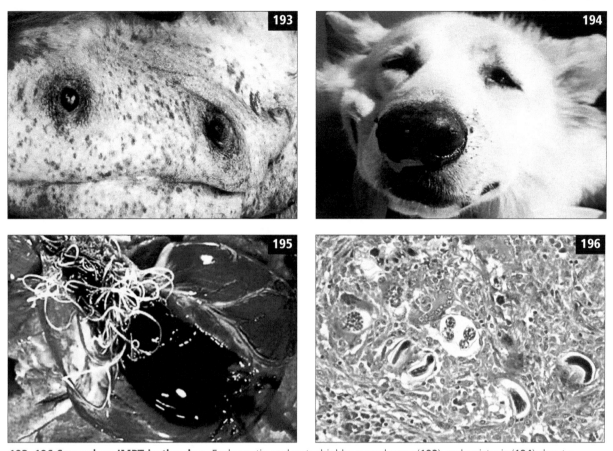

193–196 Secondary IMPT in the dog. Ecchymotic and petechial haemorrhages (**193**) and epistaxis (**194**) due to thrombocytopenia in dogs with monocytic ehrlichiosis (*Ehrlichia canis*). Intravascular parasites such as *Dirofilaria immitis* (**195**) and *Angiostrongylus vasorum* (**196**) have also been associated with IMTP in the dog. **195** shows adult *Dirofilaria* within the pulmonary artery and **196** depicts larval stages of *Angiostrongylus* within a section of lung. (Figures **193–195** from Shaw SE, Day MJ [2005] *Arthropod-Borne Infectious Diseases of the Dog and Cat.* Manson Publishing, London, with permission.)

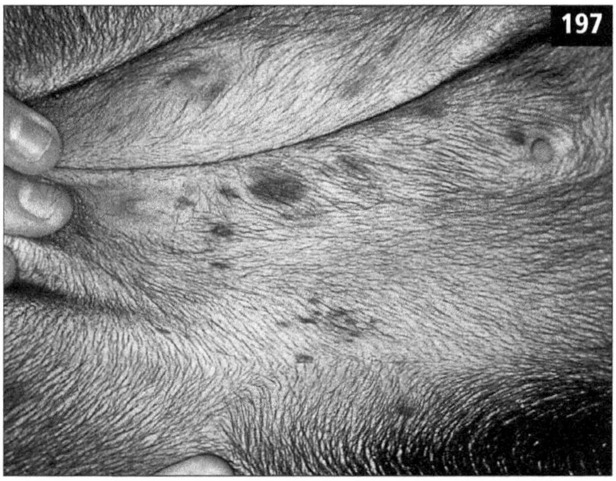

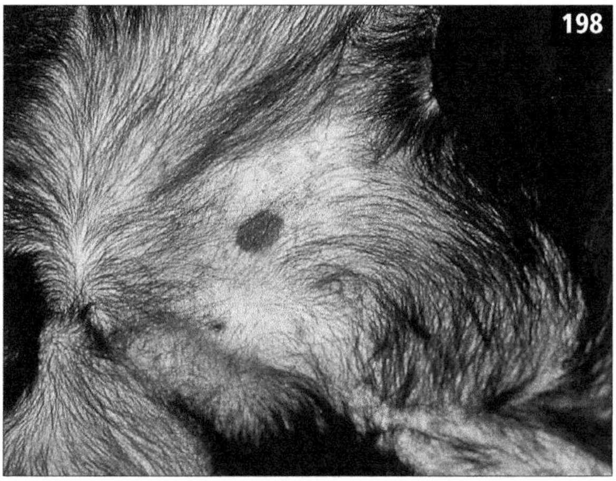

197, 198 Clinical presentation of IMPT in the dog. (**197**) Multiple petechial haemorrhages affecting the ventral abdominal skin of a dog with IMTP. (**198**) A single ecchymotic haemorrhage affecting the groin of an eight-year-old male Cocker Spaniel with IMTP. Although IMTP in this breed is most often autoimmune, in this particular dog the condition was secondary to nasal lymphoma. Neoplasia, particularly lymphoreticular neoplasia, should always be ruled out in older dogs that develop immune-mediated haematological disorders.

- Subcutaneous bruising at pressure points and ventral dependent areas.
- Hyphaema (**199**) and iridal or retinal haemorrhage.
- Gastrointestinal haemorrhage may lead to concurrent signs of acute or chronic blood loss anaemia (**200, 201**).
- There is likely to be prolonged haemorrhage after trauma, surgery or venepuncture.

Other less specific clinical signs that may sometimes be observed include:

- Weakness and lethargy.
- Mucous membrane pallor.
- Anorexia.
- Pyrexia.
- Lymphadenopathy and splenomegaly (uncommon).

Diagnosis

Haematological assessment is the first line of diagnosis in suspected IMTP (**202**). The number of circulating platelets will be reduced (normal canine reference range varies between laboratories, but is usually between 200 and 500 × 10^9/l [2 and 5 × 10^5/µl]) and often markedly so (<10 × 10^9/l [0.1 × 10^5/µl). Examination of a blood smear confirms marked thrombocytopenia (<4 platelets per ×1,000 oil immersion field) and may reveal the presence of microthrombocytes (platelet fragments derived from the immunological damage of platelets) or large 'shift platelets' (megathrombocytes) indicative of bone marrow regeneration. Examination of bone marrow is indicated in the absence of shift platelets, since megakaryocytes may be reduced in number or have cytoplasmic degeneration suggestive of autoantibody-mediated damage. Concurrent regenerative anaemia (due to haemorrhage or IMHA) and neutrophilia may be present. Neutropenia might be present if there is concurrent IMNP. Assessment of coagulation pathways (prothrombin time, activated partial thromboplastin time) will generally reveal no abnormality.

199

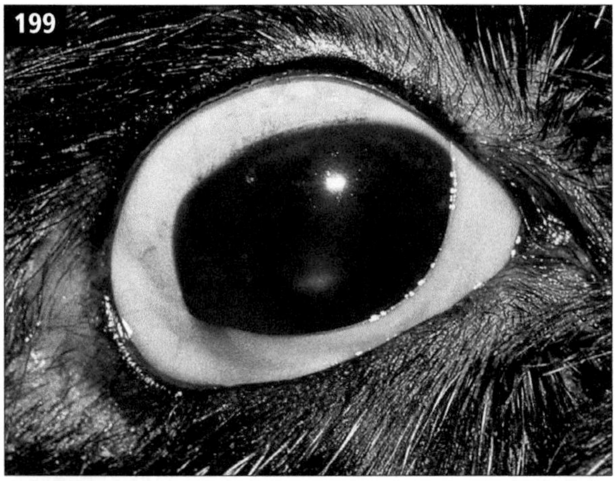

200

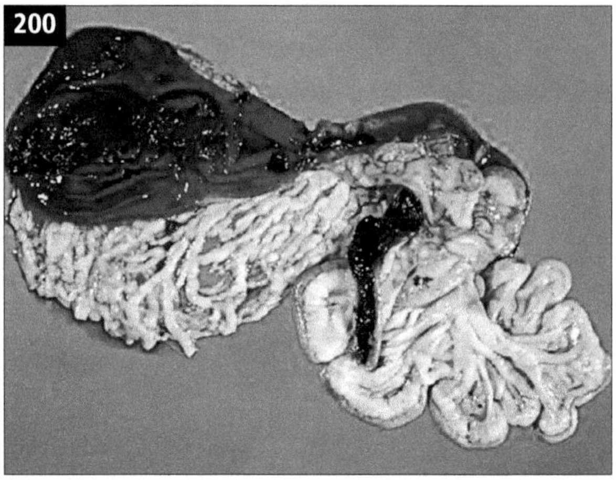

201

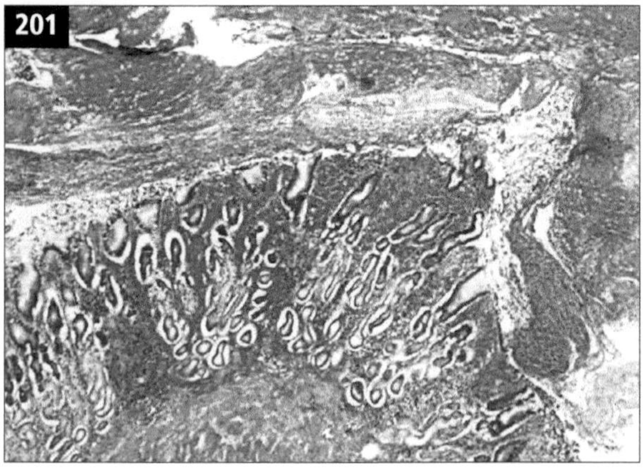

199–201 Clinical presentation of IMPT in the dog. (**199**) Hyphaema in a Cocker Spaniel with IMTP. (Photograph courtesy S.M. Crispin) (**200, 201**) Macroscopic and microscopic appearance of gastric haemorrhage in a dog that died during the acute stages of IMTP.

202

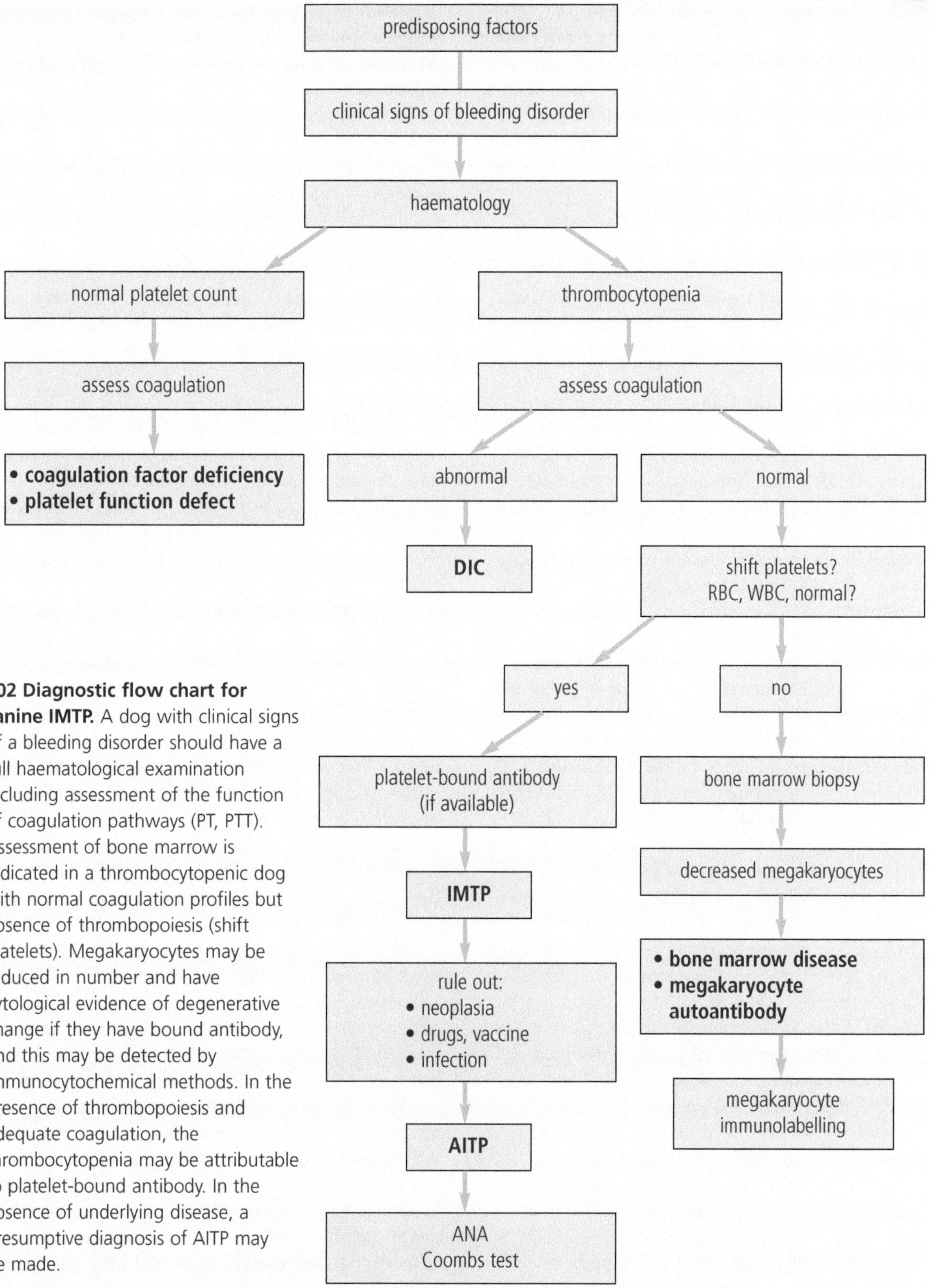

202 Diagnostic flow chart for canine IMTP. A dog with clinical signs of a bleeding disorder should have a full haematological examination including assessment of the function of coagulation pathways (PT, PTT). Assessment of bone marrow is indicated in a thrombocytopenic dog with normal coagulation profiles but absence of thrombopoiesis (shift platelets). Megakaryocytes may be reduced in number and have cytological evidence of degenerative change if they have bound antibody, and this may be detected by immunocytochemical methods. In the presence of thrombopoiesis and adequate coagulation, the thrombocytopenia may be attributable to platelet-bound antibody. In the absence of underlying disease, a presumptive diagnosis of AITP may be made.

There is no widely available 'gold standard' immunodiagnostic test for IMTP. Tests for platelet autoantibody may be available by arrangement with a specialist laboratory and may include:

- The platelet factor 3 test. The usefulness of this serum-based test is questionable and most laboratories no longer offer this assay. Serum from the thrombocytopenic patient is incubated with normal dog platelets, allowing autoantibody to bind to the platelets and damage the surface membrane. This leads to release of platelet factor 3, which enhances clotting following the addition of appropriate activation factors. The platelet factor 3 test is reported to be positive in 30–90% of dogs with AITP.
- An indirect immunofluorescence test for detection of serum platelet autoantibody (**203**).
- An indirect ELISA for serum platelet-specific antibody or direct immunoassay for platelet-bound Ig (**204**). A radioimmunoassay for the detection of platelet-bound antibody by radiolabelled staphylococcal protein A or anti-canine immunoglobulin reagents has also been described.
- Direct platelet agglutination or immunofluorescence. Platelets isolated from an affected dog may be incubated with an antiglobulin reagent (equivalent to the Coombs reagent) and scored for microscopic agglutination. Alternatively, platelet-bound IgG may be detected using fluorescein-conjugated antiserum to canine IgG. The most important recent advance in immunodiagnostic testing for canine IMTP has been the application of flow cytometry to the detection of platelet-associated antibody. This methodology appears to have good sensitivity and specificity, but access is currently limited to the few diagnostic laboratories that have a flow cytometer. One recent study has reported the application of this test to samples from 82 thrombocytopenic dogs, of which 32 tested positive. Of these 32 cases, an underlying disease was identified in 25 animals – 18 had infectious disease (ehrlichiosis, babesiosis, leishmaniosis, abscess, prostatitis/cystitis, leptospirosis or distemper), six had neoplasia (lymphoma, liver, lung or splenic neoplasia) and one was a post-transfusion reaction.
- Megakaryocyte immunofluorescence (**205**). This test is reported to be positive in 30–80% of dogs with AITP.

False-negative results may often occur with indirect or serum-based assays, as the majority of antibody will be platelet bound rather than circulating. Although direct measurement of platelet-bound antibodies would therefore be preferable, in severely thrombocytopenic patients it is difficult to isolate sufficient platelets for diagnostic purposes. Given the limitations of immunological tests for platelet autoantibody, and their general unavailability, a tentative diagnosis of AITP is often based solely on haematological findings.

Adjunct immunodiagnostic testing may be of use in some cases. Dogs with AITP may have serum ANA and, if concurrent haemolytic anaemia is suspected, a Coombs test should be performed.

Treatment

Therapy for IMTP depends on the severity of the thrombocytopenia and clinical signs. In stable patients, immunosuppressive doses of prednisolone (2–4 mg/kg p/o q24h), with or without an initial intravenous dose of injectable corticosteroid (e.g. dexamethasone 0.2 mg/kg), may be sufficient to attain an adequate platelet count (within 1–2 weeks), before tapering to a minimum maintenance dose. Glucocorticoids impair the phagocytosis of platelets, decrease autoantibody binding to platelets and eventually decrease autoantibody production. There is an additional effect on capillary endothelial cells, which increases resistance to small vessel haemorrhage. As with IMHA, other immunosuppressive drugs (e.g. azathioprine) may be included in the treatment regime in an attempt to gradually reduce autoantibody synthesis. Patients with refractory chronic IMTP may also benefit from oral danazol or ciclosporin, using the same dosing regimes as for IMHA.

Vincristine (0.02 mg/kg i/v, single dose) is used in dogs with acute or life-threatening IMTP because it affects thrombopoiesis in addition to impairing phagocytosis of platelets. A rapid and dramatic (although usually transient) rise in platelet numbers has been reported in some dogs a few days after a single dose of vincristine. Since vincristine binds avidly to platelets, the drug may be targeted to the very macrophages that destroy platelets by the intravenous administration of vincristine-loaded homologous platelets. Splenectomy, high-dose gamma globulin infusion or plasmapheresis may be considered in patients with life-threatening refractory AITP. Supportive therapy with either fresh whole blood (replacing platelets and blood lost to haemorrhage) or platelet-rich plasma may

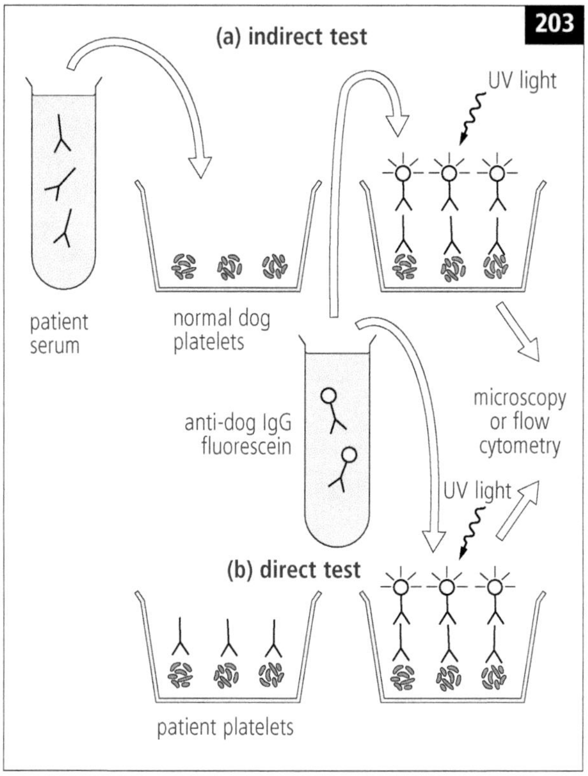

203a, b The indirect and direct platelet immunofluorescence tests. (a) In the indirect test, circulating serum platelet autoantibodies are detected by incubation with normal dog platelets and subsequent labelling by fluorescein-conjugated anti-dog IgG reagent. Binding is assessed visually by microscopy under UV light (55% of dogs with IMTP are positive) or by flow cytometry (67% of dogs with IMTP are positive). **(b)** In the direct test, platelets are harvested from the patient and the presence of *in vivo* platelet-bound antibody determined as above.

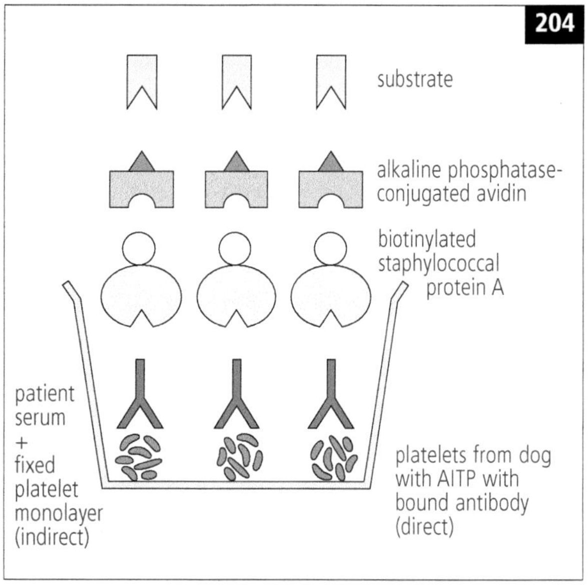

204 Immunoassay for detection of platelet-bound antibody. In the direct test, platelets from the affected dog are sequentially incubated with biotinylated staphylococcal protein A (which binds canine IgG), alkaline phosphatase conjugated avidin (which binds biotin) and an enzyme substrate that produces a colour change in positive wells of a microtitre plate. In the indirect test a monolayer of normal dog platelets is first incubated with serum from the patient. Up to 94% of dogs with IMTP have demonstrable platelet-bound antibody (direct test), but only 34% have serum autoantibody (indirect test) as determined by these assays.

205 Megakaryocyte-bound Ig in IMTP. Section of bone marrow from a cat with IMTP responsive to immunosuppressive therapy, labelled by the immunoperoxidase method for feline IgG. Brown colouration of some megakaryocytes indicates the presence of Ig and provides indirect evidence for platelet autoantibody.

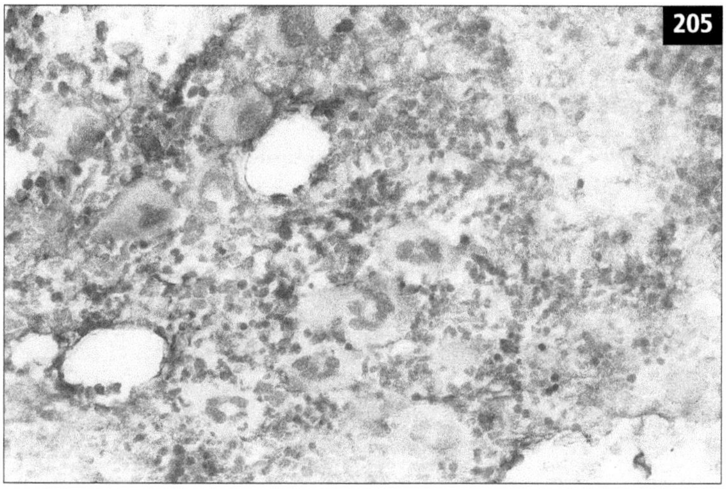

also be considered, but as platelet survival time in patients with AITP may only be a few hours, the benefits of transfusion are usually transient. Strict cage rest and minimization of potential vascular trauma (e.g. elective surgery or excessive venepuncture) may prevent life-threatening haemorrhage before immunosuppressive therapy raises platelet counts.

Prognosis

IMTP is a severe condition and approximately 30% of dogs die during the initial episode, largely from extensive gastrointestinal haemorrhage, although aggressive treatment of blood loss by whole blood transfusions may reduce mortality rates. Immunosuppressive therapy can induce recovery and remission in approximately 40% of cases, often without maintenance therapy, but recurrence (or repeated recurrence) is common. Careful monitoring of platelet numbers while gradually tapering immunosuppressive therapy will significantly reduce relapse rates. Immunosuppressive therapy should be maintained in tapered form for at least 3–6 months, and platelet numbers should be regularly monitored for at least six months after an episode.

IMMUNE-MEDIATED THROMBOCYTOPENIA IN THE CAT

IMTP is poorly characterized in the cat and most cases are likely to be secondary rather than autoimmune. Possible underlying causes include FeLV infection, vaccination, carbimazole/methimazole therapy or monocytic ehrlichiosis. Thrombocytopenia in the cat has a less severe clinical presentation than in dogs, and it may be recognized as an incidental finding on haematological examination of an animal with anaemia, lethargy, anorexia and pyrexia. Spontaneous mucous membrane or cutaneous haemorrhage may not be present, but haemorrhage can be precipitated by trauma, venepuncture or parturition (**206**). The platelet factor 3 and megakaryocyte immunofluorescence tests have been adapted for the cat; however, as IMTP in cats is usually secondary, the major emphasis of diagnostic testing should be to exclude or detect underlying disease. In one study a flow cytometric assay for the detection of platelet-bound antibodies was applied to 42 thrombocytopenic cats and 46 healthy controls. All the controls were negative, but 19 of the 42 thrombocytopenic cats had a positive test result. Only one of these 19 cats had primary idiopathic IMHA and one had Evans' syndrome, while in the remainder an underling cause was identified including fat necrosis (n = 4), FIP (n = 3), retroviral infection (n = 4), lymphoma (n = 2), leukaemia (n = 1), hepatitis (n = 1), pyelonephritis (n = 1) and hyperthyroidism (n = 1). Immunosuppressive therapy (corticosteroids) is documented to be effective and blood transfusion has been used in cats with severe haemorrhage. On rare occasions the concurrent use of corticosteroids and low doses of azathioprine (see regime described under AIHA) may be needed to control thrombocytopenia. Immune-mediated amegakaryocytic thrombocytopenia and haemolytic anaemia has been documented in a cat.

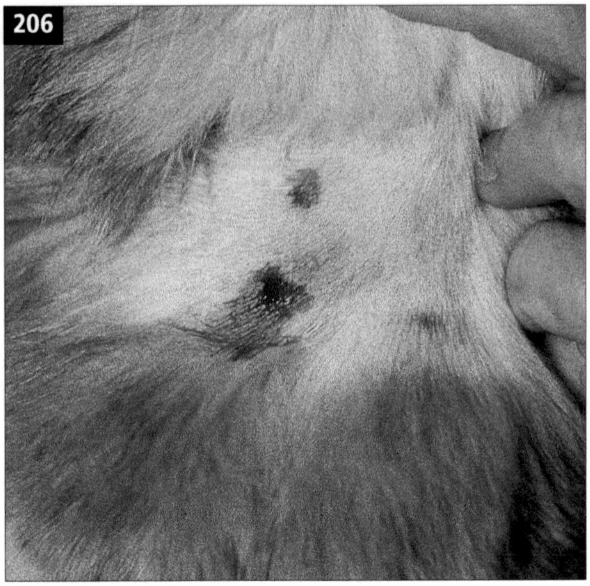

206 Clinical presentation of IMTP in the cat. Prolonged oozing of blood following jugular venepuncture in a cat with AITP. (Photograph courtesy S. Tasker.)

COLD AGGLUTININ DISEASE

Cold agglutinin disease is uncommon in the cat and dog. The pathogenesis involves intravascular erythrocyte agglutination (or haemolysis) by cold-reactive IgM antibodies, manifest clinically as ischaemic necrosis of peripheral areas (e.g. ear, nose and tail tip) following formation of microthrombi within capillary beds (**207**). The disease may be primary or associated with neoplasia, drugs or lead toxicity, and it is usually recognized during very cold weather. There will be gross

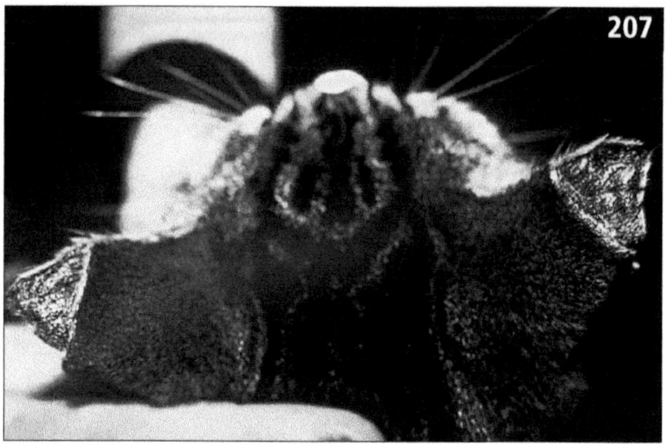

207 Clinical presentation of cold agglutinin disease. Ischaemic necrosis of ear tips in a stray, adult DSH cat following exposure to freezing weather. There was positive erythrocyte autoagglutination at 4°C. (Photograph courtesy S.E. Shaw.)

autoagglutination of a blood sample, and positive slide agglutination, on cooling to 4°C, and this will disperse upon warming to 37°C as antibody elutes from the RBCs at this temperature. A Coombs test performed at 4°C may demonstrate erythrocyte-bound IgM antibody. Response to immunosuppressive doses of glucocorticoids has been described, and affected animals should be housed in a warm environment.

IMMUNE-MEDIATED NEUTROPENIA IN THE DOG

IMNP has only recently been described in the dog and, in most instances, it occurs concurrently with either or both IMHA and IMTP. Affected dogs will be persistently neutropenic (0.0–2.0 × 10^9/l [0–2,000 cells/μl]) and, although theoretically more susceptible to infection (particularly bacterial), some dogs do not show clinical signs and are not pyrexic. Bone marrow assessment generally shows a prominent proliferating pool of neutrophils, with normal erythroid and platelet lineages (unless there is concurrent cytopenia involving these cell types). However, in some cases there is marrow neutrophil hypoplasia, suggesting that the immune-response may also potentially target these precursor cells.

The immunopathogenesis and target autoantigens in this disease have not been investigated, although in man, IMNP mechanisms include complement-mediated neutrophil cytolysis and antibody-mediated agglutination of neutrophils that are subsequently phagocytosed by macrophages. An important differential diagnosis would be the neutropenia that accompanies *Anaplasma phagocytophilum* infection (an *Ixodes* transmitted infection also known as 'granulocytic ehrlichiosis'); IMNP has also been described secondary to trimethoprim/sulphonamide or cephalosporin therapy. Anti-neutrophil antibodies have been documented in patients with IMNP, but this testing has very limited availability at the present time. Either direct or indirect immunofluorescence methodology (particularly using flow cytometry) has been used and assays for antibodies specific to myeloperoxidase and neutrophilic cytoplasmic antigen (ANCA) have been applied. It has been proposed that a diagnosis of IMNP can be made if three of the following four criteria are satisfied: (1) exclusion of other known causes of neutropenia; (2) presence of concurrent IMHA or IMTP; (3) bone marrow evaluation consistent with immune-mediated neutrophil destruction; and (4) prompt response to glucocorticoid therapy.

Dogs with IMNP have been treated with standard immunosuppressive doses of glucocorticoid (as described above), with or without concurrent azathioprine, and there appears to be relatively rapid (within ten days) rebound of circulating neutrophil levels after commencing therapy.

FELINE BLOOD GROUP ANTIGENS

The feline blood group system is characterized by expression of either the A antigen (type A; genotype *AA*, Aa^{ab} or *Ab*) or B antigen (type B; genotype *bb*), or both antigens (type AB; genotype $a^{ab}b$ or $a^{ab}a^{ab}$), on the RBC surface membrane (*Table 4*). The A allele is dominant over B and the phenotype AB is the result of a third allele allowing co-dominant expression of both A and B. The AB allele is recessive to the A allele but dominant over the B allele. Recently, a new feline blood group antigen termed 'Mik' has been identified. A proportion of type A cats appear to lack expression of the Mik blood group antigen and to have serum alloantibody specific for this molecule. In these cats, AB matched blood transfusions may lead to acute haemolytic transfusion reactions.

Blood group A is most common in the majority of geographical areas (74–100%), and groups B (0–26%) and AB (0–9.7%) are less common. Blood

Table 4: Feline blood group antigens.

Blood group	Frequency of expression	Naturally occurring alloantibody
A	Most common (74–100%)	May have weak anti-B
B	Less common (0–26%)	All have high titred anti-A
AB	Rare (0.1–9.7%)	None
Mik	Common in type A cats	Yes

Frequency data are based on a compilation of international studies.

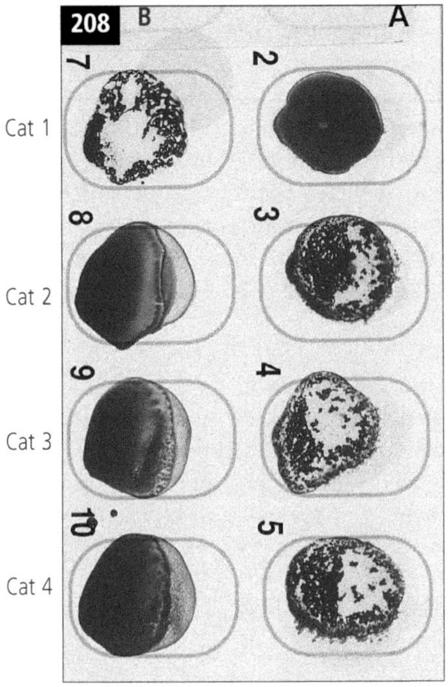

208 Card test for feline blood groups. The commercially available card test for determination of feline blood group involves placing a 50 µl volume of saline and then a 50 µl volume of whole anticoagulant blood onto each oval, mixing and incubating with gentle agitation for two minutes. The presence of agglutination is then determined. In the example shown, cat 1 is blood type B and cats 2–4 are type A. The current card also includes a negative control oval, which assesses the blood sample for the presence of autoagglutination.

group B is more prevalent amongst particular pure-bred cats including the British Shorthair, Birman and Rex (20–59%), and the Abyssinian, Persian and Somali (11–20%). All Siamese, Burmese and Tonkinese cats that have been tested are reported to be blood group A.

The incidence of spontaneously arising blood group alloantibodies is variable. All adult type B cats are reported to have a high titred IgM haemagglutinating and haemolytic (complement fixing) serum antibody to the type A antigen, and some type A cats may have low titred IgG and IgM anti-B alloantibodies. AB cats have neither alloantibody. Feline blood groups may be demonstrated by agglutination techniques involving incubation of a suspension of washed patient RBCs with heat-inactivated group-specific antiserum, with or without a source of complement. Monoclonal antibodies specific for the type A and B antigens have been produced. Type B cells can also be recognized by the ability of the B antigen to be specifically bound by the lectin *Triticum vulgaris*. Recently, a number of test kits have become available for determination of feline blood groups. The most widely used of these is a card-based test designed for in-practice use (208), but tube-based and immunochromatographic systems are also manufactured. There is good correlation between results obtained with these various test systems.

CANINE BLOOD GROUP ANTIGENS

The canine blood group antigen system is more complex than that of the cat. At least ten blood group antigens are recognized. They have a variable prevalence in the canine population (*Table 5*), although the dog erythrocyte antigen (DEA) 1 antigens are the most clinically significant. Spontaneously arising alloantibodies are less frequently observed in the dog than the cat; however, they may occur at low titres, with specificity for DEA 3, DEA 4, DEA 5 and DEA 7. DEA 4 alloantibodies have rarely caused a mild blood transfusion reaction. Spontaneously arising

Table 5: Canine blood group antigens.

Blood group	Frequency of expression	Naturally occurring alloantibody
DEA 1.1*	Common (33–45%), but recent US study of 2,500 donors reveals 0.3%	None
DEA 1.2*	Common (7–20%)	None
DEA 1.3		
DEA 1 null		
DEA 3	Rare (5–10%), but recent US study of 2,500 donors reveals 1.2%	Rare
DEA 4	Most dogs (87–98%)	Rare
DEA 5	Less common (12–22%), but recent US study of 2,500 donors reveals 0.8%	Rare
DEA 6	Most dogs	No
DEA 7*	Common (8–45%), but recent US study of 2,500 donors reveals 9.8%	Rare
DEA 8	Common	None
Dal	Rare in Dalmatians	No

*Most significant in producing clinical transfusion reactions.
Frequency data are from the USA.

alloantibodies to DEA 1.1 or 1.2 do not occur, but strong IgG haemolysins can develop in dogs sensitized by a first incompatible transfusion or following pregnancy. Recently, a new canine blood group antigen named 'Dal' has been identified in dogs of the Dalmatian breed. Dal-negative dogs may develop alloantibodies if transfused with Dal-positive blood, and this may lead to haemolytic reactions if subsequent transfusions are given. Canine blood group antigens can be recognized by *in vitro* haemagglutination techniques using a panel of specific antisera, although antisera specific for some specificities are no longer available. In many countries, canine blood typing is not widely available, but a card test for DEA 1.1 based on the use of a monoclonal antibody specific for this molecule has been developed and, recently, two tube-based assays have also been produced. One of the tube-based tests incorporates a panel of monoclonal antibodies that have been produced with specificity for canine blood group antigens, but the nomenclature used to describe the specificities of these reagents is at variance to the standard DEA blood groups. A gel column system has also been tested for detection of DEA 1.1, 3, 4, 7 and Dal.

BLOOD TRANSFUSION REACTIONS

Although transfusion reaction can occur following infusion of incompatible serum, platelets or WBCs, the compatibility of erythrocytes appears to be of greatest clinical significance in the dog and cat, and as little as 1 ml of incompatible blood may be sufficient to cause a severe reaction in an animal with alloantibodies. Transfusion reactions are uncommon in first transfusions in the dog due to the widespread prevalence of DEA 1.1 and lack of naturally occurring alloantibodies. Retrospective studies have recorded reactions in only 3% of canine transfusions.

Transfusion reactions are potentially more common in the cat (particularly in some pure breeds), as alloantibodies are relatively more frequent in occurrence and titre. The most severe reactions occur when type B cats (with anti-A antibodies) are transfused with type A blood. The milder reactions (extravascular haemolysis) that may result from transfusing type B blood into a type A cat are rarely of clinical significance, but delayed reactions may destroy the transfused RBC in 1–2 weeks (may normally survive 29–39 days), resulting in a less effective transfusion.

Transfusion reactions most frequently take the form of mild pyrexia or an episode of vomiting or facial oedema. Haemolytic reactions are less common and have a complex pathogenesis involving activation of complement, haemostatic and other inflammatory pathways. They are clinically manifest as:

- **Acute onset reaction.** The clinical features of an acute haemolytic transfusion reaction may include pyrexia, tachycardia, vomiting, dyspnoea, tremors, convulsions and acute collapse within minutes of starting the transfusion. In the cat the acute reaction is characterized by a phase of hypotension, bradycardia, cardiac arrhythmia, apnoea or hypopnoea, vomiting, diarrhoea and/or seizures, followed by a recovery phase (hours) of tachycardia and tachypnoea. In both species, haemoglobinaemia and haemoglobinuria may be present.
- **Delayed onset reaction.** Delayed onset reactions occur 3–21 days post transfusion and are usually due to extravascular removal of IgG-coated RBCs, with mild clinical signs of pyrexia and anorexia. Intravascular haemolysis (haemoglobinaemia and haemoglobinuria) is rare.

A range of non-immunological reactions may also potentially occur during blood transfusion:

- Hyperkalaemia due to leakage of potassium from RBCs during blood storage. This is a rare occurrence unless there is a massive transfusion or the recipient has pre-existing hyperkalaemia or renal failure.
- Hypocalcaemia due to the citrate used as an anti-coagulant chelating circulating calcium.
- Circulatory overload in normovolaemic patients or those with cardiac disease.
- Embolism from transfusion of clots or debris formed in the blood (or air embolism).
- Hypothermia due to administration of unwarmed blood.
- Infectious disease transferred in the blood (e.g. FeLV, FIV, FIP, ehrlichiosis, babesiosis, dirofilariasis, leishmaniosis, bartonellosis, haemoplasmosis).

Transfusion reactions can be avoided by blood typing and by performing a cross-match (**209**). In practice, unmatched first transfusion is relatively safe in the dog (provided there is no history of previous blood transfusion), but it is of much greater risk in the cat, particularly type B cats that may suffer a fatal reaction to as little as 1 ml of type

209

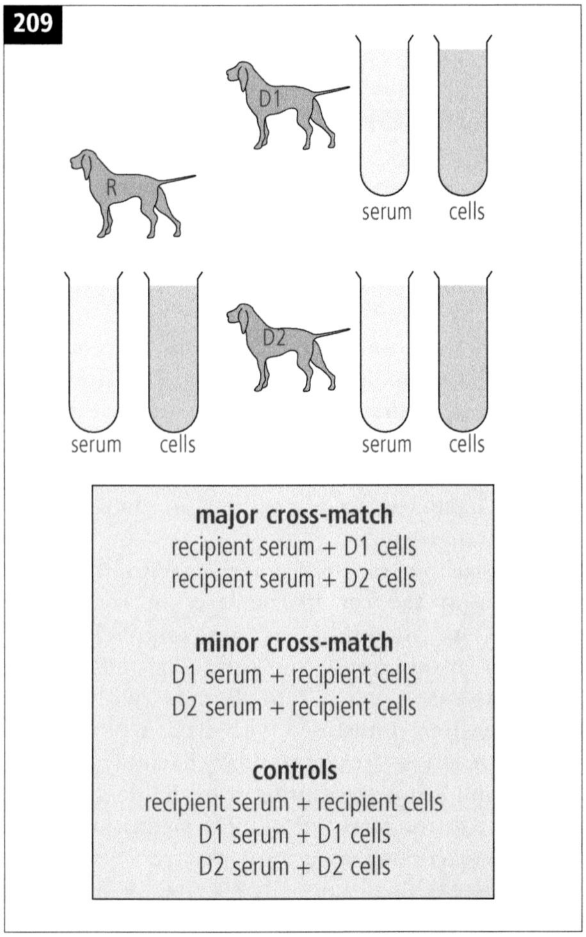

209 Cross-matching blood for transfusion. A recipient animal [R] requires a blood transfusion and two potential donors are available [D1 and D2]. Anticoagulant (EDTA) and clotted blood samples are taken from each. The cross-match can be performed using various methods, but the most important component (major cross-match) involves incubation of recipient serum with donor RBCs. The minor cross-match involves incubation of donor serum with recipient RBCs, and controls should be used for comparative purposes. A cross-match can be performed in test tubes or a microtitre tray using one volume of a 2.5% suspension of washed RBCs in saline added to an equal volume of undiluted serum. Duplicate tests can be established at different incubation temperatures (4°C, 37°C or room temperature) and, after a 30-minute incubation period, the presence of agglutination or haemolysis determined. A gel column system has also been described for canine cross-matching.

A blood. To avoid sensitization of a dog during transfusion, the optimum 'universal' donor would be negative for DEA 1.1, 1.2, 3, 5 and 7. In practice, however, typing for DEA 1.1 alone is usually sufficient, and Greyhounds are often used as blood donors due to the low frequency of DEA 1.1 and 1.2 in this breed.

BLOOD TRANSFUSION PROTOCOL

Donor animals should be healthy, vaccinated young adults and screen negative for parasitic and viral disease (e.g. babesiosis, leishmaniosis, ehrlichiosis and brucellosis in the dog; FeLV, FIV, haemoplasmosis and bartonellosis in the cat). Blood (10–20 ml/kg dog; up to 10 ml/kg cat) should not be taken more frequently than every 21 days. Blood can be collected from the jugular vein of a sedated animal into anti-coagulated bags containing citrate phosphate dextrose (CPD) or acid citrate dextrose (ACD) and may be stored at 4°C for 3–4 weeks, although if platelets or clotting factors are required, blood should be used within 12 hours of collection. The transfusion can be administered into the cephalic vein using a butterfly catheter (or via the intraosseous route if necessary) at a rate of 5–10 ml/kg/hour. Rates may be increased up to 20 ml/kg/hour in hypovolaemic patients and decreased to as low as 2 ml/kg/hour in animals with cardiac or renal disease. The volume for transfusion is calculated as:

$$\text{body weight (kg)} \times K \times \frac{(\text{desired PCV} - \text{recipient's PCV})}{\text{donor PCV}}$$

(K = 88 for dogs, 66 for cats)

A small test volume (1–3 ml) should be administered and the animal observed for signs of reaction; however, since even this volume of blood can cause fatal reactions, a test dose should not be used as a substitute for cross-matching or blood typing in at-risk patients. There is no indication for prophylactic administration of antihistamine or glucocorticoids prior to transfusion. Temperature, heart rate and respiratory rate should be monitored every ten minutes during the first 30 minutes, then every 30 minutes throughout the transfusion and at intervals for 24 hours thereafter. A transfusion should be completed within four hours.

Blood component transfusion is becoming increasingly used in veterinary medicine, but it is not routinely available in all countries. The most commonly administered fractions are packed red cells, platelet-rich plasma or plasma. Using packed red cells has the benefit of not administering excess volume to a normovolaemic patient with haemolysis. The use of platelet-rich plasma may be of short-term benefit in thrombocytopenic animals, and plasma may be used in animals with coagulopathies. Plasma that is separated and frozen within six hours of collection is termed 'fresh frozen plasma' and is a suitable source of clotting factors that will retain such activity for up to one year at a temperature of –40°C. 'Frozen plasma' is frozen more than six hours after collection and has minimal clotting factor activity, but it is used as a source of albumin. After a one-year period, fresh frozen plasma may still be used as frozen plasma.

Polymerized bovine haemoglobin has become available as an alternative to whole blood or packed RBC transfusion in emergency situations. This product has a relatively long shelf life and can provide temporary support, although standard blood transfusion is generally still required as a follow-up. The product is expensive, and one retrospective study has shown no benefit or a less successful outcome when it was used in the adjunct therapy of dogs with IMHA. Polymerized bovine haemoglobin should be used with caution in cats, as a recent retrospective study has shown that some treated animals may develop pulmonary oedema and/or pleural effusion that may be associated with the rapid infusion of a large volume of the solution.

NEONATAL ISOERYTHROLYSIS

Neonatal isoerythrolysis (haemolytic disease of the newborn) is uncommon in the cat and rare in the dog. In the cat the disease will arise when cats bearing blood group A or AB are born to type B mothers in which anti-A alloantibodies circulate and are passed to the neonate in colostrum. Such alloantibodies may be found within the serum of affected neonates within four hours of birth. Not all type A kittens born to type B queens will be affected, which may be due to variables such as the titre of alloantibody in the colostrum and the amount of antibody absorbed by the kitten.

Affected kittens may have subclinical disease or develop a severe haemolytic anaemia with jaundice, haemoglobinuria, weakness, lethargy, reluctance to suckle and death within the first few days of life. Some kittens with subclinical disease may develop tail tip necrosis 1–3 weeks post partum. The kittens will be Coombs positive. The disease can be predicted and avoided by performing blood typing or cross-matching between potential sire and dam, preventing susceptible kittens access to colostrum for at least 24 hours after birth, and foster nursing the kittens during that period. This may take the form of providing access to a type A foster queen or feeding milk replacement. It has been suggested that milk from a type A cat may be used as a colostrum replacement on the assumption that there are similar levels of IgG in these secretions. However, more recent studies have shown considerably lower concentrations of IgG in feline milk than in colostrum (see Chapter 12, p. 302). In the dog, neonatal isoerythrolysis may arise when DEA 1.1-negative bitches sensitized to DEA 1.1 (by transfusion or previous pregnancy) are mated to a DEA 1.1-positive sire.

FURTHER READING

Bianco D, Armstrong PJ, Washabau RJ (2009) A prospective, randomized, double-blinded, placebo-controlled study of human intravenous immunoglobulin for the acute management of presumptive primary immune-mediated thrombocytopenia in dogs. *Journal of Veterinary Internal Medicine* **23**: 1071–1078.

Blais M-C, Berman L, Oakley D *et al.* (2007) Canine Dal blood type: a red cell antigen lacking in some Dalmatians. *Journal of Veterinary Internal Medicine* **21**:281–286.

Brown CD, Parnell NK, Schulman RL *et al.* (2006) Evaluation of clinicopathologic features, response to treatment, and risk factors associated with idiopathic neutropenia in dogs: 11 cases (1990–2002). *Journal of the American Veterinary Medical Association* **229**:87–91.

Carli E, Tasca S, Trotta M *et al.* (2009) Detection of erythrocyte binding IgM and IgG by flow cytometry in sick dogs with *Babesia canis canis* or *Babesia canis vogeli* infection. *Veterinary Parasitology* **162**:51–57.

Fenty RK, deLaforcade AM, Shaw SP *et al.* (2011) Identification of hypercoagulability in dogs with primary immune-mediated hemolytic anemia by means of thromboelastography. *Journal of the American Veterinary Medical Association* **238**:463–467.

Forcada Y, Guitian J, Gibson G (2007) Frequencies of feline blood types at a referral hospital in the south east of England. *Journal of Small Animal Practice* **48**:570–573.

Giger U, Stieger K, Palos H (2005) Comparison of various canine blood-typing methods. *American Journal of Veterinary Research* **66**:1386–1392.

Hedwig Dircks B, Schuberth H-J, Mischke R (2009) Underlying diseases and clinicopathologic variables of thrombocytopenic dogs with and without platelet-bound antibodies detected by use of a flow cytometric assay: 83 cases (2004–2006). *Journal of the American Veterinary Medical Association* **235**:960–966.

Helmond SE, Polzin DJ, Armstrong PJ *et al.* (2010) Treatment of immune-mediated hemolytic anemia with individually adjusted heparin dosing in dogs. *Journal of Veterinary Internal Medicine* **24**:597–605.

Kessler RJ, Reese J, Chang D *et al.* (2010) Dog erythrocyte antigens 1.1, 1.2, 3, 4, 7, and *Dal* blood typing and cross-matching by gel column technique. *Veterinary Clinical Pathology* **39**:306–316.

Kjelgaard-Hansen M, Goggs R, Wiinberg B *et al.* (2011) Use of serum concentrations of interleukin-18 and monocyte chemoattractant protein-1 as prognostic indicators in primary immune-mediated hemolytic anemia in dogs. *Journal of Veterinary Internal Medicine* **25**:76–82.

Klasser DA, Reine NJ, Hohenhaus AE (2005) Red blood cell transfusions in cats: 126 cases (1999). *Journal of the American Animal Hospital Association* **226**:920–923.

Knottenbelt CM, Addie DD, Day MJ *et al.* (1999) Determination of the prevalence of feline blood groups in the United Kingdom. *Journal of Small Animal Practice* **40**:115–118.

Knottenbelt CM, Day MJ, Cripps PJ *et al.* (1999) Measurement of titres of naturally-occurring alloantibodies against feline blood group antigens in the United Kingdom. *Journal of Small Animal Practice* **40**:365–370.

Kohn B, Linden T, Leibold W (2006) Platelet-bound antibodies detected by a flow cytometric assay in cats with thrombocytopenia. *Journal of Feline Medicine and Surgery* **8**:254–260.

Kohn B, Weingart C, Eckmann V *et al.* (2006) Primary immune-mediated hemolytic anemia in 19 cats: diagnosis, therapy, and outcome (1998–2004). *Journal of Veterinary Internal Medicine* **20**:159–166.

Lanevschi A, Wardrop KJ (2001) Principles of transfusion medicine in small animals. *Canadian Veterinary Journal* **42**:447–454.

Mason N, Duval D, Shofer FS *et al.* (2003) Cyclophosphamide exerts no beneficial effect over prednisone alone in the initial treatment of acute immune-mediated hemolytic anemia in dogs: a randomized controlled clinical trial. *Journal of Veterinary Internal Medicine* **17**:206–212.

Mitchell KD, Kruth SA, Wood RD *et al.* (2009) Serum acute phase protein concentrations in dogs with autoimmune hemolytic anemia. *Journal of Veterinary Internal Medicine* **23**:585–591.

Morley P, Mathes M, Guth A *et al.* (2008) Anti-erythrocyte antibodies and disease associations in anemic and nonanemic dogs. *Journal of Veterinary Internal Medicine* **22**:886–892.

O'Marra SK, Delaforcade AM, Shaw SP (2011) Treatment and predictors of outcome in dogs with immune-mediated thrombocytopenia. *Journal of the American Veterinary Medical Association* **238**:346–352.

Perkins MC, Canfield P, Churcher RK *et al.* (2004) Immune-mediated neutropenia suspected in five dogs. *Australian Veterinary Journal* **82**:52–57.

Putsche JC, Kohn B (2008) Primary immune-mediated thrombocytopenia in 30 dogs (1997–2003). *Journal of the American Animal Hospital Association* **44**:250–257.

Ridgway J, Jergens AE, Niyo Y (2001) Possible causal association of idiopathic inflammatory bowel disease with thrombocytopenia in the dog. *Journal of the American Animal Hospital Association* **37**:65–74.

Rozanski EA, Callan MB, Hughes D *et al.* (2002) Comparison of platelet count recovery with use of vincristine and prednisone or prednisone alone for treatment for severe immune-mediated thrombocytopenia in dogs. *Journal of the American Veterinary Medical Association* **220**:477–481.

Seth M, Jackson KV, Giger U (2011) Comparison of five blood-typing methods for the feline AB blood group system. *American Journal of Veterinary Research* **72**:203–209.

Stokol T, Blue JT, French TW (2000) Idiopathic pure red cell aplasia and nonregenerative immune-mediated anemia in dogs: 43 cases (1988–1999). *Journal of the American Veterinary Medical Association* **216**:1429–1436.

Tasker S, Murray JK, Knowles TG *et al.* (2010) Coombs', haemoplasma and retrovirus testing in feline anaemia. *Journal of Small Animal Practice* **51**:192–199.

Terrazzano G, Cortese L, Piantedosi D *et al.* (2006) Presence of anti-platelet IgM and IgG antibodies in dogs naturally infected by *Leishmania infantum*. *Veterinary Immunology and Immunopathology* **110**:331–337.

Tsuchiya R, Akutsu Y, Ikegami A *et al.* (2009) Prothrombotic and inflammatory effects of intravenous administration of human immunoglobulin G in dogs. *Journal of Veterinary Internal Medicine* **23**:1164–1169.

Wardrop KJ (2005) The Coombs test in veterinary medicine: past, present, future. *Veterinary Clinical Pathology* **34**:325–334.

Warman SM, Murray JK, Ridyard A *et al.* (2008) Pattern of Coombs' test reactivity has diagnostic significance in dogs with immune-mediated haemolytic anaemia. *Journal of Small Animal Practice* **49**:525–530.

Warman SM, Helps CR, Barker EN *et al.* (2010) Haemoplasma infection is not a common cause of canine immune-mediated haemolytic anaemia in the UK. *Journal of Small Animal Practice* **51**:534–539.

Weinkle TK, Center SA, Randolph JE *et al.* (2005) Evaluation of prognostic factors, survival rates, and treatment protocols for immune-mediated hemolytic anemia in dogs: 151 cases (1993–2002). *Journal of the American Veterinary Medical Association* **226**:1869–1880.

Weinstein NM, Blais M-C, Harris K *et al.* (2007) A newly recognized blood group in domestic shorthair cats: the Mik red cell antigen. *Journal of Veterinary Internal Medicine* **21**:287–292.

Weiss DJ (2007) An indirect flow cytometric test for detection of anti-neutrophil antibodies in dogs. *American Journal of Veterinary Research* **68**:464–467.

Weiss DJ (2007) Evaluation of antineutrophil IgG antibodies in persistently neutropenic dogs. *Journal of Veterinary Internal Medicine* **21**:440–444.

Wells R, Guth A, Lappin M *et al.* (2009) Anti-endothelial cell antibodies in dogs with immune-mediated hemolytic anemia and other diseases associated with high risk of thromboembolism. *Journal of Veterinary Internal Medicine* **23**:295–300.

Wondratscheck C, Weingart C, Kohn B (2010) Primary immune-mediated thrombocytopenia in cats. *Journal of the American Animal Hospital Association* **46**:12–19.

5 IMMUNE-MEDIATED SKIN DISEASE

Michael J. Day and Susan E. Shaw

INTRODUCTION

The skin is the largest organ of the body, with well-developed innate and acquired immune defence mechanisms (**210**). The components of the cutaneous immune surveillance system include Langerhans (epidermal) dendritic cells, dermal dendritic cells and macrophages, $\alpha\beta$ and $\gamma\delta$ T lymphocytes, and other white cell populations. Epidermal keratinocytes not only provide a defensive barrier, but they are active immunological cells that can express MHC class II and adhesion molecules (e.g. ICAM-1) and can secrete immunoregulatory cytokines and chemokines including IL-1, IL-3, IL-6, IL-7, IL-8, IL-10, IFNγ, TNFα, TNFβ, TGFα, TGFβ, G-CSF, M-CSF and GM-CSF. The canine epidermis also contains anti-microbial peptides (β-defensins, cathelicidin) produced by keratinocytes and innate leukocytes. Afferent lymphatics drain to regional lymphoid tissue, which together with the cutaneous component makes up the skin-associated lymphoid tissue (SALT). Within inflamed skin, the vascular endothelium expresses a range of adhesion molecules (e.g. E selectin, ICAM-1, VCAM-1) that permits the extravasation of lymphocytes, granulocytes, mast cell precursors and monocytes (**211**).

The skin immune system is capable of mounting immune responses to cutaneous pathogens (parasitic, viral, bacterial, protozoal, algal, fungal and yeast) (**212–217**), but it can also mount inappropriate responses, which manifest as the primary cutaneous immune-mediated diseases. The skin is also a site of expression of lymphoid neoplasia (see Chapter 13, p. 330) and may have clinical changes induced by systemic immune-mediated disease (e.g. hypothyroidism [see Chapter 9, p. 243]).

210

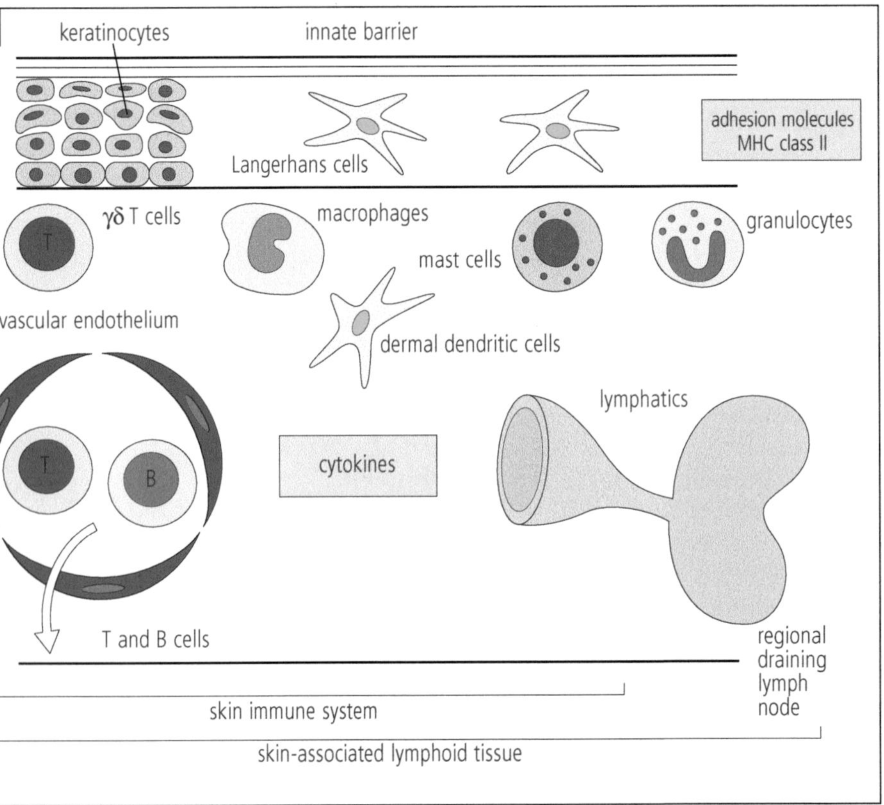

210 Skin-associated lymphoid tissue. SALT consists of the innate and adaptive skin immune system and the regional draining lymphoid tissue. Cutaneous immune surveillance is mediated by a range of immunologically active cells in the epidermis and dermis that express specific cell surface molecules and cytokines. On initiation of a cutaneous immune response, antigen-specific T and B lymphocytes, other WBCs, antibody and complement can be recruited to the site of inflammation from the bloodstream.

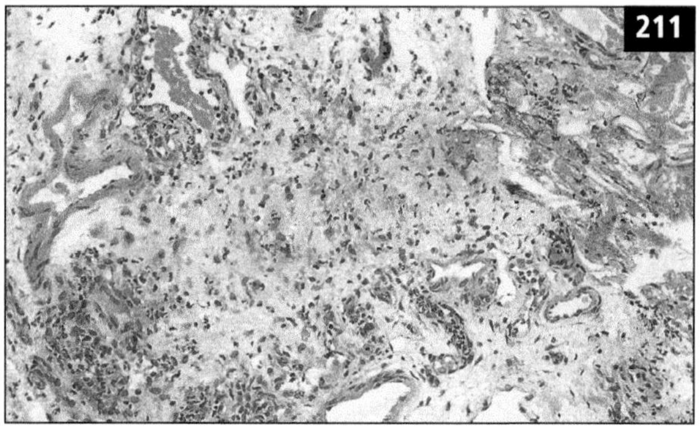

211 Neutrophil extravasation into inflamed dermis. Skin biopsy from a dog with a localized facial lesion. There is extravasation of neutrophils into oedematous dermal tissue. This is an acute inflammatory change, which is likely in response to penetration of a foreign body with associated bacteria.

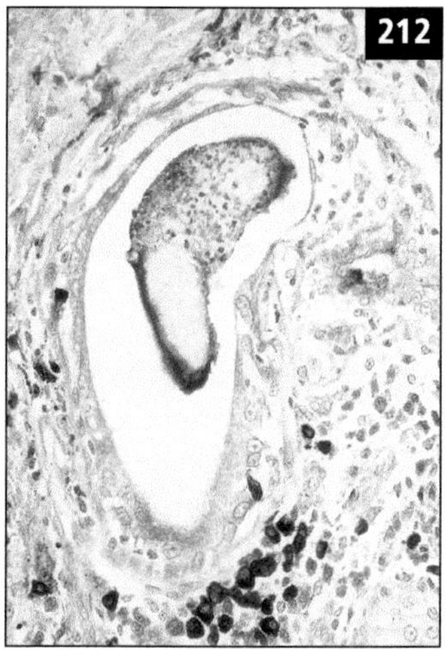

212–217 Immune response to cutaneous infection. The skin immune system is able to initiate an active response to the presence of local infectious agents. (**212**) A *Demodex* mite within a degenerate hair follicle in the skin of a dog. There is an active local infiltration of inflammatory cells, including IgA-bearing plasma cells that are marked by indirect immunoperoxidase labelling. (From Day MJ [1997] An immunohistochemical study of the lesions of demodicosis in the dog. *Journal of Comparative Pathology* **116:**203–216, with permission.) (**213**) Inflammatory cells surround a colony of *Actinomyces* bacteria, causing a localized skin lesion in a dog. (**214**) Gram stained section from the biopsy shown in **213**. (**215**) Localized furunculosis in the skin of a dog with dermatophytosis. (**216**) Hyphal forms of the dermatophyte are found within an intact hair follicle in the same skin biopsy (periodic acid-Schiff staining). (**217**) Skin biopsy from a cat with cowpox infection showing characteristic eosinophilic cytoplasmic inclusion bodies within keratinocytes.

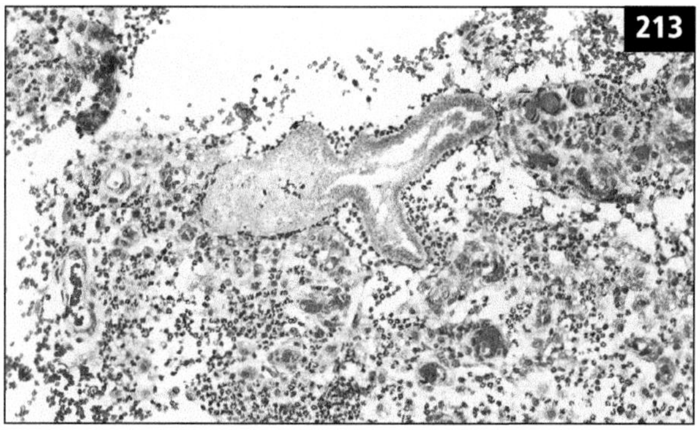

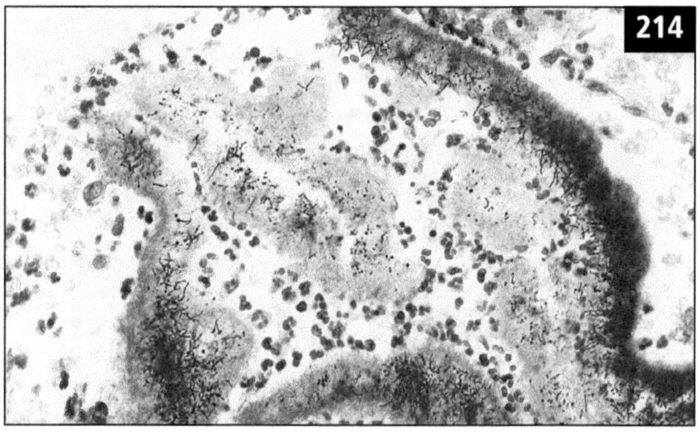

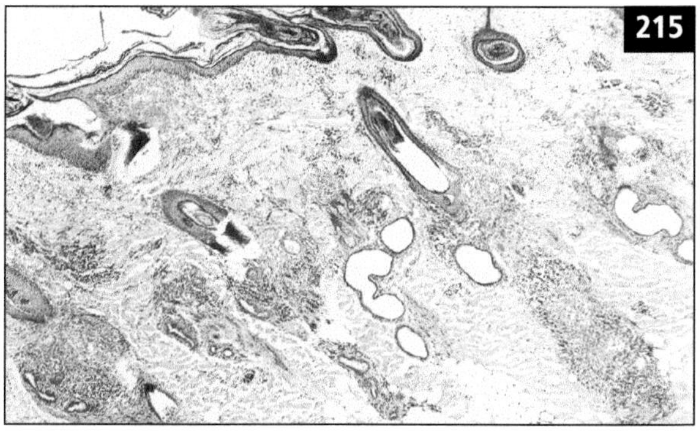

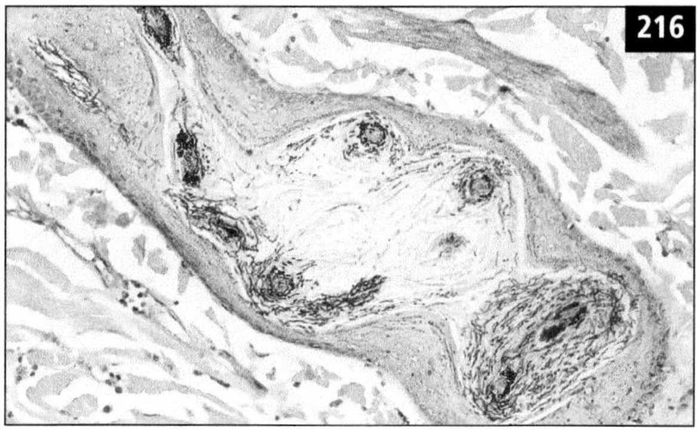

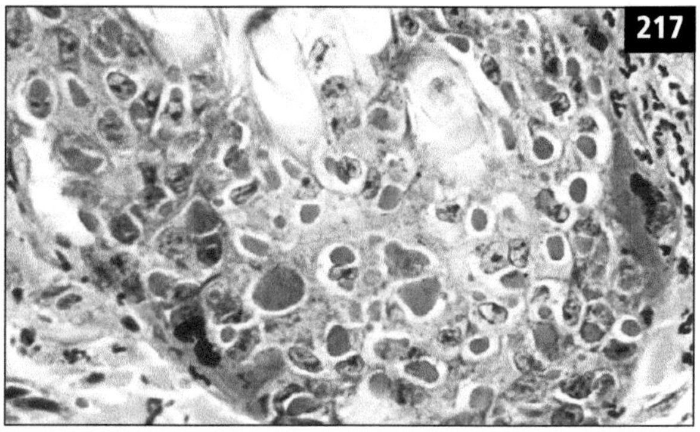

CUTANEOUS DISEASE CAUSED BY TYPE 1 HYPERSENSITIVITY

Type I hypersensitivity involves degranulation of dermal mast cells sensitized by allergen-specific IgE that is cross-linked by exposure to allergen (see Chapter 2, p. 62). Although this results in vasodilation, localized oedema and inflammation, it is pruritus that is the major clinical feature of such disease in the dog and cat. The observed lesions are largely the result of self-trauma and may be complicated by secondary *Staphylococcus pseudintermedius* and *Malassezia pachydermatis* infection. Although a range of allergens is incriminated in these disorders, including structural or metabolic components of ectoparasites, aeroallergens (dust mites, epithelia, pollens, moulds), food or drugs, the underlying immunopathogenesis is similar.

URTICARIA AND ANGIOEDEMA

Urticaria and angioedema are uncommon in the dog and cat and are an expression of immediate hypersensitivity in an individual sensitized to allergens such as drugs, vaccines, incompatible erythrocytes, plants, stinging and biting insects, or food. The clinical onset is usually acute and the lesions take the form of localized or generalized wheals, which are occasionally pruritic. In urticaria these lesions are purely dermal and may become confluent, but in angioedema (**218**), subcutaneous tissue is involved and there may be a progression to

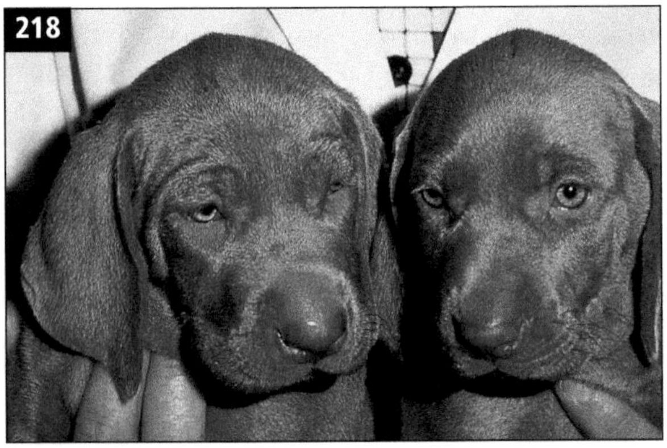

218 Angioedema. Two nine-week-old Weimaraner litter-mates. The puppy on the left developed angioedema affecting the head four hours after administration of multicomponent viral vaccine. Its sibling was unaffected.

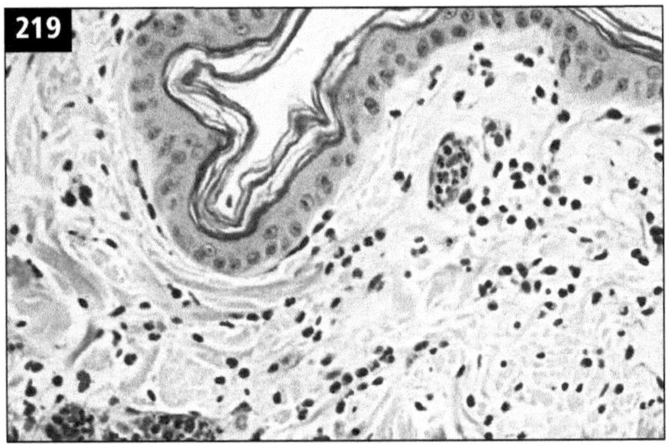

219 Urticaria. Skin biopsy from an urticarial reaction in the dog. There are mild changes including dermal oedema and infiltration of neutrophils into superficial dermis. The epidermis is of normal thickness.

Table 6: Dose rates for epinephrine in angioedema and anaphylaxis.

Species	Dose rate	Route of administration and comments
Cat	20 µg/kg of a 1:10,000 solution	I/v or i/m
Dog	20 µg/kg of a 1:1,000 solution	Diluted in 5–10 ml of normal saline; can be given i/v, intratracheal, intraosseous or intracardiac.

anaphylaxis. Histologically there is minimal change in affected skin, except for dilation of superficial dermal blood vessels, with dermal oedema and mild perivascular inflammation (**219**).

The lesions of urticaria generally persist for under 24 hours, but angioedematous lesions may be more severe and potentially life-threatening if they progress to involve the upper respiratory tract or larynx. Treatment should involve removal of any initiating agent if possible. In acute angioedema, bronchoconstriction and anaphylaxis, administration of epinephrine is required (*Table 6*). Rapid-acting soluble glucocorticoids such as methyl prednisolone sodium succinate or dexamethasone sodium phosphate may be used concurrently (*Table 7*). In cases of urticaria or less severe angioedema, glucocorticoids may be combined with short-

Table 7: Systemically administered anti-inflammatory agents used in the treatment of acute and chronic allergic diseases.

	Daily dose rate (cat)	Daily dose rate (dog)	Route of administration/ comments
Anaphylaxis, angioedema			
Methyl prednisolone sodium succinate injection	20–30 mg/kg	20–30 mg/kg	I/v for acute angioedema and anaphylaxis
Dexamethasone sodium phosphate injection	5 mg/kg	5 mg/kg	I/v for acute angioedema and anaphylaxis
Betamethasone sodium phosphate injection	0.04 mg/kg	0.04 mg/kg	I/v for acute angioedema and anaphylaxis
Allergic dermatitis			
Prednisolone tablets	1–2 mg/kg	0.5–1.0 mg/kg	P/o. Taper to alternate day administration
Methylprednisolone tablets	1 mg/kg	0.4–1.0 mg/kg	P/o. Taper to alternate day administration
Dexamethasone sodium phosphate	0.07–0.16 mg/kg	0.07–0.16 mg/kg	S/c, i/m or i/v for acute pruritus, urticaria and angioedema
Dexamethasone tablets	0.07–0.16 mg/kg	0.07–0.16 mg/kg	P/o. Not suitable for alternate day therapy
Dexamethasone suspensions (several are available)	0.04 mg/kg	0.04 mg/kg	I/m for urticaria, angioedema and short-term management of acute pruritus. S/c administration may cause leukotrichia and/or dermal atrophy over the injection site
Methyl prednisolone acetate injection	5 mg/kg	NR	I/m or S/c. S/c administration may cause leukotrichia and/or dermal atrophy over the injection site
Ciclosporin		5 mg/kg	P/o

NR: not recommended.

Table 8: Antihistamines used in allergic dermatitis, urticaria and angioedema.

Drug	Dose rate (dog and cat)	Route of administration/comments
Chlorpheniramine*	4–8 mg q8h	P/o for pruritus. Transient sedation, unpalatability
	5–10 mg/dog	I/m in angioedema, urticaria
Diphenhydramine	25–50 mg q8h	P/o. Sedation, polyphagia
Hydroxyzine	2.2 mg/kg q8h	P/o. Hyperexcitability and behaviour changes in the cat, depression and polydipsia
Clemastine	0.05 mg/kg q12h	P/o for pruritus. May cause fixed drug reaction, diarrhoea and sedation

* Only chlorpheniramine is licensed for use in dogs and cats.

acting, systemically administered H1 blockers such as chlorpheniramine (*Table 8*).

ATOPIC DERMATITIS

Pathogenesis

Atopic dermatitis (AD) may be defined as an inherited susceptibility to sensitization by environmental allergens, with the development of allergen-specific IgE antibodies that mediate cutaneous type I hypersensitivity. AD is an important disease of the dog, but remains poorly characterized in the cat. The most definitive series of papers defining pathogenic, clinical, diagnostic and therapeutic aspects of canine AD is to be found in the report of the American College of Veterinary Dermatology Task Force (see Further reading).

A range of predisposing factors is likely to underlie clinical expression of the disease:

- Genetic influence. Canine AD has a greater prevalence in particular breeds (e.g. Golden Retriever, West Highland White Terrier) and is often familial. The heritability of AD has been quantified in Labrador and Golden Retrievers by pedigree analysis. Numerous candidate genes have been proposed to be associated with human AD and one study has investigated gene linkage to the canine disease identifying some of the same genes linked to the human disease. Serum IgE concentration at 6–12 weeks of age proved not to be a predictor of the later development of AD in West Highland White Terriers. Familial atopic dermatitis has also been occasionally documented in the cat.
- AD is a disease of young dogs, with onset of clinical signs less than three years of age in 75% of cases. A similar age predisposition is suggested for the cat.
- Exposure to causative allergens is required and there is likely to be an association between magnitude of exposure and frequency of disease. A wide range of aeroallergens is incriminated, but in most studies the components of house dust (the house dust mites *Dermatophagoides pteronyssinus* and *D. farinae,* epithelia) are the dominant allergens, with fewer responses to pollens, moulds or insects (*Table 9*). There are geographical differences in the prevalence of reaction to different allergens, but in many areas reactivity to *D. farinae* is more common than to *D. pteronyssinus*. Allergen loads on the coat, and in the environment, of atopic dogs have been quantified. The immunodominant allergens of the dust mite (for atopic dogs) are high molecular weight proteins unrelated to the mite faecal allergens that are most important in human AD. Atopic dogs react strongly to a dominant 98 kDa allergen from *D. farinae*, which is a mite chitinase designated Der f15. This chitinase is expressed within cells lining the digestive tract of the mite rather than in mite faecal particles.
- In AD the allergens are more likely to be percutaneously absorbed than inhaled, and this may be permitted by a defective epidermal barrier. A recent gene expression microarray study (**374**) revealed upregulation of genes encoding molecules involved in skin barrier function and immunity. Absorbed allergen may be taken up by Langerhans cells bearing IgE associated with the low affinity IgE receptor

Table 9: Major allergens in canine atopic dermatitis. This Table summarizes data from three regional referral centres in the UK that routinely perform the IDST (using a standardized allergen source, Greer Laboratories) in the diagnosis of canine AD. The five allergen extracts most frequently giving a positive reaction are listed for each centre. The data demonstrate the importance of components of house dust, particularly epithelia and dust mites, as causative allergens of canine AD. Similar findings are reported from continental Europe and the USA; however, in Australia and the USA there is a higher prevalence of reactivity to pollen allergens. (Data from Sture GH, Halliwell REW, Thoday KL *et al.* (1995) Canine atopic dermatitis: the prevalence of positive intradermal skin tests at 2 sites in the south and north of Great Britain. *Veterinary Immunology and Immunopathology* **44**:293–308; Shaw SE, Day MJ (2000) Recent developments in atopic dermatitis of companion animals. In *Epidemiology of Atopic Dermatitis.* (ed HC Williams) Cambridge University Press, Cambridge, pp. 233–246.)

London (31 cases)	Edinburgh (87 cases)	Bristol (76 cases)
Human dander (55%)	Human dander (68%)	*D. farinae* (67%)
D. farinae (42%)	*D. farinae* (50%)	House dust (45%)
Horse epithelium (39%)	Cotton linters (39%)	*D. pteronyssinus* (41%)
T. putrescentiae (35%)	*T. putrescentiae* (36%)	Mattress dust (37%)
House dust (29%)	Horse epithelia (26%)	Mixed insect (11%)

(CD23). Experimental studies have demonstrated that allergens delivered percutaneously are more likely to trigger a Th2-dominated response.

- AD is often complicated by secondary infection (*Staphylococcus*, *Malassezia*) or flea allergy. Microbial antigens (superantigens, HSPs) may have a role in perpetuating the cutaneous immunopathology, perhaps by interaction with PRRs expressed by cutaneous dendritic cell populations. Some microbial antigens are also able to induce an IgE response, which likely contributes to the atopic state. For example, dogs with AD and *Malassezia* infection have *Malassezia*-specific serum IgE, positive intradermal test reactivity to *Malassezia* allergens and transfer of such reactivity via the Prausnitz-Kustner test. Dogs with AD appear predisposed to the development of flea allergy, suggesting a general susceptibility to the expression of Th2-driven responses. The effect of intestinal endoparasitic infection on the expression of AD has not been extensively examined.

The immunopathogenesis of AD is dominated by classical type I hypersensitivity, largely mediated by allergen-specific IgE antibodies, but reaginic IgG antibodies have been identified. These antibodies may be demonstrated associated with cutaneous mast cells, but they are also found free in the circulation or bound by circulating basophils. Allergen-specific IgG antibodies in canine serum are generally of the IgG1 or IgG4 subclass, with fewer IgG2 or IgG3 antibodies present. Recent investigations have shown that *Dermatophagoides*-specific IgE antibodies are present in similar concentration in the serum of clinically normal and atopic cats. This finding suggests either that IgE is not significant in the pathogenesis of feline AD or that functional subclasses of IgE might exist, as has been previously proposed for the dog.

In man and dogs, AD proceeds through an acute (Th2-dominated cytokine profile) phase (15–20 minutes after initiation) to an eosinophil-dominated 'late phase response' after 6–12 hours, with subsequent infiltration of lymphoid cells during the chronic stages of disease (Th1-dominated or unpolarized cytokine profile). To date, studies of cytokine involvement in canine and feline AD have been performed by assessment of cytokine mRNA expression in lesional skin biopsies or pellets of antigen-stimulated blood lymphocytes. Canine AD lesional skin has up-regulation of genes encoding IL-4, IFNγ and TNFα, but reduced transcription of TGFβ. One study has shown the presence of IL-4 protein associated with $CD4^+$ T cells in the skin of allergic cats by immunohistochemistry. In canine AD skin there is expression of mRNA encoding the chemokine TARC, which is chemoattractant for Th2 lymphocytes expressing the ligand for this molecule, CC chemokine receptor 4 (CCR4). There

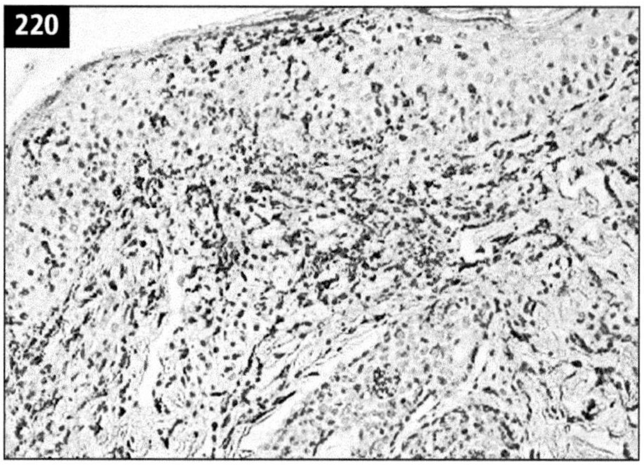
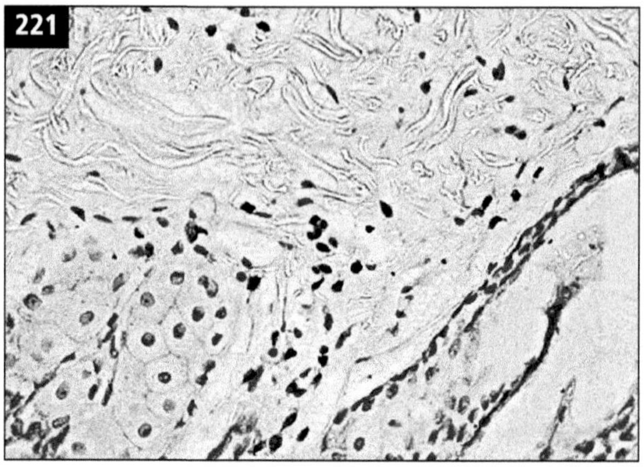

220, 221 Immunopathogenesis of atopic dermatitis. Biopsies from the lesional skin of a cat with AD. There is strong MHC class II expression by both epidermal Langerhans cells and dermal dendritic cells (**220**). Within the dermis there are numerous $CD3^+$ T lymphocytes (**221**). (Photographs courtesy K. Taglinger.)

is similar up-regulation of CCR4 mRNA in canine AD skin.

There are increased numbers of epidermal Langerhans cells (that express MHC class II and surface IgE) and dermal dendritic cells within the lesional skin of atopic dogs and cats (220). In both species there is an epidermal and dermal infiltrate of $CD4^+$ and $CD8^+$ T cells, and in dogs with AD the epidermal T cells most often express CD8 and the $\gamma\delta$ T cell receptor (221). The kinetics of these changes have been investigated in experimental models. In Beagle dogs injected intradermally with anti-IgE, skin biopsy at six hours has shown evidence of the late-phase infiltration of eosinophils together with $CD1^+$ dendritic cells and $CD3^+$ T cells. Accompanying these cellular changes was increased expression of Th2 cytokine genes (IL-5 and IL-13).

Blood lymphocytes from dogs with AD respond to stimulation with a range of crude dust mite extracts and to purified 98kD allergen from D. *farinae*. Freshly isolated blood lymphocytes from dogs with AD show elevated expression of IL-5 mRNA, but reduction in expression of IFNγ mRNA compared with cells from normal dogs.

Important information has recently been gleaned from studies of dogs allergic to pollen from Japanese cedar. Affected dogs make serum IgE responses to the major Cry j1 allergen. A panel of overlapping peptides derived from the sequence of Cry j1 has been used to stimulate blood mononuclear cells from experimentally or spontaneously allergic dogs. These studies have shown heterogeneity in the peptide responsiveness of the spontaneously allergic animals, which would suggest that any peptide-based immunotherapy for this disease must be tailored to individual dogs. Allergen-stimulated blood mononuclear cells from the experimentally sensitized dogs express genes encoding Th2 and proinflammatory cytokines consistent with the pathogenesis of AD. This model has been used to study DNA vaccination as a novel form of immunotherapy (see below).

Clinical signs

A series of major and minor criteria for the diagnosis of canine AD have been proposed (*Table 10*). The lesions of AD are largely due to pruritus and self-trauma and classically affect the face and dorsal feet, but they may extend to the ventral abdomen and flanks or become generalized (222–224). A recent study has defined breed-associated clinical phenotypes in dogs with AD. In investigative studies the clinical severity of AD is often enumerated using the 'canine atopic dermatitis extent and severity index' (CADESI). AD in cats is also pruritic and may involve the head alone or become generalized. The clinical presentation includes ulcerative facial dermatitis, symmetrical alopecia, papular dermatitis,

Table 10: Diagnostic criteria for canine atopy. A diagnosis of atopy in the dog requires that at least three of the major and three of the minor criteria defined by Willemse in 1986 be satisfied (Willemse T (1986) Atopic skin disease: a review and reconsideration of the diagnostic criteria. *Journal of Small Animal Practice* **27**:771–778). An alternative scheme proposed by Favrot in 2010 allows diagnosis of canine AD with sensitivity of 85% and specificity of 79% when five of eight criteria are statisfied. (Favrot C, Steffan J, Seewald W *et al* (2010). A prospective study on the clinical features of chronic canine atopic dermatitis and its diagnosis. *Veterinary Dermatology* **21**:23–30).

Major criteria of Willemse (at least three required)
- Pruritus.
- Facial and/or digital involvement.
- Lichenification of flexor and/or extensor surfaces of carpus or tarsus.
- Chronic or chronically relapsing dermatitis.
- An individual or family history of atopy.
- Breed predisposition.

Minor criteria of Willemse (at least three also required)
- Onset before three years of age.
- Facial erythema and cheilitis.
- Bacterial conjunctivitis.
- Superficial staphylococcal pyoderma.
- Hyperhidrosis (increased sweating).
- Positive intradermal skin test.
- Increased allergen-specific IgE or IgG subclass.

Criteria of Favrot
- Onset of signs under three years of age.
- Dog living mostly indoors.
- Glucocorticoid-responsive pruritus.
- Pruritus sine materia at onset (i.e. alesional pruritus).
- Affected front feet.
- Affected ear pinnae.
- Non-affected ear margins.
- Non-affected dorso-lumbar area.

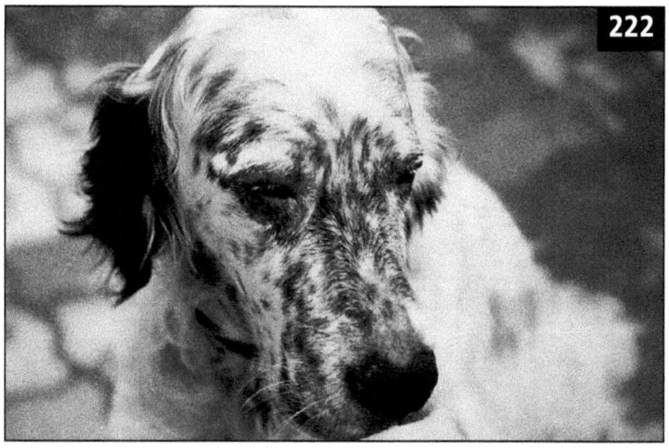

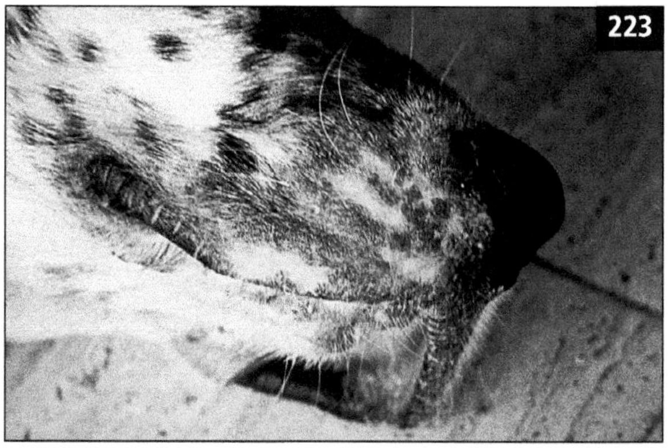

222–224 Canine atopic dermatitis. A three-year-old English Setter with severe pruritus affecting the face, axillary and inguinal regions, pinnae and dorsal aspect of the paws. Conjunctivitis (**222**) and cheilitis (**223**) are marked in this case. Alopecia, erythema and lichenification are secondary to chronic self-trauma (**224**).

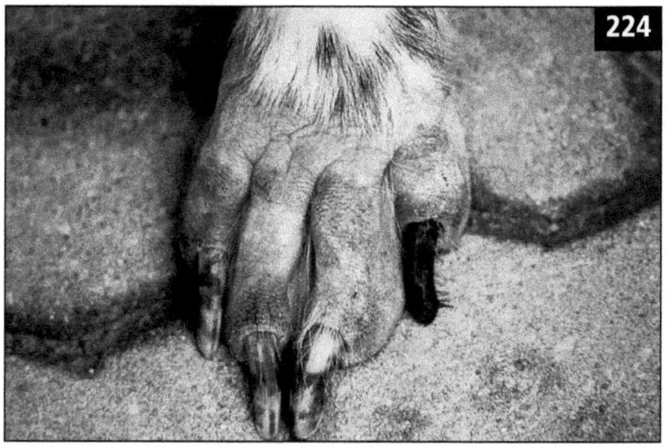

eosinophilic granuloma or combinations thereof. These are also the clinical presentations of other allergic skin diseases in the cat (225, 226).

Diagnosis

The diagnosis of AD proceeds through several stages (227). Clinical examination may reveal lesions of specific distribution in a young dog of a susceptible breed. The presence of complicating flea or food allergy should be determined by investigating the response to appropriate ectoparasite control and restriction diets. Secondary infection should be controlled by appropriate topical and/or systemic antimicrobial therapy and any immunosuppressive therapy should be withdrawn for 4–6 weeks prior to specific immunodiagnosis. The recognized 'gold standard' for immunodiagnosis of canine AD is the intradermal skin test (IDST) (228–230) using a panel of antigens (*Table 11*). Allergen preparations may vary widely in terms of antigen concentration and content. False-positive and false-negative

225

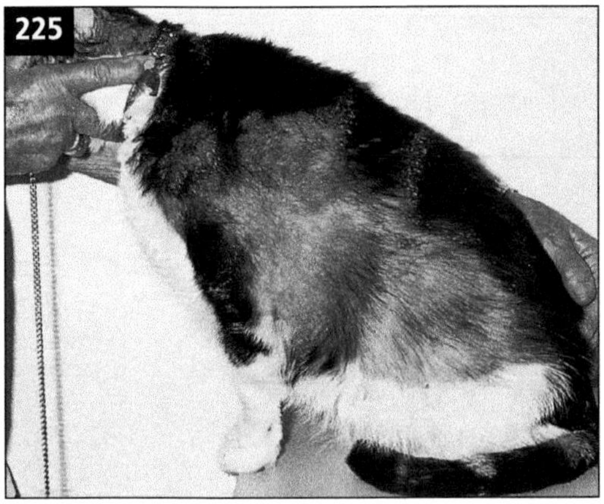

226

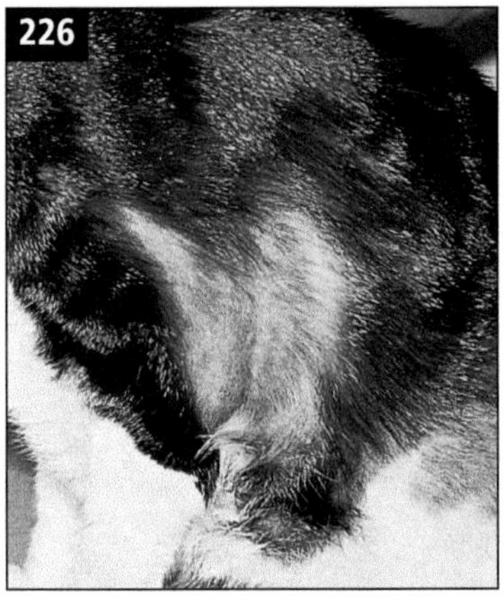

225, 226 Feline symmetrical alopecia. A five-year-old DSH cat with bilateral truncal alopecia secondary to overgrooming. The cat was unresponsive to an insecticidal trial for fleas and an eight week restriction diet. Intradermal skin testing was positive for house dust mites and several weed pollens.

227

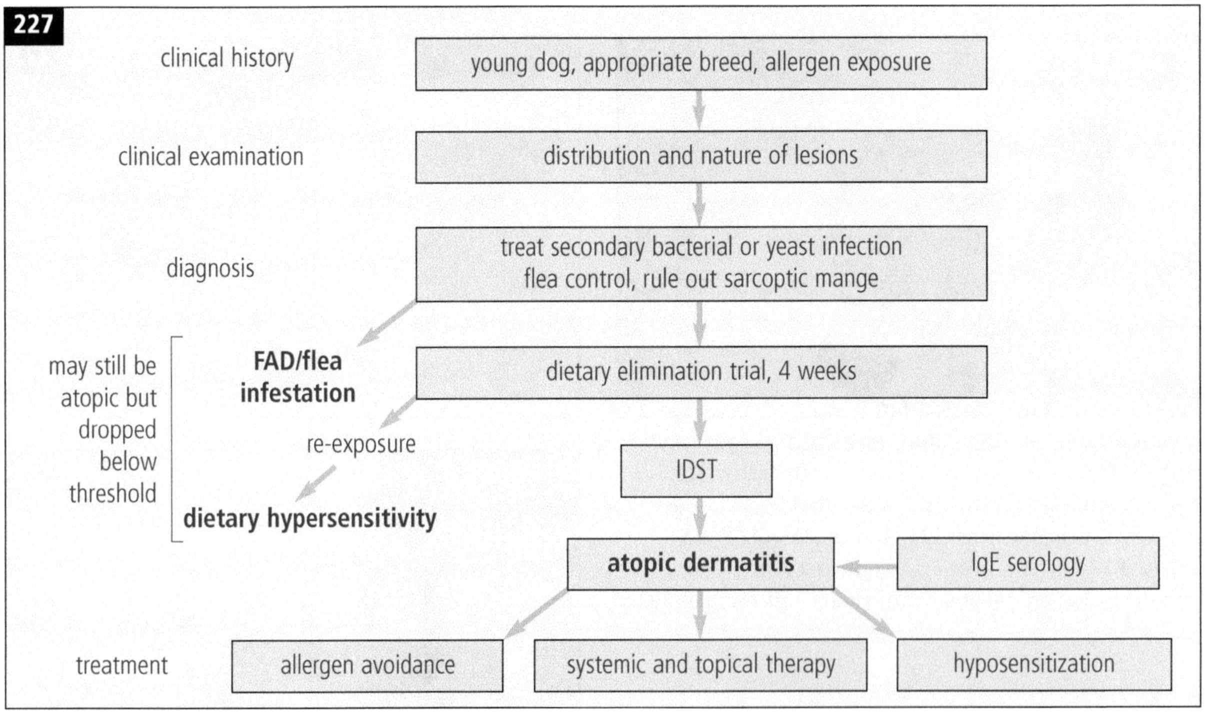

227 Diagnostic flow chart for canine atopic dermatitis. Diagnosis of canine AD should follow the sequence of events depicted in this flow chart. Flea allergy dermatitis, sarcoptic mange and dietary hypersensitivity should be ruled out before a definitive diagnosis of AD is made. Treatment may include appropriate systemic and topical measures; allergen-specific immunotherapy (ASIT) may be effective in 50–80% of cases.

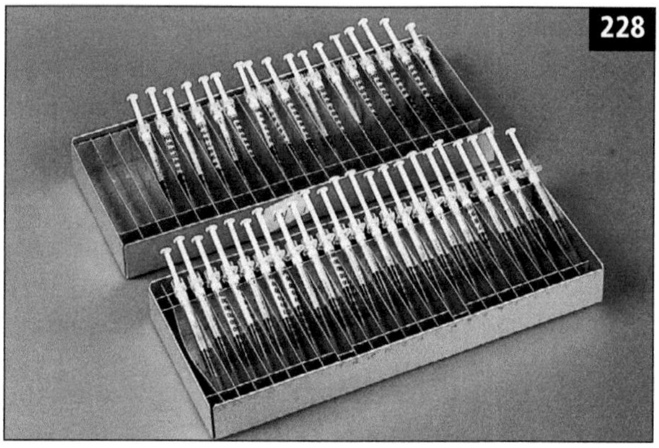

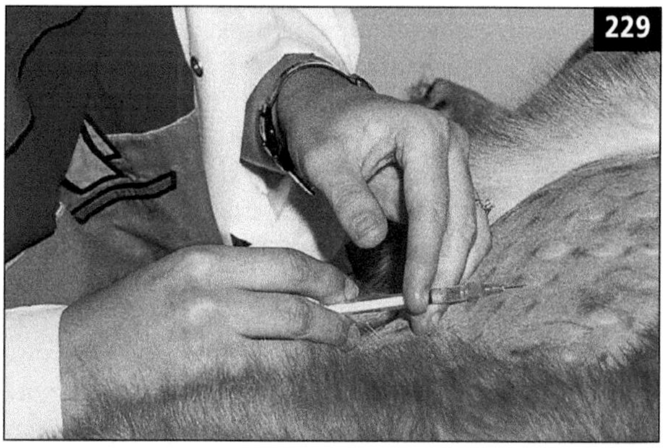

228–230 Intradermal skin testing. (**228**) Sequential intradermal injections of allergen using a 1 ml syringe and a 28 gauge needle are made into a site on the lateral thorax. The site should be carefully clipped, no chemical skin preparation used and areas of lesional skin should be avoided. (**229**) Approximately 0.05 ml of each allergen is injected. The wheal response is compared to a positive control of histamine and a negative control of sterile saline. The test is read at 15–20 minutes for immediate hypersensitivity responses; delayed reactions (8–48 hours) may be recorded as well (**230**).

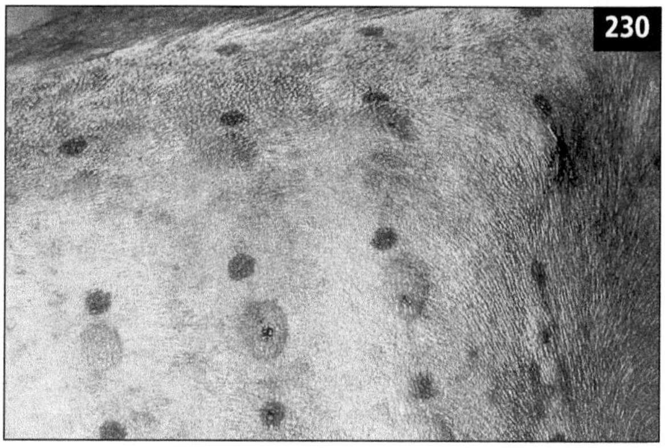

Table 11: Allergen panel for intradermal skin testing. Intradermal skin testing is generally performed using a panel of allergens such as those listed. The allergens cover the major groups of indoor and outdoor environmental allergens, dependent on the geographical location and the supplier of allergen used. Most panels include between 30–55 allergens.

Group	Allergen panel
Mites/dust group	House dust, house dust mite *(Dermatophagoides pteronyssinus)*, flour mite (*Dermatophagoides farinae*)
Epithelial group	Cat hair, human dander, horse epithelia, mixed feathers, cotton linters
Insect group	Flea (*Ctenocephalides felis*), insect mix
Mould and smut group	Mould mix (*Aspergillus* spp., *Alternaria* spp., *Penicillium* spp., *Rhizopus* spp.), smut mix (barley, oat, wheat smut)
Tree group	Privet, Scotch elm, white willow, English oak, white poplar, sycamore maple, European ash, European beech, black alder, white birch
Grass group	Italian ryegrass, quack grass, timothy grass, meadow fescue, cultivated oatgrass
Weed group	Mugwort, lambs quarter, English plantain, sheep sorrel, curly dock, dandelion, nettle, red clover

results are recognized. The IDST is also of value in the cat, but the wheals formed are generally smaller and poorly circumscribed. For this reason, a recent experimental study has reported the use of intravenous administration of fluorescein solution in assessing these reaction sites. Patch testing (percutaneous challenge with allergen) has recently been described in the dog and cat; however, it is currently restricted to the research setting, as there are practical difficulties with maintaining positioning of such patches for the appropriate period of time. Patch test sites show similar cellular infiltration to lesional atopic skin (see above) in both species.

Detection of circulating allergen-specific IgE (and IgG) antibodies by ELISA has now become widely available as an alternative diagnostic test (**231, 232**); ELISA-based, in-office screening tests for allergen groups have also been produced. Studies comparing the IDST and ELISA have suggested that there is a poor correlation, as normal (or parasitized) dogs may give false-positive reactions by ELISA, and dogs with AD may have a false-negative result, as not all mast cell-bound antibody will necessarily be circulating. In recent years, improved tests based on the use of monoclonal antibodies to IgE or identification of IgE using biotinylated FcεR1 α chain have emerged, but even these tests do not completely correlate to IDST, with sensitivity and specificity for ELISA varying between different antigens. Measurement of total serum IgE is not of use in the diagnosis of canine AD and such assays are affected by the presence of serum IgG autoantibodies specific for IgE. Normal dogs have a relatively high level of serum IgE, which varies between studies but is most recently reported as 1–41 μg/ml. This is considerably greater than human serum IgE concentration and likely reflects increased exposure to endoparasites in the dog. Dogs with AD do not have significant elevations in IgE concentration, but they may have a reduction in serum and skin surface concentration of IgA and raised serum IgG. Allergen-specific IgE (to dust mites) has been identified in both normal and atopic cats, therefore allergen-specific ELISA correlates poorly with IDST in this species. Allergen-specific IgG antibodies are also documented in cats with allergic skin disease.

An *in vitro* assay measuring histamine release following the stimulation of circulating basophils by allergen has been described, but it is not readily applicable to routine diagnosis. Similarly, responsiveness of cultured blood lymphocytes to allergen stimulation *in vitro* (see above) is a useful

231

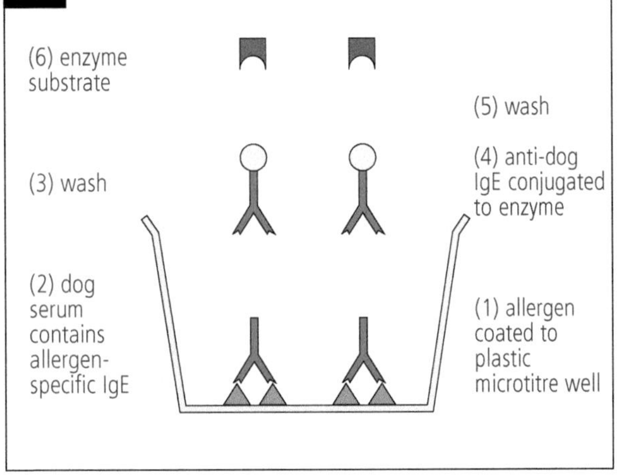

232

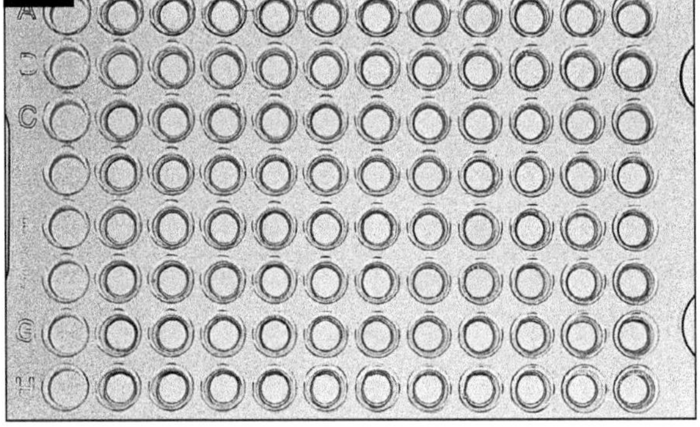

231, 232 ELISA for detection of allergen-specific IgE. (**231**) In the ELISA for allergen-specific IgE, diluted serum from the patient is added to a series of plastic microtitre wells that have been coated with individual allergens in a regional panel. After a period of incubation, unbound serum antibody is removed by washing and an enzyme-conjugated (e.g. alkaline phosphatase) antiserum specific for canine or feline IgE added. Following this second incubation the wells are again washed, before addition of enzyme substrate. Colour change after a defined interval is read spectrophotometrically using an ELISA plate reader. Positive reactions are generally defined relative to positive and negative control wells and a numerical grading system is sometimes employed. (**232**) A completed ELISA demonstrating the colour change that occurs using alkaline phosphatase as a substrate. The wells in column 1 have been left empty (plate blank) and the negative control wells are in row A (numbers 2–7).

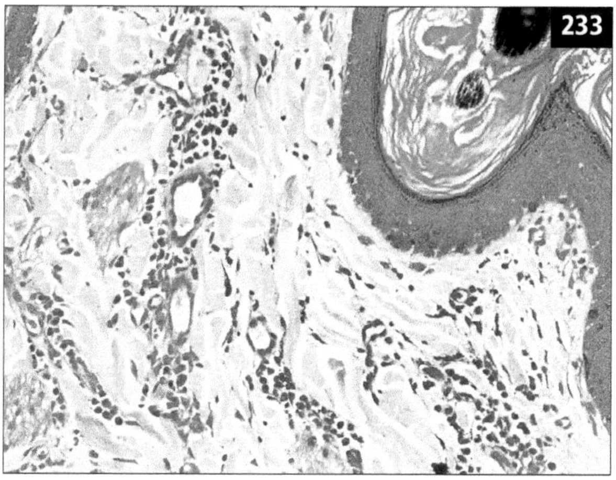

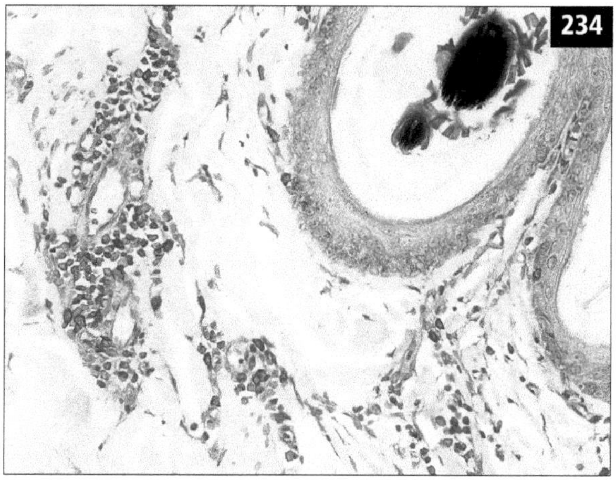

233, 234 Histopathology of canine hypersensitivity dermatitis. (**233**) Skin biopsy from a dog with hypersensitivity dermatitis demonstrating epidermal hyperplasia, hyperkeratosis, dermal oedema and superficial perivascular inflammation with prominent mast cells and eosinophils. (**234**) Mast cells in a serial section are stained by toluidine blue. (From Day MJ [1998] Mechanisms of immune-mediated diseases in small animals. *In Practice* **20**:75–86, with permission.)

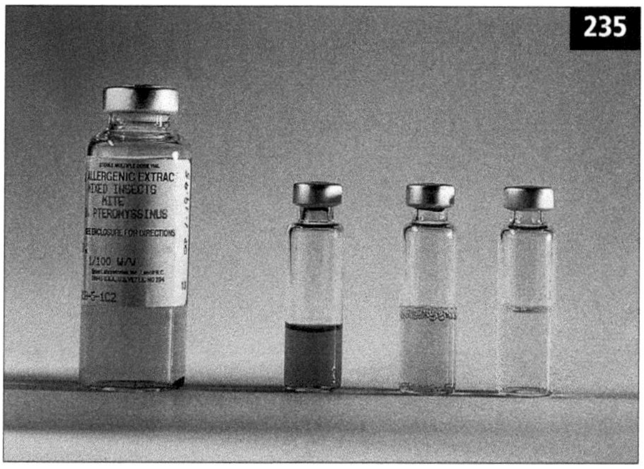

235 Allergen-specific immunotherapy for canine and feline atopic dermatitis. ASIT involves induction followed by subsequent maintenance therapy. In the induction phase, allergens are formulated based on the intradermal skin test results, and increasing doses are given over a period dependent on the protocol used. A sample protocol is illustrated (*Table 12,* p. 134). Maintenance therapy involves a booster injection of a fixed, usually maximum concentration of allergen given every 2–4 weeks depending on clinical response. Most dogs require lifelong therapy.

research tool, but such tests are not used diagnostically. Skin biopsy (233, 234) can support the clinical impression of type I hypersensitivity, but cannot distinguish between flea allergy, food allergy or atopic dermatitis.

Treatment

Therapy for AD must be individualized to the patient and depends on whether acute flares or chronic disease is being managed. Extensive guidelines are given by the international Taskforce (see Further Reading).

- For acute flares, the cause of the flare should be identified and removed if possible and treatment with non-irritating baths and topical glucocorticoids given. Oral glucocorticoids and anti-microbial therapy should be used where required.

For chronic disease, management includes

- avoidance of flare factors
- non-irritating shampoos
- essential fatty acid supplementation
- Immunomodulatory therapy involving the use of topical or oral glucocorticoids, oral ciclosporin and topical tacrolimus. Ciclosporin also appears to be an effective treatment for management of various forms of feline allergic dermatitis (eosinophilic granuloma complex [see below] or idiopathic pruritus) refractory to glucocorticoid therapy.
- Allergen-specific immunotherapy (ASIT; hyposensitization). This involves the repeated administration by subcutaneous injection of the causative allergens at increasing doses over a period of time (235, *Table 12*, p. 134).

Table 12: Allergen-specific immunotherapy sample protocol. There are numerous protocols used for allergen-specific immunotherapy (ASIT) and these are dependent on the commercial source (and nature of formulation) of the allergens used. Shown is one example that presents the principle of the induction and maintenance phases of therapy. This protocol relates to the use of the product Artuvetrin™, in which allergens are adsorbed onto aluminium hydroxide and diluted in saline. Up to eight allergens may be incorporated into the ASIT injection with this product.

Dosage during the induction period		**Dosage during maintenance period**	
Week number after start of treatment	**Dosage (ml)**	**Week number after start of treatment**	**Dosage (ml)**
1	0.2	16	1.0
2	0.4	20	1.0
4	0.6	24	1.0
6	0.8	28	1.0
9	1.0	etc.	1.0
12	1.0		

236

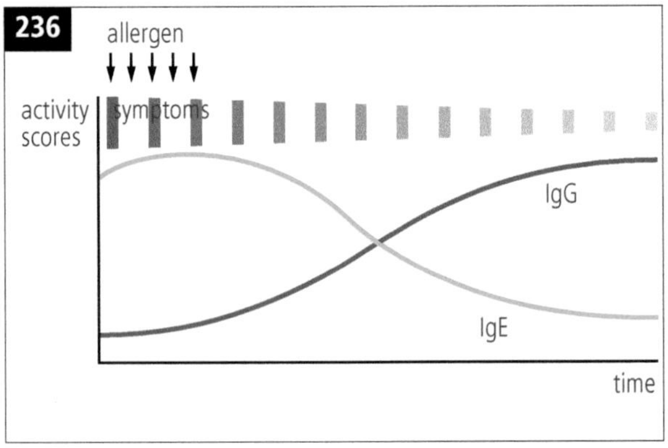

236, 237 Immunological basis of ASIT. (**236**) In ASIT there is an elevation of serum allergen-specific IgG concomitant with a presumed decrease in allergen-specific IgE. (**237**) The precise mechanism of ASIT remains poorly understood, but may involve (a) the production of allergen-specific IgG 'blocking' antibody that competes for allergen with mast-cell bound IgE, (b) an alteration in the balance between Th1 and Th2 regulatory cells, and (c) the induction of IL-10 secreting regulatory T cells.

237

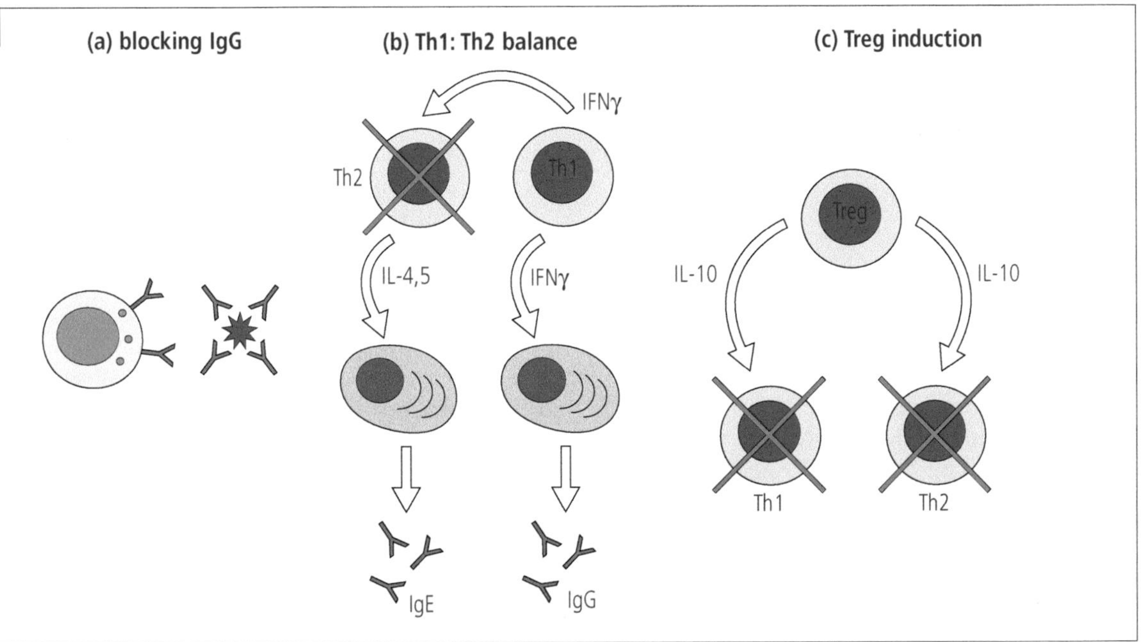

The proposed mechanism of ASIT is described in **236** and **237**. The reported efficacy of ASIT in canine AD is 50–80% (**238, 239**). Factors that decrease the chance of a successful outcome include increasing age and chronicity of clinical disease. A recent study has described induction of circulating Treg cells and increased serum IL-10 concentration in dogs subject to ASIT. Novel variations to ASIT protocols have been described including 'rush immunotherapy' (rapid administration of increasing doses of allergen every 30 minutes to achieve a maintenance dose within six hours) and the concomitant delivery of liposome-plasmid DNA complexes as a source of bacterial CpG motifs in order to skew the immune response towards Th1 immunity. Oral immunotherapy in experimentally-sensitized beagles did not have clear clinical benefit. In the model of Japanese cedar pollinosis described on page 128, experimentally sensitized dogs were injected intramuscularly five times with a plasmid containing the gene encoding Cry j1. Treated dogs showed a reduction in intradermal responses and bronchial hyper-reactivity on airway exposure. Serum allergen-specific IgE concentration was not significantly affected, but there was a reduction in the number of mast cells in airway mucosa. Long-term amelioration of clinical signs was also induced in three dogs with AD triggered by Cry j1. ASIT is also reported to be effective in feline allergic skin disease, with a successful outcome in up to 70% of cases.

- A recent study has demonstrated the efficacy of administration of commercially produced recombinant canine IFNγ (10,000 units/kg s/c given on three days per week over four weeks, with frequency of administration adjusted over a second four-week period) as a means of altering the Th2-Th1 balance in this disease. This product (Interdog®) is licensed for management of canine AD in Japan.

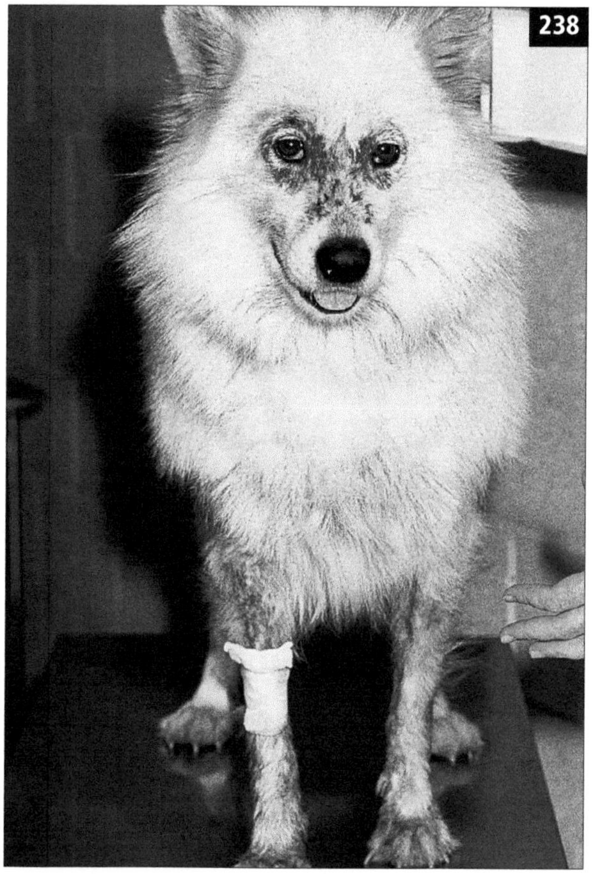

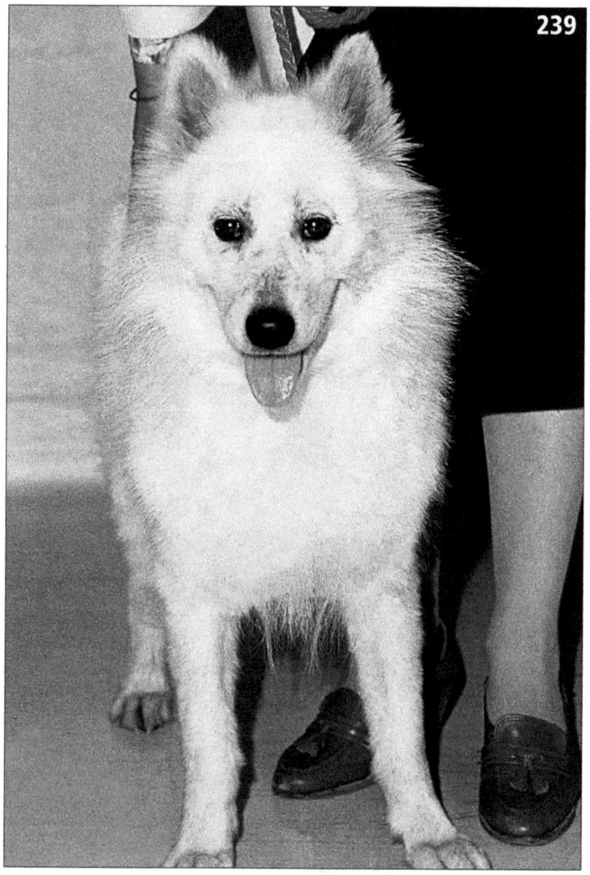

238, 239 Response to ASIT for atopic dermatitis. (**238**) A five-year-old Samoyed showing classical clinical signs of atopy. (**239**) Follow up 12 months after initiation of ASIT shows amelioration of clinical signs.

FLEA ALLERGY DERMATITIS

Pathogenesis

Flea allergy dermatitis (FAD) has a similar pathogenesis to AD. The causative allergens are components of flea saliva, which have now been cloned and sequenced. There is antigenic cross-reactivity between fleas, black ants, black flies and cockroaches, suggesting that FAD may be complicated by exposure to these insects. The Th2-regulated type I hypersensitivity pathogenesis of canine FAD has recently been proven in an experimental dog model. Allergic dogs challenged with fleas had elevation in the number of eosinophils and IgE^+ cells within skin biopsies, concurrent with increased expression of Th2 cytokine genes in biopsies and flea antigen-stimulated blood mononuclear cell cultures. It has been proposed that FAD may partially involve type III and type IV immunopathology. There is little evidence to support the former, but the possibility of a delayed reaction is suggested by histopathological studies characterizing lesional infiltrates of mononuclear cells. Alternatively, this may simply reflect the shift from Th2 to Th1 dominated immunity in chronic disease, as described above for AD. Lesional skin from cats with FAD has increased numbers of $CD4^+$ T cells and MHC class II bearing epidermal Langerhans

240
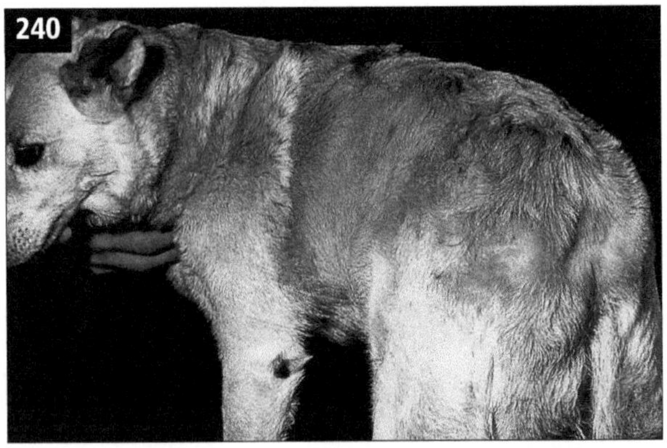

241
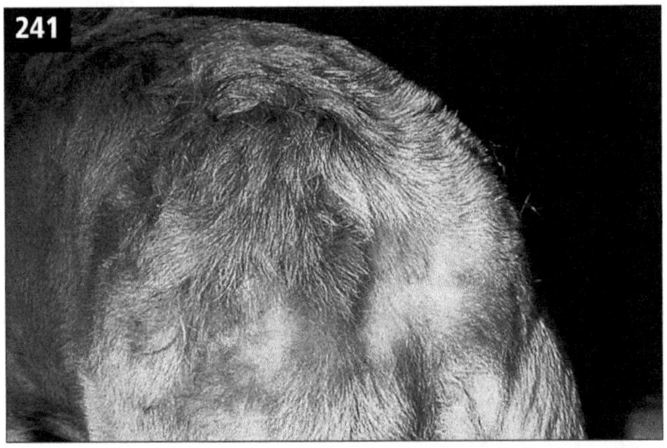

242
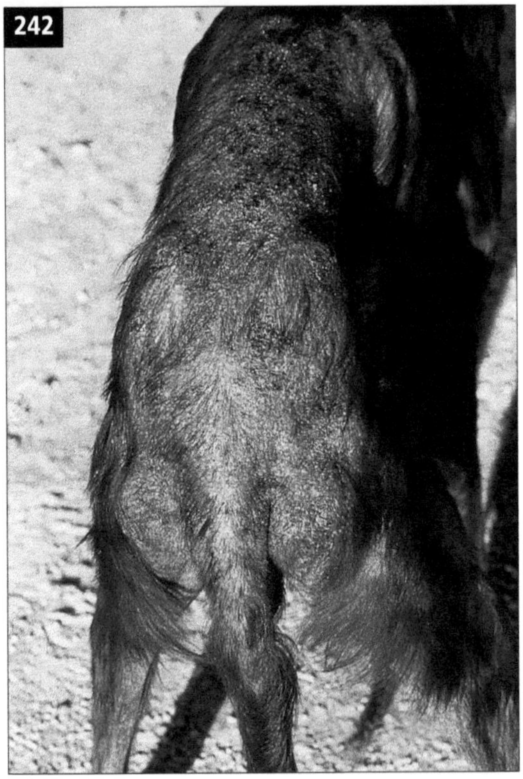

243
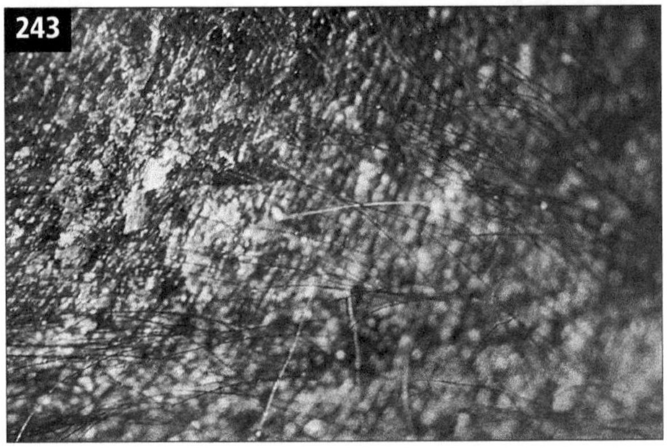

240–243 Canine flea allergy dermatitis. (**240, 241**) A six-year-old Labrador-Collie cross with acute pyotraumatic dermatitis affecting the skin of the right gluteal and tail head region. (**242, 243**) More chronic lesions of alopecia, hyperpigmentation and lichenification, classically affecting the skin of the tail head and dorsum, are illustrated in a six-year-old Irish Setter.

cells and dermal dendritic cells. A late-phase IgE-mediated reaction (8–24 hours) has also been proposed and, in an experimental challenge model, delayed type reactions at 24 and 48 hours were reported in some cats.

The most important factor predisposing to FAD is exposure to the causative agent (predominantly *Ctenocephalides felis* in the dog and cat), permitting sensitization and subsequent hypersensitivity. FAD may be seasonal (relating to hatching of flea eggs in warm temperature), but in warmer climates, or areas where central heating is common, seasonality is not necessarily a feature. Exposure to fleas does not always result in FAD, and it is suggested that some chronically exposed dogs may develop tolerance rather than hypersensitivity. Against this, a recent experimental study reported lesion development and elevation in allergen-specific IgE in dogs exposed to fleas either intermittently or continuously.

Clinical signs

The clinical signs of FAD are related largely to pruritus and self-trauma. In the dog, lesions of FAD involve the dorsal lumbosacral area and caudomedial thighs, although ventral abdominal, flank, neck or generalized lesions may occur (240–243). In the cat the syndrome most commonly associated with FAD is miliary dermatitis, although the other syndromes described for AD may occur (244, 245).

Diagnosis

Animals from environments without adequate flea control may have fleas or flea faeces within their hair coat. However, overgrooming may remove a significant proportion of adult fleas from the skin and such examination is not always rewarding. An important diagnostic procedure is determining clinical response to flea control (environmental and animal). Sensitized animals may respond to an IDST using flea allergen and have allergen-specific IgE and IgG serum antibodies. Western blotting studies have shown that serum IgE and IgG antibodies from flea allergic and non-allergic dogs react with a similar heterogeneous range of *C. felis* epitopes.

Treatment

Treatment of FAD is an integral part of diagnosis. There are an increasing number of flea control products and a description of these is beyond the scope of the present discussion. Therapy for secondary cutaneous infection using appropriate antimicrobial drugs may be necessary. In cases where pruritus is severe, short-term administration of anti-inflammatory drugs (*Table* 7, p. 125) may be required to prevent continued self-trauma. Hyposensitization using crude flea allergen has been evaluated in double-blind studies in the dog and cat and shown to be ineffective. A range of novel immunoprophylactic or immunomodulatory approaches to FAD are currently under investigation (see Chapter 16, p. 403).

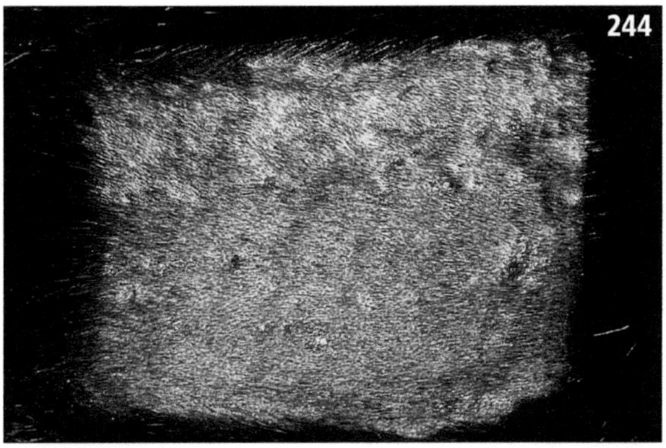

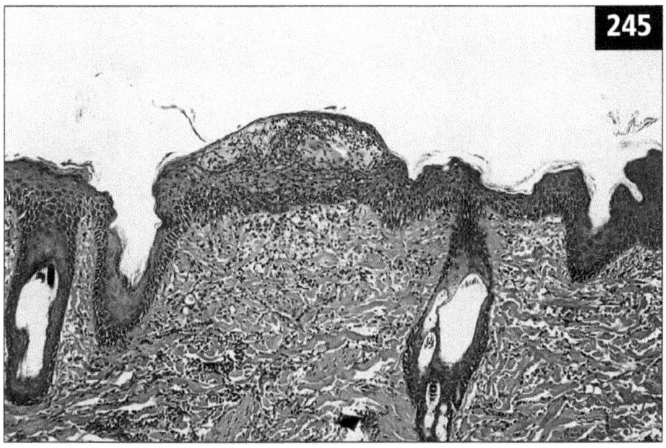

244, 245 Feline miliary dermatitis. (**244**) Papulocrustous dermatitis in a two-year-old DSH cat. Miliary dermatitis is a feline cutaneous reaction pattern commonly associated with flea allergy dermatitis. (**245**) Histopathology of the lesions in **244** shows epidermal hyperplasia with perivascular dermatitis involving eosinophilic infiltration, with eosinophil exocytosis into the epidermis and eosinophilic pustule formation. (Photographs courtesy A. Burrows.)

OTHER ARTHROPOD BITE HYPERSENSITIVITY SYNDROMES

Mosquito bite hypersensitivity

Mosquito bite hypersensitivity is documented in the cat and predominantly affects the face (nose, periorbital skin, ears) at the site of previous bites. The lesions progress from a symmetrical, erythematous eruption with papules and crusting, to the development of firm nodules, with severe ulceration and facial swelling occurring in some cases (**246**). The histological appearance is of ulceration, with dermal inflammation dominated by eosinophils. Mild collagen degeneration and eosinophilic folliculitis may occur, with some similarity to the feline eosinophilic granuloma complex. A type I hypersensitivity pathogenesis has been shown by intradermal testing of sensitized cats and Prausnitz-Kustner testing involving intradermal injection of serum from affected cats into normal animals, with subsequent challenge of the injection site by a mosquito bite. The lesions resolve when animals are housed indoors without access to mosquitoes.

Canine eosinophilic furunculosis/focal cutaneous eosinophilic granuloma

Canine eosinophilic furunculosis of the face and focal cutaneous eosinophilic granuloma may also be manifestations of arthropod bite hypersensitivity (**247**). The former is characterized by eosinophil-dominated furunculosis and small dermal foci of eosinophil degranulation and collagen degeneration. In canine eosinophilic granuloma there is collagen degeneration, with a surrounding inflammatory infiltrate composed of eosinophils and other inflammatory cell types.

Tick bites

Tick bites are likely to involve a type III/type IV hypersensitivity mechanism. These are focal lesions that have an acute erythematous/oedematous phase that progresses to a firm, nodular 'granuloma' or an area of ulceration and crusting. Histologically these lesions progress from wedge-shaped zones of necrosis and inflammation (eosinophils, lymphocytes and macrophages) to inflamed granulation tissue in the later stages (**248**).

Mite infestations

Type I hypersensitivity reactions are also part of the pathogenesis of the dermatitis caused by mite infestations. For example, type I hypersensitivity has been demonstrated in experimental and natural otitis externa caused by *Otodectes cynotis* and in infestation with *Sarcoptes scabiei* in the dog (**249**). A recent study has documented the development of serum IgE specific for *S. scabiei* in dogs experimentally infested with the mite, with epitope

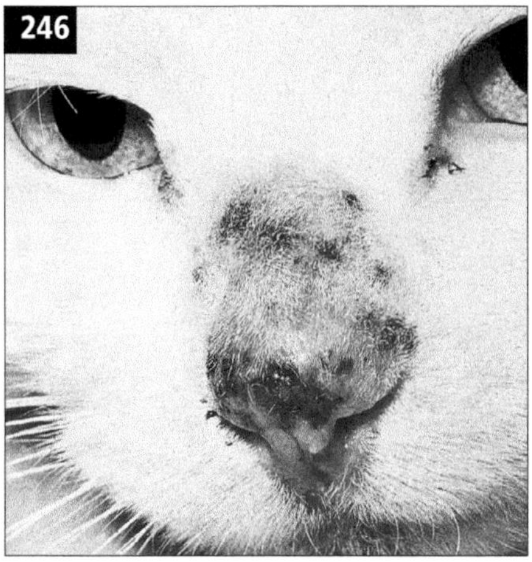

246 Arthropod bite hypersensitivity. Multifocal ulcerative lesions affecting the skin of the nasal dorsum and nasal planum in a four-year-old DSH cat. Marked swelling of the nasal and maxillary areas is present.

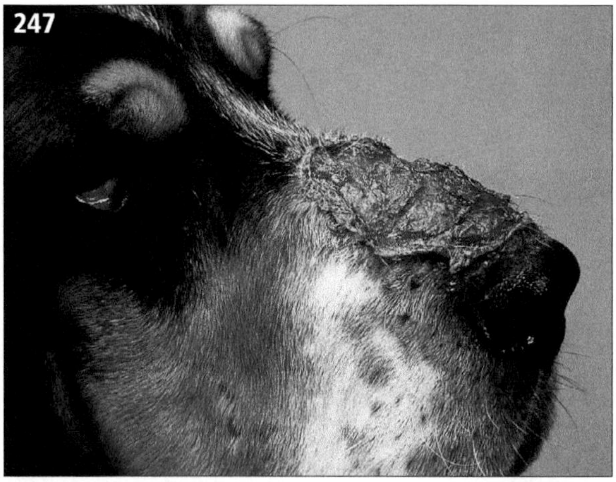

247 Eosinophilic furunculosis. Severe ulcerative lesion preceded by multifocal, coalescing papules affecting the dorsal nasal skin of a three-year-old Basset Hound. Hypersensitivity to arthropod bites was postulated to be the cause of this reaction.

spreading during the primary infestation. Interestingly, following scabicidal treatment the concentration of allergen-specific IgE increased and further epitope spreading occurred as the dead mites decomposed. On subsequent challenge there was 'self cure', which was associated with a strong and rapidly-induced IgE and IgG response.

FOOD INTOLERANCE AND DIETARY HYPERSENSITIVITY

The body may react inappropriately to ingested foodstuffs via non-immunological (food intolerance) or immunological (dietary hypersensitivity) mechanisms. Dietary hypersensitivity in the dog and cat is more often manifest as cutaneous than gastrointestinal disease (see Chapter 7, p. 206) or, less commonly, there may be both skin and gut involvement. The means by which dietary allergens are absorbed and cause intestinal or cutaneous sensitization are not fully understood. It is generally proposed that a type I hypersensitivity mechanism is involved, as food-specific serum IgE antibodies can be demonstrated. A recent study has characterized T-cell infiltration and cytokine gene expression in lesional and non-lesional skin from dogs with dietary hypersensitivity. Unlike AD, these lesions were dominated by $CD8^+$ T cells with increased transcription of genes encoding IL-4, IL-13 (Th2) and IFNγ (Th1).

The dietary allergens responsible for dietary hypersensitivity are poorly characterized and there are likely to be geographical differences dependent on the formulation of pet foods. Sensitization generally occurs over a long period of time, rather than the disease reflecting a recent dietary change. Reaction to more than one dietary protein is common.

Clinical signs

The clinical appearance of dietary hypersensitivity can mimic a range of other entities in both the dog and cat, and there are no pathognomic features. Signs may develop in a sensitized individual within minutes of exposure, but more often occur 4–24 hours post-allergen ingestion. The major cutaneous sign in the dog is pruritus, which may be associated with erythema, wheals, ulceration and crusting. Secondary infection is common. The lesions may be generalized or localized to the face, feet or ears. In the cat the presentation is of pruritus, with lesions ranging from miliary dermatitis, symmetrical alopecia and

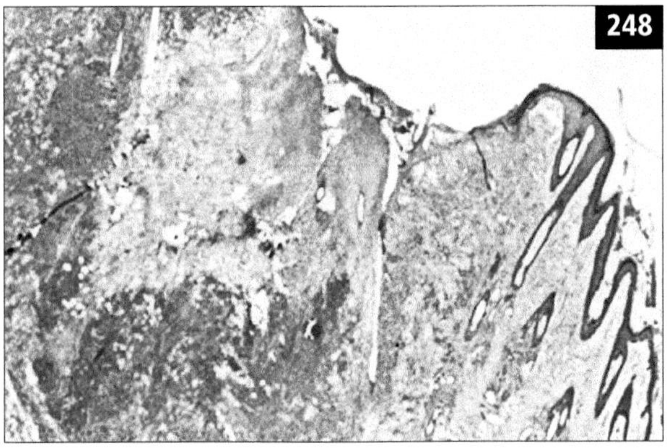

248 Tick bite. Biopsy of canine skin at the site of tick attachment. There is a central wedge-shaped zone of necrosis and ulceration surrounded by an intense lymphoplasmacytic inflammatory infiltrate. The pathogenesis of this reaction is likely to involve an hypersensitivity component. (From Shaw SE, Day MJ [2005] *Arthropod-Borne Infectious Diseases of the Dog and Cat.* Manson Publishing, London, with permission.)

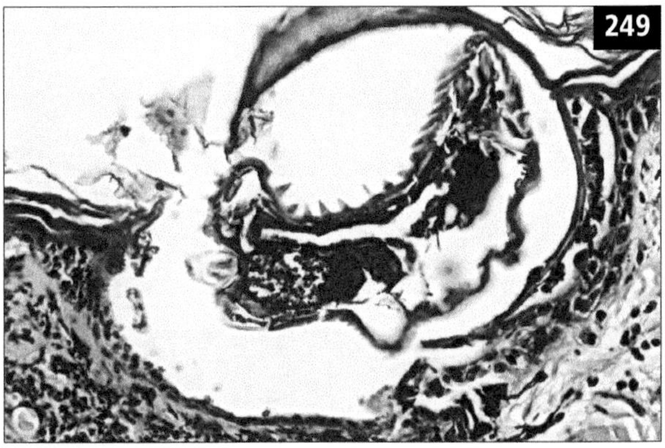

249 Sarcoptic mange. Section of skin from a dog with sarcoptic mange shows a *Sarcoptes* mite within the epidermis. Antigens derived from the mite are thought to trigger hypersensitivity reactions that play a role in the pathogenesis of the skin lesions induced by the ectoparasite.

eosinophilic granuloma to localized ulceration of the head and neck (250, 251).

Diagnosis

Diagnosis of dietary hypersensitivity involves assessment of clinical improvement (reduction in pruritus) following a restriction diet and deterioration following re-exposure. The animal is fed a diet containing a novel protein or hydrolyzed protein and carbohydrate source. The duration of the diet is controversial, but a minimum period of six weeks is usual. The diagnosis must be confirmed by reintroducing the normal diet and observing recurrence of clinical signs (usually within

250
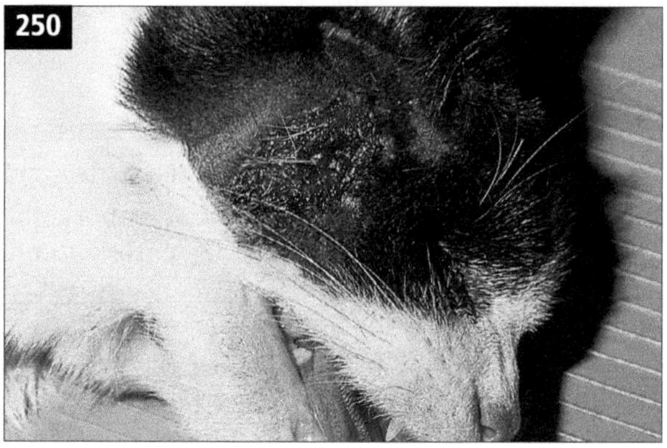

251
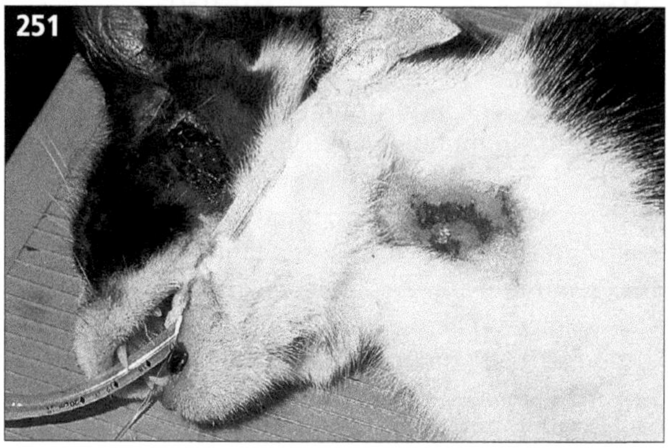

250, 251 Food allergy dermatitis. A two-year-old DSH cat with ulcerative dermatitis of the left cervical and parotid region secondary to self-trauma. The cat was unresponsive to an insecticidal trial for fleas, but responsive to a four-week restriction diet of venison. Reintroduction of the cat's original diet resulted in relapse of clinical signs within 72 hours.

252
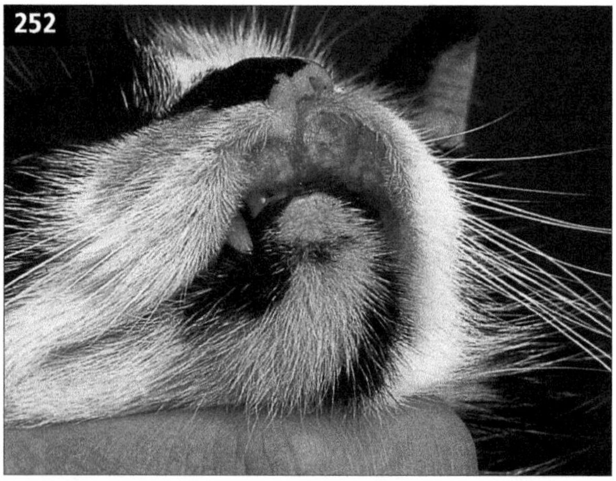

253
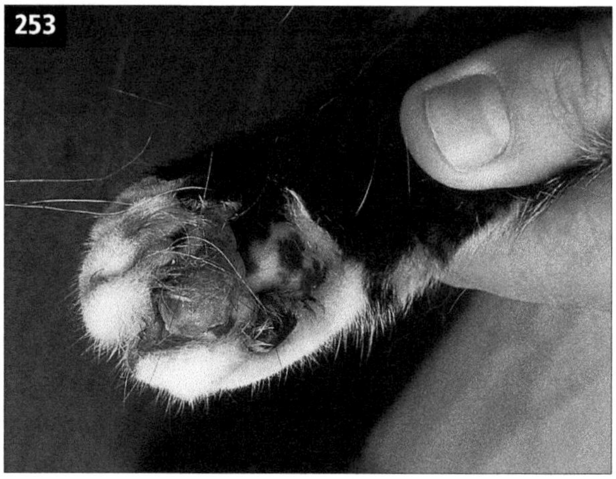

254
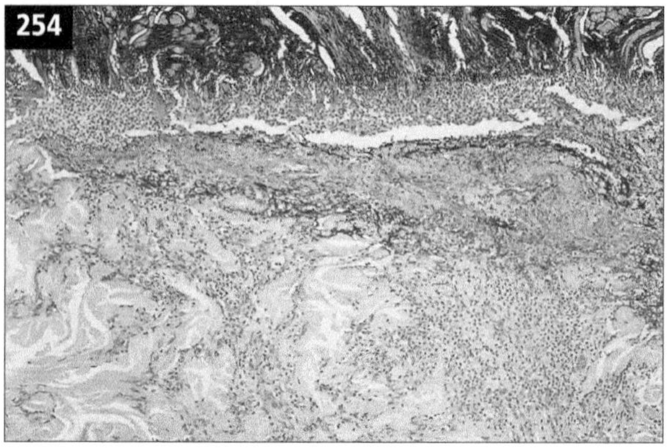

252–254 Eosinophilic (indolent) ulcer. (**252, 253**) A three-year-old semi-DLH cat with eosinophilic (indolent) ulcers affecting the upper lips and the foot pad. The cause in many cases remains obscure, but some may respond to antibiotic therapy. (Photograph courtesy H.A. Jackson.) (**254**) Eosinophilic ulcer from a four-year-old DSH cat. There is full thickness epidermal ulceration and crusting, with a mixed infiltrate of eosinophils, neutrophils and macrophages. Lymphoplasmacytic aggregates may occur chronically, but are not present in this biopsy.

12–72 hours). IDST is of no benefit. Numerous serological tests for dietary hypersensitivity are now commercially available, but there is poor correlation between the presence of allergen-specific IgE or IgG and clinical presentation of an individual case.

Treatment

The treatment of dietary hypersensitivity involves removal of the causative allergen and formulation of a nutritionally balanced replacement diet. Commercial hypoallergenic or hydrolysed protein diets are widely available. Adjunct therapy (antimicrobial, anti-inflammatory) may be required in the initial stages.

FELINE EOSINOPHILIC GRANULOMA COMPLEX

Feline eosinophilic granuloma complex (EGC) comprises three separate clinical syndromes (eosinophilic or 'indolent' ulcer, eosinophilic plaque, collagenolytic granuloma) affecting the skin and/or oral cavity; they may occur alone or concurrently. All are presumed to be reaction patterns for underlying disease, cutaneous hypersensitivity being the most common. However, identification of underlying disease may be difficult.

Eosinophilic ulcer

Eosinophilic ulcers usually occur unilaterally on the upper lip, but they can be bilateral. Lesions often have a characteristic central area of pinkish yellow tissue with a raised circumferential edge (252, 253). They occasionally affect the oral mucosa and other areas of skin. The histopathological features are shown in 254. Some cases are associated with underlying hypersensitivity, while others have been associated with infection. The true aetiology is unknown and this is illustrated by the diversity of therapeutic approach. Some cases respond to antibacterial drugs, but glucocorticoid therapy appears to be more effective (*Table 7*, p. 125). Surgical ablation, cryotherapy and radiotherapy have all been recommended for this syndrome, with variable success rates.

Eosinophilic plaque

Eosinophilic plaques occur most frequently on the abdomen and medial thighs, but they have been reported in other sites. They may be single or multiple, raised, red, often ulcerated and of varying size (0.5–7.0 cm diameter) (255–257). They frequently have a 'cobblestone' appearance. Unlike eosinophilic ulcers, these lesions are pruritic. Both blood and tissue eosinophilia are common.

255–257 Feline eosinophilic plaque. (**255**) A two-year-old DSH cat with multiple eosinophilic plaques affecting the trunk and lateral thighs. (**256**) The ulcerated tissue is pinkish yellow in colour, may be raised and is often separated from the surrounding skin by a 'rolled' edge. (**257**) The caudal aspect of the thighs is often affected. In all cases, causes of allergy (particularly fleas) should be ruled out.

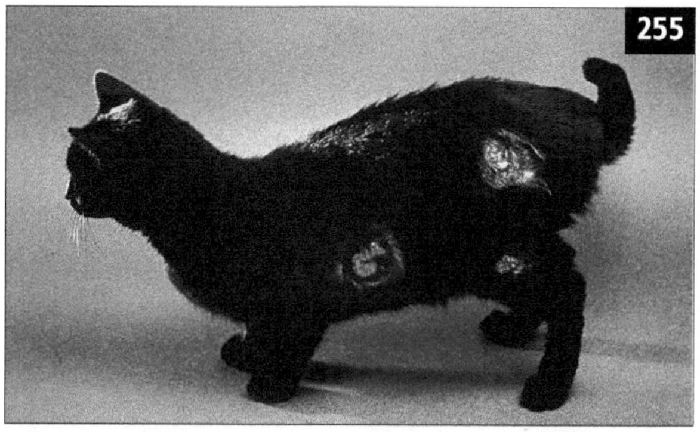

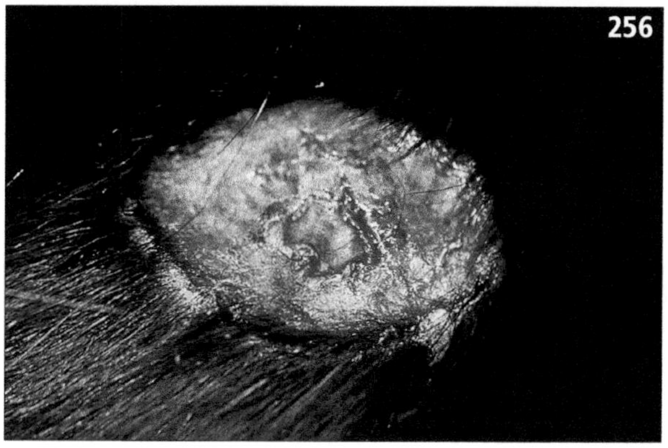

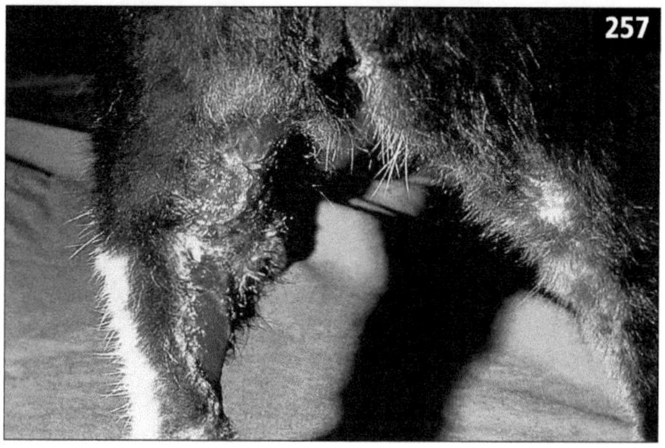

The histopathological features (**258**) are similar to those of miliary dermatitis (**245**). In cases of eosinophilic plaque, causes of allergy should be investigated thoroughly. Removal or control of the underlying cause and anti-inflammatory therapy (*Table* 7, p. 125) are recommended.

Collagenolytic granuloma (eosinophilic granuloma, linear granuloma)

These lesions most frequently occur on the caudal thighs and face (especially the chin and nose) and in the oral cavity and pharynx, although lesions affecting the footpads have also been reported (**259, 260**). Lesions affecting the thighs, trunk and oral cavity are typically raised, linear, pinkish yellow plaques, which may be pruritic. Facial and footpad lesions may be ulcerative or nodular. This is usually a disease of adult cats, but a rare form of familial granuloma complex is reported in kittens, which may regress spontaneously, except in the Turkish Van breed where the lesions persist. Tissue eosinophilia is common and blood eosinophilia may occur. Of the three lesions included in the EGC, this is the only one with 'granulomatous' pathology (**261, 262**). In common with eosinophilic ulcer, the underlying aetiology is unknown, although arthropod bites have been incriminated in some cases. Some cases respond to antibacterial therapy, but most require management with glucocorticoids (*Table* 7, p. 125).

CONTACT HYPERSENSITIVITY

An animal may develop cutaneous disease on contact with a range of chemical or biological substances. This may be simply due to the irritant nature of the substance (contact irritant dermatitis) or be due to a type IV hypersensitivity reaction (contact hypersensitivity dermatitis) (**263**). Sensitization may occur over a few weeks, but is

258
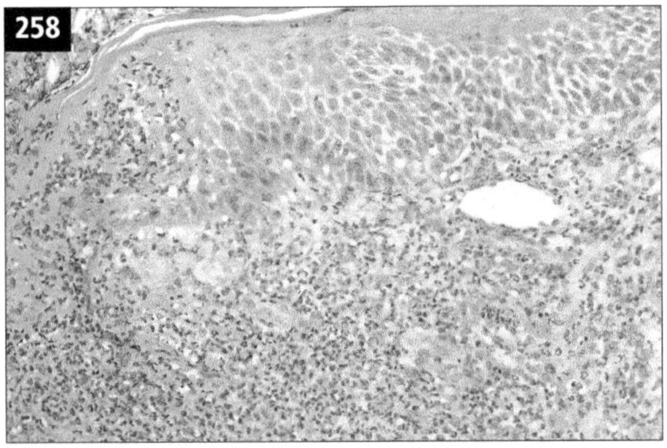

258 Feline eosinophilic plaque. Eosinophilic plaque from the inguinal region of a ten-year-old DSH cat. The epidermis is hyperplastic and spongiotic and there is an intense dermal infiltration of eosinophils, with focal eosinophil exocytosis.

259
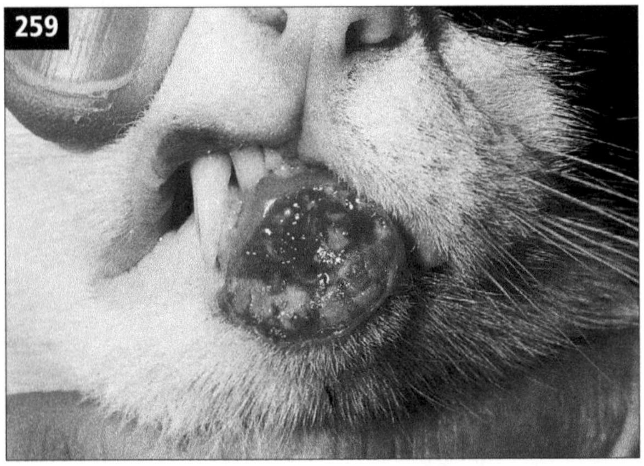

260
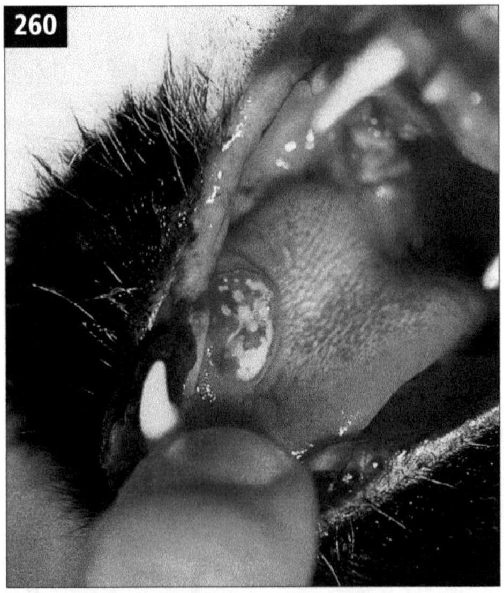

259, 260 Feline collagenolytic granuloma (linear granuloma). (**259**) Collagenolytic granuloma affecting the chin of a six-year-old DSH cat. (**260**) Collagenolytic granuloma of the oral mucous membranes and tongue of a four-year-old DSH cat. The cause in many cases cannot be determined, although causes of allergy must be ruled out.

more likely over a prolonged period of exposure. Naturally occurring contact hypersensitivity is uncommonly diagnosed in the dog, and diagnosis has rarely been supported by patch testing. Potential allergens include plants (pollens and sap), topical drugs and shampoos, synthetic substances such as furniture or carpet dyes, polishes and cleaners, rubber, plastic, leather and metal.

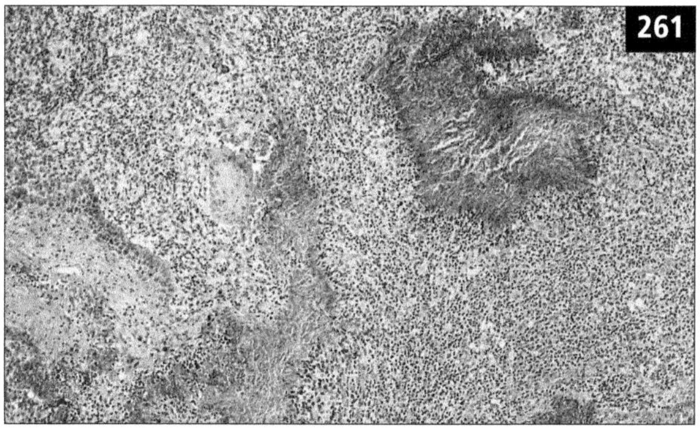

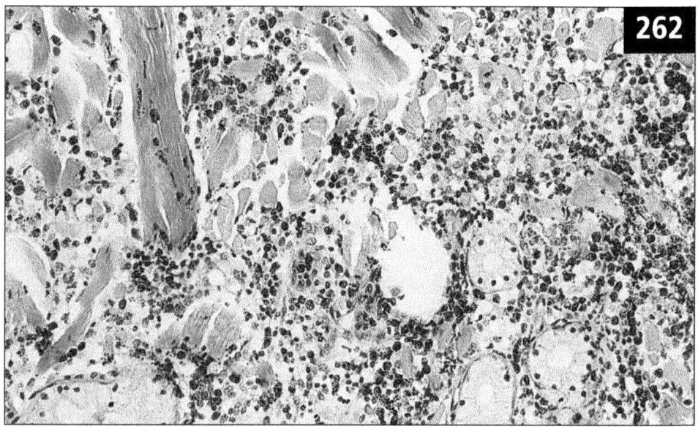

261, 262 Feline collagenolytic granuloma (linear granuloma). (**261**) Section of tongue from a three-year-old DSH cat with the oral form of collagenolytic granuloma. Large zones of eosinophilic material are surrounded by an intense infiltration of eosinophils and macrophages. It was originally proposed that the eosinophilic material was degenerate collagen, but ultrastructural studies have suggested that this comprises aggregates of degenerate eosinophils, and the alternative nomenclature of 'flame figure' has been proposed. (**262**) In this milder lesion there is some hyaline change to dermal collagen and infiltration of mixed eosinophils and macrophages.

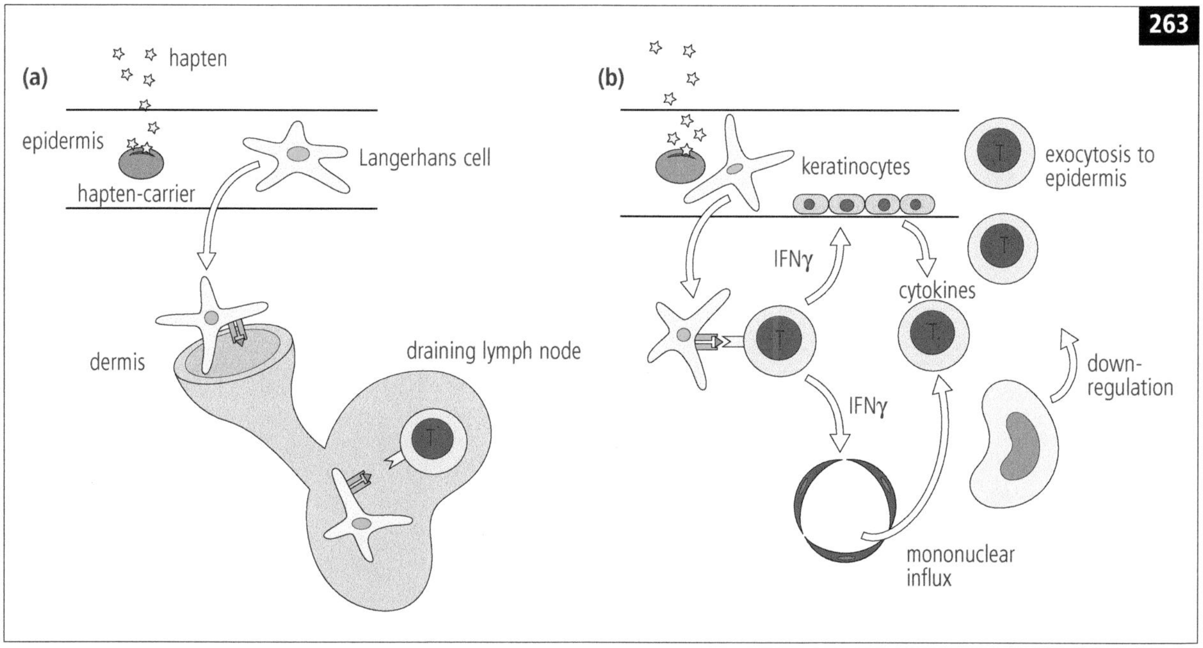

263a, b Mechanism of contact hypersensitivity. (a) During sensitization the hapten complexes with an epidermal carrier protein and is processed by epidermal Langerhans cells that migrate to the regional draining lymph node to present the antigen to CD4$^+$ T lymphocytes. **(b)** In a sensitized animal the hapten-carrier complexes are similarly processed, and antigen presentation to memory T cells occurs both within the draining lymph node and the dermis. Cytokines (IFNγ) released by activated T cells induce keratinocyte and vascular endothelial expression of MHC class II and ICAM-1 and release of pro-inflammatory cytokines (IL-1, IL-6, GM-CSF) by keratinocytes. Antigen-specific and non-antigen-specific T cells (CD4$^+$ and CD8$^+$) are attracted into the dermis and epidermis by chemokines and may bind to keratinocyte adhesion molecules. Macrophages are also attracted into the area and may release suppressive substances (e.g. prostaglandin E) that, in combination with T cell-derived cytokines (e.g. IL-10), down-regulate the response.

Clinical signs

Contact hypersensitivity presents with a defined distribution of lesions related to exposure to the allergen. It generally involves the sparsely haired surfaces of the ventral abdomen and thorax, and the limbs, tail, neck, chin, scrotum and ventral aspects of the haired areas of the paws (264–266). A localized (flea collar) or generalized (topical shampoo) distribution may occur. Pruritus is variable and a range of other lesions may be present including erythema, papules, plaques and hypo- or hyperpigmentation.

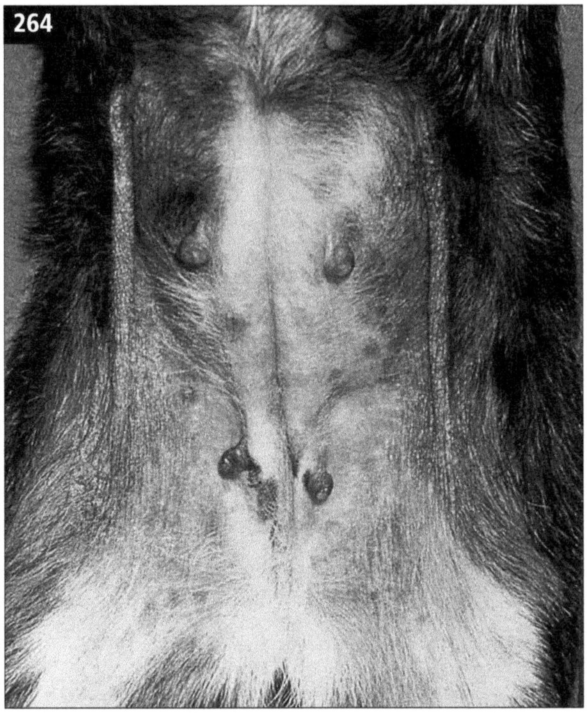

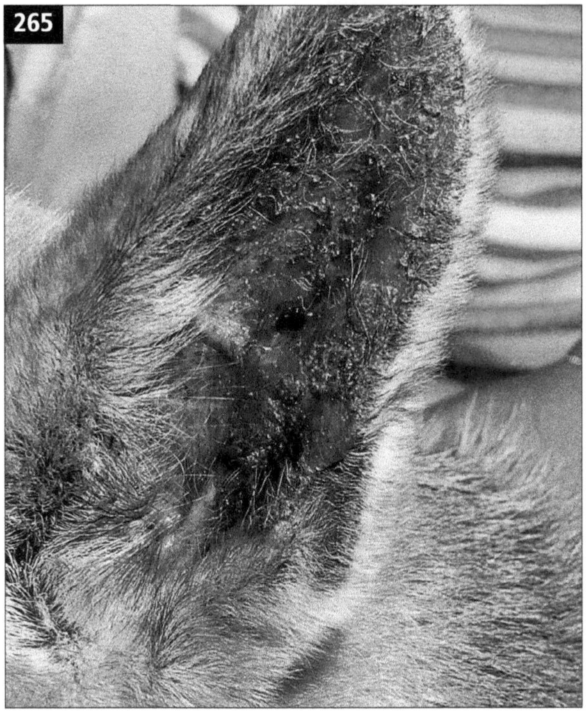

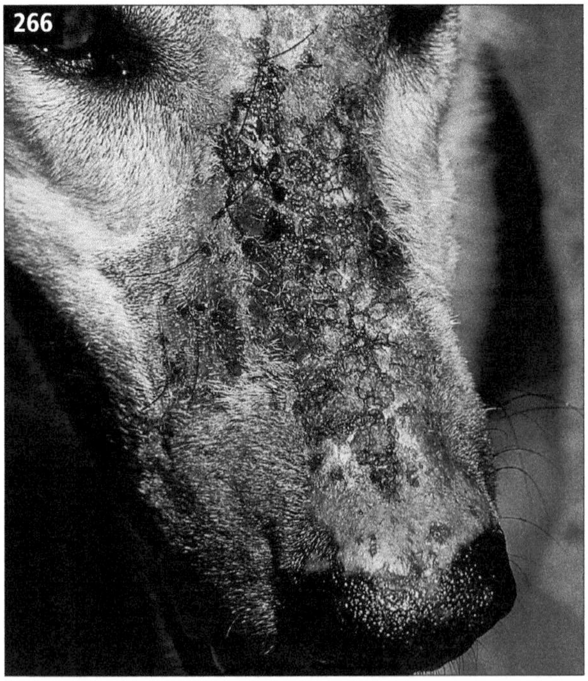

264–266 Contact sensitivity. (**264**) Contact sensitivity affecting the ventral abdomen of a five-year-old merle Collie dog. An allergic reaction to a plant of the *Grevillia* species was suspected by the owners and confirmed by recurrence of the lesions 72 hours after repeat exposure. (**265, 266**) Contact sensitivity affecting the internal aspect of the left pinna and vertical ear canal secondary to the application of a neomycin-containing topical preparation for aural and external use. The crusting, alopecic lesion affecting the haired skin of the nasal dorsum developed after the owner treated a small lesion in this area with the same preparation. The lesions regressed after drug withdrawal.

Diagnosis and therapy

Diagnosis of contact hypersensitivity is made by obtaining a clinical history of exposure and defining, by process of elimination, the causative allergen. Resolution of clinical signs following avoidance of the causative agent (for 7–10 days), with recurrence of clinical signs on re-exposure, is supportive but may not differentiate an irritant from a hypersensitivity pathogenesis. Provocative testing is theoretically required, but procedures such as patch testing (local exposure to contact allergen under a skin patch over 48 hours and then observation for 3–5 days) are difficult to perform in the dog and cat and are rarely employed. Histopathology cannot distinguish irritant from hypersensitivity contact lesions. Therapy involves avoidance of causative allergens, but anti-inflammatory drugs may be required if this is not possible.

CUTANEOUS VASCULITIS

Skin diseases with underlying dermal vasculitis are not commonly recognized in the dog and cat. Affected animals present with multiple foci of cutaneous ulceration and crusting, often of extremities such as the ear tip, nose, tail tip and footpads (267–270). The pathogenesis involves

267
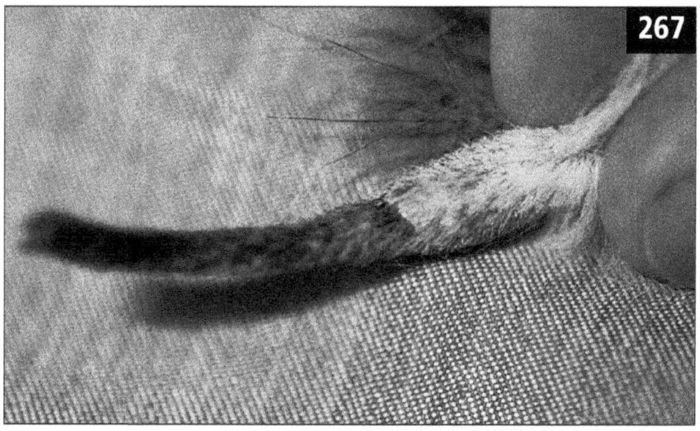

268
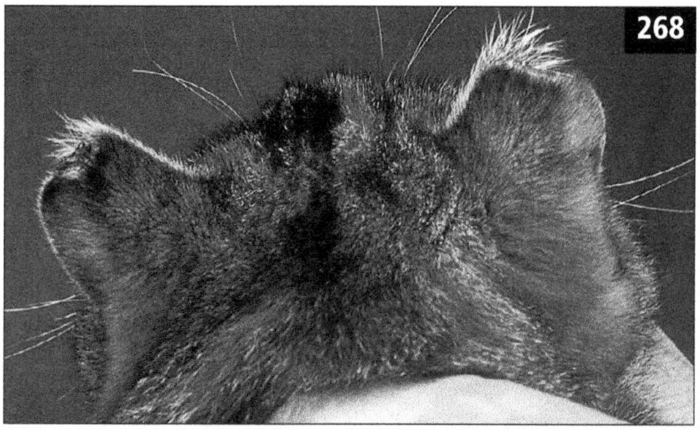

269

270
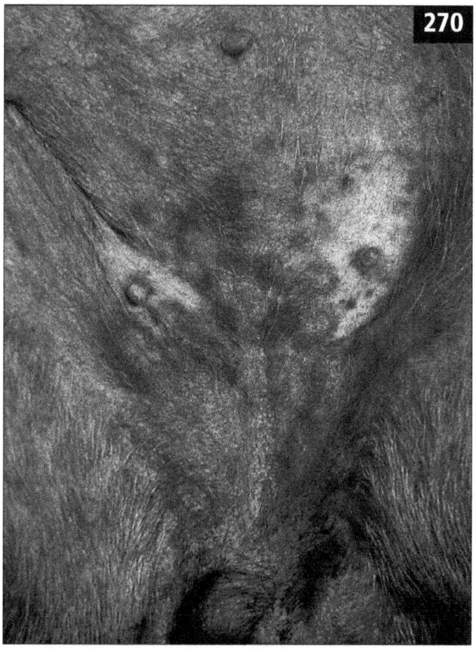

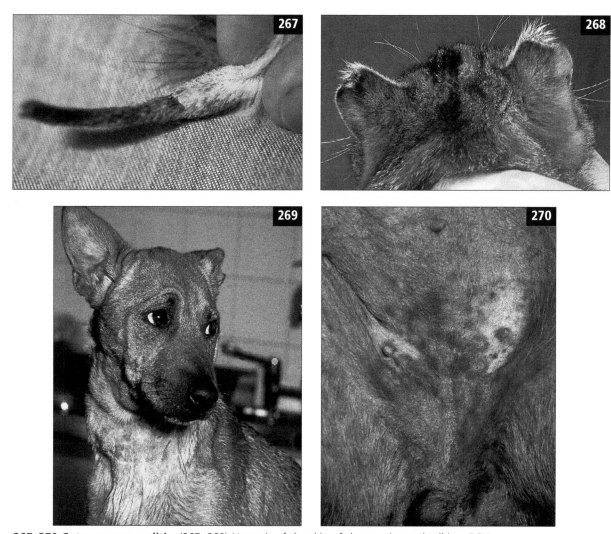

267–270 Cutaneous vasculitis. (**267, 268**) Necrosis of the skin of the ear tips and tail in a DSH cat as a consequence of vasculitis. The cause was not determined, but the cat was negative for cryoglobulins. (Photographs courtesy A.J. Shearer.) (**269, 270**) Annular haemorrhagic lesions in a four-year-old GSD-cross with acute vasculitis and septicaemia. (Photographs courtesy E.J. Hall.)

type III hypersensitivity, whereby circulating immune complexes are lodged within the small vessels of these areas of skin, initiating vasculitis and thrombosis with ischaemic necrosis of the skin supplied by the vessel. Multiple biopsies of fresh lesions may be required to identify the characteristic histopathological features (271–273).

Immunohistochemistry may demonstrate deposition of Ig and/or complement within vessel walls (155), but it is generally only of use when

271

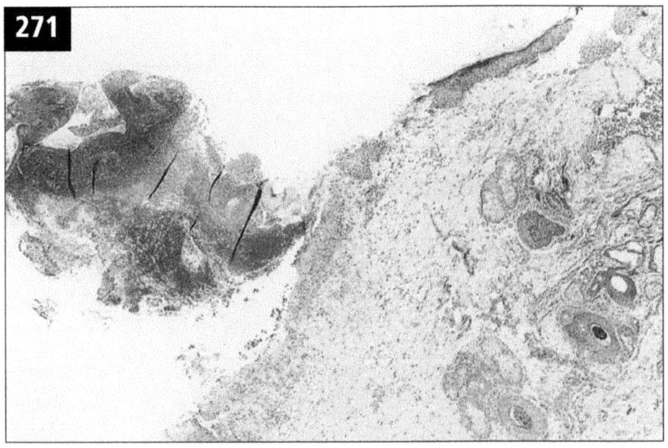

272

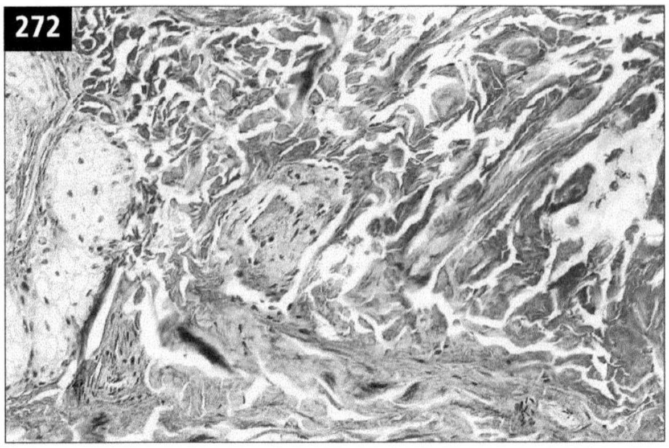

273

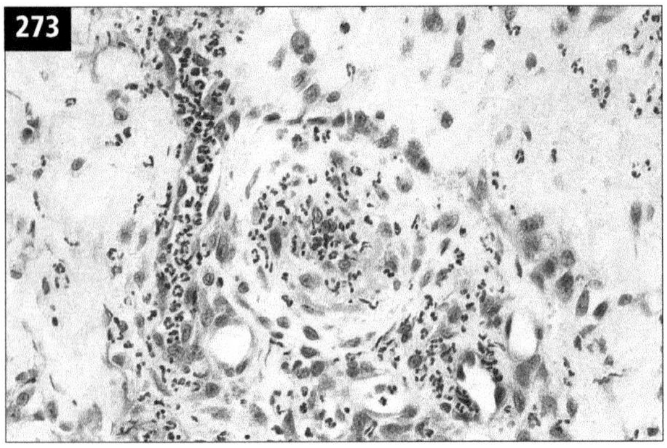

271–273 Cutaneous vasculitis. (**271**) Low power appearance of a skin biopsy from the ear of a three-year-old Dobermann with ischaemic necrosis of the margins of the pinnae. There is multifocal deep ulceration and crusting, with adjacent unaffected tissue. (**272**) Dermal blood vessels in this area have evidence of vasculitis and thrombosis. A fibrin thrombus is stained red by Martius scarlet blue. (**273**) Skin biopsy from a three-year-old GSD with immune-mediated polyarthritis (ANA positive) and ulcerative lesions of multiple footpads. There is leukocytoclastic vasculitis of dermal vessels in affected areas.

274

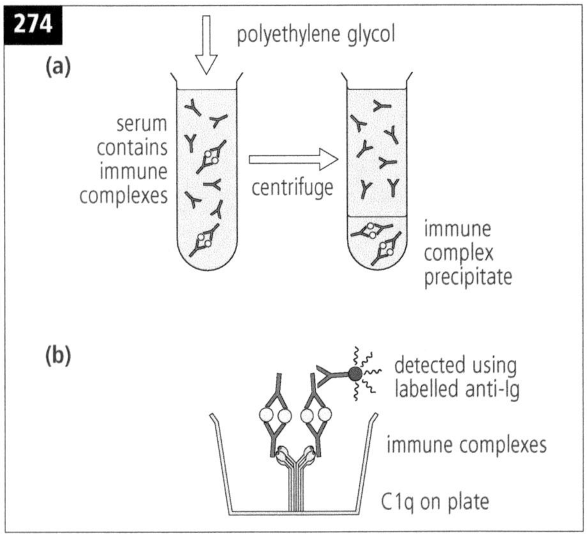

274a, b Detection of circulating immune complexes. CICs have been quantified in the serum of dogs using a variety of methods. **(a)** In the simplest method, polyethylene glycol is added to serum which, at a specific concentration, results in precipitation of complexed IgG while free IgG remains in solution. The precipitated immune complexes are separated by centrifugation, washed and redissolved in buffer. The IgG content of the immune complexes can then be determined. In a similar fashion, immune complexes have been precipitated from the serum of dogs using an equine C1q-like factor that has affinity for complexed Ig. **(b)** An alternative method relies on the affinity of immune complexes for the C1q component of complement. C1q may be attached to a solid phase such as a plastic tube or microtitre plate and immune complexes within a serum sample are taken up via the Fc region of Ig. Bound IgG is detected using radiolabelled antiserum specific for IgG. CICs have also been detected by incubating serum with a B cell lymphoma line (Raji cells) that expresses the C3 receptor, and subsequently measuring the amount of ^{125}I labelled rabbit anti-dog IgG affixed to the IgG within the complex.

lesions are less than 18 hours old. The causative antigens are rarely identified, but vasculitis may occur as part of an underlying systemic disease (e.g. infection or neoplasia). Drug administration (e.g. potentiated sulphonamides) or vaccine antigens (e.g. rabies vaccine) have been incriminated in both the dog and cat. Adjunct immunodiagnostic testing may reveal increased levels of circulating immune complexes (274), decreased serum complement (see Chapter 12, p. 294) and hypergammaglobulinaemia.

Treatment of cutaneous vasculitis involves managing the underlying cause and withdrawal of any concurrent drug therapy. Treatment with immunosuppressive (*Table 13*) or anti-inflammatory (*Table 7*, p. 125) drugs may be

Table 13: Systemically administered immunosuppressive drugs used for the treatment of immune-mediated skin diseases.

Drug	**Dose rate (cat)**	**Dose rate (dog)**	**Route of administration and comments**
Glucocorticoids			
Prednisolone	2.2–6.6 mg/kg q12h	1.0–2.0 mg/kg q12h	P/o. Taper to the lowest effective dose on alternate days
Methylprednisolone	1–2 mg/kg	1–3 mg/kg	P/o. Taper as above
Triamcinolone acetonide	0.2–0.3 mg/kg	0.2–0.3 mg/kg	I/m. For prednisolone resistant pemphigus foliaceus. S/c administration may cause leukotrichia and/or dermal atrophy over injection site
Dexamethasone	0.25 mg/cat	0.07–0.16 mg/kg	P/o. For prednisolone resistant cases
Dexamethasone sodium phosphate	5 mg/kg	5 mg/kg	Pulse therapy for resistant pemphigus foliaceus
Methyl prednisolone sodium succinate	20–30 mg/kg	20–30 mg/kg	As above
Others			
Azathioprine	NR	2.2 mg/kg q24h or q12h	In combination with glucocorticoids. Useful in management of the pemphigus group of diseases and lupus erythematosus. Use may be associated with bone marrow suppression and commensal overgrowth
Chlorambucil	0.1–0.2 mg/kg q24h or on alternate days	0.1–0.2 mg/kg q24h or on alternate days	Recommended for cats in combination with glucocorticoids. May cause bone marrow suppression and gastrointestinal disturbances

Continues on page 148

Table 13: Systemically administered immunosuppressive drugs used for the treatment of immune-mediated skin diseases. (*Continued*)

Drug	Dose rate (cat)	Dose rate (dog)	Route of administration and comments
Cyclophosphamide	NR	50 mg/m^2 on alternate days OR 1.5 mg/kg (dogs >25 kg); 2 mg/kg (dogs <25 kg); 2.5 mg/kg (dogs <5 kg)	P/o. Potent alkylating agent used alone or in combination with glucocorticoids. Use may be associated with leukopenia, haemorrhagic cystitis and gastrointestinal signs
Aurothioglucose	1 mg/kg/week	1 mg/kg/week	I/m. Clinical response to administration of gold salts may take 6–8 weeks; combination with glucocorticoids is recommended. May be associated with renal dysfunction, drug eruptions, hepatic necrosis and thrombocytopenia
Niacinamide and tetracycline		dogs <10 kg, 250 mg of each q12h; dogs >10 kg, 500 mg of each q12h	P/o. Use has not been reported in the cat
Vitamin E	400–800 IU q12h	400–800 IU q12h	P/o
Leflunomide		2–6 mg/kg q24h	P/o. Use until serum trough of 30 mg/ml for histiocytosis
Pentoxifylline		10 mg/kg q8–12h	P/o. Use for vasculitis

NR: not recommended.

required, and pentoxifylline has been used with some success. The prognosis is dependent on the severity of the underlying disease. A number of specific breed-related forms of vasculitis are described, including:

- Cutaneous vasculitis in Jack Russell Terriers.
- Vasculitis of the nasal planum in Scottish Terriers.
- Cutaneous and renal vasculopathy of racing Greyhounds.
- Familial cutaneous vasculopathy of GSDs.

PEMPHIGUS AND BULLOUS PEMPHIGOID

Pemphigus/bullous pemphigoid are considered uncommon in dogs and cats, but they have been recognized more frequently in recent years due to a greater awareness of the conditions and the use of diagnostic histopathology. There is a growing spectrum of such diseases, named for their human equivalents with which they have some common histopathological and immunological features. The diseases are characterized by the presence of a pathogenic autoantibody specific for one of the epidermal adhesion molecules. The autoantibody initiates disruption of keratinocyte cohesion, resulting in the formation of vesicles or pustules at different levels within the epidermis (pemphigus) or clefts through the basement membrane zone (BMZ) (bullous pemphigoid) (275, 276). Pemphigus foliaceus is the most common of these diseases. Pemphigus is recognized in dogs and cats with underlying diseases, particularly lymphoid

275

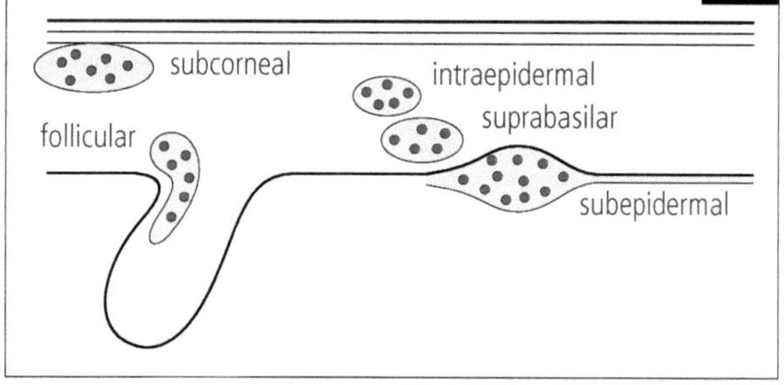

276

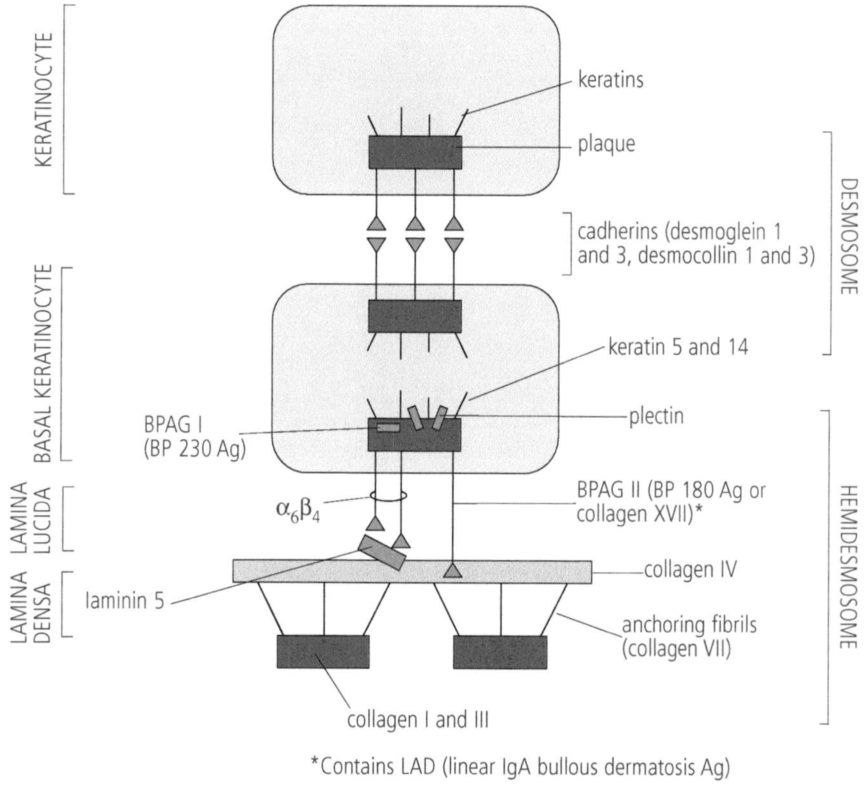

275, 276 Distribution and target antigens of vesiculobullous lesions in autoimmune skin disease. (**275**) The autoimmune skin diseases are characterized histologically by the formation of vesicles or pustules that may be subcorneal (pemphigus foliaceus, pemphigus erythematosus, pemphigus vegetans), within the external root sheath of infundibular hair follicles (pemphigus foliaceus, pemphigus erythematosus, pemphigus vegetans), suprabasilar (pemphigus vulgaris, pemphigus vegetans), intraepidermal (pemphigus vegetans, pemphigus erythematosus) or subepidermal through the lamina lucida of the BMZ (bullous pemphigoid). It has been proposed that pemphigus vegetans and pemphigus erythematosus are parts of the same spectrum of disease that should be called panepidermal pustular pemphigus. (**276**) The target autoantigens in the vesiculobullous skin diseases lie within the desmosome and hemidesmosome. The structure of these organelles and major autoantigens in man is shown.

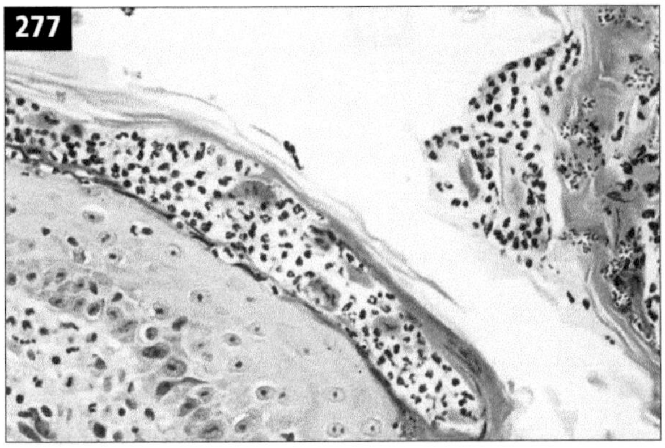

277 Pemphigus associated with underlying disease. Skin biopsy from a cat with clinical and histopathological evidence of pemphigus foliaceus. The biopsy displays a subcorneal pustule containing acanthocytes and neutrophils. Additionally, there are large numbers of *Malassezia* yeasts associated with the superficial epidermis. It is possible that in this case the pemphigus is secondary to the fungal infection, as has been described for dermatophytosis in the cat and dog. Fungi and bacteria (e.g. *Staphylococcus*) may produce proteases that cleave desmogleins causing disease that mimics pemphigus.

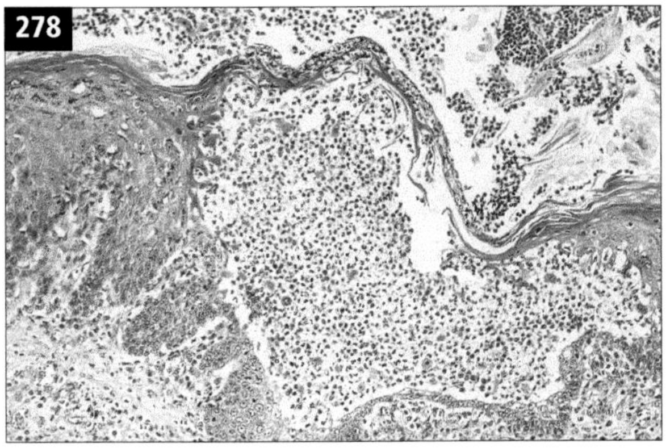

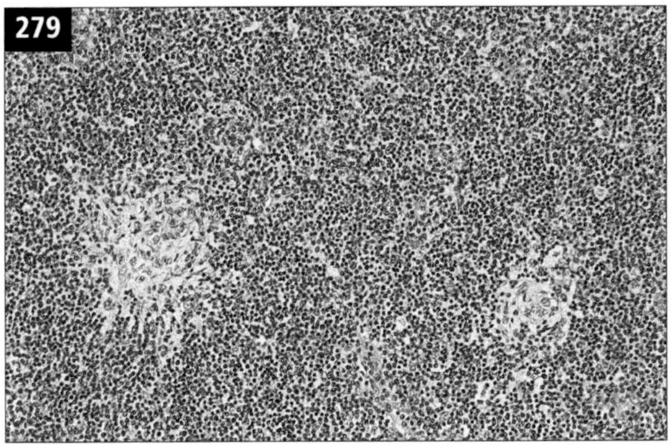

278, 279 Pemphigus associated with underlying disease. Pemphigus foliaceus is documented to occur in animals with underlying systemic neoplasia, particularly lymphoid tumours. Autoimmune disease is also recorded in animals with neoplastic or non-neoplastic thymic disease. These sections are from a seven-year-old British Black cat with generalized crusting dermatosis and subcorneal pustules characteristic of pemphigus foliaceus (**278**). On necropsy examination, multicystic thymic enlargement was identified and the histological appearance was of cystic spaces separated by densely packed aggregates of lymphocytes consistent with thymic hyperplasia (**279**). (From Day MJ [1997] A review of thymic pathology in 30 cats and 36 dogs. *Journal of Small Animal Practice* **38**:393–403, with permission.)

tumours (paraneoplastic pemphigus), infection (e.g. dermatophytosis in cats, leishmaniosis in dogs) (277) and after drug administration (278, 279).

PEMPHIGUS FOLIACEUS

Pathogenesis

Pemphigus foliaceus is a disease of middle-aged dogs, with breed predisposition for the Bearded Collie, Japanese Akita, Chow Chow, Newfoundland and Dobermann. There is one report of familial disease in two Shetland Sheepdog littermates. The specificity of the autoantibodies in pemphigus foliaceus is unknown. Preliminary investigations had suggested that the target autoantigen was the transmembrane molecule desmoglein 1 (molecular weight 148 kD), one of the cadherin superfamily of keratinocyte desmosomal adhesion molecules. However, more recent work has suggested that desmoglein 1 is only a minor autoantigen in pemphigus foliaceus, as only 6% of patient sera showed binding in an assay using the cell-expressed molecule. Examination of the distribution of serum antibody binding within substrate epidermis by indirect immunofluorescence suggests that the disease is immunologically heterogeneous, as antibody from individual patients binds at different levels of the epidermis. The pathogenesis is poorly defined, but binding of autoantibody (usually IgG) may result in:

- Physical disruption of epithelial adhesion.
- Internalization of the antigen-antibody complex, with loss of adhesion following release of urokinase plasminogen activator from keratinocytes activating the plasminogen/plasmin pathway, and proteolytic digestion of adhesion molecules.
- Complement fixation.
- Keratinocyte activation.

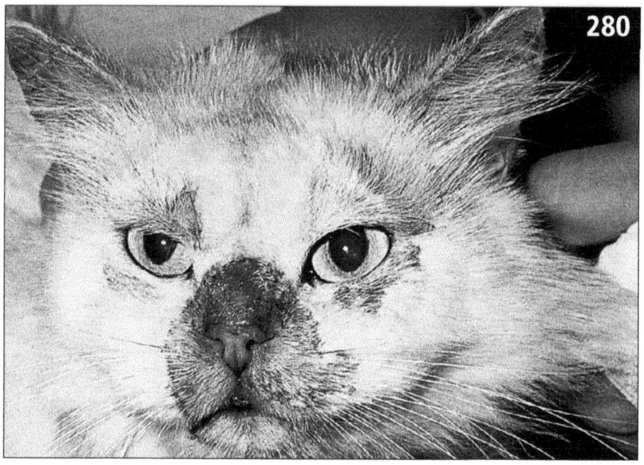

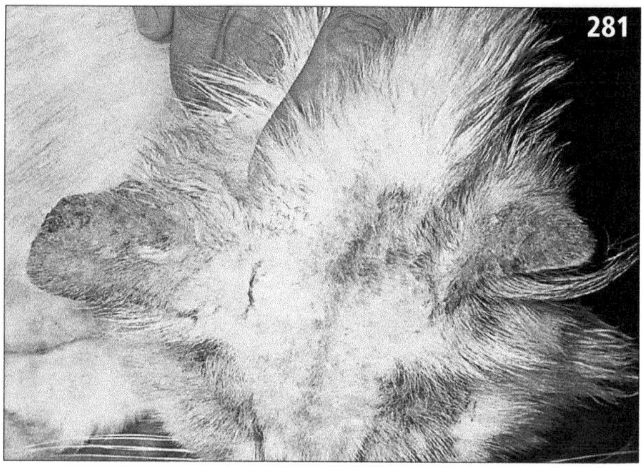

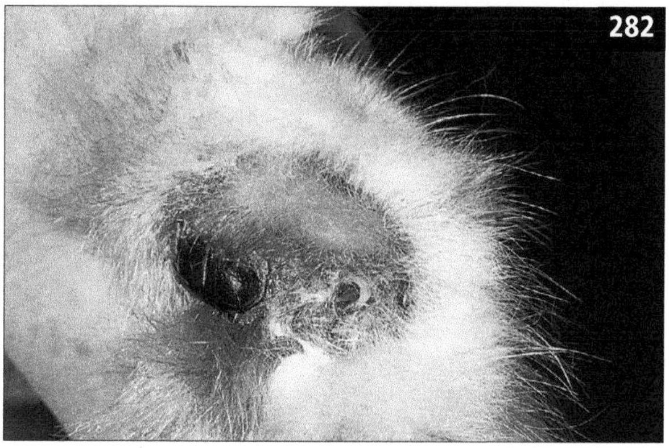

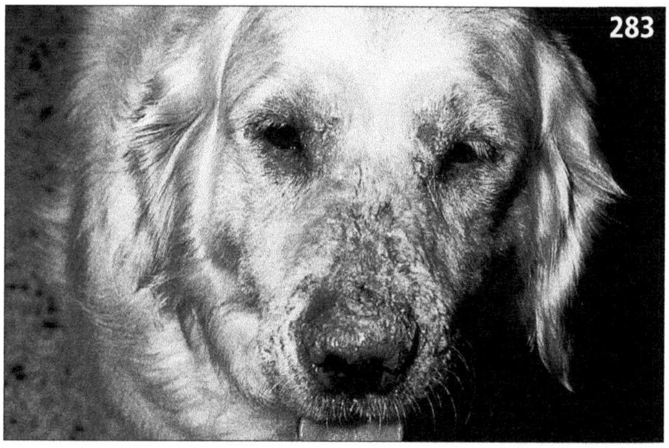

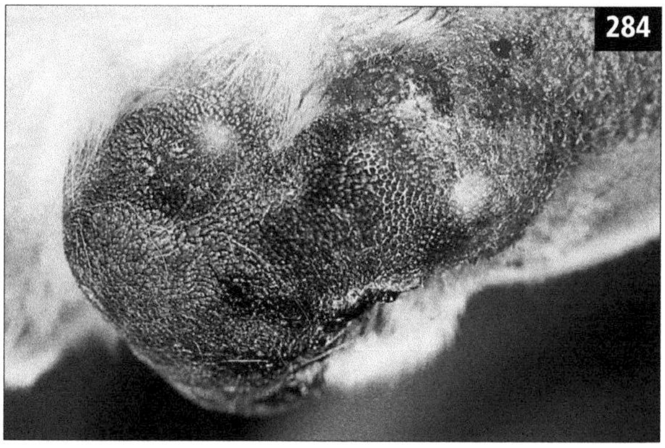

280–284 Pemphigus foliaceus. (**280, 281**) Crusting dermatitis of the face and pinnae in a six-year-old Persian cat with pemphigus foliaceus. (**282**) Paronychia is a common clinical finding in this disease in the cat. (**283**) Marked crusting of the face and pinnae with depigmentation of the nasal planum in a seven-year-old Retriever with chronic pemphigus foliaceus. (**284**) Multiple sterile pustule formation on the foot of a Great Dane with acute pemphigus foliaceus.

- Loss of cohesion between keratinocytes (acantholysis), with formation of intraepidermal, subcorneal or follicular vesicles containing individual or rafted acanthocytes.
- Chemotactic attraction of neutrophils or eosinophils into vesicular spaces to form pustules; neutrophil-derived enzymes may also contribute to acantholysis. It has recently been suggested that as neutrophil exocytosis precedes acantholysis in canine (but not human) pemphigus foliaceus, these cells may mediate lesion development rather than autoantibody.

Clinical signs

The primary lesions (sterile pustules) are rarely observed, as they are often destroyed by self-trauma, resulting in areas of crusting dermatitis with secondary bacterial infection. When present, pustules may evolve rapidly and be multiple. The classical distribution of lesions involves the face (nose, periorbital, ears) and footpads. The trunk may also be affected, but the mucocutaneous junctions (lips, rectal, vaginal) are rarely involved (280–284).

285

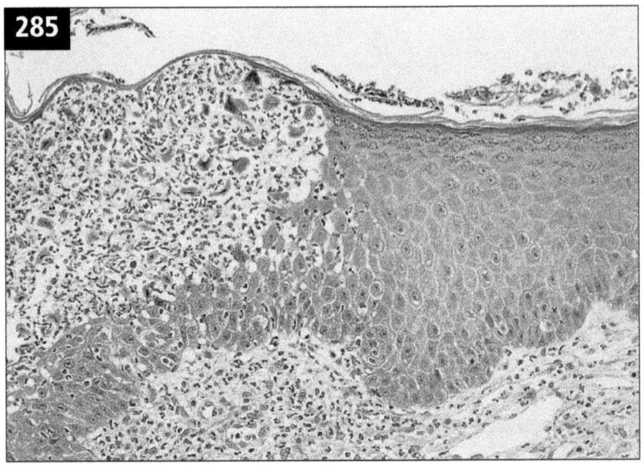

286

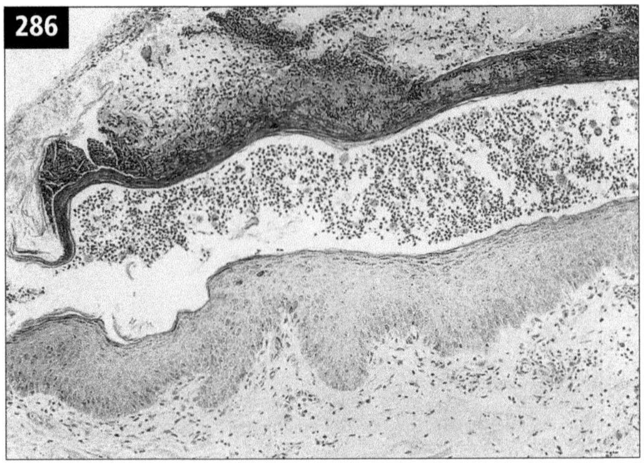

285, 286 Pemphigus foliaceus. Histopathological appearance of skin biopsies from a nine-year-old DSH cat (**285**) and a three-year-old Bernese Mountain Dog (**286**) with pemphigus foliaceus. In each case there is epidermal hyperplasia, with formation of a subcorneal pustule containing non-degenerate neutrophils (eosinophils may be found) and scattered eosinophilic acanthocytes that are sometimes adherent to the margins of the pustule. Pustules may be found in the superficial follicular epithelium (not shown). In **285** there is infiltration of the superficial dermis by mixed inflammatory cells including neutrophils and macrophages.

287

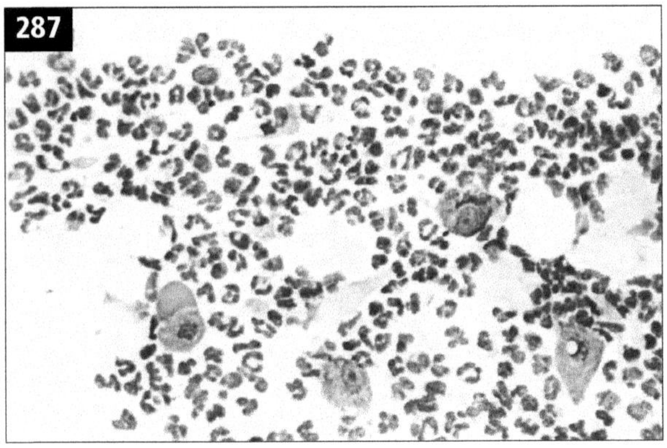

287 Pustule cytology in pemphigus foliaceus. A needle aspirate from a pustule in the skin of a dog with pemphigus foliaceus. The presence of numerous non-degenerate neutrophils and acanthocytes is typical of pemphigus foliaceus. Fewer acanthocytes would be expected in an aspirate from a pustule in superficial pyoderma. Additionally, the neutrophils would be degenerate and bacteria might be observed in the latter lesion.

Diagnosis

The distribution and nature of the lesions may be suggestive, and multiple biopsies of early lesions or the leading edge of chronic lesions may be required to demonstrate the classical histopathological features (285, 286). If pustular lesions are present, a needle aspirate and cytological examination can reveal the presence of non-degenerate granulocytes and acanthocytes (287). Differentiation from bacterial and fungal disease must be made (277).

Diagnosis can be confirmed by the use of immunofluorescence or immunoperoxidase immunohistochemical techniques to demonstrate inter-epithelial Ig and/or complement within affected skin (288–290). Immunohistochemistry may be positive in 70% of canine cases (25% of feline), but a negative result does not preclude the diagnosis in the face of clinical and histopathological evidence. False-positive reactions have been reported. IgM may be found within the epidermis of normal canine nose and footpad, and Ig may percolate non-specifically into spongiotic epidermis, giving diffuse inter-epithelial staining rather than distinct desmosomal deposition.

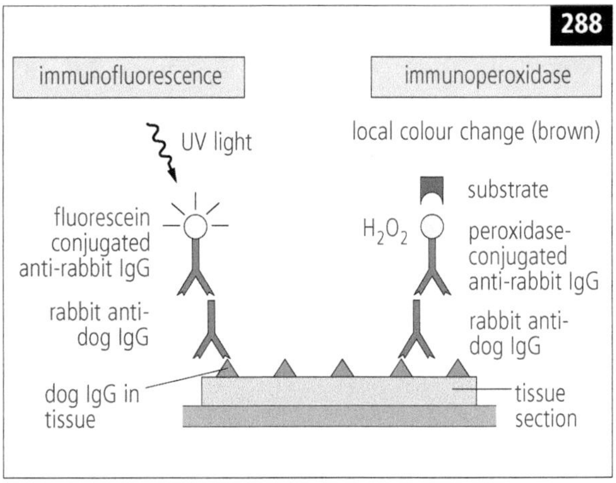

288 Immunohistochemistry in pemphigus foliaceus. Sections from a lesional skin biopsy containing Ig (in this case IgG) and/or complement within epidermis. **(a)** In immunofluorescence testing the binding of primary antibody (rabbit anti-dog IgG) is detected using a secondary antibody (anti-rabbit IgG) that has been chemically conjugated to fluorescein isothiocyanate, which will give local apple-green fluorescence under UV light. **(b)** In immunoperoxidase labelling the secondary antibody is conjugated to the enzyme peroxidase, which, in the presence of substrate (chromagen) and hydrogen peroxide, will cause local deposition of colour (brown) that can be visualized with the light microscope. The methodology shown is indirect immunohistochemistry that utilizes a 'sandwich' of antibodies. There are numerous variations on these methods; they may be more simple (e.g. use of a directly conjugated primary antibody) or more complex (e.g. use of the peroxidase-anti-peroxidase or avidin-biotin peroxidase amplification systems). In immunoperoxidase labelling the background tissue can be counterstained with haematoxylin and the tissue structure easily visualized. The sections are permanent and a specialized fluorescence microscope is not required. In contrast, in immunofluorescence labelling the tissue background is unstained and the sections will fade in a relatively short period of time.

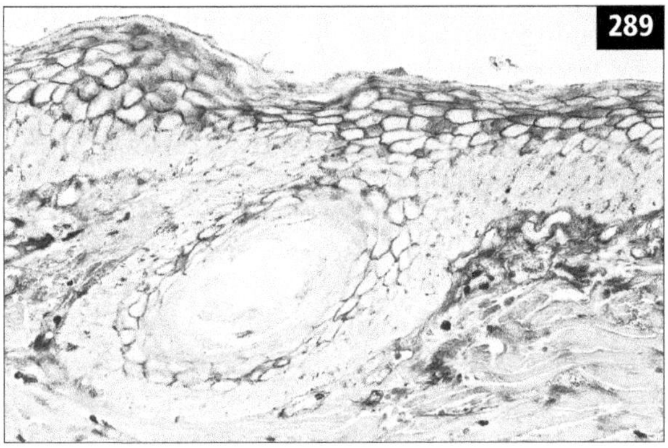

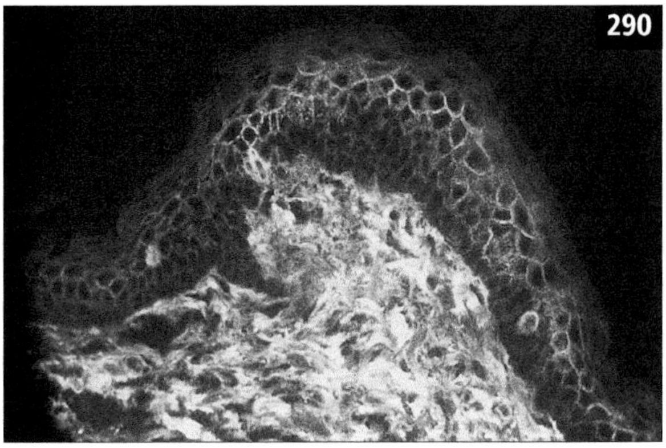

289, 290 Pemphigus foliaceus. (**289**) Immunoperoxidase labelling of a skin biopsy from the dog with pemphigus foliaceus depicted in **284**. There is deposition of IgG between keratinocytes (inter-epithelial) in the mid to superficial epidermis and between cells of the follicular outer root sheath. (**290**) Immunofluorescence labelling of a skin biopsy from a GSD with pemphigus foliaceus. There is mid-epidermal, interepithelial deposition of IgG. The fluorescence of dermal collagen is background. (From Day MJ, Penhale WJ [1986] immunodiagnosis of autoimmune skin disease in the dog, cat and horse. *Australian Veterinary Journal* **63**:65–68, with permission.)

Immunohistochemistry may be performed on snap-frozen biopsies, formalin-fixed tissue or biopsies collected into specific media (Michel's medium, Bouin's fixative). Immunofluorescence has now largely been superseded by immunoperoxidase labelling, which allows visualization of the histopathological changes in the tissue.

Although, classically, dogs with pemphigus foliaceus are negative for serum ANA (see Chapter 6, p. 176), some studies have demonstrated ANA in up to 50% of canine and 75% of feline cases. Indirect immunohistochemistry is not routinely used as a diagnostic procedure in canine pemphigus foliaceus, but it has been performed experimentally using bovine oesophagus or canine lip as a substrate.

PEMPHIGUS VULGARIS

Pemphigus vulgaris is a rare disease of the dog and cat, characterized by the formation of suprabasillar clefts and vesicles that rapidly ulcerate and become infected. The lesions are predominantly mucocutaneous, involving the mouth (tongue, palate, gingiva), lips, eyelids, nostrils, anus, prepuce and vulva (**291, 292**). Both mucosa and epidermis may be affected. Lesions of axillary and inguinal skin and footpads may be observed. Histologically the clefts are characterized by the residual basal keratinocytes remaining attached to the BMZ and having a 'tombstone' appearance (**293**). The intact primary bullae are non-inflammatory, but there is mononuclear inflammation of the superficial dermis. The classical immunohistochemical findings are of IgG and complement deposition between keratinocytes at all levels of the epidermis, and the target autoantigen is a member of the cadherin superfamily (desmoglein 3).

PEMPHIGUS ERYTHEMATOSUS

Pemphigus erythematosus is rare in the dog and cat and has traditionally been described as a 'cross-over' between pemphigus foliaceus and SLE. The disease is now considered to be a localized, photosensitive form of pemphigus foliaceus, with predominantly facial lesions. The histopathological appearance is of subcorneal pustule formation, with acantholysis. In dogs there is often a lichenoid dermal inflammation similar to that described in nasal planum lupus erythematosus; however, this has recently been suggested to be a non-specific reaction pattern in many nasal dermatoses. Serum ANA, circulating desmoglein 1 autoantibody and Ig deposition within the inter-epithelial spaces, in addition to the BMZ, are reported.

PANEPIDERMAL PUSTULAR PEMPHIGUS (PEMPHIGUS VEGETANS)

The term panepidermal pustular pemphigus has been adopted to describe cases previously classified as pemphigus vegetans. This is a rare skin disease of the dog (particularly Collies and GSDs) and may be a variant of pemphigus foliaceus. Lesions are most apparent on the trunk and the initial pustular stage may evolve into a proliferative, papillomatous phase, with concurrent pustules. The characteristic histopathological appearance is of pustule formation (containing neutrophils, eosinophils and acanthocytes) at multiple levels of the epidermis and within the follicular infundibulum.

Treatment of pemphigus disorders

Prednisolone at immunosuppressive doses (*Table 13*, p. 147) is the treatment of choice in pemphigus syndromes. Response is usually brisk, but the waxing and waning course of the disease makes response difficult to interpret. Full recovery does occur occasionally, although these are most commonly cases of drug-induced pemphigus in which the drug has been withdrawn. Relapse is not uncommon and prednisolone 'resistant' cases occur. Combination immunosuppressive therapy using prednisolone, azathioprine or cyclophosphamide is used in cases of more resistant canine pemphigus, and pulse therapy using suprapharmacological doses of prednisolone or dexamethasone has been used to 'rescue' poorly responsive cases. Feline pemphigus foliaceus is usually prednisolone responsive, but resistant cases occur and may respond to combination therapy with prednisolone and chlorambucil. Chrysotherapy has also been advocated. Treatment is usually long term, with the aim of identifying the lowest dose of drugs that will maintain remission.

In the deeper pemphigus variants, broad-spectrum antibiotic cover, using a drug of a different class to any previously administered, should be used. In addition, as considerable body surface area may be ulcerated, fluid therapy and parenteral nutrition for protein loss may be necessary. The prognosis is guarded in these cases. In pemphigus erythematosus, avoidance of ultraviolet (UV) light and vitamin E administration (*Table 13*, p. 148) is recommended, and the use of sunscreens may be indicated with localized lesions.

BULLOUS PEMPHIGOID

Bullous pemphigoid is uncommon in the dog and rare in the cat. The pathogenesis involves binding of autoantibody specific for the 'bullous pemphigoid antigen II', a glycoprotein molecule of 180 kD molecular weight (collagen type XVII) within the hemidesmosomes of the basal cells of the epidermis and the lamina lucida of the BMZ. This results in internalization of the complex and disruption of the hemidesmosome, complement fixation, keratinocyte and mast cell cytokine production, and local inflammation (neutrophils and eosinophils with matrix metalloproteinase release) disrupting the dermal–epidermal junction, with formation of sub-epidermal clefts.

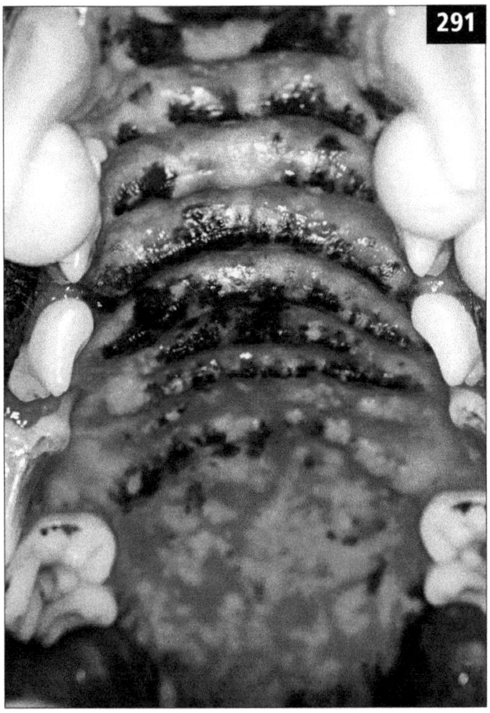

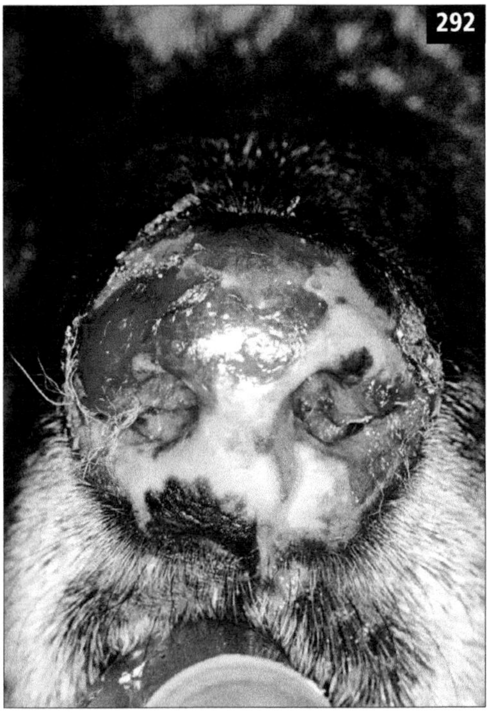

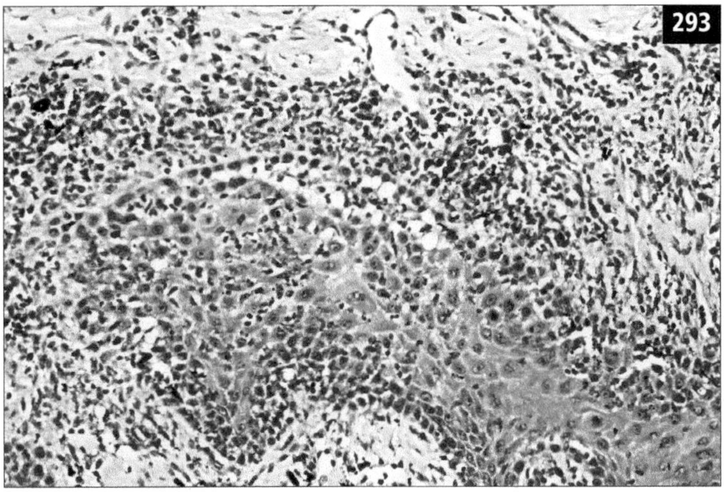

291–293 Pemphigus vulgaris. Palatal mucosa (**291**) and planum nasale (**292**) of a five-year-old male GSD with ulcerative lesions also involving the lips, scrotum, anus and footpads. (Photographs courtesy A.P. Foster.) (**293**) Biopsy from the dog in **291** displays an area of clefting above the basal layer of the epidermis, with a superficial dermal inflammatory reaction.

Clinical signs

Bullous pemphigoid has been documented more frequently in Collies and Dobermanns. The lesions most often involve the oral mucocutaneous junctions and/or skin, especially of the axilla and groin. The footpads may be affected. The primary lesion is a bulla, but these are easily traumatized and the clinical appearance is often of ulceration and epidermal collarette formation (294–297).

Diagnosis

Biopsies of early lesions are most likely to demonstrate the characteristic histopathological features (298). Electron microscopic studies may demonstrate disruption of the BMZ, with loss of hemidesmosomes and separation through the lamina lucida (299). Immunohistochemistry may demonstrate IgG (IgM or IgA) autoantibody and complement within the BMZ (300). In some cases, serum autoantibody has been demonstrated by indirect immunohistochemical labelling of salt-split substrate skin, by western blotting using epidermal antigen preparations, or by ELISA using recombinant collagen XVII peptides.

Treatment

Bullous pemphigoid may be a severe and fatal disease, but a benign, localized cutaneous variant is described. The former presentation requires aggressive combination immunosuppressive therapy (e.g. prednisolone and cyclophosphamide [*Table 13*, p. 148]), broad-spectrum antibiotic cover and fluid therapy.

OTHER SUBEPIDERMAL BLISTERING DISEASES

A number of other autoimmune subepidermal blistering diseases are now recognized in the dog:

- **Epidermolysis bullosa acquisita** is a generalized or facial ulcerative dermatitis, with subepidermal vesiculation, neutrophil inflammation and deposition of IgG, IgA and IgM specific for collagen VII within the

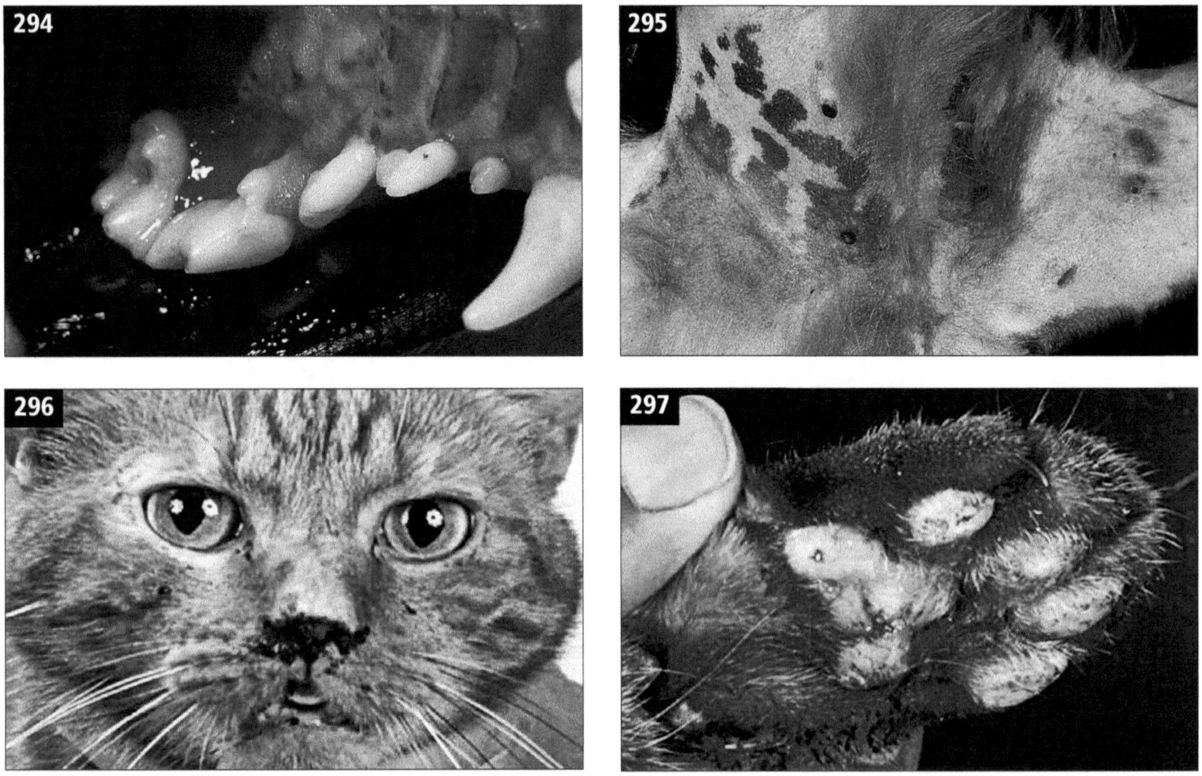

294–297 Bullous pemphigoid. (**294**) Bullae formation affecting the palatine mucosa of a six-year-old Collie-cross dog with bullous pemphigoid. (**295**) Multiple ulceration affecting the skin of the inguinal region of the same dog. (**296, 297**) A four-year-old DSH cat with erosive lesions of the oral mucosa, planum nasale, pinnae and footpads. Biopsy confirms these to be consistent with bullous pemphigoid. (Photographs courtesy S.M.A. Caney.)

hemidesmosomal anchoring fibril plaques. The prognosis is poor with generalized disease.

- **Linear IgA bullous disease** is mediated by IgA autoantibodies specific for an extracellular 120 kD molecule (LAD-1) related to collagen XVII within the BMZ. Clinical features are similar to those of bullous pemphigoid.
- **Mucous membrane pemphigoid (cicatricial pemphigoid)** is a vesicular and ulcerative disease with distribution involving the oral cavity, periocular skin, genitalia and anus. It is reported in the dog and cat and target autoantigens include the Nc16A segment of collagen XVII, collagen VII and, in one feline case, laminin-5.

CUTANEOUS LUPUS ERYTHEMATOSUS

Cutaneous lupus erythematosus (CLE) is the term now used to describe a group of immune-mediated skin diseases that likely share elements of pathogenesis. These disorders are most commonly reported in the dog. The key feature of CLE is histopathological evidence of basement membrane thickening and lymphocyte-rich interface dermatitis, with lymphocyte-mediated cytolysis (apoptosis) of basal keratinocytes. These interface changes are often accompanied by an intense lichenoid lymphoplasmacytic infiltration of the superficial dermis, which in some anatomical areas (e.g. nasal planum) may simply be a non-specific cutaneous reaction pattern. There is strong expression of MHC class II by the macrophages and dermal dendritic cells in this population. The targeting of basal cells by cytotoxic lymphocytes is consistent with a primary type IV immunopathogenic mechanism; however, immune complexes of antibody (generally IgG) and antigen with complement deposit in the BMZ between the

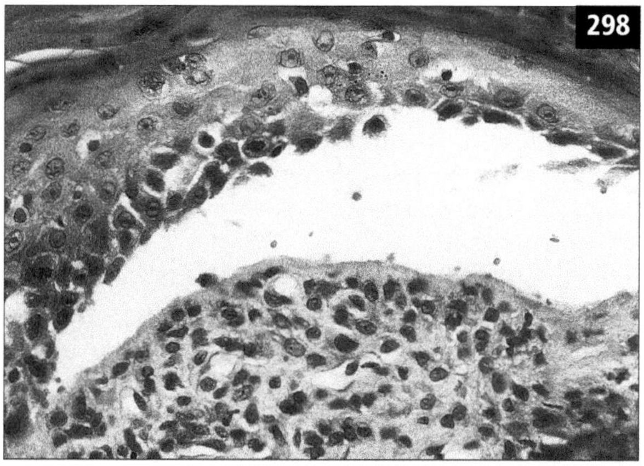

298 Bullous pemphigoid. Skin biopsy from the cat shown in **296**. There is separation of the epidermis from dermis through the BMZ. Basal epidermal cells form the roof of the cleft. There is a mixed inflammatory infiltration of the superficial dermis (macrophages, neutrophils and lymphocytes). (From Day MJ [1996] Diagnostic assessment of the feline immune system, part II. *Feline Practice* **24:**14–25, with permission.)

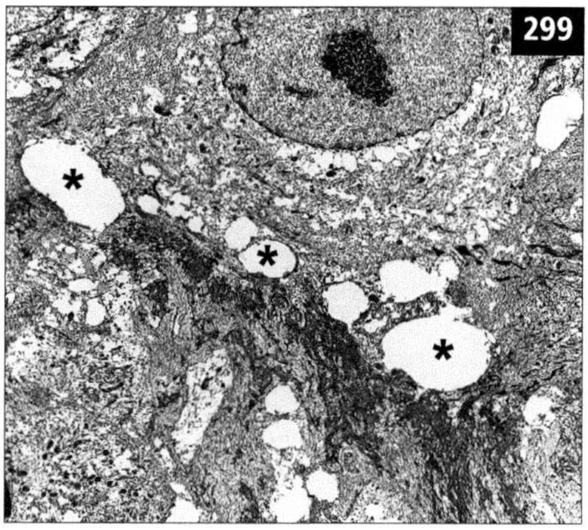

299 Bullous pemphigoid. Electron micrograph of skin from a cat with bullous pemphigoid. There are a series of vacuolar spaces (asterisks) between the upper basal epidermal cells and lamina densa of the BMZ. Higher magnification of the lamina lucida reveals disruption of hemidesmosomal structure.

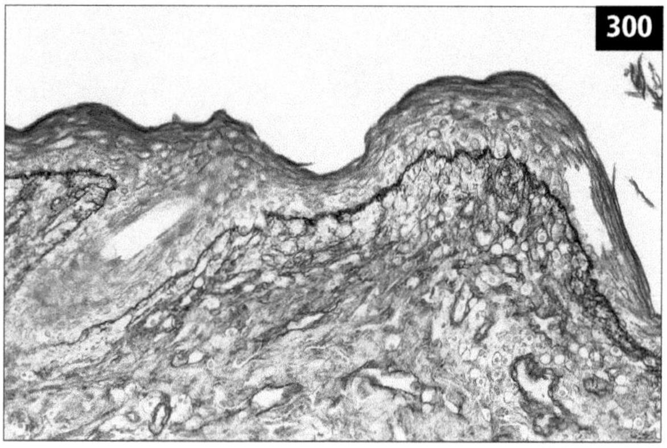

300 Bullous pemphigoid. Immunoperoxidase labelling of a skin biopsy from a cat with bullous pemphigoid. The portion of skin shown is adjacent to an area of subepidermal cleft formation and there is marked deposition of IgG within the BMZ. (From Day MJ [1996] Diagnostic assessment of the feline immune system, part II. *Feline Practice* **24:**14–25, with permission.)

epidermis and the dermis. The antigenic component of the complexes has not been characterized and it is possible that these are an epiphenomenon rather than causative of the pathology (**301**).

The canine disease once described as discoid lupus erythematosus (DLE) is not identical to the human counterpart and is therefore now termed 'nasal planum' or 'facial' lupus erythematosus. Because this disease is thought to involve the effects of UV light, it is also known as 'nasal solar dermatitis'. Nasal planum CLE is the most commonly occurring of this group of diseases. The classification CLE also includes the immune-mediated cutaneous lesions of the multisystemic autoimmune disease, SLE. The histopathological and immunological features of the cutaneous lesions of SLE are similar to those described above, but clinical lesions are more variable. The distinguishing features of SLE (see Chapter 14, p. 356) are ANA positivity and at least one other clinical manifestation of autoimmunity in addition to the skin disease.

NASAL PLANUM CLE

This entity has breed predispositions for dolicocephalic dogs including the Collie, GSD and Shetland Sheepdog. Nasal planum CLE initially presents as a depigmenting and scaling nasal lesion, with loss of the normal rough 'cobblestone' appearance of the planum nasale. Erosion and crusting then develops and the lesions extend from the planum nasale to the bridge of the nose. Lesions may also involve the periocular skin, pinnae, oral cavity and distal limbs (**302, 303**). The planum nasale is also the major site affected in the feline form of the disease.

Biopsy from the leading edge of lesions should demonstrate the characteristic histopathological features (**304**). Diagnosis is supported by the use of immunohistochemistry to identify the presence of immune complexes (IgG, rarely IgM or IgA; complement) at the BMZ (**305, 306**). Immunohistochemistry is positive in 50% of cases. Serum ANA is generally negative in dogs with CLE.

Therapy of nasal planum CLE is dependent on the severity of ulceration. In cases where there are mild clinical signs, and during times when UV light exposure is minimal, treatment with combination tetracycline/niacinamide or vitamin E (*Table 13*, p. 148) and UV blocker may be sufficient. In more severe cases, topical and/or systemic glucocorticoids at anti-inflammatory doses are used (*Table 7*, p. 125). Nasal planum CLE rarely requires high doses of prednisolone or combination immunosuppressive therapy; it is a chronic disease and long-term therapy is required. Withdrawal of therapy may be possible during winter periods in some geographic areas.

ORAL CAVITY OR MUCOCUTANEOUS CLE

Disease with histopathological features consistent with CLE may occur with this anatomical distribution.

301

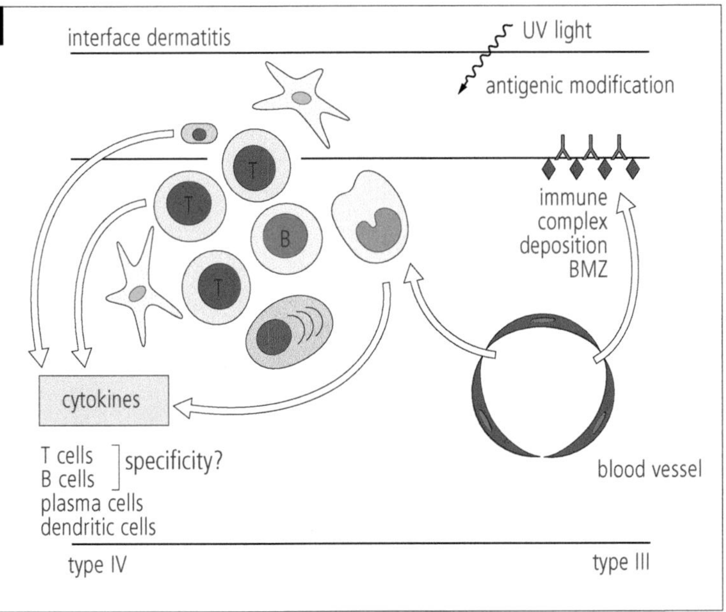

301 Cutaneous lupus erythematosus. The pathogenesis of CLE is poorly defined. The disease is exacerbated by sunlight and it has been proposed that UV light may be able to alter cutaneous antigens. There is deposition of immune complexes of Ig and complement at the BMZ (type III immunopathogenesis) and an interface inflammatory infiltration of mixed mononuclear cells, with apoptosis and hydropic degeneration of basal epidermal cells (type IV immunopathogenesis). The specificity of the infiltrating lymphoid populations is unknown; however, these cells (and keratinocytes) may be a source of cytokines that further contribute to tissue damage.

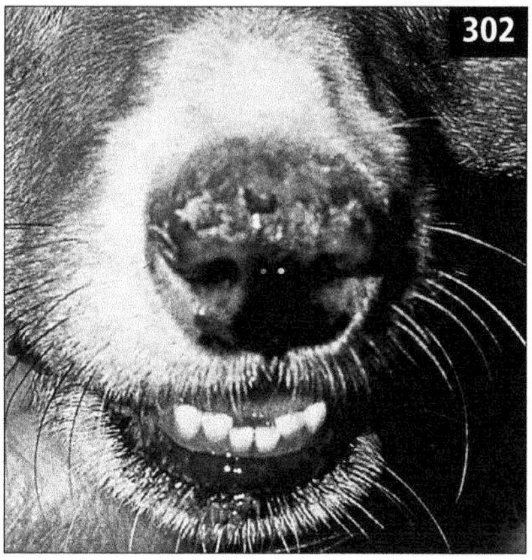

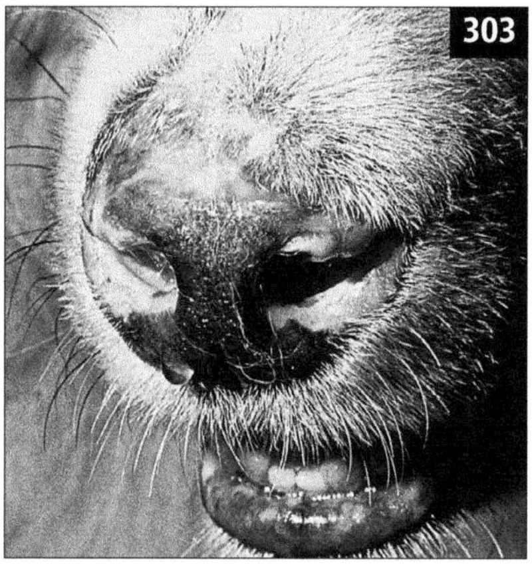

302, 303 Nasal cutaneous lupus erythematosus. (**302**) Marked depigmentation and ulceration of the nasal planum and mucosa of the nares in a three-year-old Corgi with nasal CLE. (**303**) Depigmentation and ulceration of the nasal planum and mucosa of the nares and lower lip in a seven-year-old Collie-cross with nasal CLE.

304 Nasal cutaneous lupus erythematosus. Skin biopsy from a four-year-old crossbred dog with crusting of the planum nasale. There is epidermal hyperplasia, with a lichenoid dermal infiltration of mixed mononuclear inflammatory cells with interface distribution. The BMZ is prominent. Other histopathological features (not clearly seen at low power) include the presence of individual apoptotic keratinocytes and hydropic degeneration of basal keratinocytes.

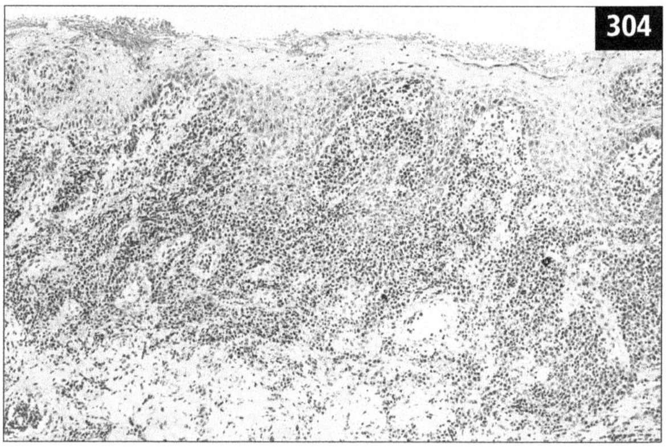

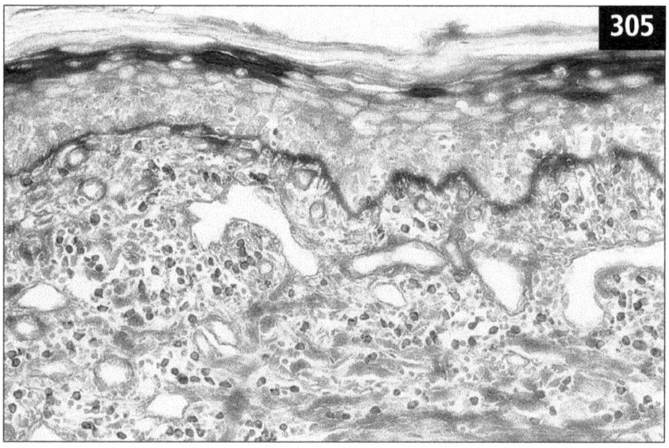

305, 306 Nasal cutaneous lupus erythematosus. (**305**) Skin biopsy from a GSD-cross with nasal CLE. There is deposition of IgG at the BMZ in this section labelled by the immunoperoxidase method. Plasma cells with cytoplasmic IgG are prominent within the interface infiltrate. (**306**) Skin biopsy from a dog with nasal CLE labelled by the immunofluorescence method for IgG. There is Ig at the BMZ and scattered IgG plasma cells throughout the dermis.

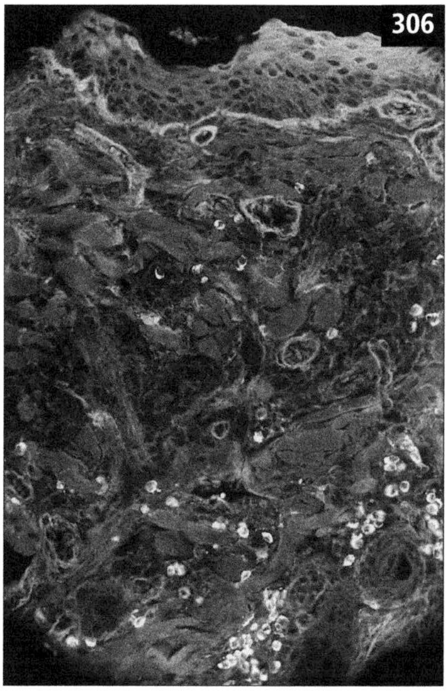

GENERALIZED CLE

Some dogs with generalized skin disease (but not concurrent systemic signs) have histological changes on biopsy that are consistent with CLE.

VESICULAR CLE OF COLLIES AND SHETLAND SHEEPDOGS

This entity was previously known as 'idiopathic ulcerative dermatosis of Collies and Shetland Sheepdogs', but it is now classified within the CLE spectrum. The disease occurs in middle-aged to older dogs of these breeds and involves the formation of vesicles and bullae that coalesce and progress to form ulcerated areas typically affecting the axillae and ventral abdomen. Less frequently, the eyelids, pinnae, oral cavity, genitalia, anus and footpads may be involved.

EXFOLIATIVE CLE OF GERMAN SHORTHAIRED POINTERS

This disease was formerly known as 'hereditary lupoid dermatosis of German Shorthaired Pointers'. It occurs in young dogs (three months to three years of age) of this breed. The lesions are scaling in nature and involve the face, ears, dorsum and trunk. More severe lesions may arise on the hocks and scrotal skin. The histopathological appearance is of lymphocytic interface dermatitis and mural folliculitis involving primarily $CD3^+$ T cells. Immunohistochemistry reveals deposition of IgG within the epidermal and follicular basement membrane. Some dogs have circulating antibody specific for hair follicle and sebaceous gland structures. This disease often responds poorly to immunosuppressive therapy and it has a guarded prognosis.

LUPOID ONYCHODYSTROPHY

This entity selectively affects the claws, which may split or crack and subsequently shed. Secondary infection commonly occurs and multiple claws are involved. The claws that regrow after shedding are dystrophic and may also be damaged and shed. Histopathological features suggestive of CLE are found in the nailbed skin and immunohistochemical studies demonstrate a mixed interface infiltrate of T and B lymphocytes, with sparse macrophages. A range of treatment protocols have been used for affected dogs, but combination doxycycline and niacinamide or tetracycline and niacinamide is reported to be efficacious.

DERMATOMYOSITIS

Dermatomyositis is uncommonly recognized in young related Collies (and Collie-crosses), Shetland Sheepdogs and Beaucerons and occasionally in other breeds. The disease is best described in the Rough-coated Collie, and the majority of information given here derives from these studies. The pathogenesis involves the formation of immune complexes before the onset of clinical signs, suggesting that immune complex deposition within tissues may initiate the lesions. Immune complex levels decrease as the disease resolves. The antigenic component of the immune complexes has not been identified, but there are differing schools of thought as to underlying pathogenesis. Some evidence exists for the direct involvement of an infectious (viral) agent, but it has also been proposed that dermatomyositis is a primary autoimmune disease related to SLE. Vaccine antigens may not be involved, as clinical signs may develop prior to vaccination. Breeding studies (Collie) have identified a strong familial tendency for this disease. The mode of inheritance has been incompletely defined, but may be autosomal dominant with variable expression. No specific association with DLA alleles has been found, but expression of DLA-D15 was associated with increased severity of disease. In the Shetland Sheepdog a recent study of 22 affected and 39 unaffected animals revealed genetic linkage to a microsatellite marker on chromosome 35.

Clinical signs

The skin lesions of dermatomyositis generally develop between seven weeks and six months of age and are characterized by alopecia, erythema, hypo- or hyperpigmentation, scaling, crusting or erosions. The distribution of lesions includes the face (periorbital, bridge of nose), oral mucocutaneous junction, pinnae, limbs, footpads and tail tip (**307–312**). Myositis develops after dermatitis and there is a correlation between the severity of the two conditions. Affected muscle groups may be reduced in size, but there may be abnormal electromyogram (EMG) tracings and histological change in grossly normal muscle. The temporalis muscle is particularly affected, but other facial muscles (masseter) and flexor/extensor muscles of the forelimbs and hindlimbs may also be involved; megaoesophagus has been recorded. The distribution of the skin and muscle lesions suggests

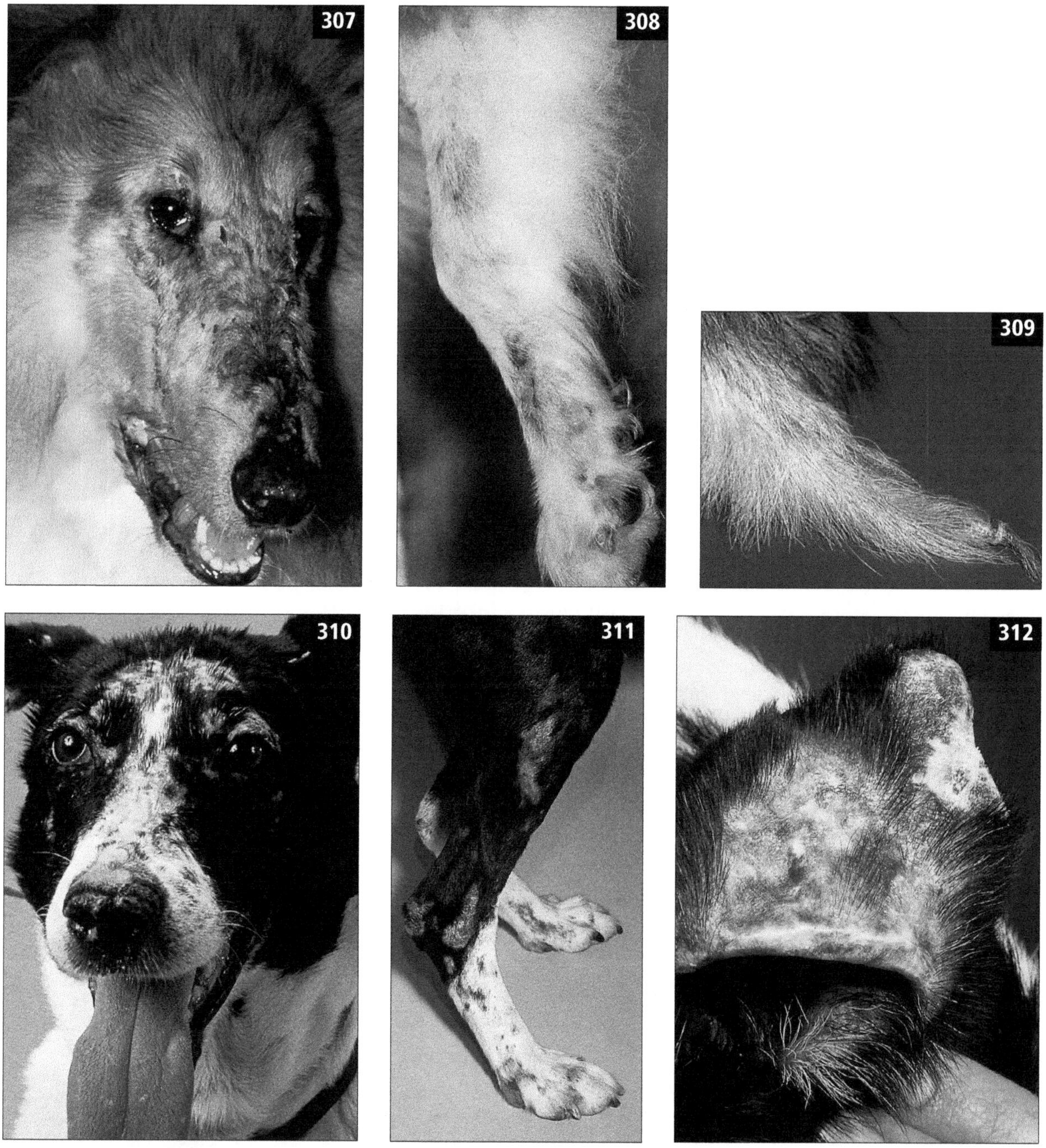

307–312 Dermatomyositis. Alopecia, ulceration and scarring of the face (**307**), left forelimb (**308**) and tail tip (**309**) of a Rough Collie with dermatomyositis. (Photographs courtesy G. Kunkle.) Alopecia, scarring and ulceration of the face (**310**) and lower hindlimbs (**311**) of a Border Collie with dermatomyositis. Necrosis of the tips of the tail and pinnae are associated with vasculitis in this case (**312**). (Photographs courtesy A.J. Shearer.)

that peripheral body temperature may have a role in the disease pathogenesis. Adult-onset disease is uncommon.

Diagnosis

An appropriate clinical presentation in a recognized breed may be supported by skin and muscle biopsy. The characteristic features of the cutaneous lesions are:

- Epidermal hyperplasia and hyperkeratosis; basal cell vacuolation; intraepidermal and subepidermal pustules are recorded in some cases.
- Mild superficial perivascular to perifollicular dermatitis, with mixed inflammatory cells and dermal melanophages.
- Dermal fibrosis with follicular atrophy may occur.
- Vasculitis may be present.

Affected muscle has evidence of myofibre abnormalities, atrophy and myositis (predominantly lymphocytes, macrophages and plasma cells), and vasculitis may be observed. Elevated creatinine phosphokinase has been documented (in the Beauceron) and EMG abnormalities have been recorded from affected muscle groups.

Immunohistochemical labelling of skin and muscle biopsies are negative. Affected dogs do not have serum ANA, but they do have elevated levels of circulating immune complexes and elevated concentration of IgG (normal serum IgM and IgA). Serum complement CH_{50} and concentrations of C2, C3 and C4 are normal.

Treatment

The clinical signs of dermatomyositis may resolve spontaneously in mildly affected dogs (with some scarring); they may be cyclic, with recurrence triggered by factors such as exposure to sunlight or oestrus. Ovariohysterectomy and avoidance of sunlight may help prevent such relapses. Treatment of more severely affected dogs with immunosuppressive doses of prednisolone may produce inconsistent clinical improvement, and vitamin E and pentoxifylline (*Table 13*, p. 148) have also been used with variable efficacy. Severely affected dogs have a poor long-term prognosis, particularly if marked atrophy of masticatory muscles, or megaoesophagus, occurs. Further breeding of parents and affected animals should be discouraged.

DERMATOUVEITIS (See Chapter 11, p. 278)

ERYTHEMA MULTIFORME AND TOXIC EPIDERMAL NECROLYSIS

Pathogenesis

Erythema multiforme (EM) and toxic epidermal necrolysis (TEN) are unusual cutaneous disorders that are reported more frequently in the dog than in the cat. The immunopathology is poorly defined and there is debate as to whether these are distinct entities or a continuum of a single disease that includes **EM minor, EM major, Stevens-Johnson syndrome (SJS), SJS-TEN overlap syndrome** and **TEN**. These conditions are often reported to be drug-related or secondary to infection or systemic

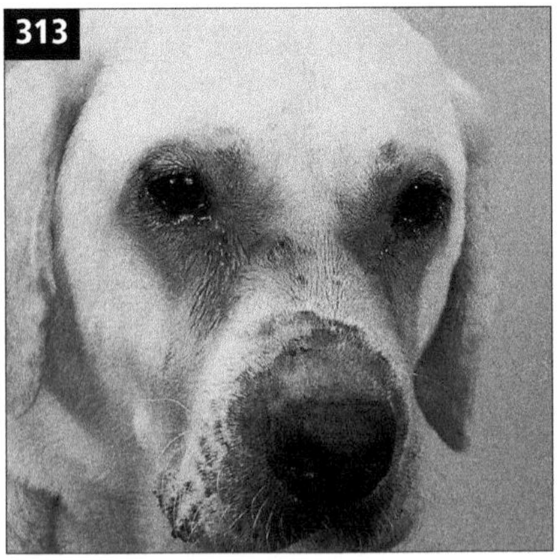

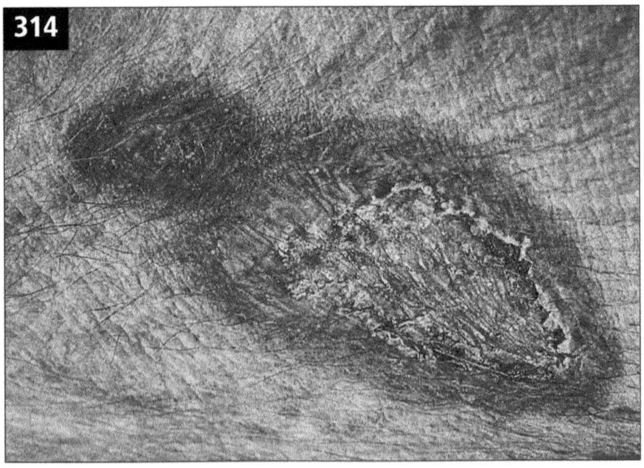

313, 314 Erythema multiforme. (**313**) Crusting lesions associated with multifocal erosion of the periocular regions, conjunctiva, perioral region and haired/non-haired skin margin of the nasal dorsum in a six-year-old Labrador with erythema multiforme of unknown cause. (**314**) Multiple annular erythematous lesions with epidermal collarette formation affecting the skin of the trunk and ventral abdomen in the same dog.

neoplasia, although recent studies have suggested that canine EM is less likely to be drug-associated than SJS, SJS-TEN and TEN. Deposition of Ig and/or complement may occur within the lesions of EM and TEN, but this may be an epiphenomenon.

Clinical signs

The clinical appearance of EM is variable and may comprise acute onset erythematous macules to papules that become confluent to form plaques. Vesiculobullous lesions may be present (**313, 314**). The cutaneous lesions of TEN are ulcerative. EM and TEN have a multifocal to generalized cutaneous or mucocutaneous distribution (**315–318**).

Diagnosis

Histopathologically the maculopapular form of EM is defined by:

- Single cell apoptosis of keratinocytes, with satellitosis of cytotoxic lymphocytes. Keratinocytes express MHC class II and other adhesion molecules that may mediate the interaction of these cells. Recent studies in affected humans have reported the key interaction between keratinocyte Fas (CD95) and the Fas ligand (CD95L) expressed by the cytotoxic T cells.

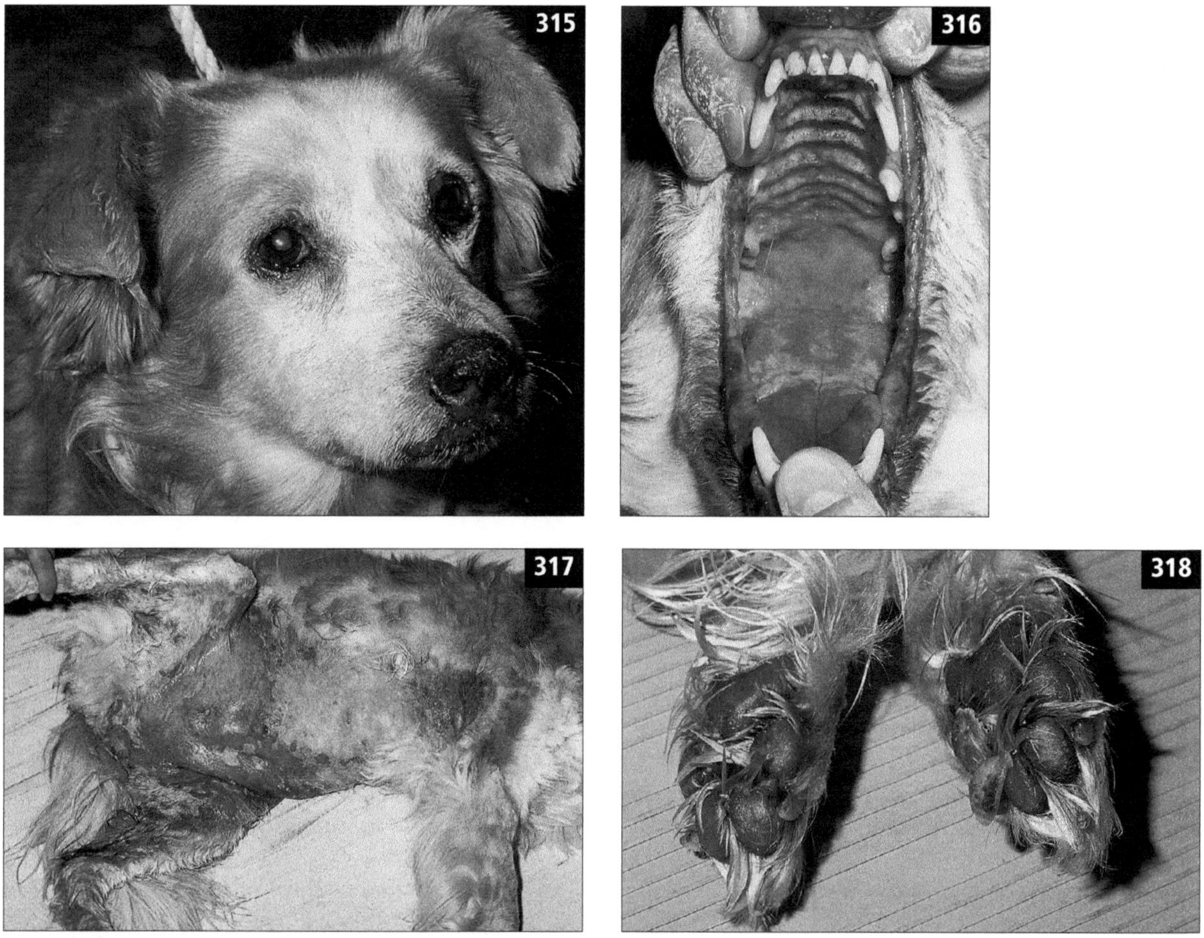

315–318 Toxic epidermal necrolysis. TEN in a ten-year-old Spaniel-cross secondary to multicentric lymphoma. (**315**) Full thickness necrosis and ulceration of the periocular skin, conjunctiva, nasal planum and skin of the philtrum. (**316**) Marked ulceration of the buccal and palatine mucosa. (**317**) Ulceration of the skin of the ventral abdomen with a positive Nikolsky's sign. (**318**) Full thickness necrosis and sloughing of the footpads.

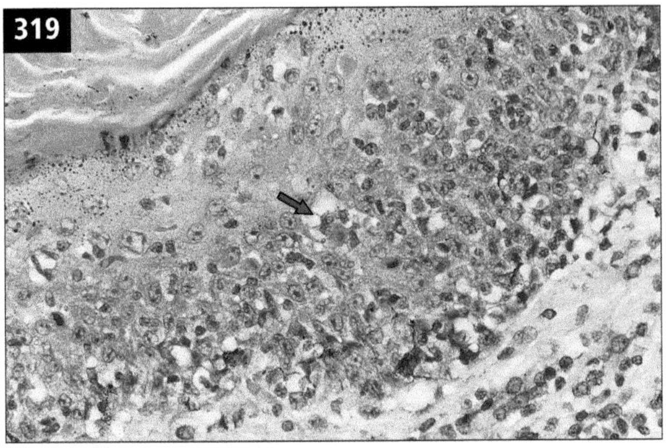

319 Erythema multiforme. Skin biopsy from a nine-year-old crossbred dog with generalized cutaneous bullae. There is an interface infiltrate of lymphocytes and macrophages with vacuolation of the basal epidermal cells. Individual to confluent apoptotic keratinocytes are prominent within the epidermis and there is satellitosis of lymphocytes around these cells (arrowed).

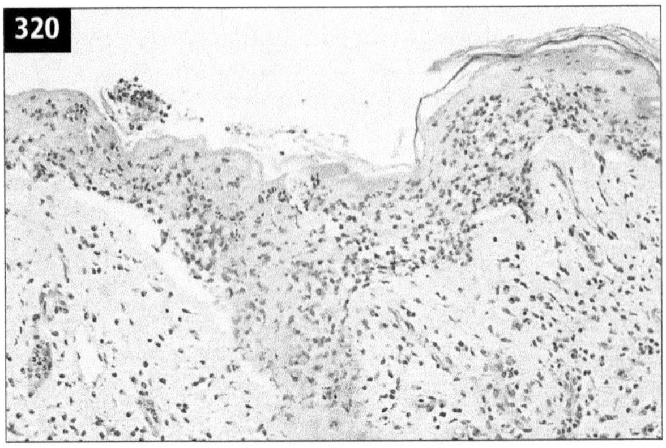

320 Toxic epidermal necrolysis. Skin biopsy from a seven-year-old Lurcher with multiple ulcerative mucocutaneous lesions. There is full-thickness, coagulative necrosis of the epidermis, with a mixed inflammatory infiltration of dermis and epidermis.

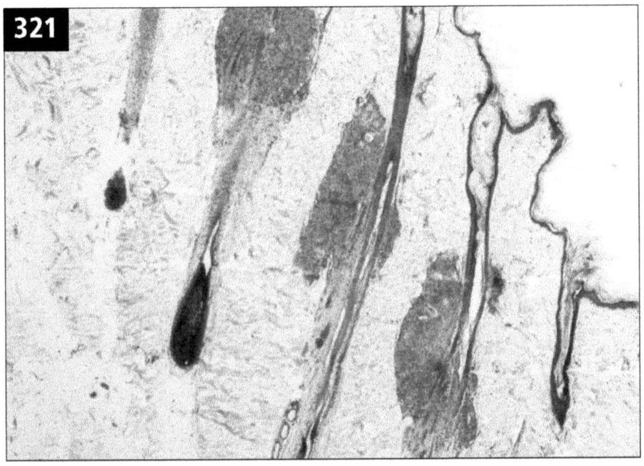

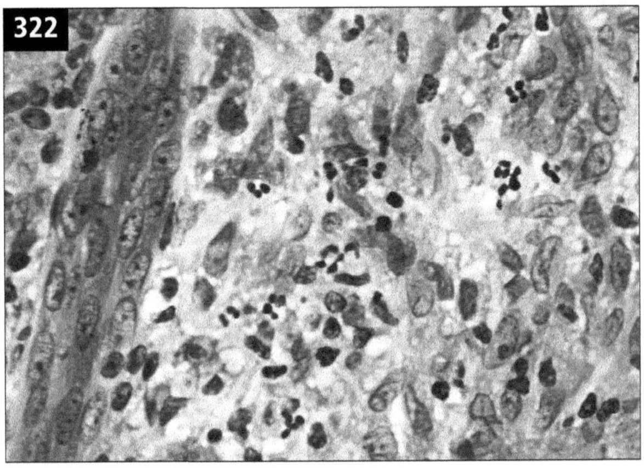

321, 322 Sebaceous adenitis. Skin biopsy from a two-year-old, neutered female Staffordshire Bull Terrier with progressive alopecia and scaling that started at six months of age. Sebaceous glands are specifically targeted and destroyed by a granulomatous inflammatory infiltrate.

- An interface inflammatory infiltrate of lymphocytes and macrophages. The lymphocytes within the epidermis and dermis of EM lesions are predominantly $CD8^+$ $\alpha\beta^+$ T cells, with fewer dermal $CD4^+$ cells and B cells (**319**).

The vesiculobullous lesions of EM are characterized by segmental full thickness epidermal necrosis and a superficial perivascular dermatitis involving lymphocytes and macrophages. The characteristic histopathological appearance of TEN is shown in **320**. Although such classical lesions are often described, it has recently been proposed that there is considerable overlap between the conditions, and histopathology should only be used to diagnose the EM-TEN spectrum rather than individual entities within it.

Treatment and prognosis

EM may be a relatively mild disease that regresses spontaneously as the underlying cause is resolved. The lesions are poorly responsive to immunosuppressive therapy. In contrast, TEN has a grave prognosis, particularly when the cutaneous lesions are extensive, with loss of fluid, electrolytes and colloid through affected skin and secondary bacterial infection. Any identified primary cause should be rectified and any concurrent medication withdrawn. The use of immunosuppressive therapy is controversial, but broad-spectrum antibiotics, analgesia, fluids, topical management and parenteral nutrition are essential. Recent reports have described the efficacy of intravenous human immunoglobulin administration (0.5–1.5 g/kg i/v over 6–12 hours) in the treatment of these disorders in some canine and feline cases. The major mechanism by which such therapy has an effect is thought to involve inhibition of the Fas-Fas ligand interaction.

SEBACEOUS ADENITIS

Pathogenesis

In this uncommon disorder there is selective destruction of the sebaceous glands by a chiefly granulomatous inflammatory infiltrate, which includes macrophages, lymphocytes, plasma cells and fewer neutrophils (**321, 322**). The lymphocytes and macrophages may also infiltrate the wall of the adjacent hair follicle isthmus. This reaction has been characterized immunohistochemically and the results suggest a cell-mediated immune mechanism based on the presence of dendritic cells, mixed $CD4^+$ and $CD8^+$ T cells (primarily expressing the αβ TCR) and fewer cells of the B lineage. Indirect immunohistochemistry, using serum from affected dogs overlaid onto normal skin substrates, has not shown the presence of sebaceous gland autoantibody, which further suggests a cell-mediated immunopathogenesis.

Clinical signs

There are recognized breed predispositions for the Vizsla, Japanese Akita, Samoyed and Standard Poodle, and possibly the Dachshund. Other affected breeds include the Old English Sheepdog, Toy Poodle, Springer Spaniel, Lhasa Apso, Boxer, Chow Chow and Collie. The disease is also reported in crossbred dogs. It is suggested than an autosomal recessive inheritance pattern occurs in the Japanese Akita and Standard Poodle. The disease is considered rare in the cat. Most dogs are young to middle-aged at disease presentation and there is no sex predisposition. The lesions are generally of scaling, follicular plugging and alopecia, but the clinical presentation varies between breeds (**323, 324**). The lesions are generally bilaterally symmetrical and particularly involve the trunk, face and pinnae. Secondary infection may occur and all of these clinical signs may relate to lack of sebum production and the presence of inflammatory infiltrates.

In long-coated breeds such as the Standard Poodle and Samoyed, the lesions characteristically appear as adherent scale, with 'frond-like' follicular keratin casts extending from dilated hair follicles. Keratin may closely adhere to the hairs. These changes are associated with areas of alopecia, predominantly over the dorsum. The lesions of the Samoyed may progress to the formation of discrete plaques. In the Japanese Akita the appearance is similar to the Standard Poodle, but with more pronounced alopecia and a greater incidence of secondary infection (bacterial folliculitis to furunculosis). Affected Japanese Akitas may also be systemically unwell (pyrexia, malaise, weight loss).

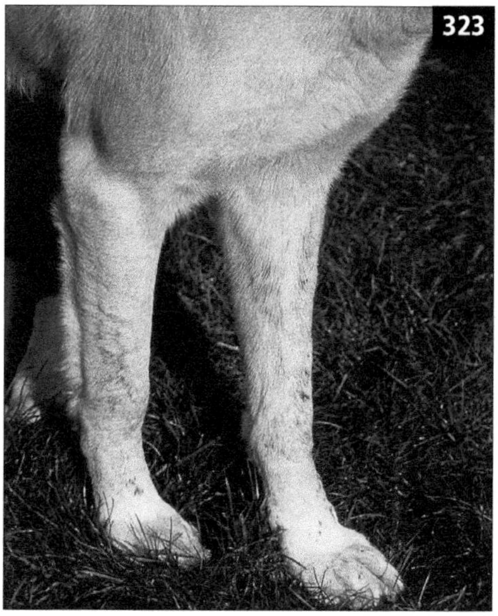

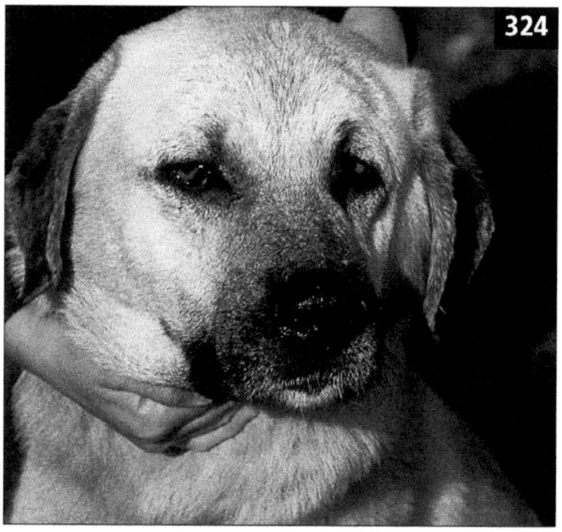

323, 324 Sebaceous adenitis. Multifocal areas of alopecia and scaling affecting the head and limbs of a four-year-old Anatolian Karabash.

In short-coated breeds such as the Vizsla and Dachshund, the clinical appearance includes truncal, focal to coalescing, firm nodular lesions and plaques, with alopecia, follicular keratin casts and adherent scale. This form of the disease is distinctly different from that described above for long-coated breeds. Cats with sebaceous adenitis also have multifocal areas of alopecia, scaling, follicular keratin casts and crusting.

Diagnosis

Skin biopsy is the definitive diagnostic test for sebaceous adenitis, and multiple samples should be collected to ascertain the involvement of multiple sebaceous glands. Histologically, in addition to the sebaceous inflammatory infiltration, there is epidermal hyperplasia, hyperkeratosis and follicular plugging ('follicular fronding'), but these changes are more pronounced in long-coated breeds. In chronic lesions the sebaceous glands will be absent and there may be no residual inflammation. Chronic lesions may also include evidence of follicular atrophy or dysplasia. As described above, in some breeds there is likely to be secondary bacterial folliculitis–furunculosis.

Treatment

The loss of sebaceous tissue may be permanent and chronic cases do not recover. Some short-coated dogs are reported to make a response to immunosuppressive glucocorticoid and retinoids have been of benefit in some affected Vizslas. High dose, oral essential fatty acids are also reported to be of benefit. There is evidence for the efficacy of ciclosporin in the treatment of this disease (5 mg/kg p/o q24h), with recurrence of lesions when therapy is withdrawn. There is also an increase in the percentage of follicles with sebaceous glands in post-treatment biopsies, suggesting some regeneration of sebaceous tissue occurs. Ciclosporin treatment should be started as early as possible in the course of disease, as animals with chronic disease may respond less effectively. Topical therapy (shampoos, baby oil) should be used in parallel.

ALOPECIA AREATA

Pathogenesis

In alopecia areata the target of the immune response is the anagen hair bulb, with infiltration of this area by lymphocytes, macrophages, plasma cells and fewer neutrophils or eosinophils (the 'swarm of bees'). Immunohistochemically the lymphocytes are a mixture of $CD4^+$ and $CD8^+$ cells (predominantly the latter) and the $CD8^+$ cells in particular are noted to directly infiltrate the bulbar epithelium. Dendritic cells also feature prominently in the infiltrates. It is proposed that the lymphoid cells mount a cytotoxic attack on bulbar epithelial cells and melanocytes, leading to apoptosis (as shown by *in situ* labelling) or hydropic degeneration of these targets. There may be peribulbar pigmentary incontinence, with prominent melanophages.

Direct immunofluorescence of lesional skin biopsies has demonstrated IgG bound to the lower hair follicles (the glassy membrane/basal lamina, the follicular papilla or medulla, the hair matrix). Indirect immunohistochemistry using serum from affected dogs overlaid onto normal skin substrates has identified autoantibody that binds to the inner and outer root sheath, medulla, matrix and precortex of anagen hair follicles. This immunolabelling corresponded in position to that produced with a monoclonal antibody specific for the structural protein trichohyalin. These observations have been extended by western blotting analysis, which identified the major autoantigens for this serological response as being of 40–60 and 200–220 kD molecular weight (MW). The higher MW molecule co-migrated with trichohyalin, as detected by use of the monoclonal antibody. Immunoprecipitation studies (using crude human hair follicle extract) confirmed that the autoantibodies in the serum of dogs with alopecia areata were able to precipitate trichohyalin from hair follicle extracts. The direct pathogenic role of these autoantibodies remains to be proven, and they may still reflect an epiphenomenon secondary to the cell-mediated attack (although antibody can be detected before the onset of alopecia in a mouse model, and such antibodies are not present in the serum of dogs with follicular breakdown due to other reasons such as demodicosis). Against this, injection of serum from dogs with alopecia areata into the clipped back of mice led to failure of hair regrowth around the injection site and the presence of telogen follicles on biopsy of this location.

Clinical signs

Alopecia areata is an uncommon disease of the dog and rare in the cat and horse. It has been suggested that there is breed predisposition for Dachshunds and GSDs, although the disease is really too uncommonly reported to clearly define such associations. There is a wide range of age of onset

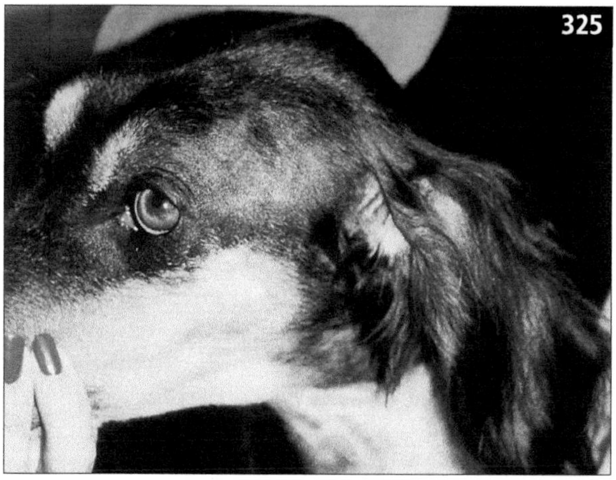

325 Lymphocytic folliculitis (alopecia areata). Partial alopecia affecting the forehead, pinnae, lateral thighs and tail tip in a five-year-old Saluki with alopecia areata. The alopecia waxes and wanes and is unassociated with signs of inflammatory skin disease.

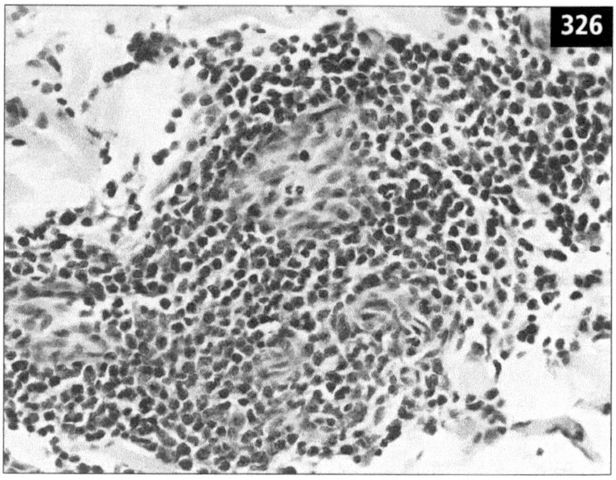

326 Lymphocytic folliculitis (alopecia areata). Skin biopsy from an 11-year-old Labrador with multifocal alopecia that progressed over a six-month period. There is selective destruction of hair bulbs by an intense lymphocytic infiltration. Apocrine and sebaceous glands are not primarily affected.

(one to 11 years, median five years) and no sex predisposition. The clinical signs relate directly to the follicular destruction and affected animals present with multifocal or bilaterally symmetrical patches of alopecia that show gradual expansion. There is a predilection to involve the hair coat of the face, and a characteristic clinical appearance is of periorbital alopecia ('goggles') (325). The neck, limbs and trunk may also be affected. In dogs with multicoloured hair coats (e.g. GSDs or Dachshunds) the disease may be restricted to hairs of one particular colour. Leukotrichia is less commonly observed and abnormalities of nail growth are rare.

Diagnosis

Definitive diagnosis is by skin biopsy, and in this disease biopsies should be collected from the centre of lesions in addition to the leading edge. The classic bulbar inflammatory lesions are described above (326). The inflammation does not (generally) involve the follicular isthmus or sebaceous gland, although in a proportion of cases the process will extend to the isthmus region. In chronic lesions the inflammation may be minimal (and predominantly lymphocytic) and follicular dysplasia or dominant telogen follicles may be prominent.

Treatment

The disease has a naturally waxing and waning course, and animals may display spontaneous recovery, with hair regrowth, after 6–24 months. The hair that regrows may be unpigmented, consistent with the proposed immune-mediated destruction of melanocytes; however, after several cycles pigmentation may be regained. The disease is relatively benign and primarily of cosmetic importance. Mild immunosuppressive therapy may be used, but evidence for its efficacy is limited by the few reported case series and complicated by the spontaneous recovery that may occur. Despite this, both response and resistance to immunosuppressive therapy is reported. Ciclosporin therapy has been reported to be effective in one case. There is no correlation between disease outcome and histopathological appearance.

PSEUDOPELADE

Pathogenesis

Psuedopelade has a similar proposed pathogenesis to alopecia areata, but it targets the mid level (isthmus) of the hair follicles rather than the hair bulb. The nature of the inflammatory infiltrates is similar to that described in alopecia areata. The folliculotropic lymphocytes are generally $CD8^+$, while those T cells located perifollicularly are a mixture of $CD8^+$ and $CD4^+$ T cells. Autoantibodies (specific for hair follicle keratins and trichohylain) are identified by western blotting or indirect immunofluorescence as described for alopecia areata. A wider spectrum of such antibodies is identified in animals affected with this disease.

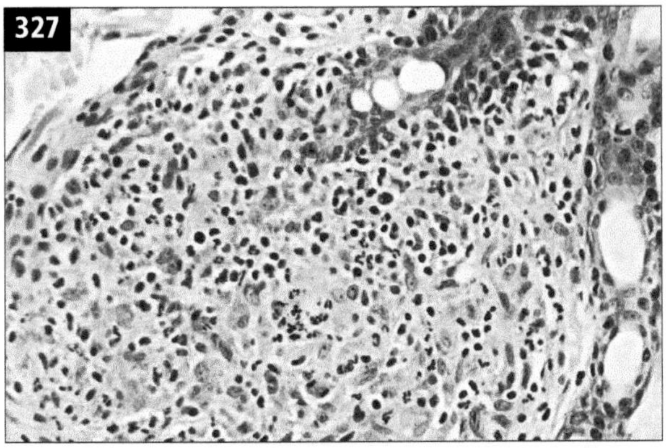

327 Granulomatous mural folliculitis. Skin biopsy from a three-year-old neutered male Labrador Retriever with a four-month history of progressive alopecia and hypopigmentation. The granulomatous inflammatory response targets the mid level of the hair follicle.

Clinical signs

Pseudopelade is a rare disease recognized in both the dog and cat (one case) and, as such, no breed, age or sex predispositions have yet been defined. The clinical presentation is of alopecia, which is usually patchy in distribution and primarily affects the trunk and limbs. In some dogs, scaling and hyperpigmentation may occur.

Diagnosis

Diagnosis is by skin biopsy and areas of maximum alopecia should be sampled. The histopathological appearance is of the isthmus inflammatory lesion described above. The hair bulbs and sebaceous glands are not generally affected. There may be degenerative change to the local follicular keratinocytes, and local pigmentary incontinence may be observed. In chronic lesions there may be minimal inflammation, with atrophic (telogen phase) follicles.

Treatment

Hair loss in pseudopelade is generally considered permanent, but limited regrowth may occur in some cases (as opposed to alopecia areata). There is no clear response to immunosuppressive therapy in affected dogs. In one reported feline case there was no response to immunosuppressive doses of glucocorticoid, but a marked response to ciclosporin (5 mg/kg p/o q12h) occurred after one month of therapy, although hair loss recommenced by three months.

CANINE GRANULOMATOUS MURAL FOLLICULITIS

This rare disorder of the dog is of presumptive immune-mediated pathogenesis, but it is often associated with drug administration (amitraz, cefadroxil, L-thyroxine and a range of topical substances). No breed, age or sex predispositions are defined. The clinical appearance is of alopecia, which may be patchy-multifocal (particularly involving the head, trunk and extremities) or, sometimes, generalized. There may be erythema, scaling and crusting, with ulceration or follicular plugging in severe cases. Focal leukoderma or leukotrichia may be present and secondary bacterial infection may occur.

Diagnosis is by skin biopsy of the areas of maximum alopecia. Histologically there is epidermal hyperplasia, hyperkeratosis and follicular keratosis. The characteristic lesion is destruction of the entire hair follicle by a pyogranulomatous inflammatory infiltrate, which also includes lymphocytes (327). Multinucleate giant cells may also be present. The inflammatory lesion may centre on the isthmus, but generally extends both to the bulb and the ostium. The sebaceous gland may also be destroyed. Apoptosis of follicular keratinocytes may be observed in regions of residual structure. Dermal inflammation may be absent, or there may be an interface lichenoid reaction with epidermal degeneration (including basal cell apoptosis). In chronic lesions there is minimal inflammation but complete absence of follicles and sebaceous glands. The clinical outcome is variable, with some dogs regrowing hair after removal of the likely causative drug.

PLASMA CELL PODODERMATITIS

Plasma cell pododermatitis is an uncommon idiopathic disorder of cats, characterized clinically by soft swelling of footpads (particularly metacarpal/tarsal) on multiple paws, which commonly become ulcerated (328, 329). Histopathologically there is an intense plasmacytic infiltration of dermal tissue (330), with other inflammatory cell types if secondary infection has occurred. Plasma cell pododermatitis in conjunction with lymphoplasmacytic gingivostomatitis or immune-mediated glomerulonephritis and serum ANA is documented. Typically, there will be a hypergammaglobulinaemia. A recent study failed to demonstrate the presence of candidate

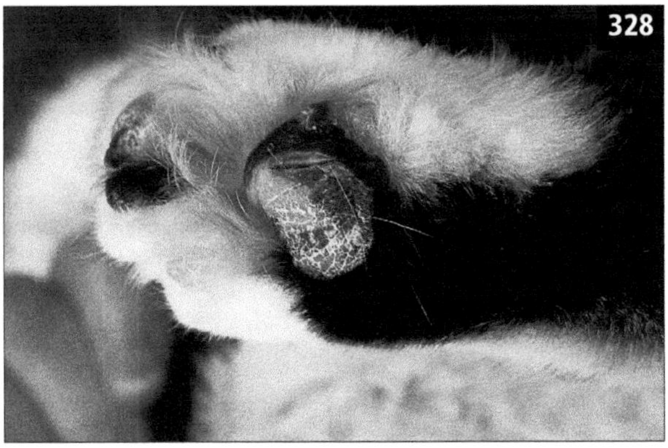

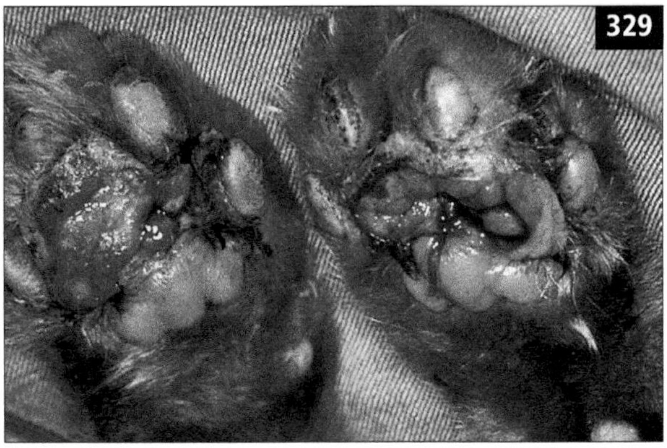

328, 329 Plasma cell pododermatitis. (**328**) Fluctuant swelling and scaling of the central pad in an acute case of plasma cell pododermatitis in a three-year-old DSH cat. (**329**) Ulceration of multiple foot pads in a five-year-old Persian cat with plasma cell pododermatitis. (Photograph courtesy The Feline Centre, University of Bristol.)

330 Plasma cell pododermatitis. Biopsy from a four-year-old DSH cat with swollen front footpads and focal pad ulceration. There is a marked inflammatory infiltrate, which consists primarily of plasma cells that occasionally contain Russell bodies.

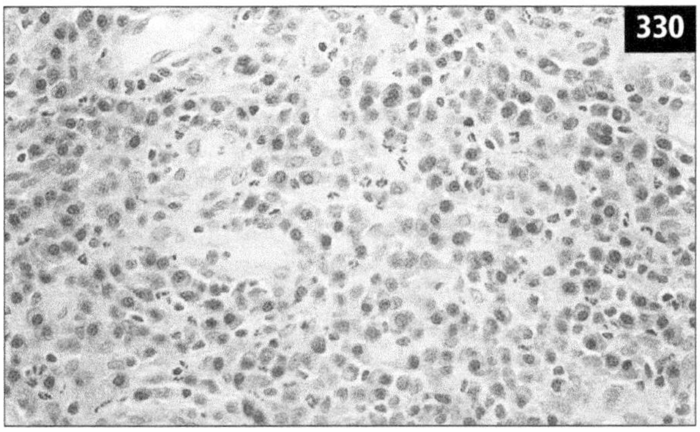

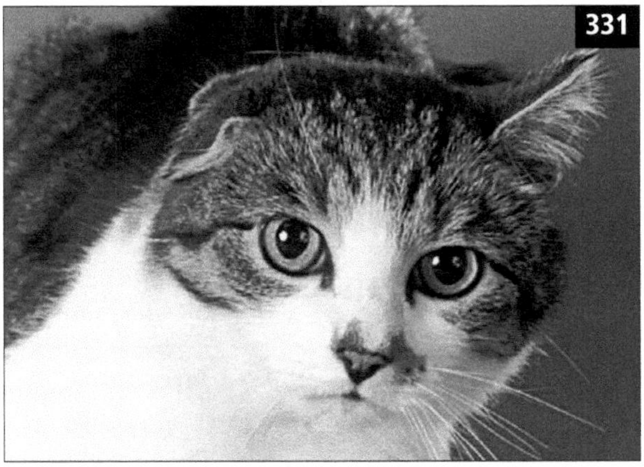

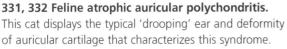

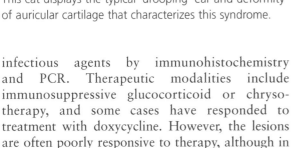

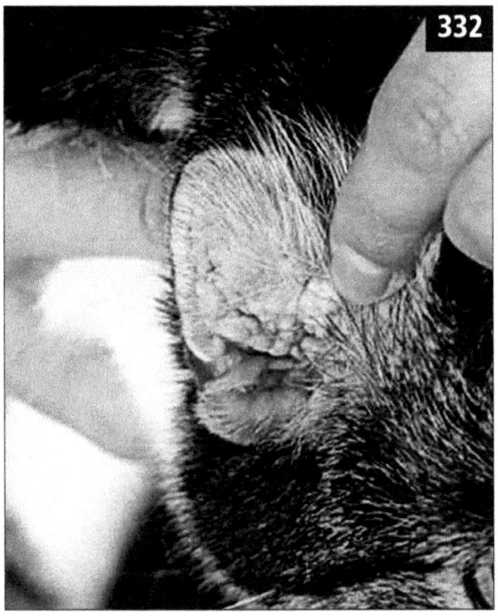

331, 332 Feline atrophic auricular polychondritis. This cat displays the typical 'drooping' ear and deformity of auricular cartilage that characterizes this syndrome.

infectious agents by immunohistochemistry and PCR. Therapeutic modalities include immunosuppressive glucocorticoid or chrysotherapy, and some cases have responded to treatment with doxycycline. However, the lesions are often poorly responsive to therapy, although in some cases spontaneous regression may occur.

FELINE ATROPHIC AURICULAR POLYCHONDRITIS

This relatively recently recognized entity classically presents with deformity of the auricular cartilage, leading to a 'drooping' appearance of the pinna (331, 332). The ear may be swollen, erythematous and painful, with evidence of self-trauma. In acute stages of the disease, affected cats may be anorexic and pyrexic. Biopsy reveals the presence of a lymphocytic to granulomatous inflammatory infiltrate of the auricular cartilage, with cartilage necrosis. There is no vasculitis and immunohistochemistry does not reveal deposition of immunoreactants. The disease has a presumed immune-mediated pathogenesis, although the target antigens and immunopathological mechanisms involved are poorly characterized. There is a homologous polychrondritis in humans, which is associated with the presence of numerous autoantibodies and involvement of cartilage in multiple anatomical locations. This form of disease is less commonly recognized in the cat (see Chapter 6, p. 190). The feline disease appears self limiting, and glucocorticoid administration does not reverse the auricular deformity.

FURTHER READING

Bettenay SV, Lappin MR, Mueller RS (2007) An immunohistochemical and polymerase chain reaction evaluation of feline plasmacytic pododermatitis. *Veterinary Pathology* **44**:80–83.

Diesel A, DeBoer DJ (2010) Serum allergen-specific immunoglobulin E in atopic and healthy cats: comparison of a rapid screening immunoassay and complete-panel analysis. *Veterinary Dermatology* **22**:39–45.

Foster AP, Knowles TG, Hotston Moore A *et al.* (2003) Serum IgE and IgG responses to food antigens in normal and atopic dogs, and dogs with gastrointestinal disease. *Veterinary Immunology and Immunopathology* **92**:113–124.

Fujiwara S, Yasunaga S, Iwabuchi S *et al.* (2003) Cytokine profiles of peripheral blood mononuclear cells from dogs experimentally sensitized to Japanese cedar pollen. *Veterinary Immunology and Immunopathology* **93**:9–20.

Hayashiya S, Tani K, Morimoto M *et al.* (2002) Expression of T helper 1 and T helper 2 cytokine mRNAs in freshly isolated peripheral blood mononuclear cells from dogs with atopic dermatitis. *Journal of Veterinary Medicine A* **49**:27–31.

Hou C-C, Day MJ, Nuttall TJ *et al.* (2006) The production of IgG subclasses against *Dermatophagoides farinae* allergens in healthy and atopic dogs. *Veterinary Dermatology* **17**:103–110.

Jackson HA, Olivry T, Berget F *et al.* (2004) Immunopathology of vesicular cutaneous lupus erythematosus in the Rough Collie and Shetland Sheepdog: a canine homologue of subacute cutaneous lupus erythematosus in humans. *Veterinary Dermatology* **15**:230–269.

Jaeger K, Linek M, Power HT *et al.* (2010) Breed and site predispositions of dogs with atopic dermatitis: a comparison of five locations in three continents. *Veterinary Dermatology* **21**:119–123.

Keppel KE, Campbell KL, Zuckermann FA *et al.* (2008) Quantitation of canine regulatory T cell populations, serum interleukin-10 and allergen-specific IgE concentrations in healthy control dogs and canine atopic dermatitis patients receiving allergen-specific immunotherapy. *Veterinary Immunology and Immunopathology* **123**:337–344.

Loewenstein C, Mueller RS (2009) A review of allergen-specific immunotherapy in human and veterinary medicine. *Veterinary Dermatology* **20**:84–98.

Lortz J, Favrot C, Mecklenburg L *et al.* (2010) A multicentre placebo-controlled clinical trial on the efficacy of oral ciclosporin A in the treatment of canine idiopathic sebaceous adenitis in comparison with conventional topical treatment. *Veterinary Dermatology* **21**:593–601.

Marsella R (2010) Tolerability and clinical efficacy of oral immunotherapy with house dust mites in a model of canine atopic dermatitis: a pilot study. *Veterinary Dermatology* **21**:566–571.

Masuda K, Sakaguchi M, Saito S *et al.* (2004) Identification of peptides containing T-cell epitopes of Japanese cedar (*Cryptomeria japonica*) pollen allergen (Cry j1) in dogs. *Veterinary Immunology and Immunopathology* **102**:45–52.

Masuda K (2005) DNA vaccination against Japanese cedar pollinosis in dogs suppresses type I hypersensitivity by controlling lesional mast cells. *Veterinary Immunology and Immunopathology* **108**:185–187.

Mauldin EA, Morris DO, Brown DC *et al.* (2010) Exfoliative cutaneous lupus erythematosus in German shorthaired pointer dogs: disease development, progression and evaluation of three immunomodulatory drugs (ciclosporin, hydroxychloroquine, and adalimumab) in a controlled environment. *Veterinary Dermatology* **21**:373–382.

Merryman-Simpson AE, Wood SH, Fretwell N *et al.* (2008) Gene (mRNA) expression in canine atopic dermatitis: microarray analysis. *Veterinary Dermatology* **19**:59–66.

Mueller RS, West K, Bettenay SV (2004) Immunohistochemical evaluation of mononuclear infiltrates in canine lupoid onychodystrophy. *Veterinary Pathology* **41**:37–43.

Mueller RS, Veir J, Fieseler KV *et al.* (2005) Use of immunostimulatory liposome-nucleic acid complexes in allergen-specific immunotherapy of dogs with refractory atopic dermatitis: a pilot study. *Veterinary Dermatology* **16**:61–68.

Nichols PR, Morris DO, Beale KM (2001) A retrospective study of canine and feline cutaneous vasculitis. *Veterinary Dermatology* **12**:255–264.

Nuttall TJ, Knight PA, McAleese SM *et al.* (2002) Expression of Th1, Th2 and immunosuppressive cytokine gene transcripts in canine atopic dermatitis. *Clinical and Experimental Allergy* **32**:789–795.

Nuttall TJ, Pemberton AD, Lamb JR *et al.* (2002) Peripheral blood mononuclear cell responses to major and minor *Dermatophagoides* allergens in canine atopic dermatitis. *Veterinary Immunology and Immunopathology* **84**:143–150.

Preziosi DE, Goldschmidt MH, Greek JS *et al.* (2003) Feline pemphigus foliaceus: a retrospective analysis of 57 cases. *Veterinary Dermatology* **14**:313–321.

Olivry T, Dunston SM, Marcy Murphy K *et al.* (2001) Characterization of the inflammatory infiltrate during IgE-mediated late phase reactions in the skin of normal and atopic dogs. *Veterinary Dermatology* **12**:49–58.

Olivry T (2006) A review of autoimmune skin diseases in domestic animals: I - superficial pemphigus. *Veterinary Dermatology* **17**:291–305.

Olivry T, Bizikova P, Dunston SM *et al.* (2009) Clinical and immunological heterogeneity of canine subepidermal blistering dermatoses with anti-laminin-332 (laminin-5) auto-antibodies. *Veterinary Dermatology* **21**:345–357.

Olivry T, Linder KE (2009) Dermatoses affecting desmosomes in animals: a mechanistic review of acantholytic blistering skin diseases. *Veterinary Dermatology* **20**:313–326

Olivry T, DeBoer DJ, Favrot C (2010) Treatment of canine atopic dermatitis: 2010 clinical practice guidelines from the International Task Force on Canine Atopic Dermatitis. *Veterinary Dermatology* **21**:233–248.

Reichler IM, Hauser B, Schiller I *et al.* (2001) Sebaceous adenitis in the Akita: clinical observations, histopathology and heredity. *Veterinary Dermatology* **12**:243–253.

Santoro D, Bunick D, Graves TK *et al.* (2010) Expression and distribution of antimicrobial peptides in the skin of healthy beagles. *Veterinary Dermatology* **22**:61–67.

Schleifer SG, Willemse T (2003) Evaluation of skin test reactivity to environmental allergens in healthy cats and cats with atopic dermatitis. *American Journal of Veterinary Research* **64**:773–778.

Taglinger K, Helps CR, Day MJ *et al.* (2005) Measurement of serum immunoglobulin E (IgE) specific for house dust mite antigens in normal cats and cats with allergic skin disease. *Veterinary Immunology and Immunopathology* **105**:85–93.

Taglinger K, Day MJ, Foster AP (2007) Characterization of inflammatory cell infiltration in feline allergic skin disease. *Journal of Comparative Pathology* **137**:211–223.

The ACVD task force on canine atopic dermatitis (2001) Special Issue. *Veterinary Immunology and Immunopathology* **81**:143–383.

Veenhof EZ, Knol E, Schlotter YM *et al.* (2011) Characterization of T cell phenotypes, cytokines and transcription factors in the skin of dogs with cutaneous adverse food reactions. *Veterinary Journal* **187**:320–324.

Vercelli A, Raviri G, Cornegliani L (2006) The use of oral cyclosporin to treat feline dermatoses: a retrospective analysis of 23 cases. *Veterinary Dermatology* **17**:201–206.

Wilhem S, Kovalik M, Favrot C (2010) Breed-associated phenotypes in canine atopic dermatitis. *Veterinary Dermatology* **22**:143–149.

Yasukawa K, Saito S, Kubo T *et al.* (2010) Low-dose recombinant canine interferon-γ for treatment of canine atopic dermatitis: an open randomized comparative trial of two doses. *Veterinary Dermatology* **21**:42–49.

6 IMMUNE-MEDIATED MUSCULOSKELETAL AND NEUROLOGICAL DISEASE

Michael J. Day and David Bennett

INTRODUCTION

This chapter describes immune-mediated diseases affecting the joints and muscles and nervous system of the dog and cat. In recent years there has been much greater understanding of the immunopathogenesis and genetic basis for many of these disorders.

IMMUNE-MEDIATED POLYARTHRITIS

The immune-mediated polyarthritidies of the dog and cat are defined by chronic synovial inflammation, failure to identify a microbial aetiology on routine culture and clinical response to immunosuppressive therapy. Although these diseases have common immunopathogenic features, they may be subdivided on the basis of clinical, radiographical, pathological and serological parameters (*Table 14*). Some entities are similar to human polyarthritis syndromes, and human nomenclature has been adapted to the canine and feline disorders. However, the classification of immune-mediated arthritis in dogs and cats is a cause of debate. There are no universally accepted criteria that define specific diseases, but

Table 14: Classification of immune-mediated polyarthritis in the dog and cat.

Dog	Cat
Erosive polyarthritis: • Rheumatoid arthritis. • Periosteal proliferative polyarthritis. *Non-erosive polyarthritis*: • Systemic lupus erythematosus. • Polyarthritis/polymyositis syndrome. • Polyarthritis/meningitis syndrome. • Arthritis of Japanese Akitas. • Amyloidosis of Chinese Shar Peis. • Polyarteritis nodosa. • Sjögren's syndrome. • Idiopathic polyarthritis: – Type I uncomplicated. – Type II reactive arthritis (associated with infection remote from joints). – Type III enteropathic arthritis (associated with gastrointestinal disease). – Type IV neoplasia related (associated with neoplasia remote from joints). • Drug-induced arthritis. • Arthritis associated with vaccination. • Lymphoplasmacytic arthritis of stifle joints. • Arthritis following microbial joint infections.	*Erosive polyarthritis*: • Rheumatoid arthritis. • Periosteal proliferative polyarthritis. *Non-erosive polyarthritis*: • Systemic lupus erythematosus. • Polyarthritis/meningitis syndrome. • Polyarteritis nodosa. • Idiopathic polyarthritis: – Type I uncomplicated. – Type II reactive. – Type III enteropathic. – Type IV neoplasia related. • Drug-induced arthritis. • Arthritis associated with vaccination. • Arthritis following microbial joint infections. • Relapsing polychrondritis.

classification of the arthropathies is important for deciding on treatment and prognosis.

The underlying aetiologies of immune-mediated arthropathies are generally unknown, although there is evidence to support the role of microbial infections. Microorganisms cannot be cultured from the joint, so these arthropathies are not examples of true infective arthritis. However, following antibiotic treatment of a bacterial arthritis, there may be residual synovitis associated with persisting bacterial antigens. An excellent example of this phenomenon occurs in human Lyme arthritis, a tick-borne disease caused by *Borrelia burgdorferi* infection. A proportion of patients have persisting arthritis after antimicrobial therapy that has rendered the joint negative for the bacterium by both culture and PCR. These 'antibiotic resistant' patients have high titred antibody specific for the outer surface protein A (OspA) of the organism and they mount strong Th1 responses to a specific peptide (amino acids 165–173) derived from the protein. Intriguingly, this peptide is identical to one derived from the sequence of the human lymphocyte function-associated antigen 1 (LFA-1), suggesting that *Borrelia*-specific T cell activity may be perpetuated by this autoantigen after elimination of the infectious agent. This is an excellent example of 'molecular mimicry' (see Chapter 3, p. 87). In canine patients as well, vector-borne agents such as *Borrelia*, *Bartonella*, *Ehrlichia* or *Leishmania* may be associated with either an infective or immune-mediated arthritis.

Studies on canine polyarthritis have also implicated the role of canine distemper virus (CDV) as an inciting cause. Western blot analyses have confirmed the presence of CDV antigens within the immune complexes precipitated from synovial fluid of dogs with immune based polyarthritis, and immunocytochemistry has shown CDV antigens within synovial macrophages of affected joints. Raised levels of CDV antibodies within the synovial fluid have also been found. This suggests that CDV antibodies are an important component of the immune complexes. The synovial fluid neutrophil count correlates with the synovial fluid CDV antibody level and the levels of CDV antibody in synovial fluid immune complexes. CDV antibody levels within synovial fluid also correlate with antibodies against a 65kD HSP, an antigen that is associated with synovial inflammation. A recent study has shown increased bacterial DNA (by PCR) within arthritic canine stifle joints. It is proposed that this microbial antigen may trigger the inflammatory events leading to synovitis.

There is increasing evidence that genetic factors are involved in susceptibility to immune-mediated arthritis, probably by permitting inappropriate immune responses to particular antigens (see Chapter 3, p. 90). In man it is thought that susceptibility to RA is associated with the presence of a conserved sequence of amino acids (QKRAA/QRRAA/RRAA) present in the third hypervariable region (3HVR) of a number of HLA-DRB1 alleles. The sequences are usually referred to as the 'RA shared epitope'. This has also been shown for the dog. Human and dog DRB1 sequences show an average 86% nucleotide homology, with the 3HVR defined at the same codons in both species. Several DLA-DRB1 alleles are associated with an increased risk for canine immune-based polyarthritis-DLA-DRB1*002, DRB*009 and DRB*018. In the 288 known human HLA-DRB1 alleles, there are 19 different amino-acid sequences found for codons 70–74 on the 3HVR, and in 52 known canine DLA-DRB1 alleles there are 12 different amino acid sequences for codons 70–74. Only five of these are found in both species – QKRAA, QRRAA, RRRAA, QRRAE and RRRAE – and the first three of these are involved in the RA shared epitope. The association of the shared epitope with RA in both species suggests that this is not a chance finding, but is due to functionality of this epitope. The 3HVR is considered to encode a functionally important part of the human DRB1 molecule influencing both affinity of peptide binding and how the T cell receptor interfaces with the MHC/peptide complex. Although the association is not totally convincing in explaining breed susceptibility, the high frequency of QRRAA/RKRAA-bearing DLA-DRB1 alleles in King Charles Spaniels, GSDs and Border Collies is interesting, since these breeds are amongst the more frequently affected with immune-based polyarthritis.

RHEUMATOID ARTHRITIS

Pathogenesis

RA is the most common form of erosive polyarthritis recognized in the dog, but it is less prevalent in cats. There is, however, an impression (at least in the UK) that canine RA has decreased in incidence over the past decade and is now a relatively uncommon diagnosis. In dogs, RA is generally a disease of middle age and there are no gender or breed predispositions. DLA genetic associations with canine RA are described in Chapter 3 (p. 92). RA is considered to be an autoimmune disorder and likely has multifactorial aetiology with a combined type III and type IV immunopathogenesis (**333**).

In the type III component of RA, immune complexes lodge within the synovium and initiate local inflammation, with degeneration of articular cartilage via release of proteolytic enzymes and cytokines from inflammatory cells and synoviocytes. Immune complexes have been identified within synoviocytes, macrophages, blood vessel walls or the synovial stroma of dogs with RA, and the concentration of immune complexes is often elevated in the serum and synovial fluid. The nature of these complexes is poorly defined, but some may contain microbial antigen, and it is of note that CDV antigen (and antibody to the virus) has been recovered from the joints of dogs with RA (see above). Additionally, RA is characterized by the presence of 'rheumatoid factor' (RF), defined as an IgM (less often IgG or IgA) autoantibody with specificity for the Fc portion of an IgG molecule. The target IgG may itself be bound to an unidentified (possibly microbial) antigen and/or be conformationally altered (perhaps by reduced glycosylation of the Fc portion). RF is found within the serum and synovial fluid of animals with RA, but it may largely originate from synovial plasma cells. Autoantibodies specific for structural components of the joint (e.g. collagen) are also recognized. These are unlikely to be the initiating cause of joint pathology, but arise subsequent to articular damage and may have a secondary role in disease pathogenesis.

The type IV component of RA is suggested by the prominent, perivascular infiltration of mononuclear cells into affected synovium (**334–337**). In the dog these include T (predominantly CD4^{+}) and B

333

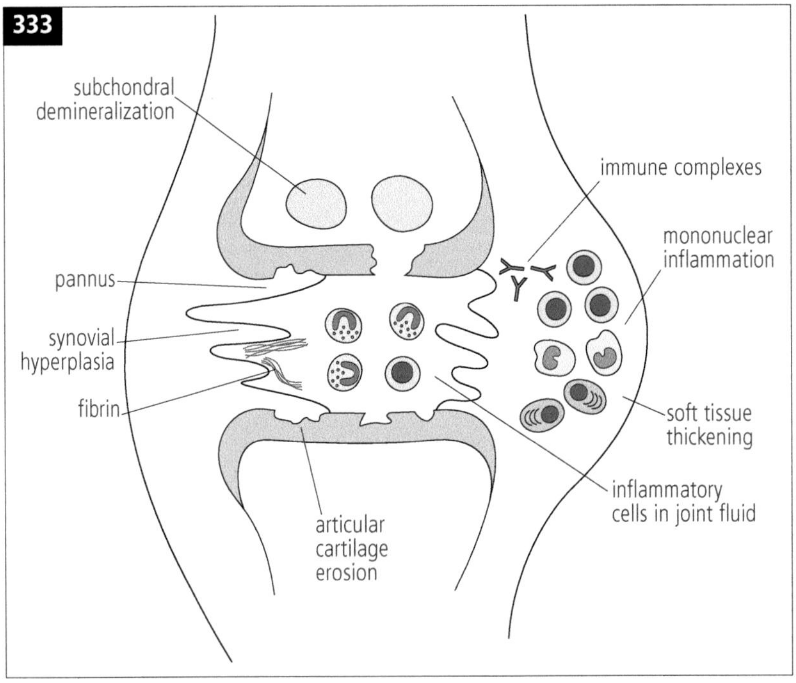

333 Immunopathogenesis of rheumatoid arthritis. RA is an autoimmune disease that involves type III and type IV immunopathogenic mechanisms. Immune complex deposition or formation within the synovial membrane leads to complement fixation and influx of inflammatory cells (chiefly neutrophils), which are found in large numbers within the synovial fluid. Synoviocyte necrosis and fibrin deposition is recognized. The type IV component of disease is characterized by an intense lymphoplasmacytic infiltration into the synovium, which is thrown up into villous folds due to synoviocyte hyperplasia and hypertrophy. The T lymphocytes (largely autoreactive), synoviocytes, neutrophils and macrophages release cytokines and enzymes that mediate degeneration of the articular cartilage and filling of the articular defects by fibrovascular granulation tissue (pannus), which extends from the synovium and may also infiltrate subchondral bone. Synovial plasma cells are a source of local antibody production. Antibodies specific for IgG (RF), articular collagen and HSPs are found within the serum and synovial fluid.

lymphocytes, plasma cells (IgG and IgM) and macrophages. There is MHC class II expression by synoviocytes and synovial dendritic cells (338). Release of cytokines and matrix metalloproteinases (MMPs) by such cells enhances inflammation and cartilage degeneration and encourages fibroblast proliferation to form the layer of granulation tissue ('pannus') that extends from the synovium to invade the articular cartilage and subchondral bone. The inflamed synovium is thrown into

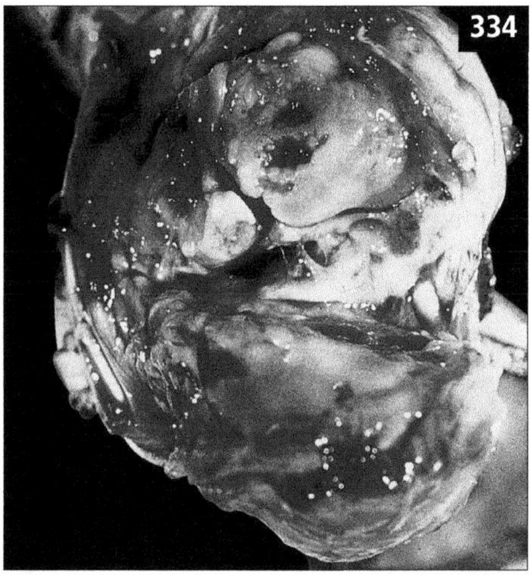

334

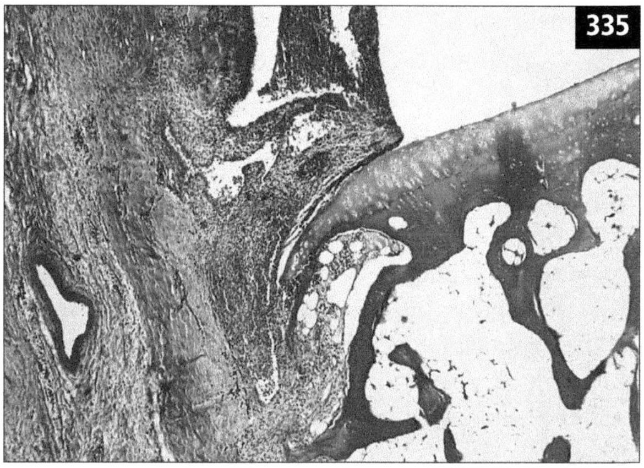

335

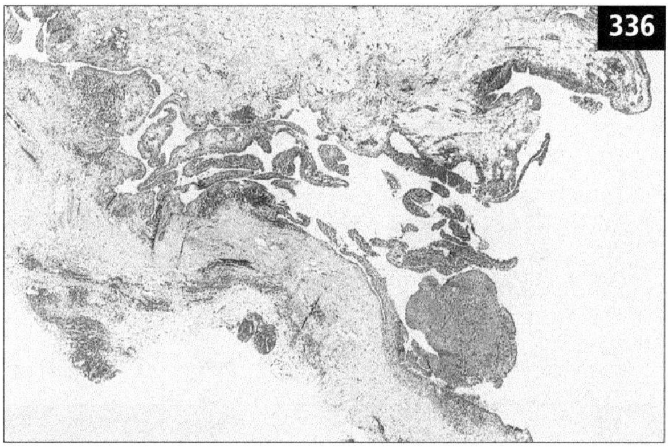

336

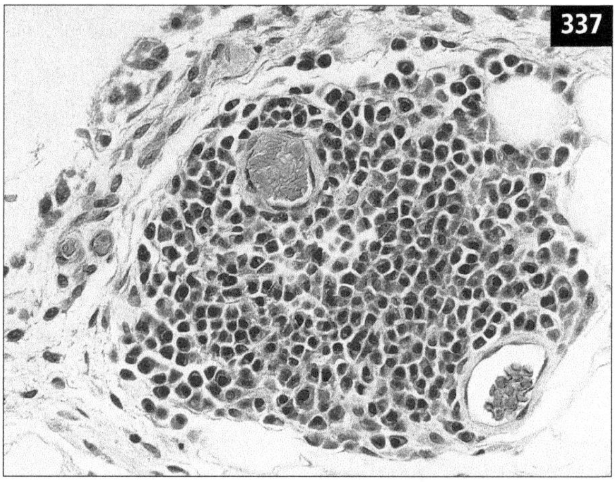

337

334–337 Pathology of canine rheumatoid arthritis. (**334**) Right carpus from a dog with RA. The synovial membrane is thickened and granulation tissue is covering the surface of the articular cartilage at the joint margins. In addition, two large cartilage defects are seen filled with granulation tissue. (**335**) Photomicrograph of a rheumatoid joint showing granulation tissue arising from the synovial membrane at the joint periphery, extending over the articular surface and forming a pannus and invading beneath the cartilage into the subchondral bone. (**336**) Synovial biopsy from an 18-month-old Bearded Collie dog with RA. There is marked villous hyperplasia of the synovial membrane, with underlying nodular aggregates of inflammatory cells. Fibrin deposition is evident on the synovial surface. (**337**) Higher power field of this synovial biopsy reveals large lymphoplasmacytic aggregates centred on blood vessels, which occasionally consist entirely of plasma cells.

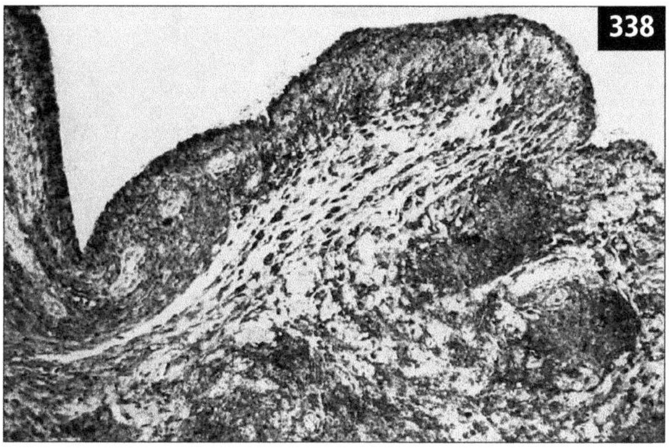

338

338 MHC class II expression in canine rheumatoid arthritis. Synovial membrane biopsy from a dog with RA demonstrating up-regulation of MHC class II. This is a common feature of all immune-mediated arthropathies, not just the rheumatoid group.

finger-like folds (villous hyperplasia). Recent studies have characterized the presence of elevated MMP-3 in the synovial fluid of dogs with RA and transcription of genes encoding IL-1, IL-8, TNFα and TGFβ by synovial fluid cells in the same animals.

The specificity of the infiltrating lymphoid cells is poorly defined. Experimental studies have suggested that many are specific for articular autoantigens (e.g. collagen), but others recognize self-'HSPs' derived from synoviocytes or chondrocytes. HSPs have a protective function in cells subjected to stress (such as heat and even inflammation) and they are involved in intracellular assembly, folding and translocation of proteins. Infective agents initiate release of HSPs by causing tissue damage. HSPs are highly conserved in nature, with a high degree of sequence homology between bacterial and mammalian HSP; therefore, although a response to HSP may appear autoimmune, it may have been initiated by prior exposure to cross-reactive bacterial HSP.

Clinical signs

In the dog, RA predominantly affects joints of the limbs, with occasional involvement of the diarthrodial intervertebral joints. The clinical history is of gradual onset or relapsing lameness, with generalized stiffness that is worse after rising from a period of rest. The clinical presentation is of bilaterally symmetrical polyarthritis and there may be pain, reduced movement, soft tissue thickening, heat and crepitus of affected joints. In some cases there may be subluxation or deformity of carpal and/or tarsal joints and joints of the digits (339–342). These cases represent the deforming type of the disease, which has a particularly poor prognosis. The deformities can occur with

339

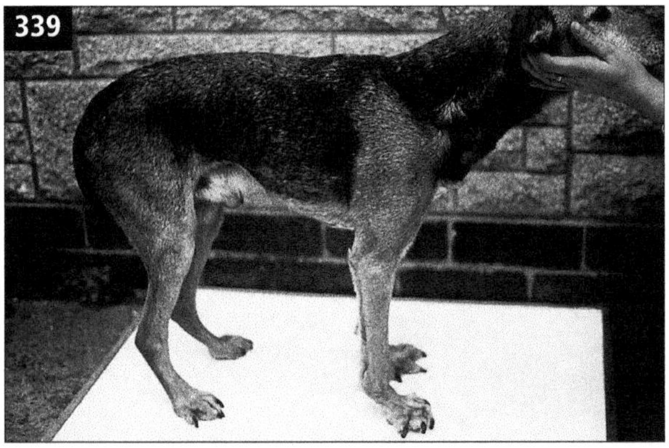

340

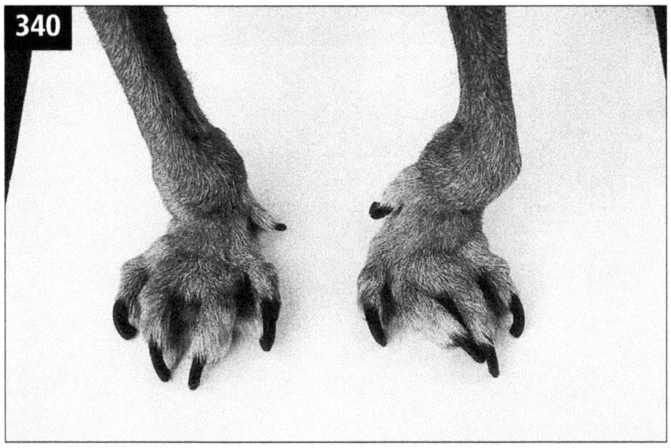

341

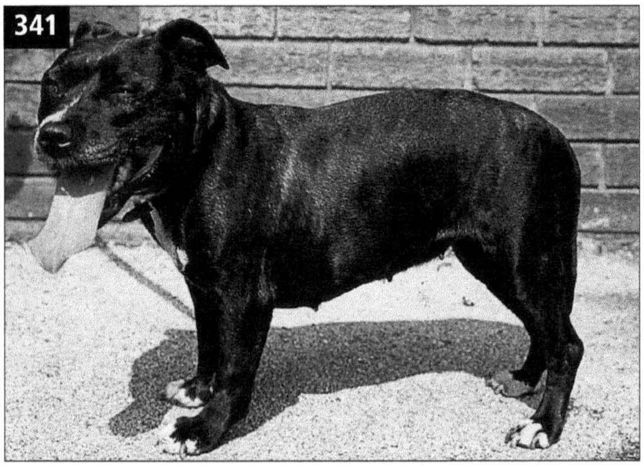

342

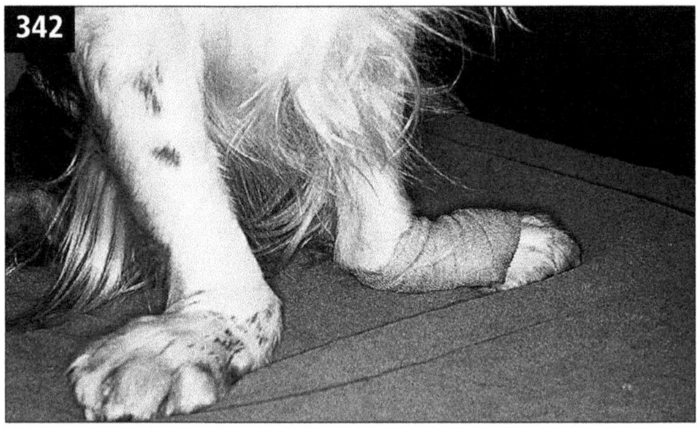

339–342 Clinical presentation of rheumatoid arthritis in the dog. (**339**) An eight-year-old crossbred dog with RA of the deforming type. (**340**) A closer view of the front feet of this dog showing swelling and deformity of the carpal and metacarpophalangeal joints. (**341**) A five-year-old Staffordshire Bull Terrier with RA of the non-deforming type. Although the joints were thickened, with synovial effusions and erosive changes evident on radiography, joint instability and deformity are not present. (**342**) A four-year-old Cavalier King Charles Spaniel with deforming RA. The carpal joints have collapsed, causing lateral angulation of the forefeet and a palmigrade posture. The bandages on the feet are to prevent excoriation. Pain was not a significant feature.

surprising speed, the joints changing from apparent normality to severe subluxation within a matter of days. There may occasionally be lethargy, pyrexia, anorexia or peripheral lymphadenopathy, and intercurrent respiratory or gastrointestinal disease is sometimes present. The range of clinical signs is similar in feline RA.

Diagnosis

The diagnostic criteria for RA in the dog and cat are adapted from those defined for humans (*Table 15*) and diagnosis involves a range of clinical and laboratory procedures (**343**). The nature of the arthritis and the extent of joint involvement can be determined by synovial fluid analysis and radiography. The radiographic features may be

Table 15: Diagnostic criteria for rheumatoid arthritis.

- Stiffness.
- Pain or tenderness on motion of at least one joint.
- Swelling of at least one joint.
- Swelling of one other joint within three months.
- Symmetry of joint swelling.
- Subcutaneous nodules.
- Erosive changes on joint radiographs.
- Serological test positive for rheumatoid factor.
- Abnormal synovial fluid.
- Characteristic histological changes in synovium.
- Characteristic histological changes in subcutaneous nodules (poorly defined in dogs and not reported in cats; may not be the same as human nodules).

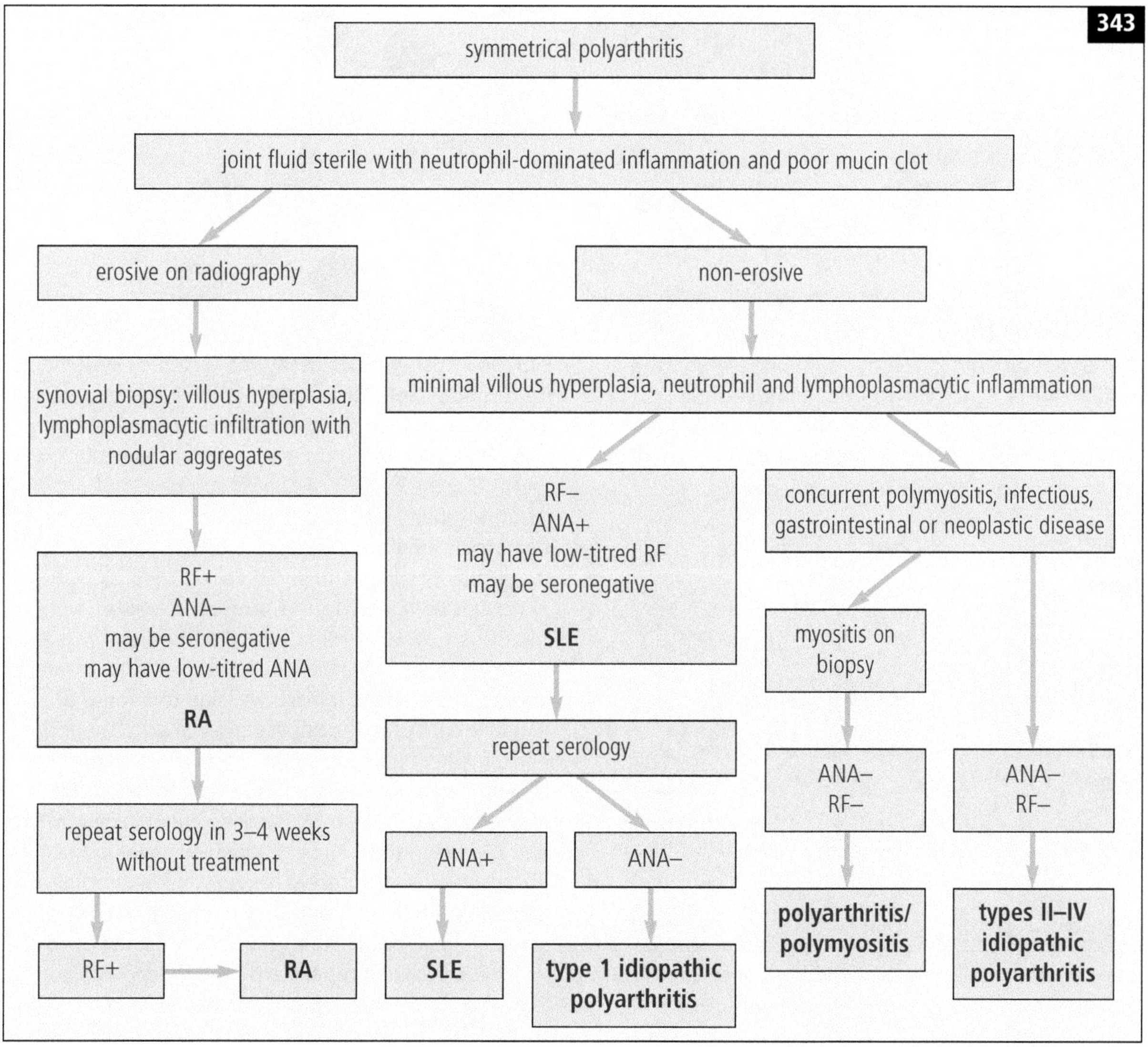

343 Diagnostic flow chart for canine immune-mediated polyarthritis.

complicated by secondary osteoarthritic change, but include:

- Increased periarticular soft tissue with focal calcification.
- Synovial effusion.
- Widening or collapse of joint spaces.
- Loss of mineral from epiphyses or intra-articular bones.
- Subchondral foci of rarefaction; irregular or eroded joint margins.
- Periosteal new bone formation.

Laboratory investigation occasionally reveals leukocytosis or leukopenia, and most patients have a lowered serum albumin:globulin ratio. A sample of joint fluid should be obtained for bacterial culture, examination of mucin clot formation (usually poor), enumeration of inflammatory cells and cytological examination. The synovial fluid will generally have 6–90 × 10^9 white cells/l (6,000–90,000 white cells/µl), the majority of which will be neutrophils, with occasional macrophages, lymphocytes or plasma cells (**344**). Synovial biopsy may reveal the changes described above.

Assays for serum (and/or synovial fluid) RF and serum ANA should be performed. The results of these tests must be interpreted carefully, as both serum RF and serum ANA are non-specific autoantibodies that may be present at low titre in

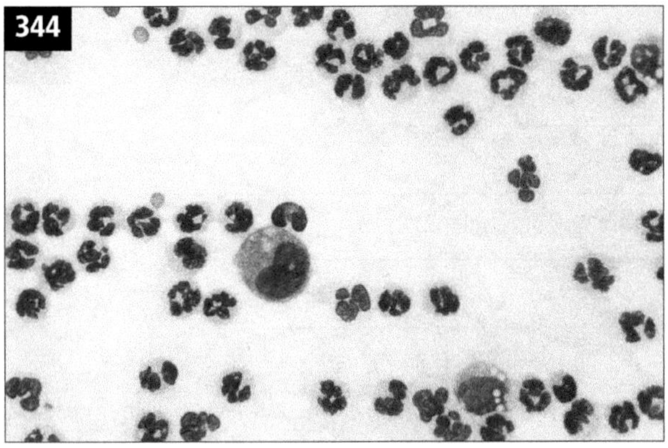

344 Synovial fluid cytology in immune-mediated polyarthritis. Synovial fluid from a five-year-old DSH cat with immune-mediated polyarthritis. The fluid is markedly cellular and the infiltrate is dominated by non-degenerate neutrophils with occasional macrophages.

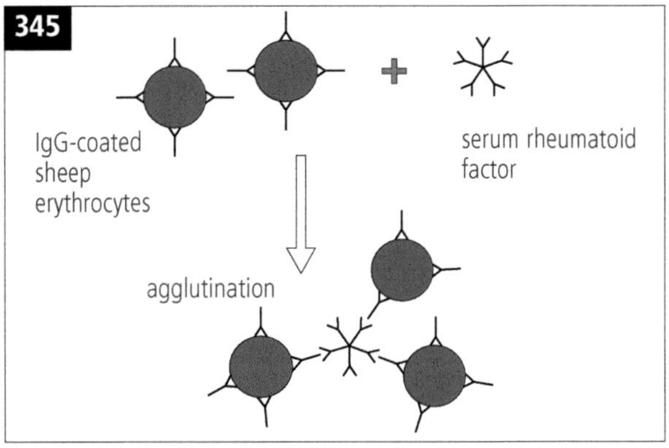

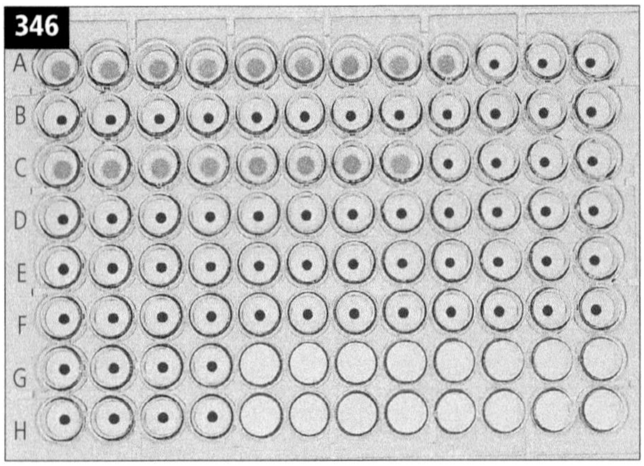

345, 346 Rose-Waaler assay for serum or synovial fluid rheumatoid factor. (**345**) In the Rose-Waaler assay for RF, a suspension of sheep RBCs are coated (sensitized) by a sub-agglutinating dose of rabbit or canine antibody specific for sheep RBCs. A control suspension of non-sensitized sheep RBCs is also prepared. Patient serum is heat inactivated by incubation at 56°C for 30 minutes (to destroy complement) and serially diluted (from 1 in 2) in phosphate-buffered saline across the wells of a microtitre tray. Similar titrations of positive and negative control sera are made. An equal volume of sensitized sheep RBCs is added to each well and to a series of negative control wells containing saline only. The test is performed in duplicate, so that each serum sample is also titrated against non-sensitized sheep RBCs. The antibody-coated sheep RBCs will be agglutinated by RF and the serum titre can be determined. (**346**) In this assay, serum from a patient (rows A and B), a positive control serum (rows C and D) and a negative control serum (rows E and F) have been serially diluted across the plate from a starting dilution of 1/2 in column 1. Rows G and H are a saline control. Sensitized sheep RBCs are added to rows A, C, E and G and non-sensitized sheep RBCs to rows B, D, F and H. This animal has a clinically significant RF titre of 512. The positive control serum has a titre of 256. (From Day M.J. [1996] Diagnostic assessment of the feline immune system, part II. *Feline Practice* **24:**14–25, with permission.)

the serum of clinically normal dogs and cats or animals with a wide range of chronic inflammatory (including osteoarthritis), infectious or neoplastic diseases. In classical RA the patient should have high titred RF but be negative for ANA. However, only approximately 70% of dogs with erosive polyarthritis that otherwise satisfy the criteria for RA will be seropositive for RF, and occasional cases will have a significant titre of ANA in addition to RF. RF may be detected by the Rose–Waaler test (**345**, **346**) or by ELISA (**347**).

Serum ANA is detected by indirect immunofluorescence or immunoperoxidase techniques (**348–350**). The titre of ANA and the pattern of

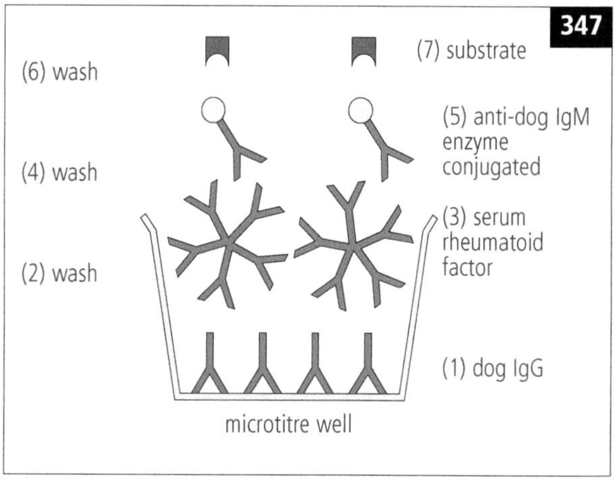

347 Detection of serum or synovial fluid rheumatoid factor by ELISA. The wells of microtitre trays are coated with a source of purified canine IgG (1). Unbound IgG is removed by washing (2) and the wells incubated with appropriately diluted patient serum or synovial fluid (3). RF will recognize the Fc portion of the IgG molecule, which may be conformationally altered by binding to the plastic of the well. After washing to remove unbound protein (4), RF is detected using an enzyme-conjugated antiserum with specificity for canine IgM (5). Unbound conjugate is removed by washing (6), and an enzyme substrate added to cause a colour change in positive wells (7). IgA RF can be detected by substitution of an enzyme-labelled antiserum specific for canine IgA at step (5).

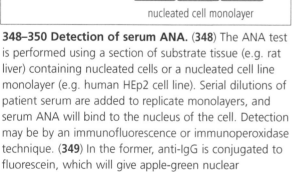

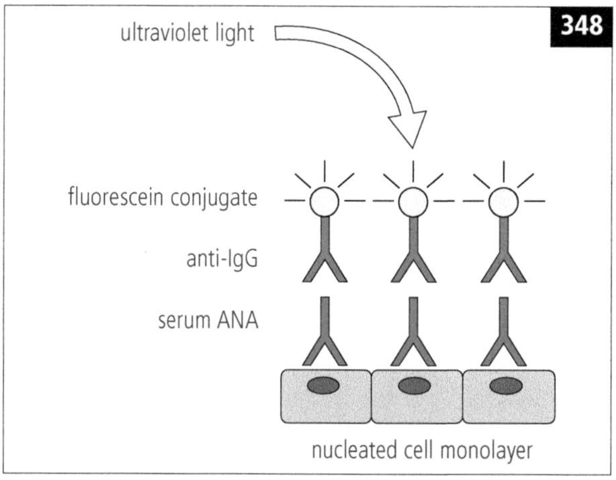

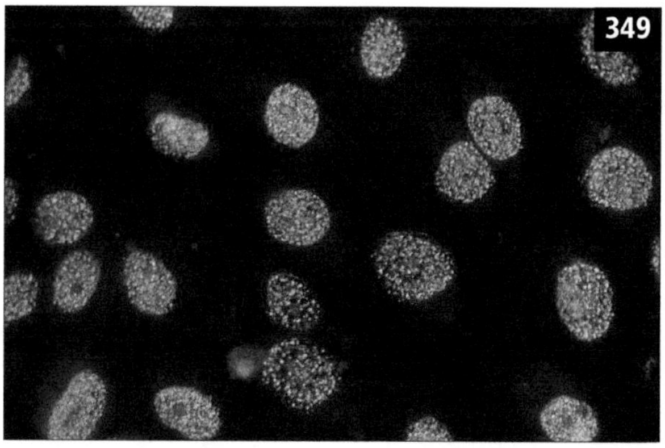

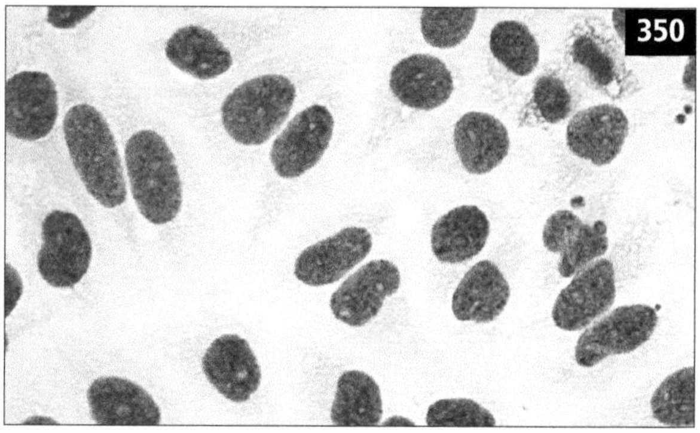

348–350 Detection of serum ANA. (**348**) The ANA test is performed using a section of substrate tissue (e.g. rat liver) containing nucleated cells or a nucleated cell line monolayer (e.g. human HEp2 cell line). Serial dilutions of patient serum are added to replicate monolayers, and serum ANA will bind to the nucleus of the cell. Detection may be by an immunofluorescence or immunoperoxidase technique. (**349**) In the former, anti-IgG is conjugated to fluorescein, which will give apple-green nuclear fluorescence under UV light (speckled nuclear pattern). (From Day M.J. [1996] Diagnostic assessment of the feline immune system, part II. *Feline Practice* **24:**14–25, with permission.) (**350**) In the immunoperoxidase method the anti-IgG is conjugated to peroxidase, which will cause brown nuclear colour change when incubated with enzyme substrate and hydrogen peroxide (homogenous nuclear pattern).

nuclear labelling are recorded (351). There are associations between these patterns and specific diseases of man, but such associations are not yet widely recognized for the dog and cat. One recent study has suggested that homogenous nuclear labelling is related to the presence of multisystemic autoimmunity, whereas speckled labelling is associated with musculoskeletal disease. In this study, only dogs with speckled nuclear staining had evidence of precipitating antinuclear antibodies in gel diffusion testing (see below). Moreover, four distinct precipitin patterns were recognized, suggesting that these ANA positive dogs might be sub-grouped on the basis of this reactivity. The 'LE cell' test no longer has a place in the diagnosis of immune-mediated disease.

ELISA, radioimmunoassay, immunoprecipitation or western blotting may be used to demonstrate the presence of serum antibody specific for different constituents of the nucleus including native DNA, histone proteins and extractable nuclear antigens (Sm and ribonucleoprotein [RNP]). Although such antibodies are recognized in dogs with polyarthritis, their clinical significance is not understood and the assays are not widely available. ANA specificity differs between dogs and humans. Dogs appear to lack autoantibody to double-stranded DNA, but have other reactivities not seen with human sera (e.g. for the glycoprotein hnRNPG). In contrast, the pattern of reactivity to the Sm and RNP antigens is relatively conserved between the two species.

351

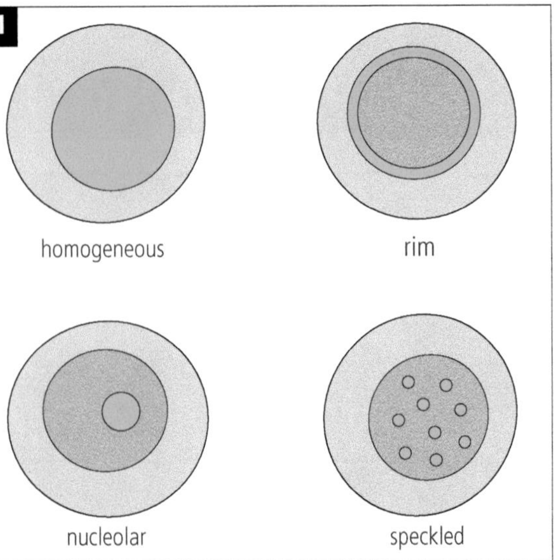

351 ANA patterns. Mixed patterns may occasionally occur.

Treatment and prognosis

RA carries a poor prognosis. The erosive changes visible radiographically indicate severe joint damage. Although treatment can help affected animals, residual lameness or stiffness must be accepted. There are two main approaches to treatment:

- Analgesic and/or anti-inflammatory drugs to improve quality of life.
- Immunosuppressive treatment (prednisolone and/or cytotoxic drugs) to slow disease progression.

The latter is generally used if there is clinical and/or radiographic evidence of severe disease or if the animal has systemic illness in addition to lameness. Treatment protocols using corticosteroids and the common cytotoxic drugs are discussed below.

Gold therapy (chrysotherapy) is sometimes used to treat RA. The exact mode of action is unknown, although gold may be immunosuppressive. Gold is classed as a slow-acting anti-rheumatic drug (SAARD) and can be given by intramuscular injection (sodium aurothiomalate) at a dose rate of 0.5 mg/kg once weekly for six weeks. The dose can be repeated after 2–3 months. Before embarking on a course of gold therapy, a small test dose should be given to check for adverse reactions. The intramuscular injections can be uncomfortable, and an oral preparation is available (Auranofin, given at 0.05–2.0 mg/kg q12h). This is less toxic than the injectable form, but commonly causes diarrhoea due to an osmotic effect on the gastrointestinal tract. Gold is slow acting, therefore low dose prednisolone is generally given at the same time. Since gold is potentially toxic, there should be regular clinical assessment and haematological examination, ideally every 7–14 days. Response to therapy is determined by clinical assessment and synovial fluid cytology.

A combination of methotrexate and leflunomide has been used in the cat with apparent success. The methotrexate dose is given once weekly and, on the day it is given, the total dose of 7.5 mg is divided into three 2.5 mg amounts and given at eight-hourly intervals. The leflunomide dose of 10 mg is given orally each day. Once significant clinical improvement has occurred, the dose of methotrexate is reduced to 2.5 mg once weekly and the dose of leflunomide to 10 mg twice weekly. Leflunomide causes preferential arrest of T cell proliferation and methotrexate, being an analogue to folic acid, is a cytotoxic drug. Leflunomide can cause hepatotoxicity, haematotoxicity and allergic reactions. Methotrexate is also potentially hepatotoxic.

Anti-cytokine therapy has become very popular in human rheumatology for treating RA (see Chapter 16, p. 398). These agents include Infliximab^{TM}, which is a neutralizing monoclonal antibody specific for TNFα, recombinant IL-1 receptor antagonist, which inhibits the actions of IL-1, and Etanercept^{TM}, which is a soluble TNFα receptor fusion protein that inhibits the actions of TNFα. These agents are powerful anti-inflammatories and they also inhibit matrix metalloproteinase production. They are generally used in combination with methotrexate and, as well as producing clinical improvement, reversal of radiographical erosions has been documented. To date these so-called 'biological agents' have not been developed for veterinary patients, but there is certainly potential application.

Surgical treatments are described for RA, although they are of limited application. Arthrodesis of diseased joints or replacement of damaged ligaments in unstable joints has been attempted with limited success. Synovectomy can afford temporary relief, particularly if a single joint is predominantly affected, and patellectomies and other excision arthroplasties have been undertaken. Restricted exercise and removal of stress factors are important adjuncts to treatment.

PERIOSTEAL PROLIFERATIVE POLYARTHRITIS

Periosteal proliferative polyarthritis predominantly occurs in the cat and is rare in dogs. It is characterized by production of extensive periosteal new bone around and beyond joints, chronic synovitis and (usually) erosion of articular cartilage and subchondral bone (352, 353). The hocks and carpi are most often affected, but the absence of joint instability and deformity helps distinguish the

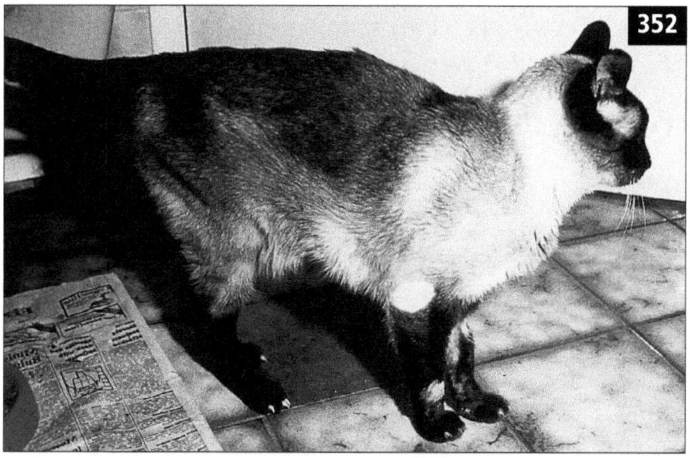

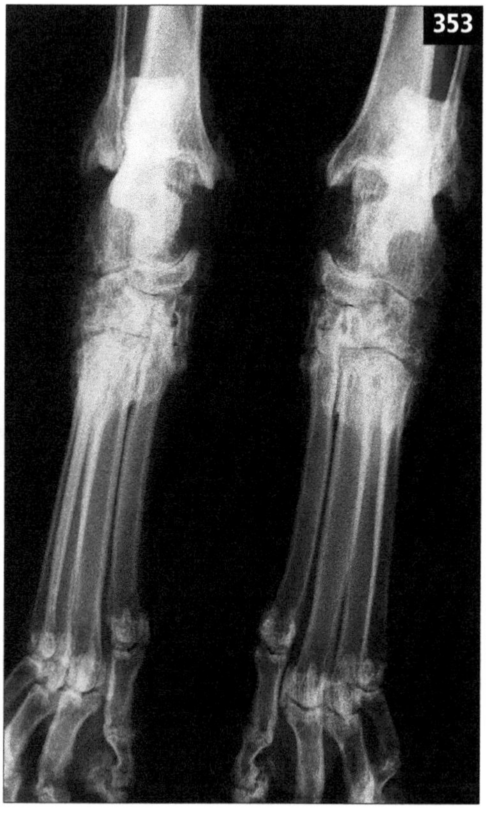

352, 353 Feline periosteal proliferative polyarthritis. (**352**) A five-year-old neutered male Siamese cat with periosteal proliferative polyarthritis. The carpi and hocks were particularly affected. The cat had a very stiff gait, was reluctant to jump and suffered recurrent episodes of pyrexia and anorexia. (**353**) Craniocaudal radiograph of the hock joints of an eight-year-old male DSH cat with periosteal proliferative polyarthritis. Note the extensive new bone deposits.

condition from RA. Bony erosions may be seen at the attachment of tendons and ligaments (erosive enthesiopathy). Affected cats may have pyrexia, malaise and generalized stiffness, with swollen joints and peripheral lymphadenopathy. Laboratory features are similar to those in RA, but serum RF or ANA are not present. Synovial biopsy demonstrates neutrophil infiltration of superficial areas, with deep lymphoplasmacytic inflammation. The immunopathogenesis is poorly understood, but synovial immune complex deposition may be involved. The isolation of feline foamy virus (previously feline syncytium-forming virus) from affected joints appears not to be relevant, as this virus can be isolated from normal feline joints.

The prognosis is generally poor, as the disease tends to progress and lameness is likely to persist. Short courses of prednisolone at anti-inflammatory doses may be given in severe disease. Chrysotherapy has been used to treat feline periosteal polyarthritis, but gold is particularly toxic in cats and monitoring is essential. If diagnosis is reached in the early stages, immunosuppression with corticosteroids or cytotoxic drugs can be undertaken. Euthanasia is necessary where quality of life has become unacceptable.

SYSTEMIC LUPUS ERYTHEMATOSUS

The multisystemic autoimmune disease SLE is described in Chapter 14. However, it is relevant to consider this condition here as polyarthritis is the most consistent clinical feature of SLE in the cat and dog and, although not the commonest, it is the most cited example of non-erosive, immune-mediated polyarthritis in these species (**354**).

Pathogenesis

The immunopathogenesis of joint disease in SLE involves synovial immune complex deposition. The content of these complexes is poorly defined, but some may comprise nuclear material complexed with antinuclear antibody. Microbes, particularly viruses, have been implicated in the causation of SLE in humans and in dogs and cats. Immune complexes may be found within the synovial lining, macrophages and blood vessel walls of dogs with SLE. The synovitis is similar to that of RA, but the synovial hyperplasia is not villous and there is a greater proportion of neutrophils within the infiltrate (**355**).

Clinical signs

The diagnostic criteria for canine SLE are discussed in Chapter 14. The clinical history is of either gradual or acute onset generalized stiffness. The polyarthritis is usually bilaterally symmetrical and although soft tissue swelling and joint pain may be recognized, it can sometimes be difficult to identify affected joints on clinical examination (**356**, **357**). Cats with polyarthritis as part of SLE usually have acute onset generalized discomfort and stiffness, but again it may be difficult to determine the involvement of specific joints on clinical

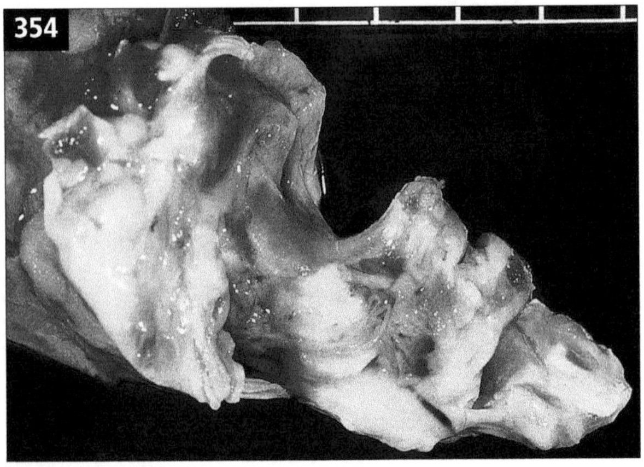

354 Canine SLE. Right elbow joint from a dog with SLE. The synovial membrane is thickened and discoloured. The articular cartilage shows no obvious pathology. This appearance is typical of all the non-erosive, immune-mediated arthropathies.

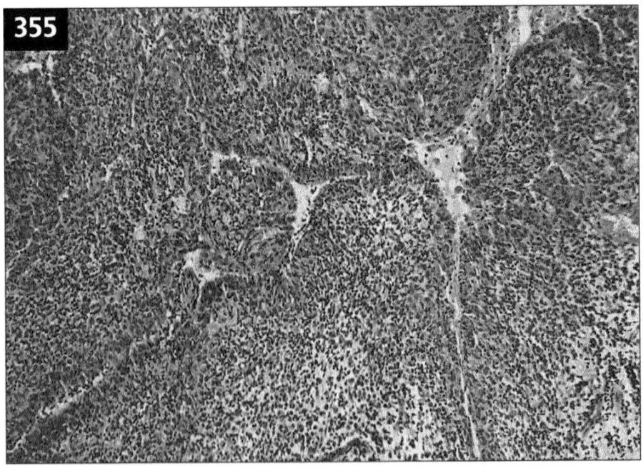

355 Canine SLE. Synovial membrane biopsy taken from the stifle joint of a dog with SLE. There is an extensive inflammatory infiltrate consisting of both polymorphonuclear and mononuclear cells.

examination (358). Clinical signs relating to involvement of other body systems are to be expected.

Diagnosis

The diagnostic process should include radiography, examination of joint fluid (poor mucin clot formation and neutrophil-dominated inflammation of the order of 10–220 × 10^9 cells/l [10,000–220,000 cells/μl]) and synovial biopsy. Classically, there will be a high titred serum ANA in the absence of RF, but in some cases both autoantibodies will be demonstrated. Circulating immune complexes (see Chapter 5, p. 146) may be detected and reduced serum concentration of complement C3 and C4 is documented in dogs with ANA-positive, non-erosive polyarthritis.

Treatment and prognosis

The prognosis for SLE is always guarded because of its multisystemic nature, and it becomes unfavourable if renal involvement develops. SLE should be treated aggressively by immunosuppression (high doses of corticosteroids or cytotoxic drugs). The use of these drugs is discussed later in this chapter.

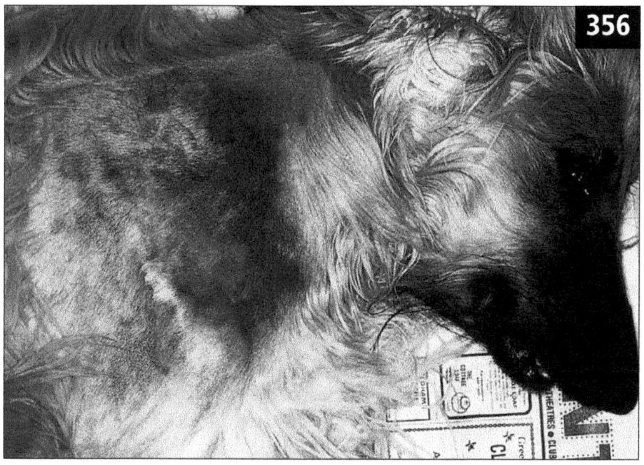

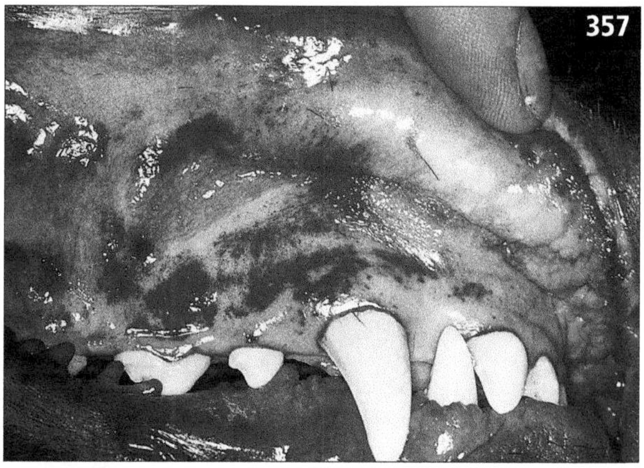

356, 357 Canine SLE. (**356**) A two-year-old Afghan Hound with SLE. The dog is recumbent because of severe, multiple joint pain associated with a polyarthritis. There is also a haemorrhagic discoloration of the skin following a subcutaneous injection. Bleeding occurred because of severe thrombocytopenia. This dog had serum ANA and immune complex deposition within the synovium and at the BMZ of the dermoepidermal junction. (From Bennett D. [1987] Immune-based nonerosive inflammatory joint disease of the dog. 1. Canine systemic lupus erythematosus. *Journal of Small Animal Practice* **28**:871–889, with permission.) (**357**) Oral mucosa of a dog with thrombocytopenia associated with SLE. This dog also had a polyarthritis and severe proteinuria, possibly associated with glomerulonephritis. (From Bennett D. [1984] Autoimmune disease in the dog. *In Practice* **6**:74–86, with permission.)

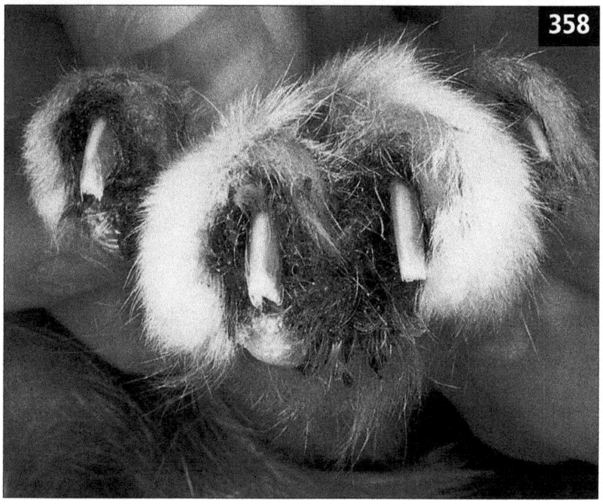

358 Feline SLE. A three-year-old neutered female DSH cat with polyarthritis and cutaneous manifestations of SLE. Paronychia was present in all four feet and small, circumscribed crusty lesions were present on the ventral surface of the body wall.

CANINE POLYARTHRITIS/POLYMYOSITIS SYNDROME

In this form of non-erosive polyarthritis the radiographic and immunopathogenic features of the joint disease are similar to those of SLE. Clinical examination reveals swelling and pain on palpation of major limb joints (carpi, hocks, stifles, elbows) and there may be pyrexia and generalized lymphadenopathy (359). Analysis of synovial fluid reveals a white cell count of 20–80 × 10^9/l (20,000–80,000/μl) dominated by neutrophils, and poor mucin clot formation.

Affected dogs also have muscle atrophy, pain and contracture, which is often generalized, involving muscles of the limbs, spine and skull. It may be difficult to distinguish between joint and muscle pain on clinical examination. Muscle biopsy reveals myofibre degeneration and infiltration of neutrophils, macrophages, lymphocytes and plasma cells. There may be leukocytosis and hypergammaglobulinaemia, but serum ANA is negative. Concentrations of creatine kinase (CK), lactate dehydrogenase, aspartate aminotransferase and aldolase in the blood are often increased. Electromyography may show focal areas of spontaneous activity in affected muscles.

Aggressive immunosuppression is indicated for polyarthritis/polymyositis. Cytotoxic drugs are most often used, in combination with low dose corticosteroids. There may be remission of disease; however, some animals have residual lameness due to muscle fibrosis and contracture. In other cases, low grade muscle and joint inflammation persists, and low dose corticosteroids may be necessary to maintain quality of life.

POLYARTHRITIS/MENINGITIS SYNDROME

This syndrome is recognized in the Weimaraner, German Shorthaired Pointer, Boxer, Bernese Mountain Dog, Newfoundland and Japanese Akita, and is also reported in the cat. Affected animals present with stiffness and neck pain (360) and sometimes nervous signs. They are negative for serum ANA. The arthritis is symmetrical and

359

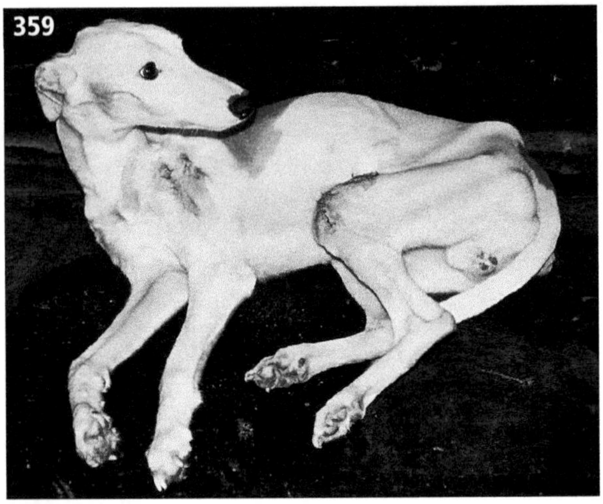

359 Canine polyarthritis/polymyositis. A two-year-old Whippet with polyarthritis and polymyositis. This animal was unable to stand and walk. (From Bennett D. [1987] Immune-based nonerosive inflammatory joint disease of the dog. 1. Canine systemic lupus erythematosus. *Journal of Small Animal Practice* **28:**871–889, with permission.)

360

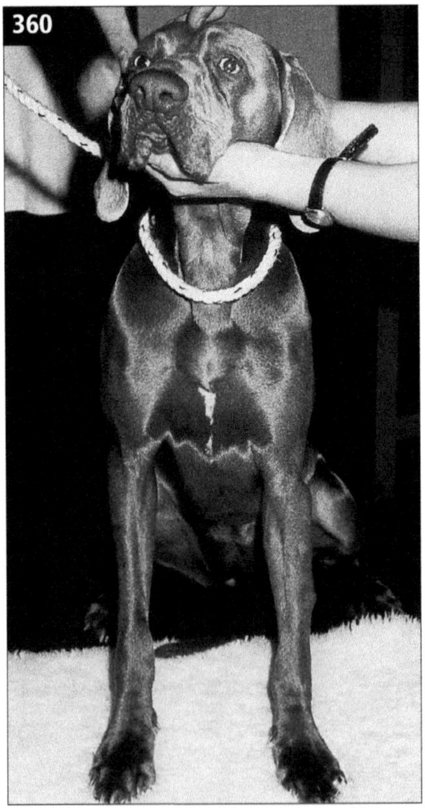

360 Canine polyarthritis/meningitis. A one-year-old Weimaraner with polyarthritis and meningitis. In addition to joint pain, neck pain was an obvious feature.

non-erosive, and is confirmed by synovial fluid analysis and synovial biopsy. Cerebrospinal fluid shows increased protein, white cells and CK levels, consistent with central nervous system (CNS) inflammation. The prognosis is usually good, as such cases respond to immunosuppressive doses of corticosteroids, but relapse can occur at any time. Some cases may be associated with polyarteritis, and the condition in the Japanese Akita is further discussed below because of the poor prognosis.

POLYARTHRITIS OF ADOLESCENT JAPANESE AKITAS

Affected Japanese Akitas are usually less than one year old and present with polyarthritis, peripheral lymphadenopathy and systemic illness (pyrexia, lethargy, inappetence) (**361**). Meningitis may also be present, as may other organ involvement, giving some resemblance to SLE. However, serum ANA is not found. Anaemia and leukocytosis are common laboratory findings. These dogs have a poor prognosis, since response to anti-inflammatory and immunosuppressive drugs is generally poor. Use of these drugs in immature animals is more likely to have side-effects. Euthanasia is often necessary on humane grounds.

FAMILIAL RENAL AMYLOIDOSIS OF CHINESE SHAR PEIS

These dogs present with episodes of fever and swelling of one or both hocks and, occasionally, other joints, although seldom with a polyarthritis (**362**). The joints can be normal between attacks, which are often at 4–6 week intervals. The condition is often referred to as 'Shar Pei fever' or 'Shar Pei hock'. There is synovitis of varying severity, and enthesiopathies are seen, most often as bony proliferation at the attachments of ligaments and tendons. The age of onset is variable; the condition may affect young puppies or adults.

A mutation upstream of the gene encoding hyaluronan (HA) on chromosome 13 is associated both with the excessive deposition of HA within the dermis of Shar Peis (giving the 'wrinkled' skin

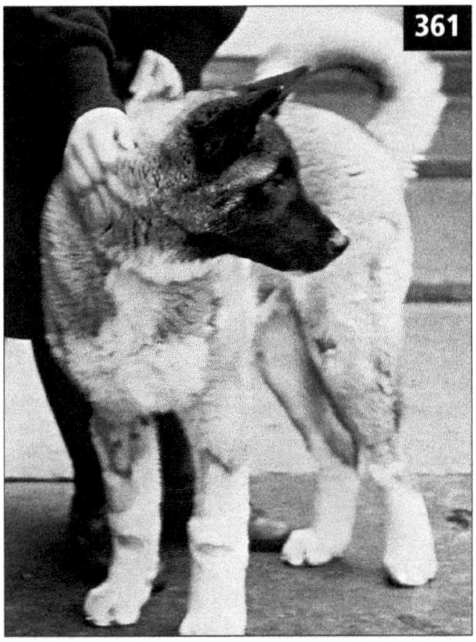

361 Polyarthritis of the Japanese Akita. A seven-month-old Japanese Akita with polyarthritis. This dog also developed metaphyseal osteopathy. The prognosis for polyarthritis in juvenile Akitas is very poor. Euthanasia of this dog was necessary, since response to treatment was incomplete.

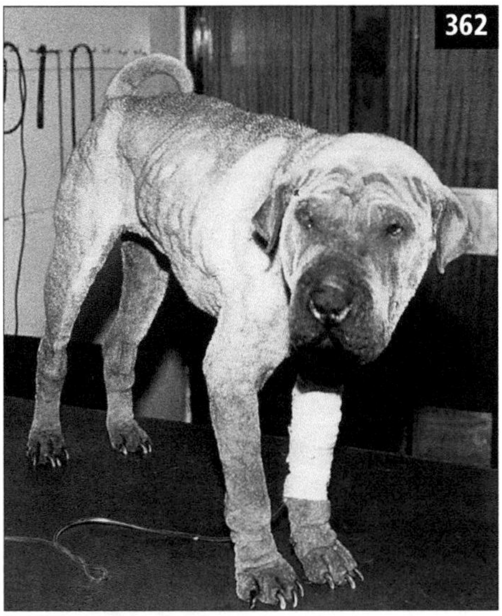

362 Familial renal amyloidosis of Shar Peis. A Chinese Shar Pei with amyloidosis. This dog suffered episodic attacks of arthritis for several years. It is now in renal failure, secondary to amyloidosis.

phenotype) and with Shar Pei fever. HA is thought to trigger innate immunity and lead to sterile fever and inflammation.

Amyloid deposition (amyloid A) occurs in several organs, but renal and hepatic amyloidosis is the most significant and eventually results in renal and/or hepatic failure (363), generally between 1.5–6 years of age, so the disease carries a poor prognosis. Some dogs have elevated levels of serum amyloid A and IL-6. Amyloid deposits can often be seen in renal and hepatic biopsies. The attacks of arthritis and pyrexia generally resolve within 24–48 hours without treatment; however, the use of non-steroidal anti-inflammatory drugs (NSAIDs) (e.g. meloxicam) helps control pain and pyrexia. Colchicine (0.03 mg/kg p/o q24h) on a continuous regime has been used in some cases. This drug does not prevent pyrexia/arthritis, but it does have anti-amyloid properties, although it is not clear whether it reduces the incidence or severity of amyloidosis.

POLYARTERITIS NODOSA

This is most often a multisystemic disease (see below), but polyarthritis or pauciarthritis is a common feature. If polyarteritis is seen in a biopsy of synovium or other tissue, in the absence of serum ANA, a clinical diagnosis of polyarteritis nodosa is justified. Meningitis and myositis are often seen in combination with the arthritis, so there is overlap with the syndromes discussed above. Attacks of arthritis are often cyclical, although persistent signs can occur. Affected animals are often pyrexic, depressed and stiff. Meningitis produces extreme neck pain, which may be the only obvious symptom. In some young animals (e.g. Beagles) the prognosis is good, with spontaneous recovery as the animal matures. Treatment is by immunosuppression (high dose corticosteroids or cytotoxic drugs) and clinical remission can be achieved, although adult dogs may relapse at any time.

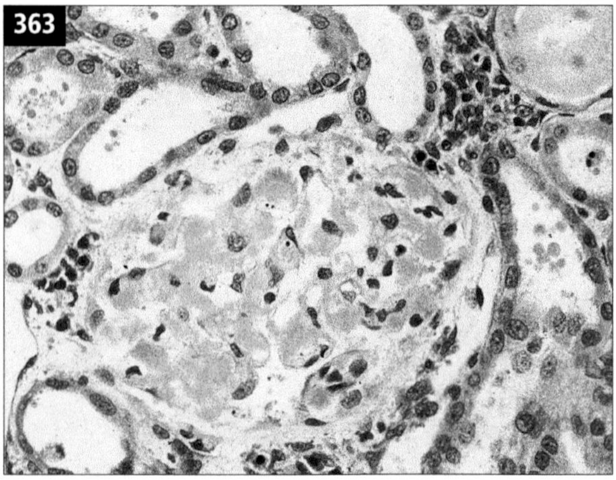

363 Familial renal amyloidosis of Shar Peis. A renal biopsy showing amyloid deposition within the glomerulus (Congo red stain).

SJÖGREN'S-LIKE SYNDROME

In human rheumatology, both primary and secondary forms of Sjögren's syndrome are recognized. In the secondary form there is evidence of accompanying RA or other connective tissue disease. The clinical presentation of this autoimmune syndrome is of keratoconjunctivitis sicca (KCS) (see Chapter 11, p. 272) in combination with xerostomia (dry mouth), due to lymphocytic infiltration and destruction of the lacrimal and salivary glands. Although KCS is well-documented in the dog, true Sjögren's-like syndrome is rare. Only two dogs satisfying the criteria for diagnosis of this disease have been formally reported in the literature (with one further report as part of a case series). However, there may be some 'overlap syndromes' in which dogs presenting with apparently uncomplicated KCS have serological changes related to connective tissue disease (e.g. ANA and RF), or in which dogs with KCS have another concomitant autoimmune disease such as hypothyroidism, RA, diabetes mellitus, chronic active hepatitis or autoimmune skin disease. The two affected canine patients were part of an experimental breeding colony of dogs with SLE.

It has been suggested that canine primary Sjögren's-like syndrome may be underdiagnosed. Dogs presenting with primary KCS have been shown to have subclinical histopathological changes in salivary gland tissue, and some dogs with KCS that are evaluated for parotid duct transposition also have a degree of xerostomia. One study of 50 dogs with KCS identified ten animals as having evidence of xerostomia. All dogs presenting with polyarthritis should have their tear production regularly assessed using the Schirmer test in order to check for the complication of secondary Sjögren's-like disease.

A single case of Sjögren's-like syndrome has been reported in a two-year-old cat that presented with dysphagia, weight loss, ocular signs (blepharospasm and conjunctival hyperaemia), enlargement of salivary glands and 'tacky' oral mucous membranes with food debris within the mouth.

The treatment of KCS is discussed in Chapter 11. A combination of local ocular (e.g. ciclosporin) and systemic immunosuppressive/anti-inflammatory therapy can be used. Tear substitutes are also an important part of disease management.

IDIOPATHIC POLYARTHRITIS

Pathogenesis

Idiopathic polyarthritis is the most common presentation of immune-mediated arthritis in the dog and cat. Animals with idiopathic polyarthritis do not, at least initially, satisfy the diagnostic criteria for the entities described above. Affected animals most commonly have joint disease alone (type I) or joint disease in association with infectious disease of other body systems (type II; reactive arthritis), gastrointestinal disease (type III; enteropathic arthritis) or neoplastic disease of other body systems (type IV; arthritis of malignancy). The immunopathogenesis most likely involves synovial immune complex deposition, and the complexes in types II, III and IV disease may involve microbial or tumour antigens. It has been suggested that type I disease may in some cases be triggered by vaccination, and the detection of distemper antigens in synovial immune complexes in some dogs adds support to this concept. In most cases there is synovial hyperplasia, which is occasionally villous. The inflammatory infiltrates consist of lymphocytes, plasma cells and neutrophils, and fibrin deposition and vasculitis are recorded.

Clinical signs

The presentation of idiopathic polyarthritis in dogs is similar to other forms of immune-mediated arthritis. The clinical features include overt lameness or stiffness after rest or exercise, joint pain, soft tissue thickening, synovial effusion, heat or crepitus (**364–366**). There may be periods of remission and relapse.

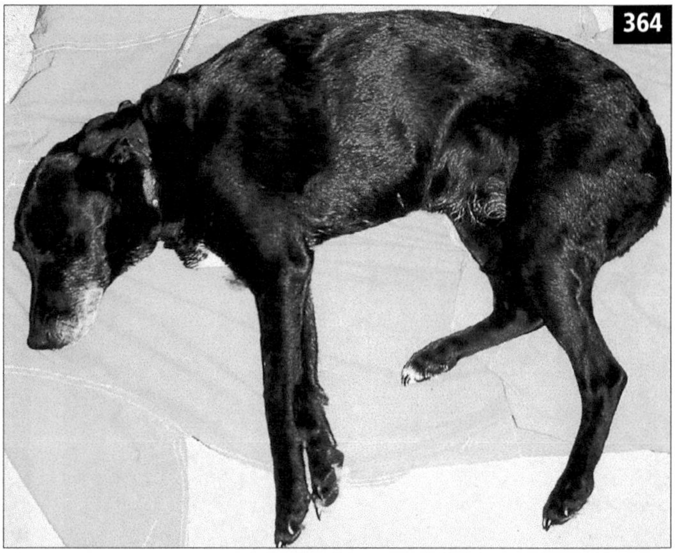

364

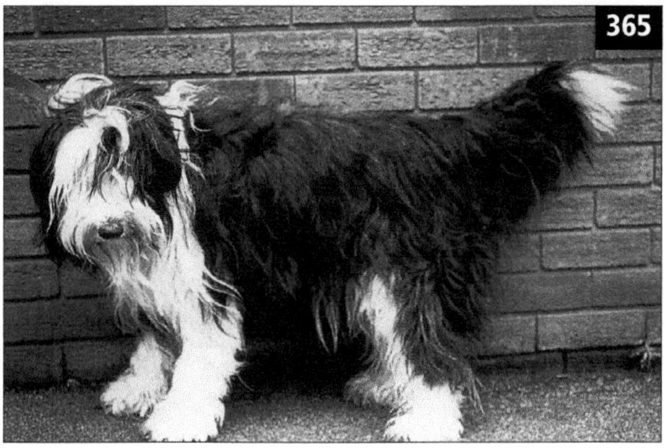

365

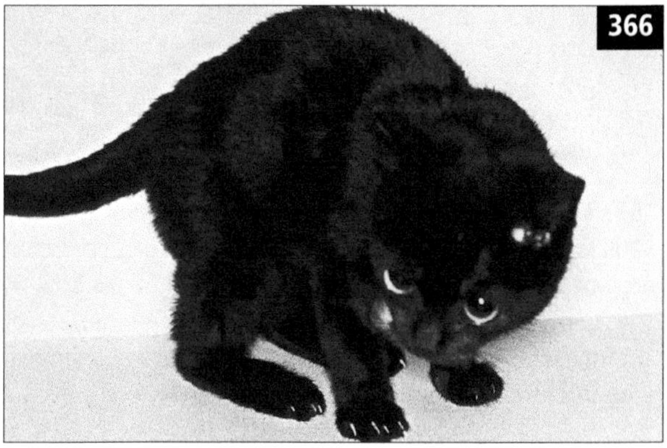

366

364–366 Idiopathic polyarthritis. (**364**) A four-year-old dog with an acute onset, non-erosive idiopathic type I polyarthritis. This dog has severe joint pain and was unable to stand or ambulate. (**365**) A Bearded Collie with ulcerative colitis and non-erosive polyarthritis, a probable example of type III idiopathic polyarthritis (enteropathic arthritis). (**366**) A young cat with polyarthritis and myeloproliferative disease confirmed by bone marrow biopsy. This is an example of an idiopathic type IV polyarthritis (the arthritis of malignancy).

Diagnosis

Radiographically the lesions are non-erosive, with soft tissue swelling and synovial effusion, and, sometimes, periosteal new bone formation may be seen (**367, 368**). Synovial fluid has poor mucin clot formation and neutrophil-dominated inflammation ($3–100 \times 10^9$ cells/l [3,000–100,000 cells/μl]). Additionally, animals with idiopathic polyarthritis generally have signs of systemic illness. Both leukocytosis and leukopenia are recorded, and most dogs have elevated serum globulin. Serum ANA or RF are generally absent; however, occasional cases have low titred autoantibodies. Some cases of type I polyarthritis in the dog progress to erosive rheumatoid disease and require reclassification at a later stage.

Treatment and prognosis

The prognosis for type I polyarthritis is generally good. Most cases respond to immunosuppressive therapy; however, some fail to respond completely and may need continuous low dose corticosteroid treatment to maintain quality of life. Other animals may go into remission, but relapse at any time.

The drug of choice for immunosuppressive therapy is prednisolone (2–4 mg/kg q24h for 2 weeks, then gradually tapered over 3–4 months). There is generally a marked response within a few days, but therapy must be maintained for several weeks in order to prevent relapse. Response to therapy can be judged by clinical examination or by repeating synovial fluid analysis (two weeks after commencing therapy) of one or more joints that were initially sampled for diagnosis. If the cell count has fallen below 4×10^9/l (4,000/μl), and most cells are mononuclear, the prognosis is reasonably good. If relapse occurs after finishing prednisolone therapy, the treatment regime can be repeated.

Cytotoxic drugs are indicated if the animal relapses while receiving corticosteroid treatment, if there is poor response to corticosteroid therapy alone, or if there are repeated relapses after cessation of therapy. Cytotoxic drugs are SAARDs; they are combined with low dose (anti-

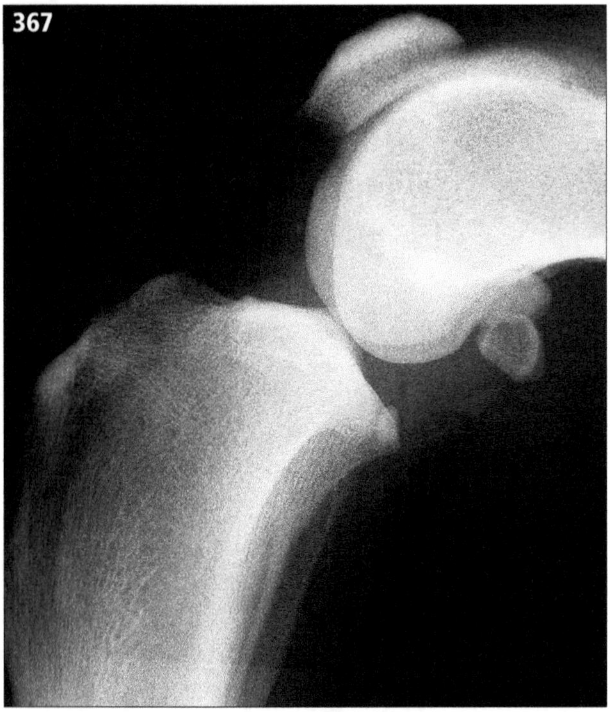

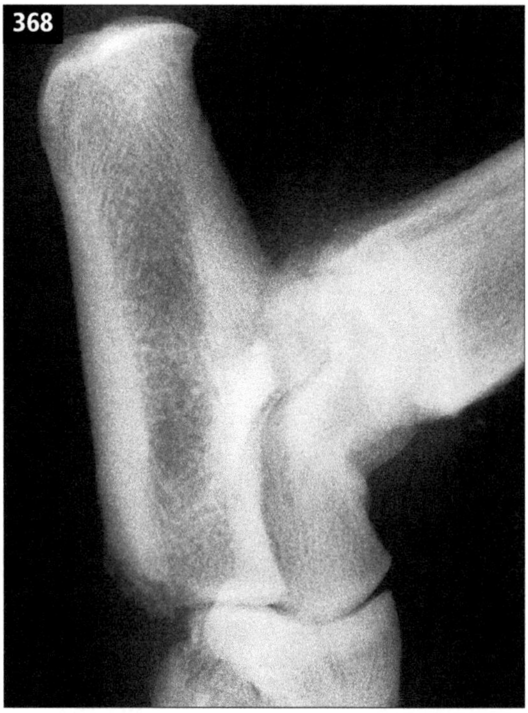

367, 368 Idiopathic polyarthritis. (**367**) Lateral radiograph of right stifle joint showing loss of intrapatellar fat pads and distension of the caudal joint capsule, consistent with marked synovial effusion. No bony changes are present. (**368**) Lateral radiograph of hock joint showing increased soft tissue density around the tarsocrural joints, consistent with synovial effusion. No bony changes are present. The lack of bony change is typical of all non-erosive immune-mediated polyarthropathies. Soft tissue changes are usually the only feature and these may not be easily seen in certain joints or with mild cases.

inflammatory) prednisolone (0.25–0.5 mg/kg q24h), which reduces joint inflammation and pain and improves the animals' quality of life while the cytotoxic drugs take effect. The cytotoxic drug of choice for immune-mediated arthritis is cyclophosphamide (1.5 mg/kg for dogs <30 kg; 2.0 mg/kg for dogs 15–30 kg; and 2.5 mg/kg for animals less than 15 kg [including cats]). The drug is given on four consecutive days of each week, although it can be used on alternate days or every third or fourth day depending on the dosage. Cyclophosphamide is usually given for 3–4 months, but prolonged therapy is not recommended as bladder toxicity may develop. Urine samples should be regularly tested for blood. The presence of significant haematuria is an indication for cessation of therapy. Haematology should also be monitored every 7–14 days and, if the white cell count falls below 6×10^9/l (6,000/μl) or platelets below 125×10^9/l (125,000/μl), the dose should be reduced by a quarter. If the white cell count falls below 4×10^9/l (4,000/μl) or platelets below 100×10^9/l (100,000/μl), the drug is discontinued for two weeks and then recommenced at half the original dose. There is substantial anecdotal evidence that the use of levamisole (3–7 mg/kg p/o every other day) in addition to cyclophosphamide and low dose corticosteroids can improve the possibility of successful remission. Levamisole should not be used for longer than four months.

If cyclophosphamide therapy is unsuccessful, or if immunosuppressive treatment is needed for more than four months, azathioprine is generally used (2 mg/kg every other day, alternating with low dose prednisolone also used every other day). Bone marrow suppression is more likely with thiopurines and may occur within 4–6 weeks of therapy (cyclophosphamide takes several months). There has been limited experience with the use of ciclosporin in the treatment of type I polyarthritis, but when used as monotherapy this agent has not proven efficacious. A recent report has indicated that monotherapy with leflunomide (3–4 mg/kg p/o q24h) for a minimum period of 6 weeks is an effective alternative treatment for immune-mediated polyarthritis.

If remission is achieved with cytotoxic drugs but relapse occurs subsequently, the previously successful regime can be repeated as often as necessary. If remission is not achieved, or relapses become common or occur shortly after finishing immunosuppressive therapy, the latter should not be repeated and low dose corticosteroid treatment should be used to maintain quality of life. Because of the associations between immune-mediated polyarthritis and CDV antigens referred to above, all dogs that have suffered immune-mediated polyarthritis should not receive distemper booster inoculations unless antibody titres are significantly low. Booster vaccinations should never be given if the dog is on immunosuppressive therapy.

Some cases of mild, type I polyarthritis will have spontaneous remission within a day or two, without treatment. NSAIDs may be used to relieve joint pain and pyrexia while the diagnosis of immune-mediated polyarthritis is being confirmed. Immunosuppressive treatment should not be instigated until other diagnoses (e.g. bacterial endocarditis) have been ruled out.

Treatment of type II idiopathic polyarthritis is directed towards controlling the infection and if this is successful, the arthritis should resolve spontaneously. Occasionally, low dose corticosteroids are used in combination with antimicrobial therapy to help resolve the arthritis.

Treatment of type III idiopathic arthritis concentrates on controlling the gastrointestinal disease. Low dose corticosteroids may provide relief from arthritis while the gastrointestinal problem is being treated, but corticosteroids may sometimes be appropriate for both the intestinal and joint disease.

The prognosis for type IV idiopathic arthritis depends on the prognosis for the tumour. In cats, myeloproliferative disease is the most common association, and the bone marrow of cats with non-erosive polyarthritis should be examined if there is no response to treatment.

DRUG INDUCED ARTHRITIS

Drug-induced vasculitides (see Chapter 5, p. 145) are increasingly recognized in dogs and are reported in the cat. Polyarthritis is one feature of such reactions, which may also involve fever, lymphadenopathy or cutaneous lesions. Antibiotics are most commonly incriminated, particularly sulphonamides, lincomycin, erythromycin, cephalosporins and penicillins. The most prevalent syndrome occurs in Dobermanns given sulphadiazine-trimethoprim; they may develop polyarthritis, glomerulonephritis, focal retinitis, polymyositis, skin lesions, fever, anaemia, leukopenia and thrombocytopenia. Diagnosis is made on the basis of worsening clinical signs while on therapy and rapid improvement after drug withdrawal. Occasionally, low dose corticosteroid therapy aids recovery.

ARTHRITIS ASSOCIATED WITH VACCINATION

Immune-mediated polyarthritis can follow vaccination, most commonly 5–7 days after primary vaccination of kittens (**369**). The calicivirus component is incriminated and calicivirus antigens have been identified within synovial macrophages in affected joints. The lameness is generally transient, lasting 24–48 hours, and further episodes after subsequent inoculations are unlikely. There is evidence that calicivirus is a feline joint pathogen and a cause of viral arthritis characterized by joint pain, stiffness, overt lameness and pyrexia. Some field strains of calicivirus may also produce an immune-mediated arthritis, similar to that produced by vaccine strains.

Polyarthritis following primary vaccination is also reported in puppies that develop transient lameness. Treatment of transient, vaccine-associated polyarthropathy is seldom required, although NSAIDs can be given. Some cases of rheumatoid and idiopathic polyarthritis become apparent within three weeks of vaccination (see above), although this does not necessarily imply an aetiological association.

LYMPHOPLASMACYTIC ARTHRITIS OF STIFLE JOINTS

This form of canine arthritis affects both stifles and is characterized by intense lymphoplasmacytic synovitis and synovial hyperplasia, which may be villous. There is no clear evidence that this disease is primary immune-mediated in nature.

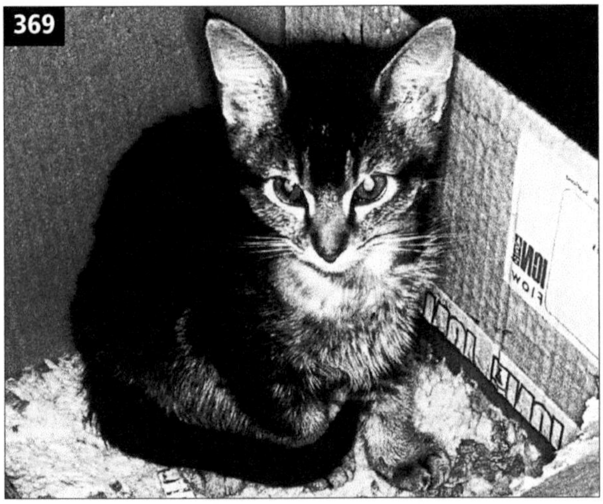

369 Vaccine-associated arthritis. This kitten developed lameness five days after its first vaccination. This is an example of polyarthritis associated with vaccination.

ARTHRITIS FOLLOWING MICROBIAL JOINT INFECTIONS

Immune-mediated arthritis as a sequela to bacterial arthritis, and the possibility of such disease following *Borrelia* or calicivirus infection, has been discussed above. Bacterial endocarditis is an important condition to consider when dealing with a suspected case of immune-based polyarthritis. It can lead to both a true infective polyarthritis and/or an immune-mediated polyarthritis, and affected dogs can have high levels of circulating ANA and RF. Such dogs usually have a cardiac murmur and ultrasonography will generally reveal the vegetative endocarditis lesion. Ophthalmological examination may reveal retinitis and/or retinal haemorrhages.

RELAPSING POLYCHONDRITIS

This is a rare disease reported in the cat (see also Chapter 5, p. 169) and yet another term taken from human rheumatology. Relapsing polychondritis is characterized by episodic attacks of inflammation of hyaline and elastic cartilaginous structures including the ears, nose and laryngotracheal and articular cartilage, as well as the organs of special sense. It is thought to be an autoimmune response against cartilage, based on these cardinal features, the observed association with other conditions such as vasculitis, the presence of cartilage inflammation on biopsy, the demonstration of anti-collagen antibodies and a therapeutic response to corticosteroid therapy. It is reported mainly in middle-aged cats and auricular chondritis is the single most common manifestation. This may show as erythema, swelling, alopecia, crusting and pruritus of the pinnae, with curling of the ear margins. Involvement of articular cartilage leads to non-erosive inflammatory polyarthritis and lameness. Involvement of the laryngeal and tracheal/bronchial cartilages causes respiratory signs and inflammation of the heart valves can lead to valvular incompetency. Corneal opacification has also been reported in the cat. Dapsone has been used as a treatment (1 mg/kg p/o q24h).

MYOSITIS

Primary myositis is uncommon in the dog and rare in the cat. Four forms of immune-mediated myositis are documented in dogs: masticatory muscle myositis (MMM), extraocular myositis (EOM), dermatomyositis (DM) and polymyositis (PM).

MASTICATORY MUSCLE MYOSITIS

MMM is the most prevalent form of myositis in the dog. It involves the temporal, masseter and pterygoid muscles of the head, and presents clinically with symmetrical wasting of these muscle groups, pain on opening the mouth, restricted jaw movement and difficulty in eating (370). There may be mild elevation in serum CK and electromyographic abnormalities may be detected.

Canine masticatory muscles have a unique type 2M myofibre composition, which may explain their apparently selective involvement in these disorders. Autoantibodies specific for these 2M myofibres may be demonstrated in affected dogs. Biopsy reveals degenerative change in muscle fibre bundles, with fibrosis and inflammation. The infiltrate may be predominantly eosinophilic during the acute phase of disease (371) or during periods of relapse, whereas in chronic stages or periods of remission the lesions are dominated by lymphocytes and plasma cells (372, 373). This spectrum of histological change was once considered to

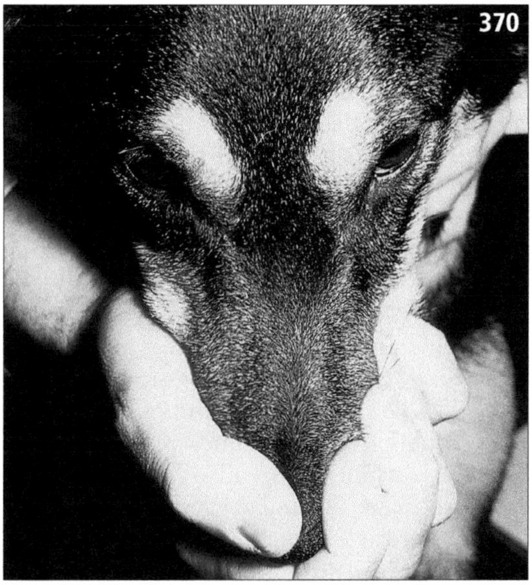

370 Canine masticatory myositis. A dog with atrophic myositis. Initially the temporal muscles become swollen and painful with the acute inflammatory phase. Very soon the muscles atrophy and fibrous contracture can result. This case shows obvious temporal muscle atrophy.

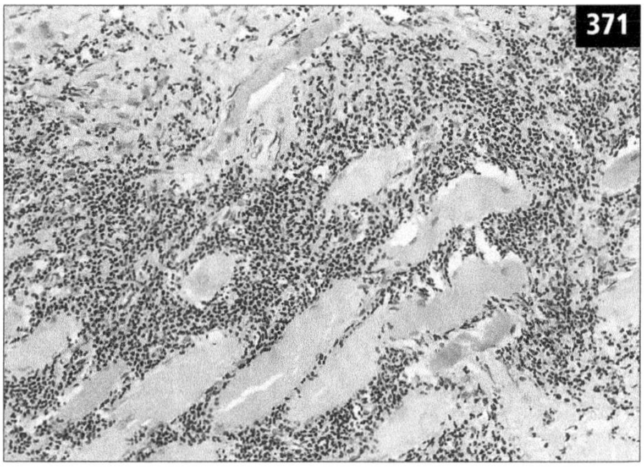

371 Canine masticatory myositis. Muscle biopsy from a three-year-old GSD with swelling of the temporal muscle. There is an intense infiltration of eosinophils, with focal lymphoplasmacytic aggregates associated with degeneration of muscle fibre bundles.

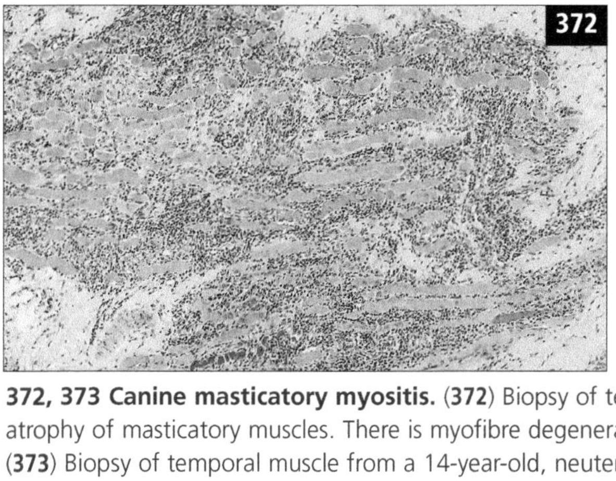

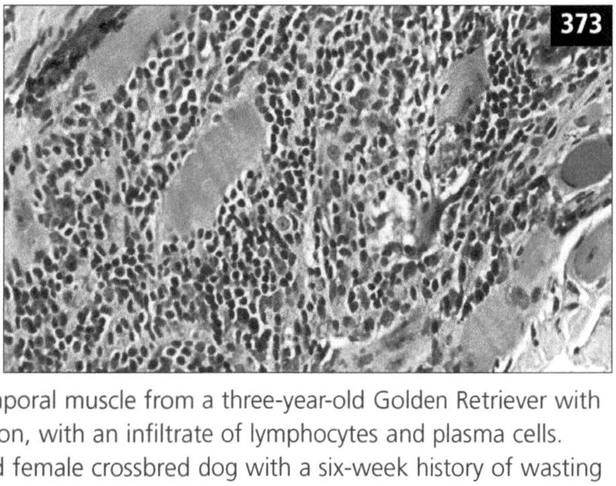

372, 373 Canine masticatory myositis. (**372**) Biopsy of temporal muscle from a three-year-old Golden Retriever with atrophy of masticatory muscles. There is myofibre degeneration, with an infiltrate of lymphocytes and plasma cells. (**373**) Biopsy of temporal muscle from a 14-year-old, neutered female crossbred dog with a six-week history of wasting of the temporal muscles. The dog has elevated serum creatinine kinase and abnormalities on EMG examination. This high power view shows intense infiltration of lymphocytes and plasma cells, with loss of myofibres.

represent distinct diseases (eosinophilic myositis and atrophic myositis), but this concept has now altered and MMM is discussed as a single entity. Recent studies have suggested that MMM is primarily humorally mediated. The infiltrating leukocytes have a largely perivascular distribution, and B lymphocytes dominate over macrophages, dendritic cells and T lymphocytes on immunohistochemical analysis of the lesions. Moreover, $CD4^+$ T cells are greater in number than $CD8^+$ cells and both $\alpha\beta$ and $\gamma\delta$ TCR expression is found.

Treatment is by the administration of prednisolone (1–2 mg/kg p/o q12h) until normal jaw function is attained and the serum CK normalizes. The dose should then be tapered to achieve the lowest possible alternate day maintenance dose, which should be maintained for 4–6 months. Azathioprine may be added to this regime if there is a poor response or concern over glucocorticoid side-effects. Forced stretching of the fibrotic muscles under general anaesthesia, followed by jaw exercises and immunosuppressive therapy, is an alternative approach. Care is required not to create a jaw fracture.

EXTRAOCULAR MYOSITIS

In this form of myositis, clinical signs (bilateral exophthalmos related to muscle swelling) are related to the extraocular muscles, with sparing of masticatory and limb musculature. There are no autoantibodies to type 2M fibres, so the immune response may involve a target antigen unique to this muscle group. Golden Retrievers may be predisposed to EOM. CK may be mildly elevated and muscle biopsy should reveal mononuclear inflammatory infiltration restricted to the extraocular muscles. Therapy is as described for the other forms of myositis (see above).

DERMATOMYOSITIS

DM is described fully in Chapter 5 (p. 160).

POLYMYOSITIS

Canine PM involves muscles of the head, trunk and limbs and occurs most frequently in large breed dogs (e.g. Newfoundlands and Boxers). The clinical signs are similar to those of polyarthritis/polymyositis and these connective tissue disorders may be related. Affected dogs may display stiff gait, muscle pain and weakness, exercise intolerance, muscle swelling or atrophy, and regurgitation/difficulty swallowing if the disease involves the pharyngeal or oesophageal muscles. Occasionally, dogs with PM may have associated neoplasia (bronchogenic carcinoma, myeloid leukaemia, tonsillar carcinoma and others). Affected dogs may have elevation of serum CK and abnormalities on electromyography. Muscle biopsy reveals myofibre degeneration and lymphoplasmacytic infiltration, and serum ANA and anti-sarcolemmal antibodies are documented. In contrast to MMM, immunohistochemical investigation of the lesions of PM suggests that this is a T cell-mediated pathology. The infiltrates are primarily endomysial and perimysial and there is invasion of non-necrotic muscle fibres. The infiltrates are dominated by $CD8^+$ T cells that principally express the $\alpha\beta$ TCR.

In both PM and MMM there is marked expression of MHC class II by the infiltrating leukocytes and also by stromal cells. In both diseases there is evidence of myofibre regeneration histologically and immunohistochemically by expression of the developmental myosin heavy chain molecule. In both diseases, real-time RT-PCR studies have shown enhanced expression of mRNA encoding TGFβ, eotaxin-2 and -3 and the receptor for these chemokines CCR3. TGFβ protein expression has also been shown immunohistochemically and suggests a role for this molecule in fibrosis and muscle regeneration.

Recent investigations have examined gene expression profiles by microarray analysis in MMM and PM (374). In both diseases there is up-regulation of genes involved in innate immunity (pertaining to macrophage and dendritic cell function), B cell activity and inflammation. In MMM, genes of the complement pathways, in addition to those encoding molecules involved in fibrosis and immunoregulation, were also activated.

The medical management of PM is as described above for MMM. Adjunct care may include elevation of the feeding/drinking position (with oesophageal muscle involvement) and provision of adequate exercise to prevent additional steroid-induced muscle atrophy.

FELINE MYOSITIS

Myositis is rare in the cat. Myositis affecting masticatory and limb musculature, in addition to myocardium, is reported in cats with thymoma.

374 Gene microarray analysis. Microarray provides a means of analysing the expression of many genes within a tissue sample. In the first stage of the procedure, mRNA is extracted from control and diseased samples and reverse transcribed to complementary DNA (cDNA). A fluorescent label is incorporated into the cDNA, in this example a red label with the cDNA from normal tissue and a green label for diseased tissue cDNA. The samples of cDNA are then mixed and hybridized to the surface of a 'gene chip'. This contains large numbers of gene sequences from the genome of the species under consideration, each of which is located within a tiny 'spot' on the chip. As an example, commercially available canine gene chips currently contain in the order of 20,000 gene sequences. After hybridization, the chips are scanned with lasers able to activate the red and green dyes and the emission of fluorescence is recorded. A single merged image is created for computer analysis. Where the gene is expressed in only normal tissue the spot will be red. In contrast, gene expression related to only diseased tissue will result in green fluorescence. A yellow spot reflects gene expression that occurs in both normal and diseased tissue.

374

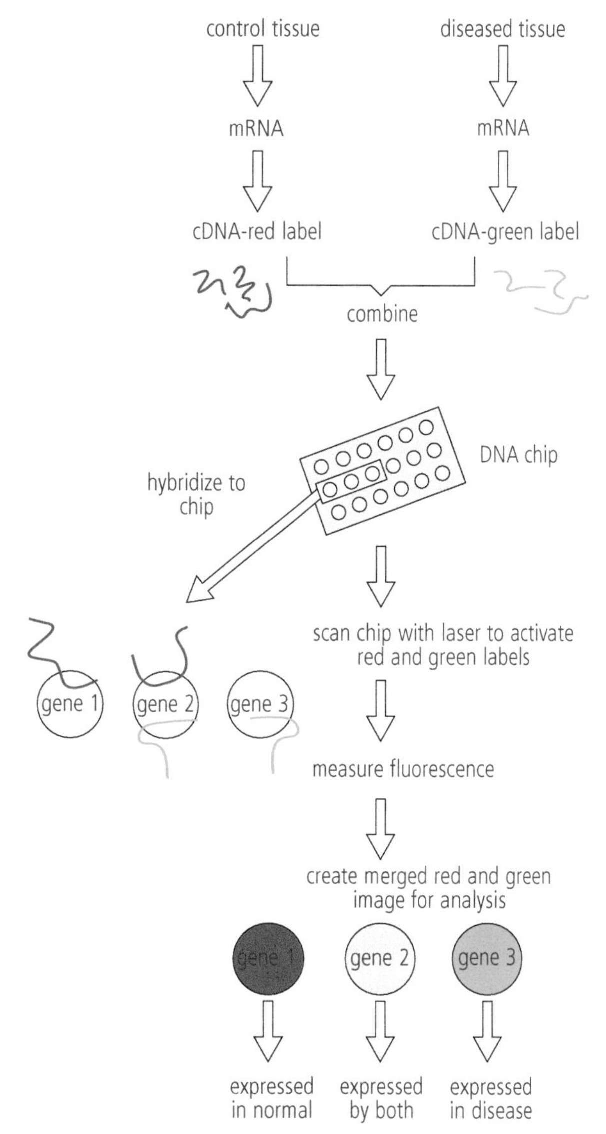

MYASTHENIA GRAVIS

Myasthenia gravis (MG) is documented in the dog and cat and may have a range of presentations. A congenital, inherited form occurs in young Jack Russell Terriers, Springer Spaniels and Fox Terriers and is characterized by deficiency of AChRs in the motor end-plate of the neuromuscular junction in the absence of autoantibody specific for AChRs. Acquired canine MG may be a primary autoimmune disease or it may occur in association with thymoma (or other tumours) (see Chapter 14, p. 364), hypothyroidism, hypoadrenocorticism or other autoimmune diseases. Purebred dogs at greatest risk of developing acquired MG include Japanese Akitas, the Terrier group, Scottish Terriers, German Shorthaired Pointers and Chihuahuas. Familial disease has been reported in the Newfoundland. The age of onset of acquired MG in the dog and cat is usually 3–5 years, although dogs as young as seven weeks may be affected.

Pathogenesis

The immunopathogenesis involves autoantibody specific for the AChR (375). Autoantibodies to the muscle protein titin and the ryanodine receptor are also identified in myasthenic humans and dogs with thymoma. It has been proposed that the autoimmune response in MG is initiated in the thymus (thymic myoid cells express surface AChR and neoplastic thymic epithelia may express a titin epitope), and that autoreactive T cells escape negative selection and are exported to secondary lymphoid tissue where they induce autoantibody production. Lymph node cells from a myasthenic dog spontaneously produced IgG AChR autoantibody when cultured *in vitro*.

Clinical signs

The presentation of acquired MG may take one of four clinical forms:

- **Generalized MG** involves generalized skeletal muscle weakness (including oesophageal and pharyngeal weakness), which is precipitated by exercise.
- **Focal MG** affects only oesophageal and pharyngeal musculature and generally presents as megaoesophagus (**376**), which may lead to aspiration pneumonia.
- Dogs with **acute fulminating MG** present in acute collapse, with weakness of respiratory musculature.
- **Paraneoplastic MG** is that form of disease which occurs in association with neoplastic disease.

Diagnosis

Diagnosis is made by observing rapid reversal of clinical signs following administration of a test dose of anticholinesterase drugs:

- Intravenous edrophonium: cat 2.5 mg/kg; dog 0.11–0.22 mg/kg, 5 mg maximum.
- Intramuscular neostigmine: 0.01–0.1 mg/kg.
- Pre-treatment with atropine (0.05 mg/kg) in each case.

However, the test may be negative where the available AChR content is markedly reduced, such as in dogs with acute onset collapse. There may be a decremental response of motor evoked potential during repetitive stimulation of nerves on electromyography. Immunohistochemistry may

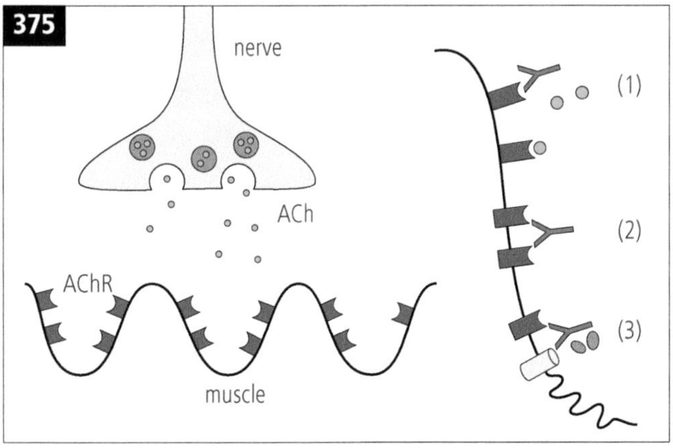

375 Myasthenia gravis. During a normal nerve impulse, acetylcholine is released at the motor end-plate and diffuses across the neuromuscular junction to bind to AChRs on the muscle. This initiates the opening of ion channels and results in muscular contraction. In myasthenia gravis, autoantibodies specific for the AChRs inhibit this process by (1) blocking the AChRs and preventing binding of ACh; (2) cross-linking AChRs, causing receptor internalization and degradation; and (3) fixing complement, causing lytic damage to the post-synaptic membrane.

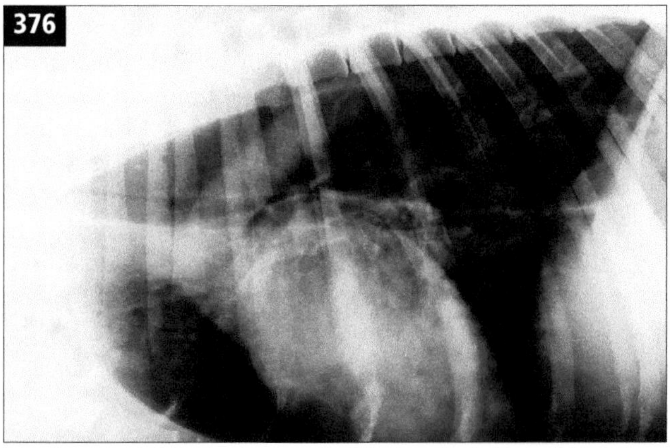

376 Myasthenia gravis. Lateral thoracic radiograph showing an air-filled oesophagus. This represents megaoesophagus associated with myasthenia gravis.

demonstrate deposition of IgG at the neuromuscular junction of affected muscle, and serum AChR autoantibodies can be demonstrated by indirect immunohistochemistry using sections of normal muscle. The current 'gold standard' for diagnosis is the demonstration of serum AChR autoantibodies by radioimmunoassay (377). Serum ANA is not found in canine or feline acquired MG.

Treatment

The therapeutic approach to canine MG includes:

- Administration of anticholinesterase drugs to prolong the action of available acetylcholine (e.g. pyridostigmine bromide 1–3 mg/kg p/o q8 or 12h).
- Administration of low dose glucocorticoid in the absence of optimum response to anticholinesterase (prednisolone 0.5 mg/kg p/o q48h). Immunosuppression is not widely applied in this disease, but small numbers of dogs have been treated with glucocorticoids with or without azathioprine, ciclosporin or mycophenolate mofetil.
- Elevation of feeding position or placement of a PEG tube if oesophageal dilation is present.
- Supportive care in acute fulminating MG.
- Management of any underlying disease (e.g. thymoma).
- Spay intact females to avoid disease exacerbation by oestrous or pregnancy.
- Avoid drugs that may affect neuromuscular transmission and vaccination that may exacerbate disease.

377

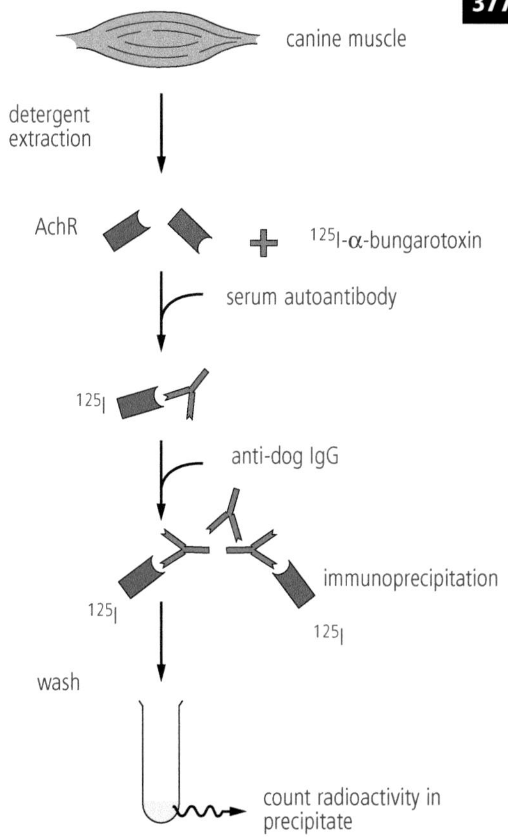

377 Immunoprecipitation radioimmunoassay for detection of AChR autoantibodies. AchRs are extracted from canine muscle by detergent solubilization and labelled with ^{125}I-α-bungarotoxin, which specifically binds to the AchR. Serum from the patient is incubated with radiolabelled AchRs and autoantibody will bind to the receptor molecule. The complexes are precipitated from solution by the addition of antiserum specific for canine IgG and the amount of radioactivity in the precipitates is counted. Titres are expressed as moles of ^{125}I-α-bungarotoxin binding sites per litre of serum.

Monitoring the success of treatment may be performed clinically and by using the serum AChR antibody titre, which reduces in clinical remission.

MYASTHENIA GRAVIS IN THE CAT

MG is rare in the cat; however, both congenital and acquired forms are recognized. Acquired MG is recognized most frequently in Abyssinian and Somali cats. Feline MG may be either generalized (but without megaoesophagus) or focal (with megaoesophagus and dysphagia in the absence of generalized weakness). Generalized MG may occur in the presence of a cranial mediastinal mass (thymoma or cystic thymus). The diagnostic methods are similar to those described for the dog, with the 'gold standard' being detection of serum AChR autoantibody.

POLYNEURITIS

Immune-mediated polyneuritis is uncommon in the dog and cat. The best defined condition is acute onset polyradiculoneuritis (Coonhound paralysis), which is associated with preceding exposure to racoons. The disease may be transmitted experimentally by racoon saliva, but a causative agent is not identified. A similar disease may arise after rabies vaccination, but many cases are idiopathic. These conditions are thought to be immune-mediated and involve demyelination, axonal degeneration and inflammation of ventral

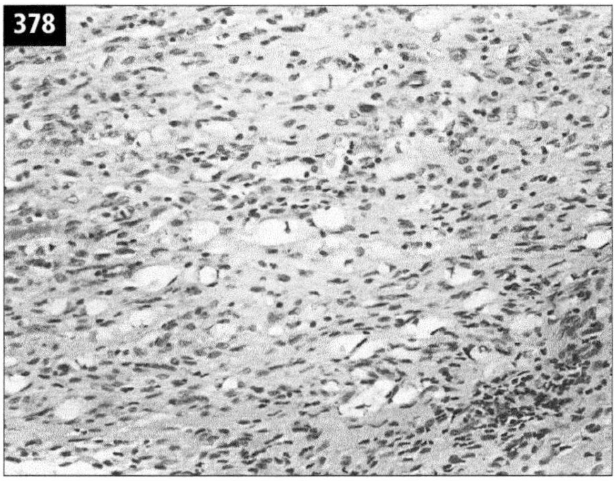

378 Polyneuritis. Section of brachial plexus nerve from a two-year-old DSH cat with Horner's syndrome and fore- and hindlimb paralysis. There is mixed mononuclear infiltration into the nerve, with evidence of demyelination.

roots of the spinal cord and peripheral nerves (378). There may be abnormalities on nerve conduction studies. Clinical signs develop 7–10 days after exposure to the initiating stimulus (when apparent), and take the form of ascending, flaccid paralysis progressing to quadriplegia and muscle atrophy. There is no cerebral involvement and affected dogs remain alert. Animals that do not die from respiratory paralysis may recover with symptomatic nursing, and there is no documented benefit from glucocorticoid therapy.

A chronic, relapsing form of polyradiculoneuritis is recognized in the dog and cat and is characterized by a longer clinical course and asymmetry in the severity of quadriplegia. Nerve biopsy reveals demyelination, axonal degeneration and lymphoplasmacytic infiltration.

DEGENERATIVE MYELOPATHY OF GSDs

Degenerative myelopathy (progressive myelopathy, chronic degenerative radiculomyelopathy) is predominantly recognized in older GSDs, although the Pembroke Welsh Corgi, Boxer, Rhodesian Ridgeback and Chesapeake Bay Retriever may be affected. There is loss of hindlimb proprioception, progressing to hindlimb ataxia and eventual paraplegia over a period of 6–12 months. Atrophy of hindlimb and pelvic musculature occurs, and in late stages of the disease there may be involvement of the forelimbs (379).

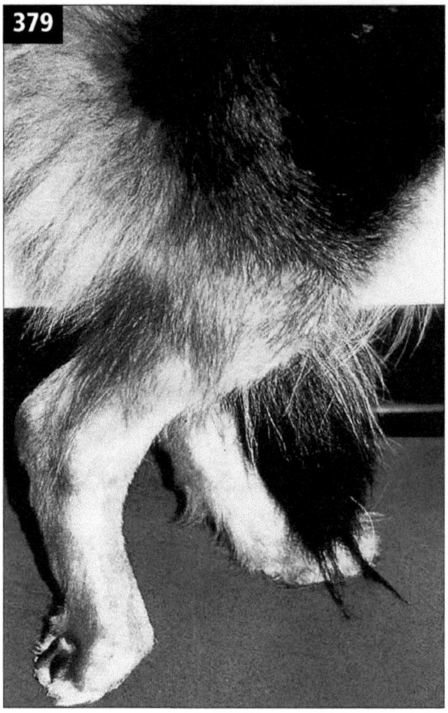

379 Degenerative myelopathy of GSDs. A ten-year-old GSD with chronic degenerative radiculomyelopathy. Notice the failure to return the knuckled paw to its correct position, indicating severe proprioceptive loss.

There is extensive demyelination and axonal degeneration, which begins in the thoracolumbar spinal cord and may progress to other locations in the cord. The disease was believed to have an immune-mediated pathogenesis based on:

- Raised circulating immune complexes.
- Depressed response of blood lymphocytes to mitogen stimulation, and failure of such cultures to respond to stimulation with myelin basic protein.
- Increased IgG concentration in cerebrospinal fluid (CSF).
- Deposition of IgG and C3 within blood vessels and areas of demyelination in affected spinal cord.

However, a recent study of affected Pembroke Corgis revealed a mutution in the gene encoding superoxide dismutase 1 protein (SOD1) as occurs in the homologous human disease amyotrophic lateral sclerosis(ALS). Although there is no specific treatment for this condition, a recent study has shown increased survival time when patients are provided with controlled, daily physiotherapy.

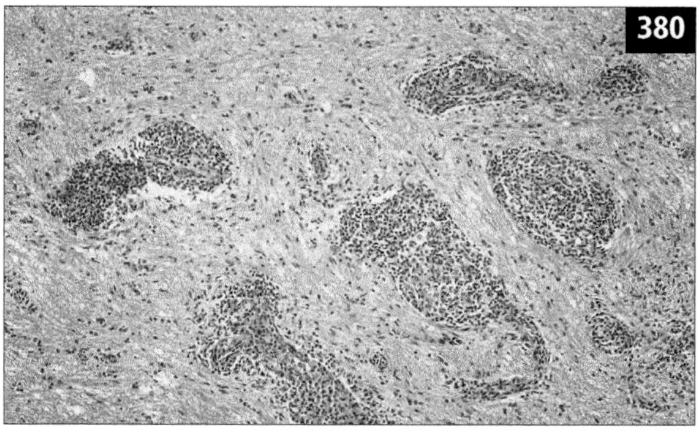

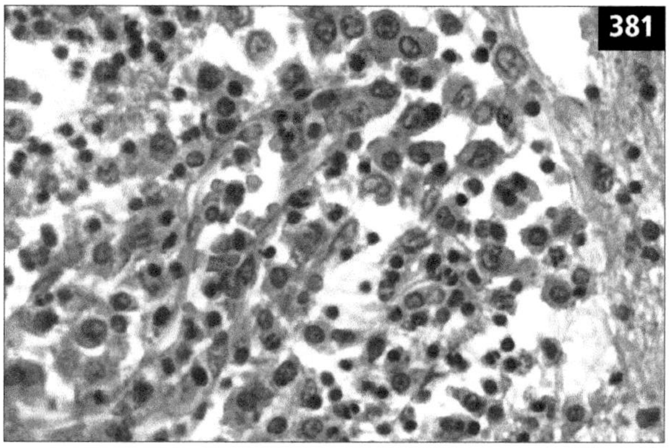

380, 381 Granulomatous meningoencephalitis. (**380**) Section of brain from a four-year-old West Highland White Terrier with a five-month history of progressive lameness and ataxia. There are multiple foci of granulomatous inflammation throughout the white matter of the brain. (**381**) High power view shows localized malacia, with an intense infiltrate of macrophages with fewer lymphocytes and occasional granulocytes.

GRANULOMATOUS MENINGOENCEPHALITIS

Granulomatous meningoencephalitis (GME) is an idiopathic CNS disease. It is characterized histologically by perivascular cuffing with macrophages, giant cells, lymphocytes and plasma cells and focal macrophage-dominated granulomas, with patchy distribution throughout the white matter of the brain and spinal cord and within the meninges (380, 381). Immunohistochemical investigations have revealed a dominance of T lymphocytes and MHC class II expressing macrophages within the inflammatory foci. The lesions are not associated with CDV, rabies virus or *Toxoplasma* antigens, and PCR investigation of lesional tissue has not revealed molecular evidence for the involvement of a range of other potential pathogens although in a recent study *Bartonella* DNA was detected in 1/6 cases. An immune-mediated pathogenesis is therefore proposed.

The greatest prevalence is amongst toy breeds and terriers. A range of non-specific neurological signs may be observed dependent on the areas of CNS affected, and the disease may be classified as focal, disseminated or ocular. The most useful diagnostic procedure is analysis of CSF, in which there may be elevated protein (0.4–1.0 g/l [0.04–0.1 g/dl]) and numerous macrophages and lymphocytes (5–11 × 10^9 cells/l [50–11,000 cells/μl]), but these findings are not specific for GME. There may be temporary improvement with glucocorticoid treatment and improved outcome with concurrent procarbizine, but the disease is progressive and most dogs die or are euthanazed within six months of initial presentation. Ciclosporin has been successfully used as an alternative immunosuppressive in the treatment of focal or ocular disease. Radiation therapy has been reported to extend survival time in dogs with focal (forebrain) GME.

NECROTIZING MENINGOENCEPHALITIS

The lesions of GME are distinct from the idiopathic necrotizing meningoencephalitis (NME) (Pug dog encephalitis) reported in young Pugs or Maltese with seizures, ataxia and depression and CSF lymphoid pleocytosis. The mononuclear inflammatory infiltrates of Pug dog encephalitis are less angiocentric and involve both grey and white matter, particularly of the cerebrum. There is a marked reactive astrogliosis and CSF autoantibody to glial fibrilliary acidic protein has been recently identified. PCR studies have failed to demonstrate an infectious aetiology. The genetic basis of this disease is discussed in chapter 3.

NECROTIZING LEUKOENCEPHALITIS

A third syndrome, necrotizing leukoencephalitis (NLE), is described in the Yorkshire Terrier, Chihuahua and Shih-Tzu. Clinically, NME and NLE are regarded as a continuum of the same disease process, but these entities may be distinguished by the histological distribution of lesions. In NLE the cerebral cortex and meninges are spared and there is targeting of the white matter of the proventricular cerebrum and thalamocortex. The proposed aetiopathogenesis of NLE is as described above for NME, with no evidence of an infectious causation thus far described.

GREYHOUND MENINGOENCEPHALITIS

This breed-restricted disease has only been documented in Ireland. It affects young (less than one year old) Greyhounds, which develop a range of either acute or insidious onset neurological signs. The lesions are of lymphoplasmacytic meningitis, with gliosis, gemistocytosis and mononuclear cell perivascular cuffing in the cerebral cortex, brainstem and proximal cervical spinal cord. The disease is regarded as idiopathic and PCR testing has not consistently identified a range of candidate viral or protozoal pathogens. Gene expression microarray has revealed upregulation of a set of 21 genes mostly related to immune function.

POLYARTERITIS NODOSA

Polyarteritis nodosa (panarteritis, periarteritis nodosa) is characterized by widespread necrotizing inflammation of small to medium sized arteries, sometimes associated with thrombosis and tissue infarction. The inflammatory infiltrates (macrophages, lymphocytes and plasma cells) form nodular aggregates around affected vessels (382, 383). On necropsy, haemorrhages may be recognized in association with arteries of the cervical spinal cord meninges, mediastinum and heart (coronary vessels). A more restricted form of arteritis is recognized in dogs with polyarthritis (384). Polyarteritis nodosa is rare in cats, but it may have a similar presentation (involving kidney, liver, pancreas, lungs, meninges and muscle) and must be distinguished from the vascular pathology of FIP infection.

382

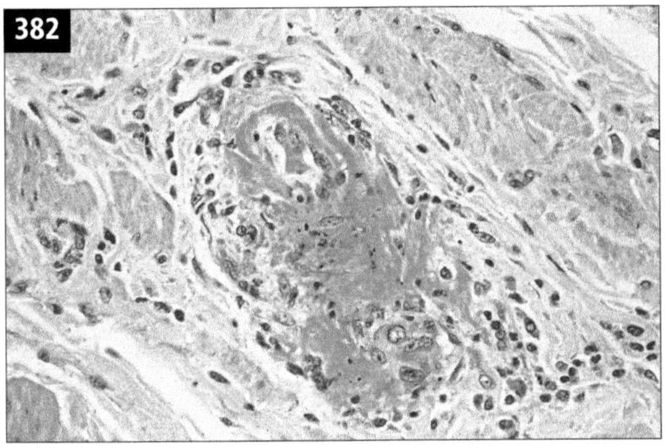

383

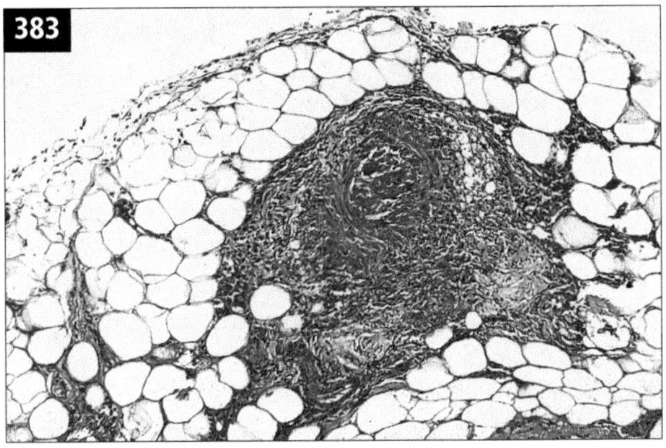

382, 383 Polyarteritis. (**382**) Section of bladder mucosa from a six-year-old Labrador Retriever with widespread fibrinoid necrosis and inflammation of small to medium-sized arteries. The degenerative vessels shown are associated with local fibrin deposition and a mixed inflammatory aggregate. (**383**) Synovial membrane biopsy from a dog with polyarteritis nodosa. There is inflammation of the arterial wall and a nodular aggregate of mononuclear cells around the affected vessel.

384

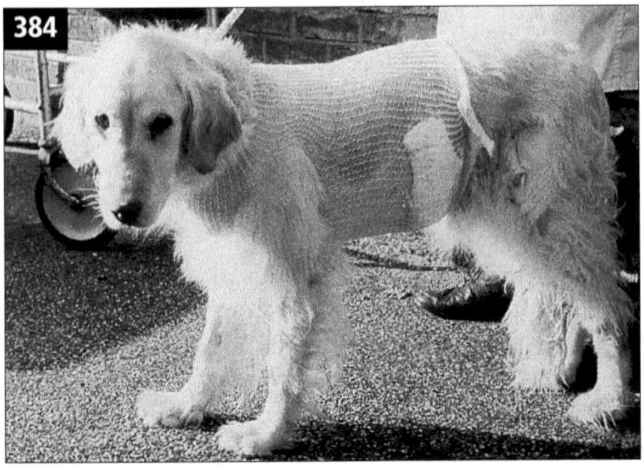

384 Polyarteritis nodosa. A two-year-old Golden Retriever with polyarteritis nodosa. This dog suffered from polyarthritis, with severe systemic illness and anorexia. A gastrostomy tube has been inserted for nutritional support.

STEROID-RESPONSIVE MENINGITIS-ARTERITIS

Steroid-responsive meningitis-arteritis (SRMA) is a localized form of canine arteritis that may occur in any breed, but most often arises in young adult, large breed dogs. Clinical signs include pyrexia, neck pain and stiff gait. There is generally leukocytosis and examination of the CSF reveals non-septic neutrophil pleocytosis and elevated protein concentration. The disease may be chronic and recurrent in nature. SRMA has a proposed immune-mediated pathogenesis, based on:

- The relapsing, remitting nature of the disease.
- Failure to identify infectious agents within the lesions.
- Temporary clinical response to immunosuppressive doses of glucocorticoids.
- Depressed response of blood lymphocytes to mitogen stimulation *in vitro*.
- Elevated levels of IgG, IgM and IgA within the CSF.
- IgG, IgM and IgA plasma cells within the infiltrates.
- Elevated serum IgA concentration.
- Elevated circulating immune complexes.
- Low T:B cell ratio in blood and CSF and increased CD4:CD8 ratio in blood.
- Deposition of IgA, but not immune complexes, within the vascular lesions.
- A Th2 (IL–4) bias in cytokine profile of blood and CSF leukocytes.
- Increased expression of genes encoding matrix metalloproteinases by CSF leukocytes.

The diagnostic hallmark of the disease is an elevation in serum and CSF IgA concentration, and this increased IgA synthesis may have a role in the pathogenesis of the disease. Although a range of autoantibodies to CNS proteins is recognized in affected dogs, such antibodies are also found in animals with a range of other CNS diseases and are thus regarded as an 'epiphenomenon' rather than a primary cause of disease. SRMA may be recognized concurrently in dogs with immune-mediated polyarthritis (see above). Treatment is by long-term, tapered, immunosuppressive glucocorticoid therapy (oral prednisolone), which leads to clinical improvement and remission from disease. Successful therapy is associated with reduction in CSF pleocytosis, but there is persistence of elevated serum and CSF IgA concentration.

FURTHER READING

Adamo FP, O'Brien RT (2004) Use of cyclosporine to treat granulomatous meningoencephalitis in three dogs. *Journal of the American Veterinary Medical Association* **225**:1211–1216.

Awano T, Johnson GS, Wade CM *et al.* (2009) Genome-wide association analysis reveals a *SOD1* mutation in canine degenerative myelopathy that resembles amyotrophic lateral sclerosis. *Proceedings of the National Academy of Sciences USA* **106**:2794-2799.

Barber RM, Li Q, Diniz PPVP *et al.* (2010) Evaluation of brain tissue or cerebrospinal fluid with broadly reactive polymerase chain reaction for *Ehrlichia*, *Anaplasma*, spotted fever group *Rickettsia*, *Bartonella*, and *Borrelia* species in canine neurological diseases (109 cases). *Journal of Veterinary Internal Medicine* **24**:372-378.

Cizinauskas S, Jaggy A, Tipold A (2000) Long-term treatment of dogs with steroid-responsive meningitis-arteritis: clinical, laboratory and therapeutic results. *Journal of Small Animal Practice* **41**:295–301.

Clements DN, Gear RNA, Tattersall J *et al.* (2004) Type I immune-mediated polyarthritis in dogs: 39 cases (1997–2002). *Journal of the American Veterinary Medical Association* **224**:1323–1327.

Coates JR, Barone G, Dewey CW *et al.* (2007) Procarbizine as adjunctive therapy for treatment of dogs with presumptive antemortem diagnosis of granulomatous meningoencephalitis: 21 cases (1998–2004). *Journal of Veterinary Internal Medicine* **21**:100–106.

Daly P, Drudy D, Chalmers WSK *et al.* (2006) Greyhound meningoencephalitis: PCR-based detection methods highlight an absence of the most likely primary inducing agents. *Veterinary Microbiology* **118**:189–200.

Evans J, Levesque D, Shelton GD (2004) Canine inflammatory myopathies: a clinicopathologic review of 200 cases. *Journal of Veterinary Internal Medicine* **18**:679–691.

Gerber B, Crottaz M, von Tscharner C *et al.* (2002) Feline relapsing polychondritis: two cases and a review of the literature. *Journal of Feline Medicine and Surgery* **4**:189–194.

Greer KA, Daly P, Murphy KE *et al.* (2010) Analysis of gene expression in brain tissue from greyhounds with meningoencephalitis. *American Journal of Veterinary Research* **71**:547-554.

Hansson-Hamlin H, Lilliehöök I, Trowald-Wigh G (2006) Subgroups of canine antinuclear antibodies in relation to laboratory and clinical findings in immune-mediated disease. *Veterinary Clinical Pathology* **35**:397–404.

Hansson-Hamlin H, Ronnelid J (2009) Detection of antinuclear antibodies by the Inno-Lia ANA update test in canine systemic rheumatic disease. *Veterinary Clinical Pathology* **39**:215-220.

Hegemann N, Wondimu A, Ullrich K *et al.* (2003) Synovial MMP-3 and TIMP-1 levels and their correlation with cytokine expression in canine rheumatoid arthritis. *Veterinary Immunology and Immunopathology* **91**:199–204.

Hegemann N, Wondimu A, Bohn B *et al.* (2005) Cytokine profile in canine immune-based polyarthritis and osteoarthritis. *Veterinary and Comparative Orthopaedics and Traumatology* **18**:67–72.

Jacques D, Cauzinille L, Bouvy B *et al.* (2002) A retrospective study of 40 dogs with polyarthritis. *Veterinary Surgery* **31**:428–434.

Kohn B, Garner M, Lubke S *et al.* (2003) Polyarthritis following vaccination in four dogs. *Veterinary and Comparative Orthopaedics and Traumatology* **16**:6–10.

Lowrie M, Penderis J, McLaughlin M *et al.* (2009) Steroid responsive meningitis-arteritis: a prospective study of potential disease markers, prednisolone treatment, and long-term outcome in 20 dogs (2006-2008). *Journal of Veterinary Internal Medicine* **23**:862-870.

Olsson M, Meadows JRS, Truve K *et al.* (2011) A novel unstable duplication upstream of *HAS2* predisposes to a breed-defining skin phenotype and a periodic fever syndrome in Chinese shar-pei dogs. *PLOS Genetics* **7**:e1001332.

Salvadori C, Peters IR, Day MJ *et al.* (2005) Muscle regeneration, inflammation, and connective tissue expansion in canine inflammatory myopathy. *Muscle and Nerve* **31**:92–198.

Schatzberg SJ, Haley NJ, Barr SC *et al.* (2005) Polymerase chain reaction screening for DNA viruses in paraffin-embedded brains from dogs with necrotizing meningoencephalitis, necrotizing leukoencephalitis, and granulomatous meningoencephalitis. *Journal of Veterinary Internal Medicine* **19**:553–559.

Schwab S, Herden C, Seeliger F *et al.* (2007) Non-suppurative meningoencephalitis of unknown origin in cats and dogs: an immunohistochemical study. *Journal of Comparative Pathology* **136**:96–110.

Schwartz M, Puff C, Stein VM *et al.* (2010) Marked MMP-2 transcriptional up-regulation in mononuclear leukocytes invading the subarachnoid space in aseptic suppurative steroid-responsive meningitis-arteritis in dogs. *Veterinary Immunology and Immunopathology* **133**:198-206.

Schwartz M, Puff C, Stein VM *et al.* (2011) Pathogenetic factors for excessive IgA production: Th2-dominated immune response in canine steroid-responsive meningitis-arteritis. *Veterinary Journal* **187**:260-266.

Schwartz Z, Zitzer NC, Racette MA *et al.* (2011) Are bacterial load and synovitis related in dogs with inflammatory stifle arthritis? *Veterinary Microbiology* **148**:308-316.

Shelton GD, Ho M, Kass PH (2000) Risk factors for acquired myasthenia gravis in cats: 105 cases (1986–1998). *Journal of the American Veterinary Medical Association* **216**:55–57.

Shelton GD, Hoffman EP, Ghimbovschi S *et al.* (2006) Immunopathogenic pathways in canine inflammatory myopathies resemble human myositis. *Veterinary Immunology and Immunopathology* **113**:200–214.

Smith BE, Tompkins MB, Breitschwerdt EB (2004) Antinuclear antibodies can be detected in dog sera reactive to *Bartonella vinsonii* subsp. *berghoffii*, *Ehrlichia canis*, or *Leishmania infantum* antigens. *Journal of Veterinary Internal Medicine* **18**:47–51.

Webb AA, Taylor SM, Muir GD (2002) Steroid-responsive meningitis-arteritis in dogs with non-infectious, nonerosive, idiopathic, immune-mediated polyarthritis. *Journal of Veterinary Internal Medicine* **16**:269–273.

7 IMMUNE-MEDIATED ALIMENTARY DISEASE

Michael J. Day and Edward J. Hall

GASTROINTESTINAL IMMUNOLOGY

The immune system of the gastrointestinal tract has been considered briefly in Chapter 1. In recent years, extensive immunological and molecular studies have enabled considerable advances in our understanding of immune parameters within the normal canine and feline intestine and have defined alterations in these parameters that characterize immune-mediated alimentary diseases.

The normal intestine may be considered to have three distinct immunological 'compartments':

- The **organized lymphoid aggregates** (e.g. the Peyer's patches, isolated gastric and intestinal lymphoid follicles and mesenteric lymph nodes with lymphatic and vascular drainage). These foci are generally considered inductive sites, where immune responses to antigen are triggered. Following activation, antigen-specific lymphocytes undergo recirculation and final recruitment back into the intestinal lamina propria through the interaction between homing receptors (e.g. $\alpha_4\beta_7$) and vascular addressins (e.g. MAdCAM1) (385).
- The **intestinal lamina propria,** which is rich in individual scattered lymphocytes, plasma cells and APCs (macrophages and dendritic cells), in addition to occasional eosinophils and mast cells. The lamina propria lymphocytes (LPLs) are generally considered as 'effector cells' that have undergone activation and recirculation and are capable of immune responsiveness (386).
- The **epithelial compartment**, consisting of the enterocytes and the intraepithelial lymphocytes. Enterocytes likely have much broader function than simply providing a barrier between the intestinal lumen and the lamina propria. These cells may be able to process and present antigen as they express MHC class II. In addition, enterocytes may produce a wide range of cytokines and other soluble mediators. The intraepithelial lymphocytes (IELs), which chiefly express the $\gamma\delta$ TCR, have been discussed in Chapter 1.

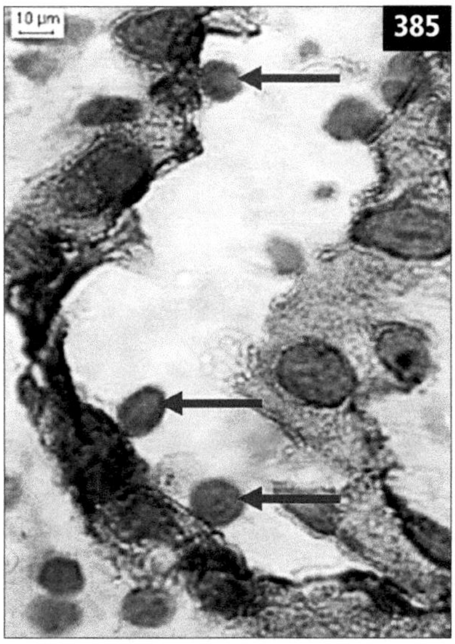

385 Lymphocyte recirculation in canine gut. Canine intestinal lamina propria labelled for the gut vascular addressin molecule MAdCAM. Marginated lymphocytes are present within the lumen of the vessel (arrowed). (From German AJ, Hall EJ, Moore PF *et al.* [1999] Analysis of the distribution of lymphocytes expressing the $\alpha\beta$ and $\gamma\delta$ T cell receptors and expression of mucosal addressin cell adhesion molecule-1 in the canine intestine. *Journal of Comparative Pathology* **201**:249–263, with permission.)

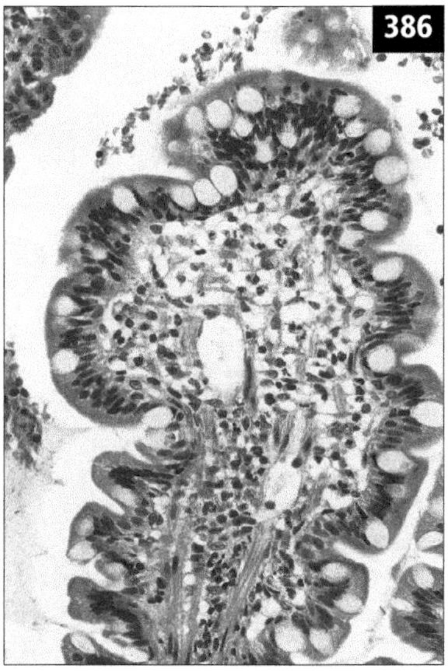

386 Epithelial and lamina propria compartments of the canine gut. Section of normal canine villus demonstrating enterocytes, goblet cells, intraepithelial lymphocytes and a mixed population of lamina propria lymphocytes (haematoxylin and eosin).

These various compartments are broadly similar across mammalian species, with occasional unique species characteristics. The lamina propria of both dogs and cats is rich in T lymphocytes (**387**) and plasma cells. In both species, $CD4^+$ T cells (**388**) dominate over $CD8^+$ T cells (**389**), and in the dog (where appropriate reagents are available) it has been shown that the LPLs preferentially express the αβ TCR. Plasma cells of the IgA class dominate the lamina propria of both dogs and cats (**390**) and there are also significant numbers of IgG cells, with fewer IgM plasma cells. The distribution of T cell subsets and plasma cells varies slightly within the villus-crypt unit and at different levels of the intestine (duodenum, jejunum, ileum and colon). The lamina propria is also rich in APCs that express MHC class II (**391**). These often have distinct dendritic morphology, and in the cat the dendritic processes of subepithelial dendritic cells have been observed to penetrate the enterocyte barrier (between enterocytes) to undertake sampling of antigen from the luminal surface. There are appreciable numbers of eosinophils within the normal lamina propria (**392**) and a distinct population of mast cells, which lie in an arcade immediately beneath the villus epithelium and

387

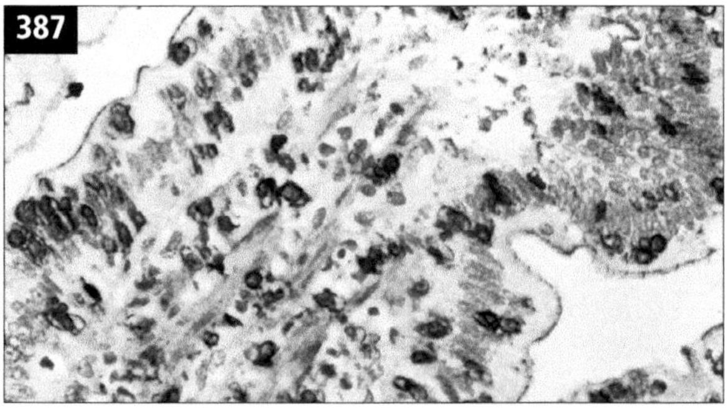

387 T lymphocytes in feline epithelium and lamina propria. Section of feline villus labelled using an antiserum specific for the CD3 molecule that identifies both intraepithelial and lamina propria T cells. (From Waly N, Gruffydd Jones TJ, Stokes CR *et al.* [2001] The distribution of leucocyte subsets in the small intestine of normal cats. *Journal of Comparative Pathology* **124:**172–182, with permission.)

388

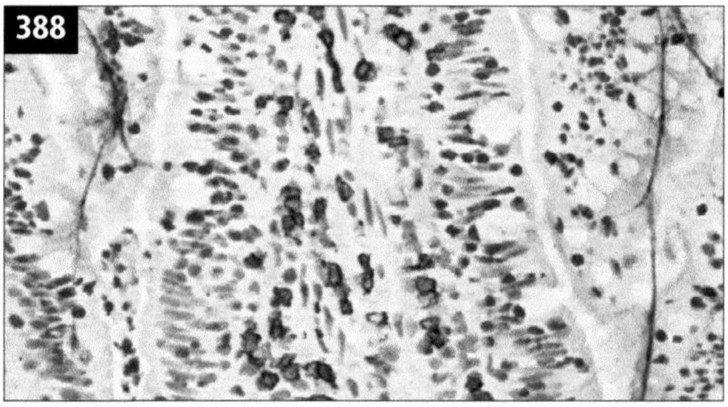

388 CD4 T cells in feline intestine. Section of feline villus labelled for CD4 demonstrates that these cells are predominantly located in the villus lamina propria. (From Waly N, Gruffydd Jones TJ, Stokes CR *et al.* [2001] The distribution of leucocyte subsets in the small intestine of normal cats. *Journal of Comparative Pathology* **124:**172–182, with permission.)

389

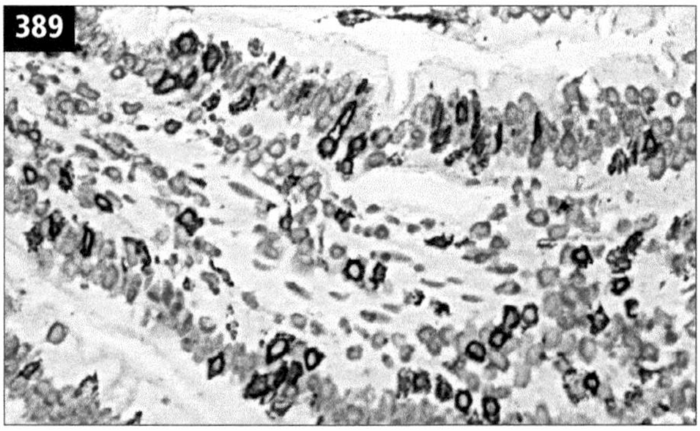

389 CD8 T cells in feline intestine. Section of feline villus labelled with antiserum specific for CD8. The majority of intraepithelial lymphocytes are $CD8^+$ and there are numerous positively stained cells within the villus lamina propria. (From Waly N, Gruffydd Jones TJ, Stokes CR *et al.* [2001] The distribution of leucocyte subsets in the small intestine of normal cats. *Journal of Comparative Pathology* **124:**172–182, with permission.)

390

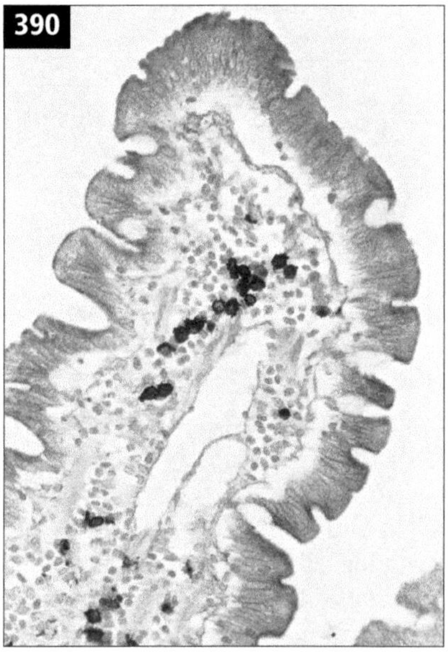

390 IgA plasma cells in canine villus. Section of normal canine villus labelled using an antiserum specific for IgA. Plasma cells bearing cytoplasmic IgA are found in greater proportion to IgG and IgM plasma cells in the intestinal lamina propria.

adjacent to small capillaries in this area.

The epithelial compartment of both species has also now been well characterized. IELs are present in relatively greater numbers in the cat than in the dog. One interpretation of this finding might be that it reflects a greater microbial load within the small intestine of cats, although there is dispute as to whether there is a significant quantitative difference between the canine and feline intestinal microflora. In both species the IELs are predominantly $CD8^+$ T lymphocytes. Immunohistochemistry has confirmed dominant γδ TCR expression by canine IELs (**84**). A major species difference lies with MHC class II expression by enterocytes. In the dog this appears to be constitutive, with both membrane and cytoplasmic class II expression recognized that is strongest in crypt epithelium or epithelium overlying Peyer's patches (**63**). In contrast, in the cat the enterocytes do not normally express MHC class II, although this may be induced during intestinal disease.

Molecular studies have characterized the expression of mRNA encoding a range of cytokines and chemokines in normal canine and feline intestinal mucosa (**393**). In general terms the normal intestinal mucosa of both species expresses a range of Th1-related (e.g. IFNγ, IL-12, IL-18),

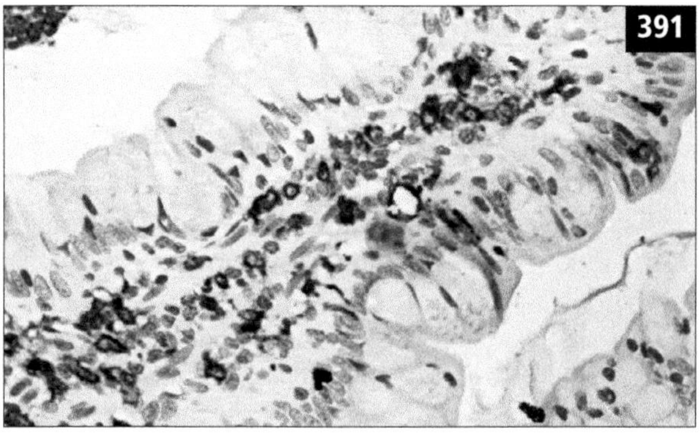

391 MHC class II expression in feline intestine. Section of feline villus labelled for MHC class II delineates populations of lamina propria cells with the cytological appearance of macrophages and dendritic cells. (From Waly N, Gruffydd Jones TJ, Stokes CR *et al.* [2001] The distribution of leucocyte subsets in the small intestine of normal cats. *Journal of Comparative Pathology* **124:**172–182, with permission.)

392 Lamina propria eosinophils. Section of normal canine villus demonstrating scattered eosinophils within the lamina propria (Sirius red stain).

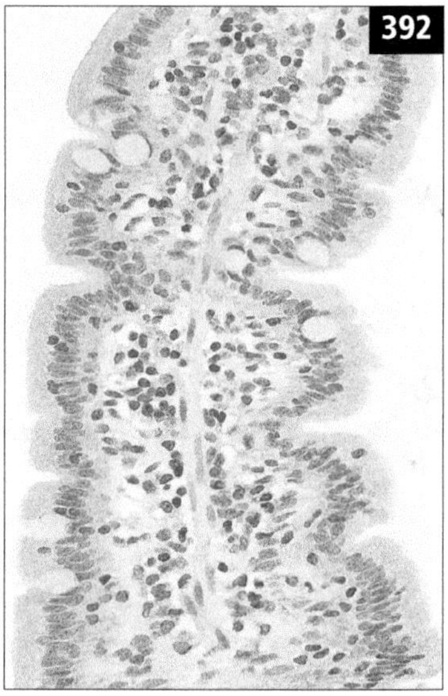

393 Cytokine gene expression in canine intestine. Expression of mRNA encoding a panel of cytokines was determined in duodenal tissue from eight normal dogs. A range of transcripts are present, with those encoding IL-18, TGFβ and TNFα being most abundant. (Data from Peters IR, Helps CR, Calvert EL *et al.* [2005] Cytokine mRNA quantification in histologically normal canine duodenal mucosa by real-time RT-PCR. *Veterinary Immunology and Immunopathology* **103:**101–111.)

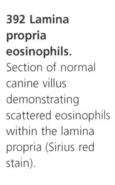

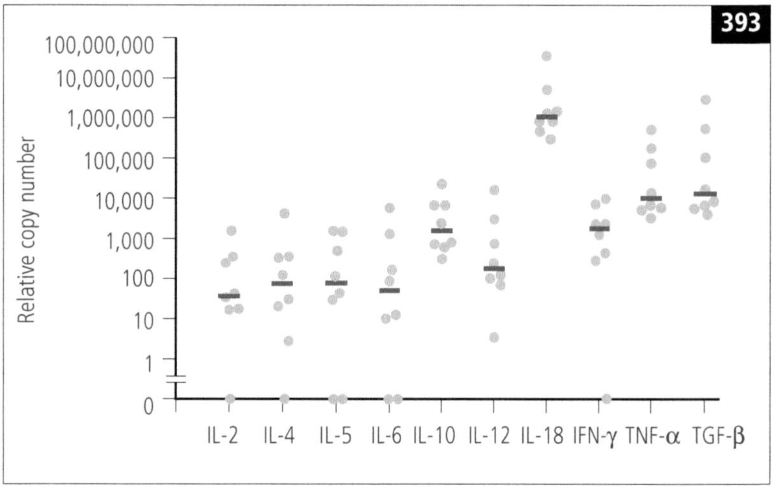

pro-inflammatory (e.g. TNFα) and immunoregulatory (e.g. IL-10, TGFβ) cytokines. A dominance of Th1 cytokines might not have been predicted in a mucosal site chiefly protected by IgA antibody, but this finding is consistent with the cytokine profile (Th1 dominated) that occurs in humans and experimental rodents.

In functional terms, mucosal sites such as the intestine display a fine balance between responsiveness and immunological tolerance. The gut is continuously bombarded by a plethora of antigens (e.g. derived from food or luminal microflora), which may be 'sampled' by the mucosal immune system, with a range of possible outcomes:

- The antigen may be recognized as foreign (e.g. a pathogenic nematode, bacterium or virus) and a local protective immune response mounted. There is some evidence that antigens that stimulate an active local immune response may be sampled via the M cells overlying Peyer's patches of the small intestine.
- The antigen may be ignored by the gut immune system, with the induction of local and/or systemic tolerance. This phenomenon is represented by the classical experimental demonstration of 'oral tolerance', whereby the immune system fails to respond to systemic challenge with an antigen to which it has been previously exposed via the intestine. The development of immunological tolerance is now recognized as being an active rather than a passive event. The antigen under question must be processed and presented, and activation of T cells occurs that underpins the tolerance response. It is most likely that oral tolerance is mediated by regulatory cells, in particular the Th3 regulatory population that is characterized by production of TGFβ. That such immune responses occur during the process of tolerance induction is supported by the common finding of serum IgG and IgA antibodies to dietary antigens that occur in the circulation of normal individuals. It is suggested that antigen that is transferred across the enterocyte barrier (e.g. of the villus) is more likely to induce a tolerance response.
- Continued exposure (sensitization) to antigen may induce an inappropriate hypersensitivity response (e.g. dietary hypersensitivity).

It is likely that the 'default' immune response of the gut is towards tolerance, and that a range of factors such as the physical form and dose of antigen, the type of PRRs engaged on the surface of dendritic cells and the location of antigen exposure (e.g. Peyer's patch or villus) may modulate this baseline response towards a protective or hypersensitivity reaction.

IMMUNE-MEDIATED GASTROINTESTINAL DISEASE

This chapter is concerned with the primary immune-mediated disorders that affect the alimentary system (*Table 16*). Given that the intestinal tract contains the greatest concentration of immunological tissue in the body, it is not surprising that immune-mediated disease of the alimentary system is common in both the dog and cat. Although we are learning more of the immunopathogenesis of these disorders, these entities are still often regarded as idiopathic. They are generally described as distinct clinical and pathological entities, but some may fall within a single disease spectrum with common aetiology. For example, although antibiotic responsive diarrhoea (ARD) and idiopathic inflammatory bowel disease (IBD) are both considered individual diseases, both disorders are likely reflections of an abnormal intestinal immune response to bacterially-derived antigens. To this end, some current research studies investigate 'chronic enteropathy' in mixed populations of dogs with IBD, ARD and dietary hypersensitivity, making it difficult to associate findings with a specific entity. This applies to current investigations of TLR expression and genetic associations with TLR gene polymorphisms, intestinal dendritic cell numbers and cytokine gene expression.

Table 16: Immune-mediated alimentary disease of the dog and cat.

- Feline gingivostomatitis.
- Dietary hypersensitivity.
- Gluten enteropathy of Irish Setter dogs.
- Protein-losing enteropathy/nephropathy of Soft Coated Wheaten Terriers.
- Antibiotic responsive diarrhoea.
- Inflammatory bowel disease:
  - Lymphoplasmacytic enteritis.
  - Eosinophilic gastroenteritis.
  - Granulomatous enteritis.
  - Lymphoplasmacytic colitis.
  - Histiocytic ulcerative colitis (now considered infectious).

FELINE GINGIVOSTOMATITIS

Pathogenesis

The aetiopathogenesis of feline gingivostomatitis is unknown, but the condition is often considered to represent an inappropriate immune response to oral microflora. Feline calicivirus is frequently isolated from the lesions and there is often serological evidence of infection by FeLV and FIV, which may contribute to a multifactorial pathogenesis via systemic immunosuppression. A role for anaerobic bacteria has been suggested and serological responses have been demonstrated towards the gram-negative *Porphyromonas* spp. In contrast, a causative role for dietary allergens has not been defined.

Clinical signs

The disease has greatest prevalence in purebred cats and is not necessarily associated with dental disease. The spectrum of clinical changes includes:

- Dysphagia, halitosis, weight loss, inappetence and ptyalism.
- Focal or diffuse inflammation of the gingival and buccal mucosa, the glossopalatine arches (fauces) and the palatine and lingual mucosa.
- Chronic lesions may become proliferative (394), ulcerated and infected.

Diagnosis

Histologically the lesions are characterized by intense cellular infiltration, which is most often lymphoplasmacytic, although neutrophils, eosinophils and macrophages may be present (395). There may be hyperplasia or ulceration of the overlying epithelium. The lymphoid populations within the normal and affected feline oral mucosa have been characterized immunohistochemically. Affected cats generally have elevated serum concentrations of IgG, IgM and IgA. In contrast, there is elevation in the concentration of IgG and IgM (but not IgA) in saliva. Lesional tissue displays elevated expression of genes encoding the cytokines IL-2, IL-4, IL-6, IL-10, IL-12 and IFNγ, consistent with a mixed immunological reaction involving Th1, Th2 and regulatory populations.

Treatment and prognosis

There is no standard therapy for feline gingivostomatitis. Reported treatments include:

- Maintenance of oral hygiene and dental health.
- Radical extraction of all teeth.
- Dietary management.
- Metronidazole (10–20 mg/kg p/o q12h).
- Type I interferon (see Chapter 16, p. 398) has been given as adjunct therapy by subgingival and subcutaneous administration.
- Levamisole as an immunomodulator (see Chapter 16, p. 396).
- Glucocorticoids (methylprednisolone acetate 20 mg s/c every 3 weeks; dexamethasone 0.1–0.2 mg/kg p/o q24h).
- Gold salts (1 mg/kg i/m weekly, for not more than 20 weekly injections; the first 2 injections are test doses of 1 and 2 mg; a CBC should be performed regularly).
- Progestagens (megestrol acetate 1 mg/kg p/o every other day).

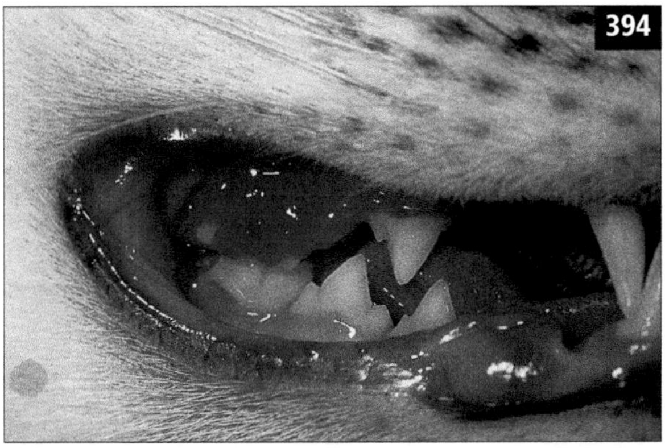

394 Feline gingivostomatitis. Typical proliferative gingival lesion in a cat with lymphoplasmacytic gingivitis. (Photograph courtesy A.H. Sparkes.)

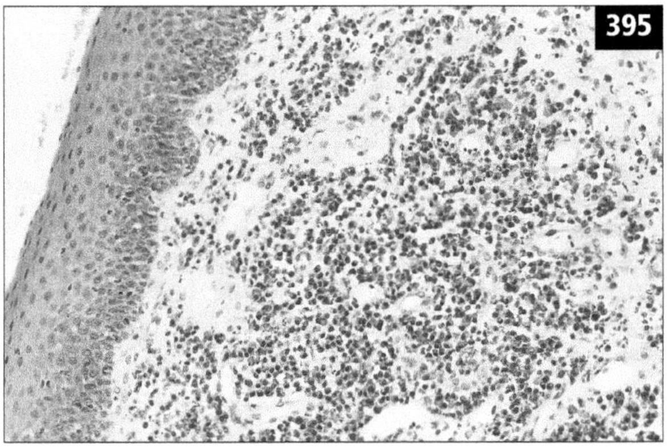

395 Feline gingivostomatitis. Section of gingiva from an eight-year-old neutered male DSH cat with severe proliferative gingivitis. There is epithelial hyperplasia, with an intense inflammatory infiltration of subepithelial tissue that is dominated by plasma cells.

- Other immunosuppressive drugs (e.g. azathioprine 0.3 mg/kg p/o every other day; chlorambucil 0.1–0.2 mg/kg p/o q24h). A recent study has reported clinical improvement in some cats with the use of ciclosporin.
- Topical application of bovine lactoferrin has been suggested to be of clinical benefit.

A recent clinical trial has compared the efficacy of several long-term (six months) treatment modalities by assessing the ability to alter clinical lesion severity scores and some immunological parameters. All cats in the trial underwent initial dental treatment (scale, polish, and extraction where necessary) and a course of metronidazole and spiramycin. Following this initial therapy, four treatment groups were established. These four groups were administered either methylprednisolone, sodium aurothiomalate, metronidazole and spiramycin, or oral hygiene products. The most significant improvement in measured parameters was obtained in cats administered glucocorticoids.

DIETARY HYPERSENSITIVITY

Pathogenesis

In some individuals, particular dietary components may cause immunological sensitization and subsequent hypersensitivity. True dietary hypersensitivity must be distinguished from dietary intolerance, whereby ingestion of a particular food results in intestinal disturbance by non-immunological means (toxic, pharmacological, metabolic, idiosyncratic). The immunological basis of dietary hypersensitivity is poorly understood, but is thought to involve predominantly a type I mechanism, although hypersensitivity types III and IV have been incriminated. The most common dietary components incriminated as causative of food allergy in the dog include beef, chicken, milk, eggs, corn, wheat and soy. A similar range of proteins induce feline dietary hypersensitivity (beef, wheat and corn gluten). It is uncommon for any one animal to react to more than two specific dietary allergens. The antigenic components of food that are most often involved are protein or glycoprotein molecules, which are stable in the presence of heat, acid or digestive enzymes. There may be greater accessibility of allergen to gut-associated lymphoid tissue (GALT) in the presence of mucosal immunodeficiency (e.g. IgA deficiency) or damage to the tight junctions of enterocytes. Intestinal biopsies from animals with dietary hypersensitivity may have eosinophilic or lymphoplasmacytic infiltration of the lamina propria, suggesting overlap with the syndromes of IBD described below. Limited studies of the phenotype of lymphoid subpopulations, and cytokine mRNA expression, in the intestinal mucosa of dogs with proven food allergy has shown no significant differences compared with control mucosa.

An experimental model of canine food allergy has been developed by subcutaneously immunizing inbred, high IgE-producing dogs with food antigen extracts in adjuvant during the neonatal period. The dogs also receive routine vaccination during this time. These dogs develop food-specific serum IgE and positive skin tests and show an immediate hypersensitivity reaction to injection of food extract into the gastric mucosa during gastroscopy. There is also a late phase gastric response characterized by an eosinophil and mononuclear cell infiltration. This model has been used to study the effects of feeding chemically or genetically modified proteins to allergic individuals. Further experimental challenge studies have been conducted with colonies of dogs that have spontaneously developed food allergy.

Clinical signs

Food allergy in the dog and cat most frequently presents as cutaneous disease (see Chapter 5). It has been estimated that 1% of the canine population may suffer from dietary hypersensitivity and that up to 10% of dogs with dermatological disease may be affected, although AD and FAD are far more common causes of pruritic skin disease. Approximately 30–50% of cases develop clinical signs at under one year of age, and in general the onset of disease is not related to a recent dietary change, but involves foodstuffs to which there has been long-term exposure. In only a small proportion (estimated to be 10–15%) of cases is dietary hypersensitivity recognized as a cause of primary gastrointestinal disease, with clinical signs that may include vomiting, diarrhoea, weight loss and abdominal discomfort. Concurrent dermatological and gastrointestinal manifestations are occasionally recognized. Additionally, there is anecdotal evidence to suggest that dietary hypersensitivity may occasionally manifest as CNS disease, characterized by seizures or behavioural abnormalities, as respiratory disease involving asthma-like attacks or rhinitis (with conjunctivitis) or, rarely, as musculoskeletal or urinary tract disease.

Diagnosis

The diagnosis of dietary hypersensitivity is made by demonstrating a positive response to feeding an exclusion diet based on a novel protein and carbohydrate source. The diet is given as the sole source of food for a minimum of three weeks, although there are suggestions that a ten-week trial is required to document every case. Exclusion diets have restricted antigen diversity and may be home-cooked. Similar commercial diets are often termed hypoallergenic, as they are also highly digestible, thereby reducing not just the antigenic diversity but also the antigenic load. Recently, a range of diets based on hydrolysed protein have become available. The protein in these diets has been extensively degraded such that the size of the protein molecules is insufficient to cross-link IgE on the surface of mast cells, and thereby prevent mast cell degranulation. If there is a positive response to an exclusion diet, the diagnosis is confirmed by showing relapse when challenged with the original diet and remission when 'rescued' with the exclusion diet.

Intradermal, gastroscopic and colonoscopic testing with food allergens has been reported and, although rarely undertaken, the latter two procedures likely have greater utility than skin testing. Serological testing is now widely available, but the few published studies of this modality have suggested that this is an unreliable diagnostic procedure, as many normal dogs and dogs with non-hypersensitivity alimentary disease will have serum IgG and IgE antibodies specific for dietary proteins. Similarly, normal cats will make serum IgG and IgA responses to dietary antigens. Serum IgG and IgE antibody specific for bovine proteins may also be induced following vaccination with viral vaccine that incorporates residual traces of bovine serum used in the cell culture system for viral propagation. The use of Doppler ultrasound examination of coeliac and cranial mesenteric arteries after dietary provocation has recently been reported, the suggestion being that the intestinal inflammatory response involves increased blood flow to this organ. At the research level, *in vitro* basophil degranulation or lymphocyte stimulation assays have been described.

Treatment

Treatment is by feeding a diet that avoids the offending antigen(s). Glucocorticoid therapy may be indicated in the initial stages of management in order to control the observed clinical signs.

PROTEIN LOSING ENTEROPATHY/ NEPHROPATHY OF THE SOFT COATED WHEATEN TERRIER

This complex breed-specific disorder is thought to have an immunopathogenesis involving dietary hypersensitivity. Affected dogs may initially develop dietary hypersensitivity, with an intestinal inflammatory response that weakens the tight junctions between enterocytes and permits absorption of high levels of luminal antigen. This antigen in turn combines with circulating immunoglobulin and may deposit within the glomerulus, leading to secondary immune complex glomerulonephritis.

The evidence for dietary hypersensitivity in this disorder is provided by dietary challenge studies in which vomiting, diarrhoea and pruritus develops in susceptible dogs fed chicken or corn, and the fact that affected dogs sometimes make a clinical response following dietary modification. Moreover, gastroscopic testing has demonstrated local reactions to milk, lamb, wheat and chicken. Finally, affected dogs develop raised concentrations of faecal (but not serum) allergen-specific IgE on dietary challenge.

GLUTEN-SENSITIVE ENTEROPATHY

Irish Setters with a familial sensitivity to wheat protein (gluten-sensitive enteropathy) have been described. The trait is inherited in an autosomal recessive fashion. In these dogs, clinical signs of inappetence, poor weight gain or weight loss, and chronic intermittent diarrhoea are manifest by 7–10 months of age when a diet containing wheat is fed (**396**). There is histological evidence of villus atrophy and increased numbers of IELs and goblet

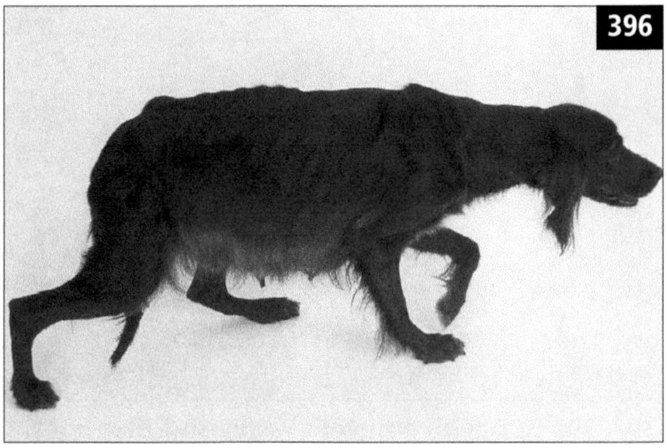

396 Gluten enteropathy in Irish Setters. Irish Setter affected with gluten-sensitive enteropathy; the dog is significantly underweight, with prominent ribs.

cells, but increased cellularity of the villus lamina propria is variably observed. The increased number of IELs is likely to be a marker for disease rather than directly associated with intestinal damage. Exposure to dietary wheat is associated with specific loss of brush border alkaline phosphatase and aminopeptidase N activity, but other brush border enzymes are unaffected. These changes are accompanied by ultrastructural abnormalities of the brush border microvilli. Treatment is by feeding a diet that excludes wheat gluten and related proteins in barley, oats and rye. Rice and maize (corn) are suitable cereal substitutes.

ANTIBIOTIC RESPONSIVE DIARRHOEA

Pathogenesis and clinical signs

ARD is a relatively new designation for the disorder previously known as small intestinal bacterial overgrowth (SIBO). There is a clear distinction between these two entities. SIBO describes the presence of elevated numbers of bacteria within the small intestine, although precisely how many bacteria define an elevation is widely debated. One proposal for the dog is that numbers greater than 10^5 colony-forming units of bacteria per ml of duodenal juice is consistent with SIBO. In some individuals, SIBO may be secondary to intestinal ileus or hypomotility, impaired production of gastric acid, partial intestinal obstruction or exocrine pancreatic insufficiency (EPI). However, in the majority of dogs there is no underlying cause recognized and SIBO is considered idiopathic. The overgrowth predominantly involves anaerobes (e.g. *Clostridium, Bacteroides*); aerobic overgrowth (e.g. *Escherichia coli*) is less common. Recently, a new molecular approach to investigation of intestinal microflora has been introduced. Amplification by PCR of bacterial 16S ribosomal DNA and separation of amplicons by denaturing gradient gel electrophoresis (DGGE) allows assessment of the diversity of the microflora within a sample of duodenal juice. These studies have shown marked qualitative differences between the microflora of different dogs, but relative consistency when the same dog is sampled on more than one occasion.

Many dogs with SIBO have chronic, intermittent, small bowel diarrhoea and weight loss, but SIBO need not be a cause of clinical signs or histopathological change in the intestinal mucosa. Moreover, SIBO need not always be ameliorated by antibiotic therapy. In contrast, ARD literally describes a dog with chronic diarrhoea in which the clinical signs respond to antibiotic therapy. A dog with ARD need not necessarily have SIBO in the same way that a dog with SIBO need not have ARD. It has been suggested that ARD may be particularly linked to infection with enteropathogenic *Escherichia coli* (EPEC), but

397

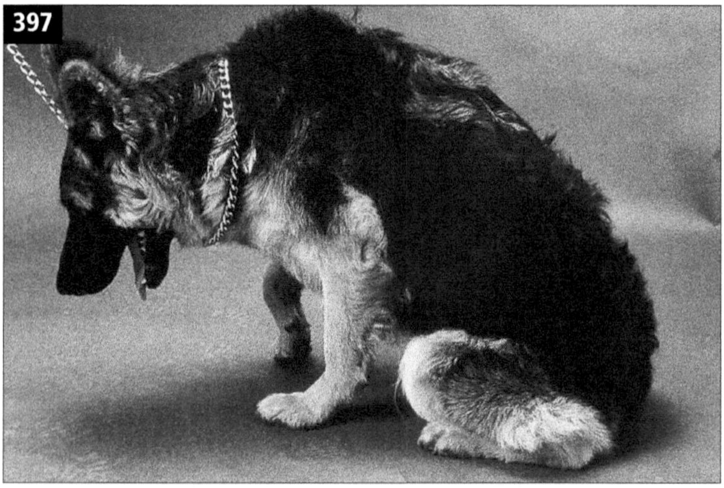

398

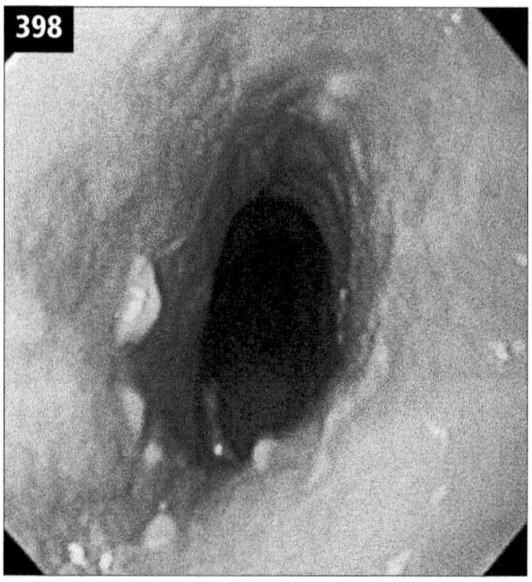

397, 398 GSD with antibiotic responsive diarrhoea. (**397**) A ten-month-old female GSD with idiopathic ARD. The dog was stunted and underweight; signs of chronic diarrhoea, polyphagia and coprophagia were controlled with oral oxytetracycline administration. (**398**) On endoscopic examination the duodenal mucosa appeared grossly normal. with no evidence of inflammation. Bile-stained mucus is seen adherent to the surface.

many clinically normal dogs are also known to harbour EPEC. ARD is also likely to exist in the cat; however, it has been poorly defined, as the proximal intestinal microflora of the healthy cat is suggested to be numerically greater than other species and may normally include anaerobes.

GSDs appear particularly susceptible to ARD, and underlying mucosal immunodeficiency is thought to predispose to this condition (**397, 398**). GSDs with ARD may have reduced concentration of IgA in serum, duodenal juice or duodenal explant culture supernatant (**399, 400**). Some studies have also suggested that dogs of this breed may have low concentration of faecal IgA relative to other breeds, particularly when repeat faecal samples are examined over time from one individual. In contrast, affected GSDs have no abnormality in the number of IgA plasma cells within intestinal lamina propria (**401**). These findings suggest that there may be reduction in local synthesis or secretion of IgA rather than lack of IgA-producing cells; however, there is no breed difference in expression of genes encoding the IgAα heavy chain, the polymeric Ig receptor or the joining (J) chain within intestinal tissue (**10**). Moreover, there is no defect in expression of genes encoding cytokines involved in

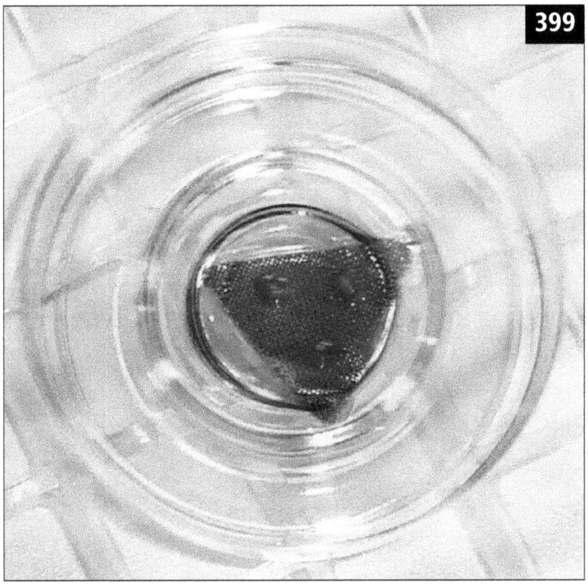

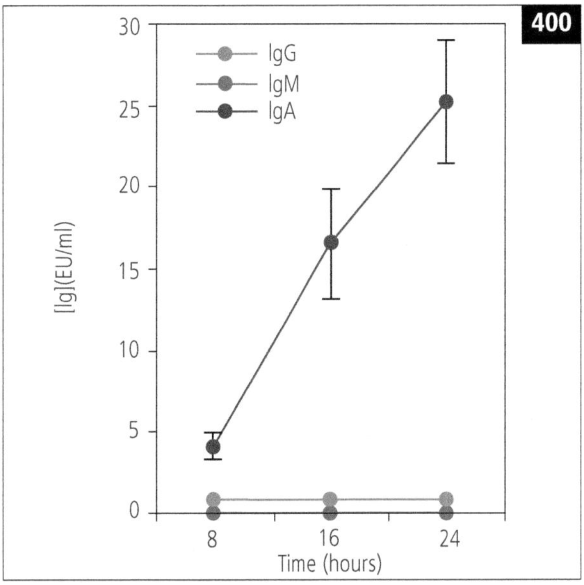

399, 400 Low IgA secretion by GSD duodenal explants. (**399**) These endoscopic pinch biopsies of duodenal mucosa can be cultured for up to 72 hours and the release of protein into the culture supernatant measured over the same period. (**400**) In normal (non-GSD) dog explants, there is clear release of IgA over the first 24 hours of culture. When duodenal explants from GSDs are compared with those obtained from dogs of other breeds, there is significantly reduced secretion of IgA into the culture fluid surrounding the GSD explants. (Data from German AJ, Hall EJ, Day MJ [2000] Relative deficiency in IgA production by duodenal explants from German Shepherd Dogs with small intestinal disease. *Veterinary Immunology and Immunopathology* **76:**25–43.)

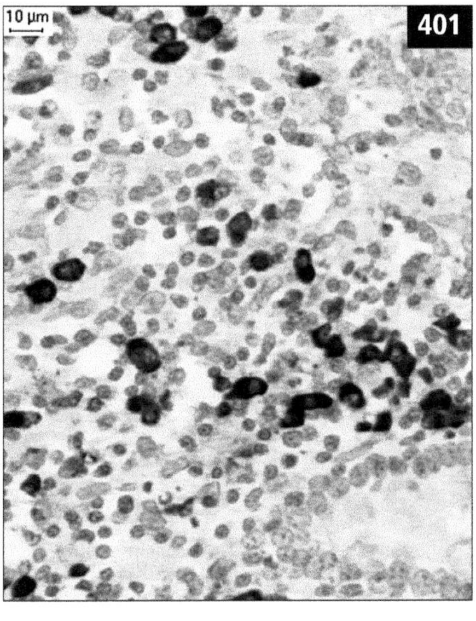

401 Normal lamina propria IgA plasma cells in a GSD. An endoscopic biopsy of duodenal mucosa from a GSD labelled to show IgA plasma cells by immunohistochemistry. The number of these cells is normal, although a matched biopsy from this dog failed to secrete normal quantities of IgA into culture supernatant when incubated in the explant culture system.

the regulation of IgA synthesis (e.g. TGFβ) within the intestinal mucosa of GSDs. As IgA is a key candidate for intestinal immunodeficiency in this breed, this aspect of the GSD immune system continues to be investigated. The recent observation of homogeneity in IgA allotypic variant usage in this breed (see Chapter 1, p. 15) may suggest that GSDs selectively express a particular functional subtype of IgA that may underlie their susceptibility to mucosal disease. Genetic analysis has shown association between GSD enteropathy and SNPs in genes encoding TLR-4 and -5, but these studies do not separate dogs with ARD from other chronic enteropathies.

The spectrum of histological appearance in ARD ranges from normal (in most cases) to mild villus atrophy with lymphoplasmacytic infiltration of the lamina propria and increased IELs. Immunohistochemical evaluation has defined elevated numbers of IgA plasma cells and $CD4^+$ T cells in the lamina propria of duodenal biopsies from dogs with ARD. The latter appearance suggests overlap with the IBDs described below, and ARD could either be a consequence or a cause of enteric inflammation. In human IBD, and in induced experimental models of intestinal inflammation, there is failure of tolerance to intestinal microflora as blood lymphocytes respond vigorously to *in vitro* stimulation with antigenic extracts of autologous intestinal flora, whereas lymphocytes from normal individuals respond only to heterologous, not autologous, flora.

Despite the absence of histological change in many cases, there may be alterations in enterocyte number or function, resulting in malabsorption. Ultrastructural lesions of the brush border have been observed and lipid may accumulate within the cytoplasm of enterocytes. In aerobic overgrowth there may be reduction in brush border alkaline phosphatase activity.

Diagnosis

The diagnosis of ARD may involve:

- Bacteriological culture (or molecular analysis) of small intestinal fluid, usually obtained by endoscopy.
- Histopathological examination of endoscopic biopsies of small intestine.
- Assay of serum trypsin-like immunoreactivity (TLI) to rule out EPI.
- Identification of reduced serum vitamin B_{12} (due to reduced absorption following bacterial binding of B_{12}) and elevated serum folate (due to synthesis by bacteria and jejunal absorption). However, although this pattern of changes has good specificity for detecting increased duodenal bacterial numbers, it has poor sensitivity (5%) and does not correlate with the response to antibiotics. Therefore, measurement of serum folate and B_{12} cannot be used to diagnose this condition.
- Similarly, measurement of serum total unconjugated bile acids (TUBA) (elevated in serum due to deconjugation of secreted bile acid by bacteria within the intestinal lumen and absorption of the bile acid) has not been proven to have diagnostic utility in this disorder.
- Analysis of breath excretion of metabolites (e.g. hydrogen) produced by the bacteria following fermentation of a fed carbohydrate source.

Treatment and prognosis

If ARD is secondary to an underlying cause, treatment is directed towards this problem and adjunctive antibiotic therapy is used. However, treatment of idiopathic ARD primarily involves the use of broad-spectrum antibiotics. In the UK, oxytetracycline (10–20 mg/kg p/o q8h) is the antibiotic of first choice because of its spectrum of activity, relatively low cost and apparent efficacy. Suggested alternatives are tylosin (10 mg/kg p/o q8h) or amoxicillin (10 mg/kg p/o q8–12h). Metronidazole (10–20 mg/kg p/o q8–12h) can also be effective, but whether this is due to the antibacterial or immunomodulatory effects of the drug is unknown.

As an adjunct to antibiotics, feeding a highly digestible, reduced fat diet can decrease production of diarrhoeogenic bacterial metabolites such as deconjugated bile salts and hydroxy fatty acids. If cobalamin malabsorption is severe, parenteral supplementation (250–500 µg s/c once weekly until serum concentrations normalize) is indicated. Initially, antibiotics are given for a 4–6 week period, although failure to produce any improvement within two weeks necessitates re-evaluation of the diagnosis and a possible change of antibiotics. Relapse may occur on cessation of antibiotics and, in the absence of any underlying cause, is an indication for continued antibiotics. Some animals may require lifelong treatment, although an empirically reduced dose of antibiotics may control clinical signs. In other cases there is improvement with age. Thus the prognosis for cure is guarded, but good control is generally possible.

IDIOPATHIC INFLAMMATORY BOWEL DISEASE

IBD is a poorly defined syndrome of the dog and cat and includes a group of chronic intestinal disorders characterized by inflammatory infiltration of the lamina propria in the absence of a primary cause (e.g. infection, neoplasia). IBD has been subdivided into a number of clinical or histopathological entities (*Table 16*, p. 204), which form a spectrum of disease that most likely overlaps with dietary hypersensitivity and ARD. The aetiopathogenesis of IBD is likely to be multifactorial and involve genetic background, altered intestinal immunoregulation, enhanced intestinal permeability and exposure to specific microbial or dietary antigens. Distinct differences in the duodenal mucosa-adherent microbiota are found in dogs with IBD compared with normal dogs by molecular analysis of the microbiome.

The clinical presentation of IBD involves chronic vomiting, diarrhoea, weight loss and anorexia, and the general diagnostic approach to such cases is summarized in **402**. Other diagnostic correlates have been recently evaluated. For example, assessment of intestinal permeability was examined by intragastric administration of lactulose, rhamnose, xylose, 3-0-methylglucose and sucrose with collection of a six-hour urine sample for determination of various sugar ratios. Such measures did not, however, correlate with clinical or histopathological severity

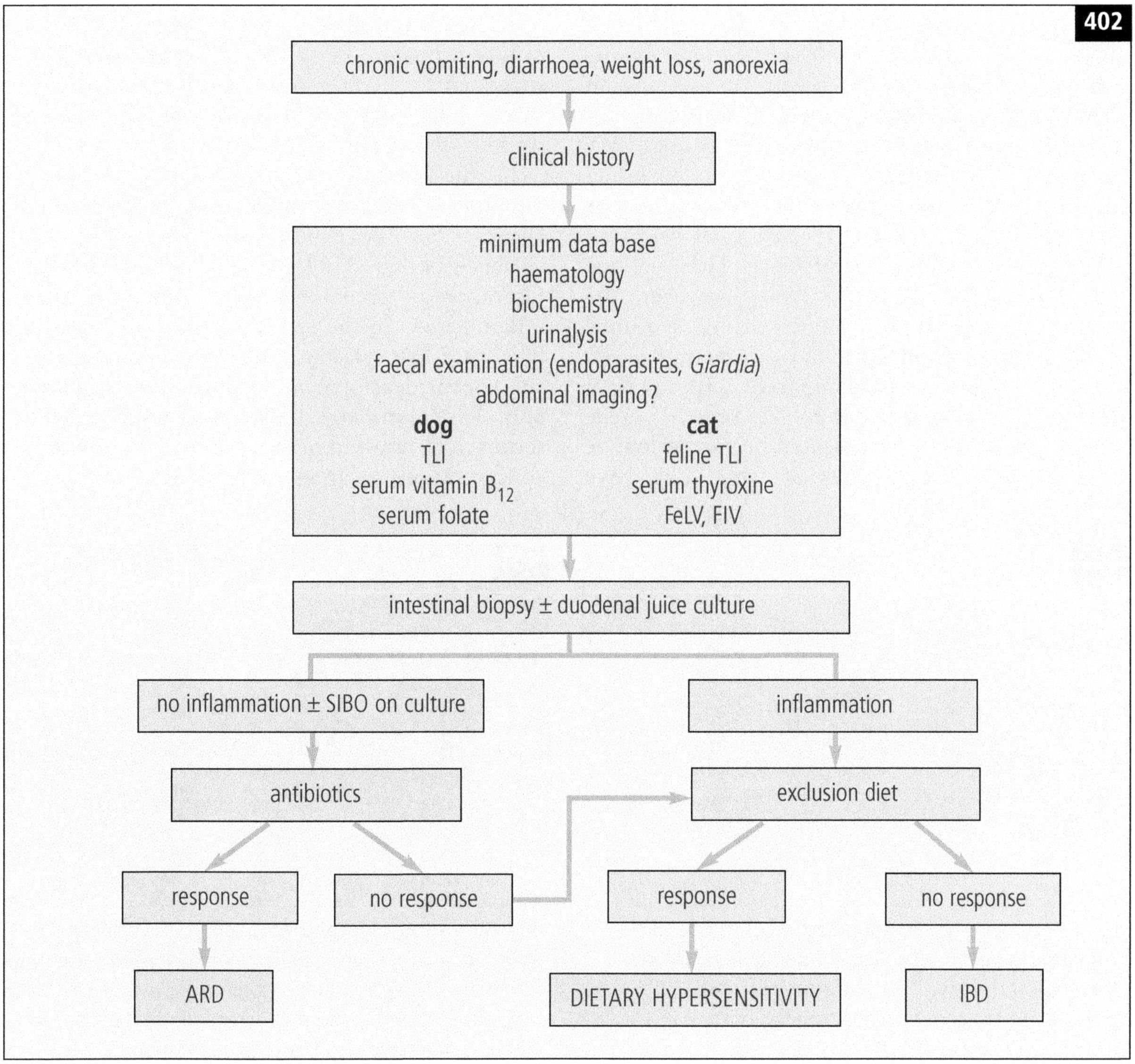

402 Diagnostic flow chart for inflammatory bowel disease.

of disease. In contrast, elevation of serum-derived faecal α_1-proteinase inhibitor (α_1-PI) correlates well with the presence of a protein-losing enteropathy, of which IBD is the most common cause. Although a non-specific marker of inflammation, dogs with IBD also show elevation of serum C-reactive protein. Similarly, one study has shown that the presence of serum perinuclear anti-neutrophil cytoplasmic antibodies (pANCA) and antibodies specific for the yeast *Saccharomyces cerevisiae* may be useful markers for the presence of intestinal inflammatory disease. Clinical scoring indices for the severity of both canine and feline inflammatory bowel disease have been developed.

LYMPHOPLASMACYTIC ENTERITIS

Pathogenesis and clinical signs

No specific aetiology for lymphoplasmacytic enteritis (LPE) has been identified, but an immune-mediated pathogenesis has been proposed and an inappropriate response to microbial and/or dietary antigens may be involved. Molecular studies have examined the expression of genes encoding numerous cytokines in intestinal biopsies from dogs and cats with IBD. Using conventional gel-based RT-PCR, early studies suggested a Th1 cytokine bias in affected mucosal tissue; however, the subsequent application of more sensitive real-time RT-PCR methodology failed to confirm any specific cytokine profile bias compared with normal intestine. Increased TLR-2, -4 and -9 gene expression has been documented by this technique in dogs with LPE. Studies of feline LPE have suggested elevation in mRNA expression for proinflammatory and Th1 cytokines (IL-1, IL-6, IL-8, IL-12, IL-18 and TNFα) in addition to immunoregulatory cytokines (IL-10, TGFβ). The number and composition of mucosa-associated bacteria alters in cats with IBD, with numbers of Enterobacteriaceae, *E. coli* and *Clostridium* spp. correlating with mucosal architectural changes and cytokine gene expression. In both the cat and the dog, LPE has been observed to precede the onset of, or be present adjacent to, alimentary lymphoma (403, 404). It is often very difficult to distinguish histopathologically between severe LPE and emergent lymphoma, particularly in the cat. The application of immunohistochemistry or molecular testing for clonality (see Chapter 13, p. 324) can help distinguish between these possibilities.

There is no well-defined breed predisposition for canine primary LPE, although some studies have suggested that GSDs and Labrador Retrievers are susceptible (405–407). There are some breed-specific variants of LPE.

In the Basenji, an hereditary syndrome of 'immunoproliferative enteritis' is characterized by chronic diarrhoea and wasting, sometimes with chronic gastritis; skin lesions including necrosis and ulceration of pinnal margins; lymphoplasmacytic inflammation of the small intestine, with elevated IgA and IgG plasma cells; hypoalbuminaemia; subsequent development of alimentary lymphoma; and hypergammaglobulinaemia with elevated serum concentration of IgA, but no elevation of IgA concentration within intestinal fluid.

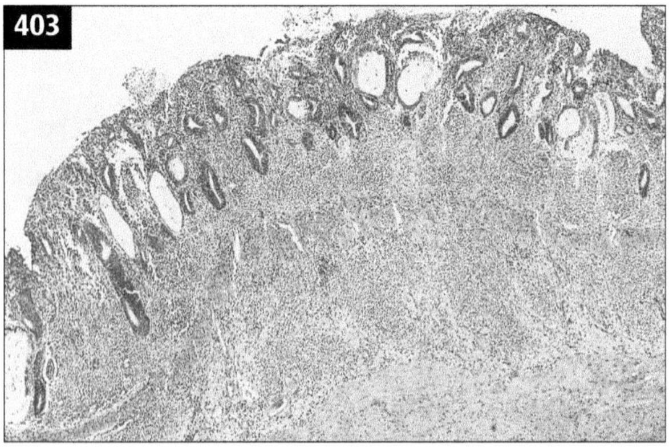

403 Alimentary lymphoma. Section of duodenum from a ten-year-old Jack Russell Terrier with vomiting, diarrhoea and weight loss. On gross necropsy examination there was no abnormality, but there was microscopic evidence of diffuse infiltration of alimentary lymphoma throughout the duodenum and jejunum.

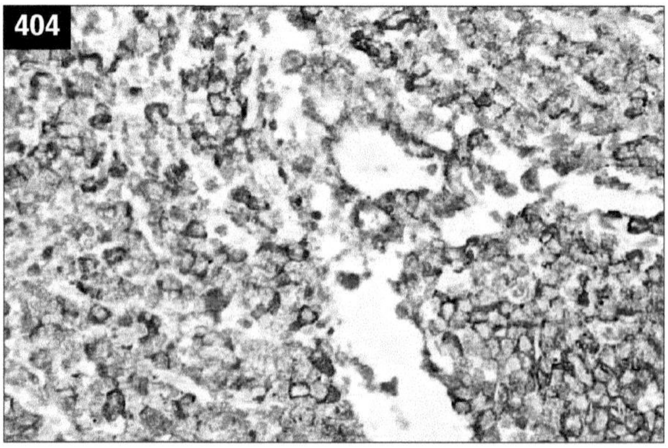

404 Alimentary lymphoma. Section of small intestine from a cat with alimentary lymphoma labelled for CD79a expression. There is a monomorphic population of small B lymphocytes infiltrating the lamina propria consistent with B cell neoplasia rather than inflammation.

Similarly, the Norwegian Lundehund is predisposed to a diarrhoeal syndrome, which again likely overlaps with LPE. A recent study has more fully evaluated the biochemical changes in the enteropathy of this breed, which include elevation in faecal α_1-PI, elevated serum folate and reduced vitamin B_{12}.

In the cat, LPE is characterized by weight loss, vomiting, diarrhoea and anorexia (**408**) and may be associated with chronic pancreatitis and

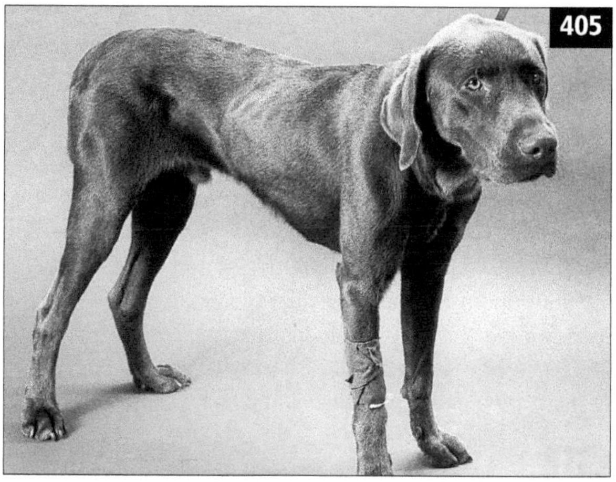

405 Canine lymphoplasmacytic enteritis. An 18-month-old chocolate Labrador Retriever with LPE showing evidence of severe weight loss associated with chronic malabsorption.

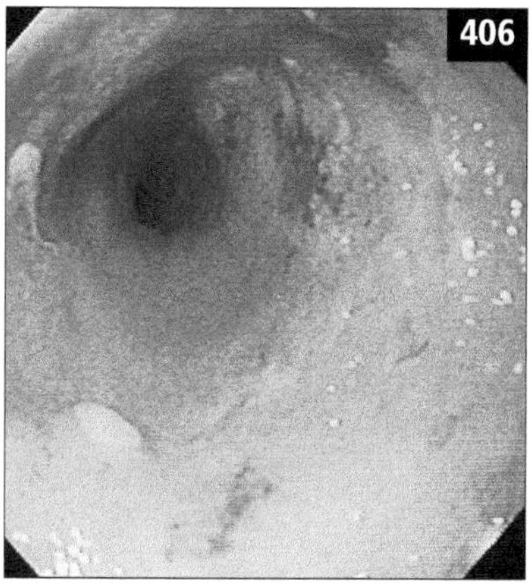

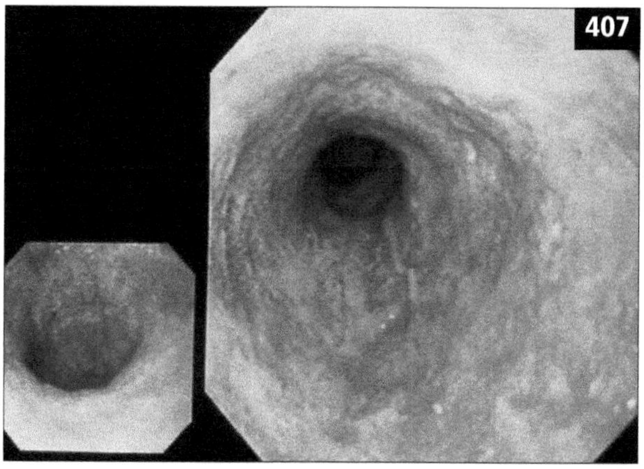

406, 407 Endoscopic appearance of the duodenum in lymphoplasmacytic enteritis. (**406**) A six-year-old Golden Retriever with chronic diarrhoea and weight loss. The mucosa appears rough and irregular and it was very friable when biopsied. Areas of haemorrhage where the endoscope has abraded the mucosa are noted. The duodenal papilla is visible in the foreground. The signs were successfully controlled with prednisolone. (**407**) An eight-year-old Springer Spaniel with a protein-losing enteropathy and consequent hypoproteinaemia and ascites. Mucosal irregularity and friability is marked, and treatment with both prednisolone and azathioprine was required to control signs.

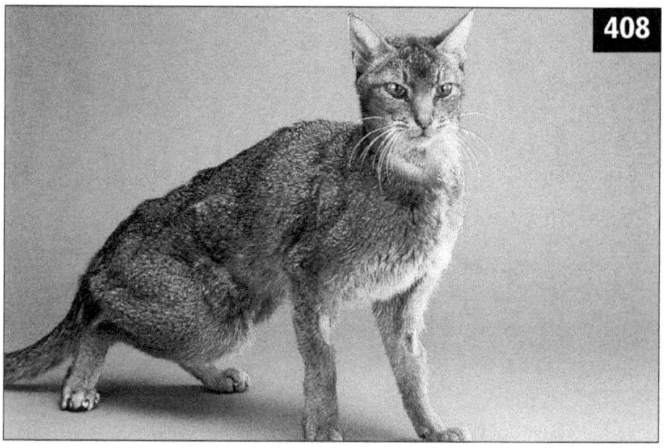

408 Feline lymphoplasmacytic enteritis. An adult Abyssinian cat with LPE showing signs of chronic vomiting, diarrhoea and weight loss. (Photograph courtesy A.H. Sparkes.)

409

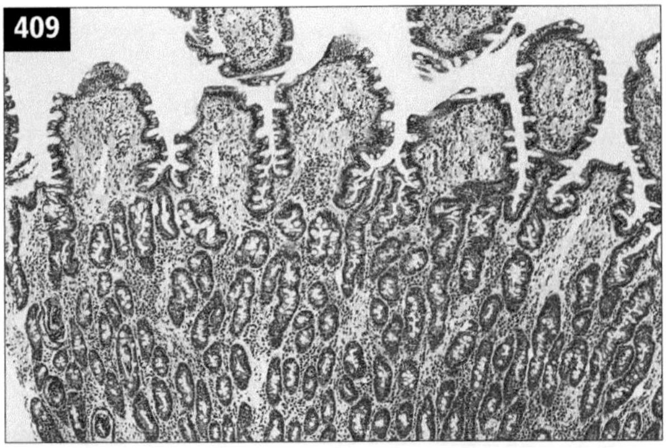

410

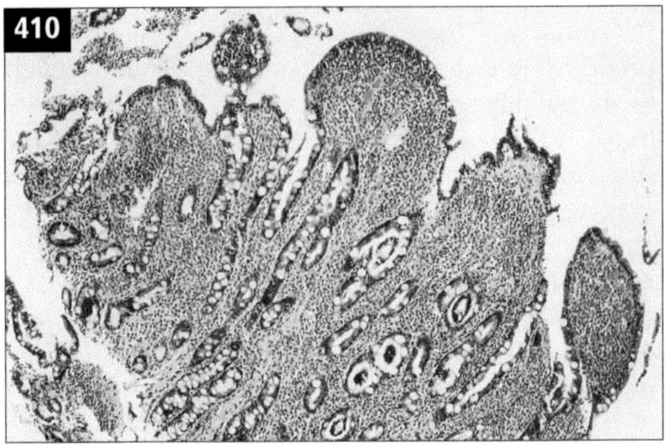

409, 410 Canine lymphoplasmacytic enteritis. (**409**) Endoscopic biopsy of duodenum from a five-year-old Miniature Dachshund with gross inflammation of the intestinal mucosa on endoscopy. There is evidence of villus atrophy and prominent infiltration of lymphocytes and plasma cells into the lamina propria between crypts. (**410**) Endoscopic biopsy of duodenum from a seven-year-old Golden Retriever with chronic diarrhoea, anorexia, weight loss and hypoproteinaemia. The duodenum was thickened and irregular on endoscopic examination. There is microscopic evidence of villus atrophy, with attenuation and inflammation of mucosal epithelium and an intense infiltration of the villus lamina by lymphocytes and plasma cells.

411

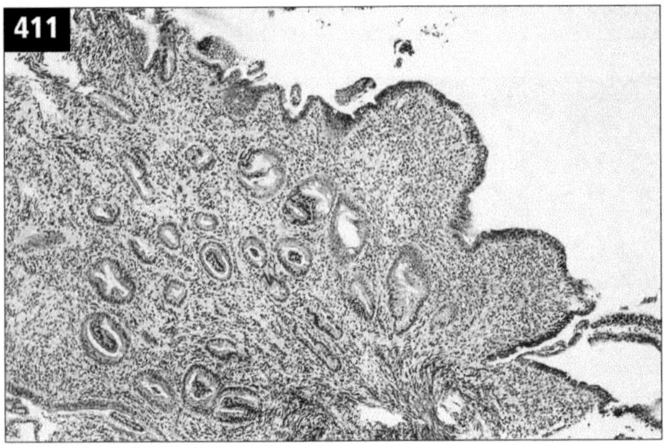

411 Feline lymphoplasmacytic enteritis. Endoscopic biopsy from a ten-month-old Bengal kitten with chronic diarrhoea and poor growth since birth. There is marked villus atrophy and intense lymphoplasmacytic infiltration of the lamina propria.

cholangiohepatitis ('triaditis'). There are no breed predispositions and older cats may be more frequently affected.

Diagnosis

LPE is characterized histopathologically by combinations of the following morphological changes:

- Villus atrophy and fusion.
- Epithelial attenuation, necrosis or ulceration.
- Crypt hypertrophy to dilatation, with crypt abscesses (although these latter may occur in normal mucosa).
- Lamina propria fibrosis.

Although LPE would also classically be defined by an infiltration of lymphocytes and plasma cells (with neutrophils, eosinophils and macrophages) into the villus lamina propria, between the crypts and occasionally into the submucosa (**409–411**), there is growing consensus that such infiltration is of less significance than the structural abnormalities defined above. The WSAVA Gastrointestinal Standardization Group has recently defined a standard for the histological assessment of such lesions. Although it may be difficult clearly to define infiltration by subjective assessment of haematoxylin and eosin stained sections, quantitative immunohistochemical studies have shown significant differences in subpopulations of lymphoid cells within the mucosa. Specifically, dogs with IBD have elevated numbers of lamina propria $CD3^+$ and $CD4^+$ T cells, IgG plasma cells, macrophages and neutrophils. Additionally, there are increased numbers of $CD3^+$ intraepithelial T lymphocytes in such patients (**412**). There is reduced apoptosis (caspase 3 expression) of lymphocytes within the

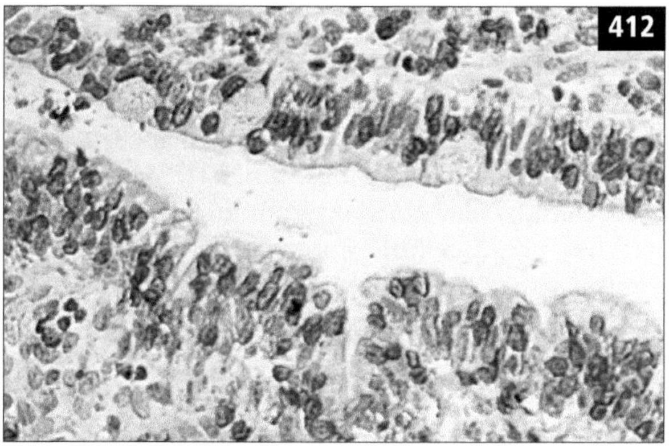

412 Canine lymphoplasmacytic enteritis. Section of small intestine from a dog with LPE immunolabelled to show the distribution of $CD3^+$ T lymphocytes. There are many more intraepithelial cells present than in normal canine intestine. (From German AJ, Hall EJ, Day MJ [2001] Characterization of immune cell populations within the duodenal mucosa of dogs with enteropathies. *Journal of Veterinary Internal Medicine* **15:**14–25, with permission.)

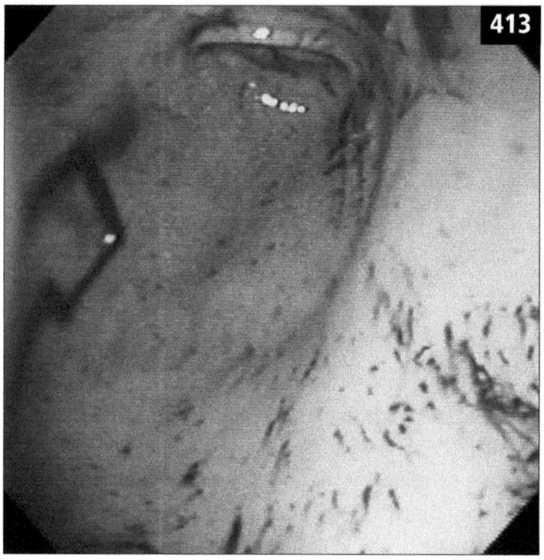

413 Eosinophilic enteritis. Endoscopic view of the fundus of the stomach from a six-year-old male Boxer with eosinophilic gastroenteritis that displayed intermittent haematemesis and diarrhoea. Numerous haemorrhagic linear erosions are present in the gastric mucosa of the antrum.

villi of dogs with IBD. In contrast, in feline LPE there are no significant elevations in the number of various leukocyte subsets, but MHC class II expression by enterocytes is induced (whereas it is constitutive in the dog and does not significantly elevate in LPE).

Treatment and prognosis

LPE may be associated with intestinal conditions such as giardiasis or dietary hypersensitivity, which should be treated. Antibiotics may be indicated if the inflammatory infiltrate represents a response to luminal bacteria, and metronidazole (10–20 mg/kg p/o q8–12h) may be effective because of its dual action. Idiopathic IBD is treated with immunosuppressive drugs. A hypoallergenic or hydrolysed protein diet may also be helpful in case management. The feeding of a 'sacrificial protein' during the initial phase of severe mucosal inflammation has been proposed as a means of preventing development of hypersensitivity to the staple diet, but the value of this approach remains unproven. The use of diets containing prebiotics or probiotics, or altered n3:n6 fatty acid ratios, may be considered a logical adjunct to management of immune abnormalities in LPE, although no controlled trials of their efficacy in this context have been published.

Prednisolone is the immunosuppressive drug of first choice and is given initially at a dose of 2–4 mg/kg p/o divided daily. After 2–3 weeks of treatment and clinical improvement, the dose is tapered (over a 3–6 month period) until either the minimum dose necessary to control signs is reached or the patient remains in remission without treatment. The chances of control are high, but complete remission is uncommon. Failure to respond to prednisolone or the development of side-effects necessitates use of more potent, steroid-sparing immunosuppressives; for example, azathioprine (in dogs 1–2 mg/kg p/o q24h initially, reducing to every other day; in cats 0.3 mg/kg p/o q24h maximum). Locally active steroids such as budesonide, beclomethasone and fluticasone are currently being evaluated as alternative therapies. The efficacy of ciclosporin (5 mg/kg p/o q24h) as an immunosuppressive agent has been evaluated in canine IBD, but the clinical response to this drug has been equivocal.

EOSINOPHILIC GASTROENTERITIS

Eosinophilic gastroenteritis may affect any breed of dog and is characterized by chronic vomiting, diarrhoea (small and/or large bowel) and weight loss (413). Haematemesis, melaena and haematochezia are often noted. The inflammatory infiltrate is dominated by eosinophils (**414–416**) and circulating eosinophilia is sometimes present. The pathology may be focal or diffuse, involving all levels of the gastrointestinal tract from stomach to rectum. The infiltration of eosinophils is generally accompanied by lymphocytes and plasma cells and may extend from the mucosa through to the serosa. There may be villus atrophy or mucosal ulceration. Endoparasite antigens have been proposed as a cause of stimulation of the intestinal immune system. Canine eosinophilic colitis is defined as a distinct entity, but likely overlaps with both eosinophilic gastroenteritis and lymphoplasmacytic colitis (LPC).

Eosinophilic enteritis is rare in the cat. It may be a primary disease or a manifestation of **feline hypereosinophilic syndrome**, characterized by circulating eosinophilia, eosinophil hyperplasia within bone marrow, and eosinophilic infiltration of skin, myocardium, liver, spleen, intestine, mesenteric lymph nodes and kidney. The clinical presentation of such cats may include vomiting, diarrhoea, anorexia and weight loss. A similar idiopathic hypereosinophilic syndrome has been documented in Rottweiler dogs, where it is associated with marked elevation in serum IgE concentration.

The presence of an eosinophilic mucosal infiltrate may reflect a parasitic problem or dietary hypersensitivity, so treatment with fenbendazole and an exclusion diet are indicated. In the absence of response to either procedure, immunosuppressive treatment as for LPE may be used, although the response to treatment tends to be slightly poorer.

GRANULOMATOUS ENTERITIS

Granulomatous enteritis occurs in the dog and cat as focal inflammation of the terminal ileum, colon and associated mesenteric lymph nodes. The infiltration is generally transmural, with villus

414

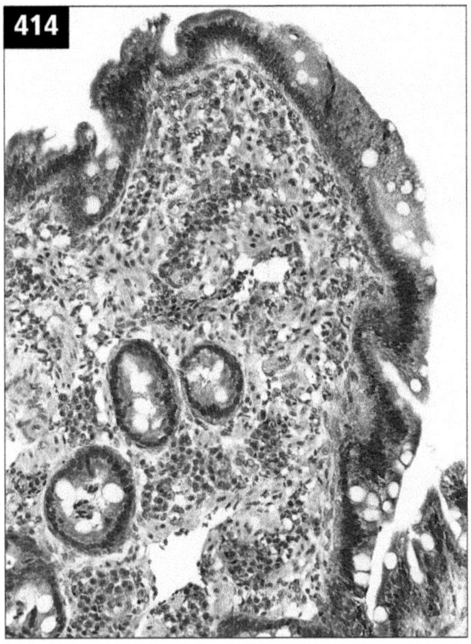

415

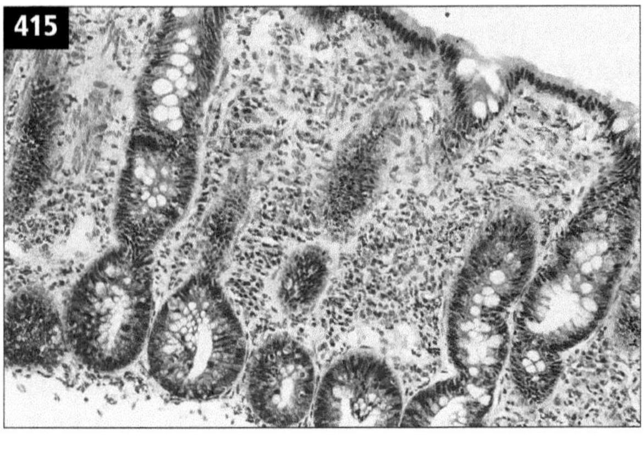

416

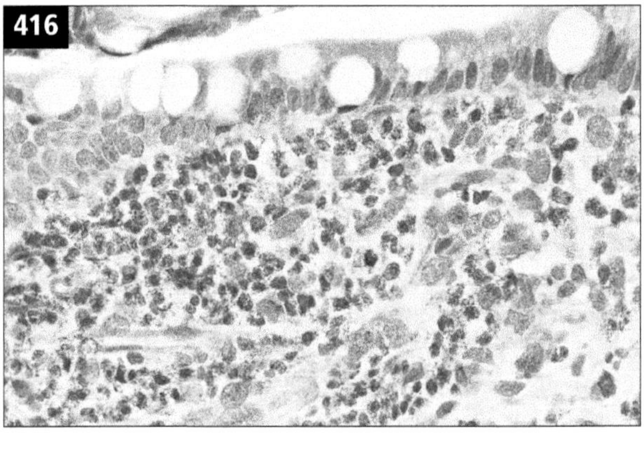

414–416 Eosinophilic enteritis. Endoscopic biopsies from a two-year-old English Setter with chronic intermittent vomiting and diarrhoea and fresh blood in the faeces. There is an inflammatory infiltration of duodenum (**414**) and colon (**415**) that is dominated by eosinophils, with numerous lymphocytes and plasma cells. (**416**) Sirius red staining highlights the eosinophil infiltration of duodenum.

atrophy, crypt hypertrophy or mucosal ulceration; diffuse or focal infiltration of macrophages, with fewer giant cells, neutrophils, eosinophils, lymphocytes and plasma cells (**417**); areas of necrosis and fibrosis; and reactive hyperplasia of mesenteric lymph nodes, with granulomatous foci and sinus histiocytosis.

The disease is idiopathic and microorganisms (e.g. *Mycobacterium*) are rarely identified. In the cat, primary granulomatous enteritis must be distinguished from the predominantly serosal lesions caused by FIP virus. Empirical treatment with glucocorticoids and other immunosuppressive agents has been recommended, but so few cases have been reported that the efficacy of treatment has not been evaluated. Generally, the prognosis is considered poor.

LYMPHOPLASMACYTIC COLITIS

LPC is an idiopathic disease that is uncommon in the dog and rare in the cat; it is most often part of LPE. Clinical features include diarrhoea and tenesmus, with blood and mucus in the faeces. The lymphoplasmacytic nature of the lesions may only be apparent during chronic disease, and during the acute stages there may be a dominance of neutrophils (**418**). There may be attenuation of mucosal epithelium with reduced goblet cells, in addition to glandular hyperplasia and dilation that may lead to the formation of crypt abscesses. Dogs with LPC have a greater proportion of IgA plasma cells in the colonic mucosa than normal dogs, and there is overexpression of mRNA encoding IL-2 and TNFα as measured by conventional RT-PCR. LPC occurs commonly in the GSD and it has recently been suggested that there is an association between colitis and anal furunculosis in this breed.

LPC may be treated with the same range of antibiotics (oxytetracycline, metronidazole, tylosin) and immunosuppressive agents (prednisolone, azathioprine) used for ARD and LPE. In addition, locally active 5-aminosalicylate derivatives can be used as anti-inflammatory agents, although their safety margin in cats is low. Novel delivery systems of 5-ASA (mesalazine) to the colon have been devised to avoid small intestinal absorption and consequent renal toxicity, but they have only been tested in humans. Administration per rectum is the most direct method, but this is not practical in dogs and cats; delayed-release oral preparations are available (e.g. PentASA) but may not be safe. Conjugation of 5-ASA to a sulphonamide residue in sulphasalazine (Salazopyrin, 15–30 mg/kg p/o

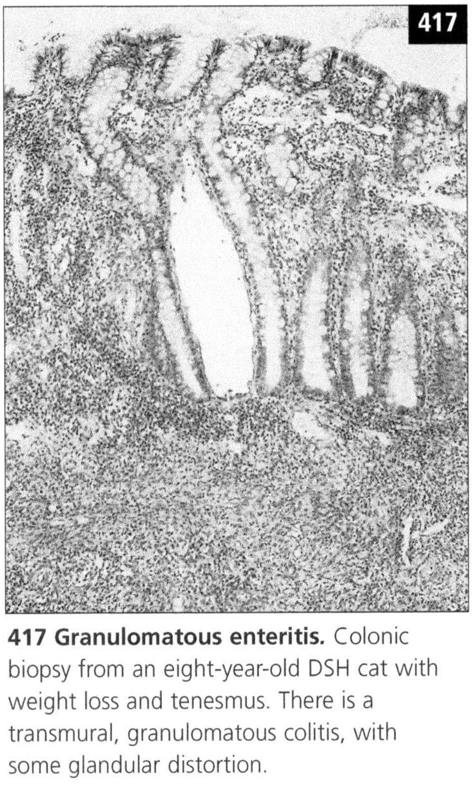

417 Granulomatous enteritis. Colonic biopsy from an eight-year-old DSH cat with weight loss and tenesmus. There is a transmural, granulomatous colitis, with some glandular distortion.

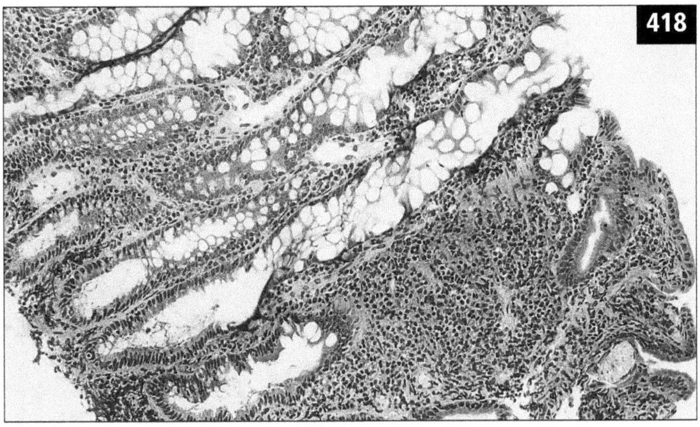

418 Lymphoplasmacytic colitis. Colon biopsy from a ten-year-old DSH cat with a two-year history of diarrhoea and weight loss. The loss of mucosal epithelium is likely an artefact of processing, but there is glandular hyperplasia with an intense lymphoplasmacytic infiltration into the lamina propria.

q12h) enables passage through the small intestine and colonic release of 5-ASA by bacterial cleavage of the diazo bond. Similar cleavage of two 5-ASA residues conjugated together in olsalazine (Dipentum, 10–20 mg/kg p/o q12h) reduces the incidence of the side-effect KCS seen with Salazopyrin. Approximately 70% of cases of LPC are reported to respond to treatment and not to relapse. Simultaneous feeding of an exclusion diet has been shown to reduce drug requirement and relapse rates in dogs and cats with LPC.

HISTIOCYTIC ULCERATIVE COLITIS

Histiocytic ulcerative colitis (HUC) is recognized chiefly in young (less than two year old) Boxers (and rarely in the French Bulldog) that present with weight loss and large bowel diarrhoea with blood and mucus. There is a severe, transmural and ulcerative colitis characterized histologically by a macrophage-dominated infiltration that may also involve colonic lymph nodes. The precise aetiology was, until recently, unknown. The observation of large cytoplasmic vacuoles in many macrophages, containing material stained by periodic acid-Schiff (**419, 420**), led to the proposal that there might be defective lysosomal function in these cells, allowing accumulation of partly digested phospholipid membranes within the cytoplasmic compartments. Although traditional methodology did not reveal a microbial aetiology for HUC, recent molecular studies have suggested a microbial causation, and attaching and invading *E. coli* (AIEC) have been identified within the mucosal inflammatory lesions by fluorescent *in situ* hybridization. Immunohistochemical evaluation of the lesions of HUC reveals an elevation in lamina propria IgG$^+$ plasma cells, CD3$^+$ T cells and cells expressing the myelomonocytic antigen L1. There is strong MHC class II expression by the infiltrating inflammatory population and the overlying enterocytes (**421**). A similar

419
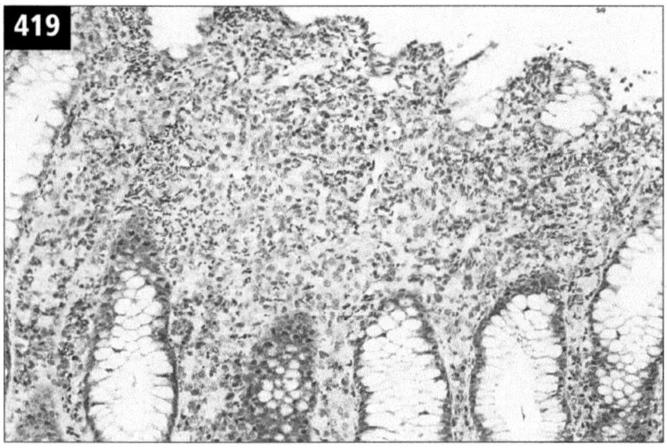

420
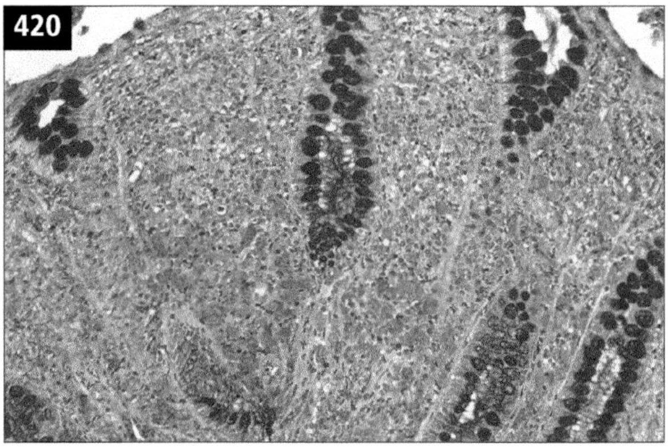

421
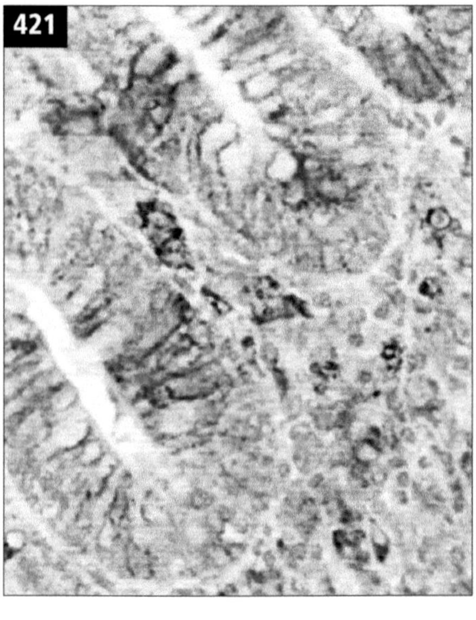

419–421 Histiocytic ulcerative colitis. (**419**) Colon biopsy from a three-year-old female Boxer with chronic intermittent diarrhoea, haematochezia and weight loss. The mucosa was thickened and friable on endoscopic examination. There is marked infiltration of the lamina propria by a mixed population dominated by macrophages, with evidence of glandular distortion. (**420**) PAS-stained section demonstrates diffuse cytoplasmic staining of the infiltrating macrophages. (**421**) Section of colon from a Boxer with HUC showing strong expression of MHC class II by cells infiltrating the lamina propria and the overlying epithelium. (From German AJ, Hall EJ, Kelly DF *et al.* [2000] An immunohistochemical study of histiocytic ulcerative colitis in Boxer dogs. *Journal of Comparative Pathology* **122:**163–175, with permission.)

pathology has been recognized in the cat, but this is rare and may be associated with FIP infection.

Traditionally, HUC has been considered an untreatable condition with a grave clinical prognosis. Previous studies have reported that diarrhoea may improve with antibiotic treatment of the secondary bacterial invasion of ulcerated mucosa, but that there is no histological improvement. However, more recent case series have shown both clinical and histological response to antimicrobial therapy with enrofloxacin.

CANINE ANAL FURUNCULOSIS

Anal furunculosis is a chronic debilitating disorder of the dog involving perianal ulceration, inflammation and sinus tract formation (**422, 423**). The majority of reported cases have occurred in GSDs that may have concurrent deep pyoderma or intestinal disease. A genetic association has recently been shown for affected GSDs (see Chapter 3, p. 92). This combination of diseases in a breed known to have defective mucosal immunity (see Chapter 12, p. 302) has led to the proposal that anal furunculosis is an immune-mediated condition, and recent reports have demonstrated amelioration of lesions following a variety of immunosuppressive regimes. These include treatment with glucocorticoids (prednisolone 2 mg/kg daily for 2 weeks, then 1 mg/kg daily for 4 weeks, then 1 mg/kg on alternate days) or ciclosporin (7.5–10 mg/kg q12h for 1 week, then 5–7.5 mg/kg q12h continued for 8–20 weeks). Ciclosporin has also been used to effect at lower doses in conjunction with concurrent ketoconazole administration (2–4 mg/kg ciclosporin q24h plus 8–10 mg/kg ketoconazole q24h given for up to 16 weeks) (see Chapter 16, p. 394). In many dogs there is a dramatic and rapid response to ciclosporin therapy and lesions reduce to a size where they are much more amenable to surgical excision. Reliance on ciclosporin therapy alone, however, may lead to recurrence of the lesions in time. Topical application of 0.1% tacrolimus ointment as sole treatment, or in

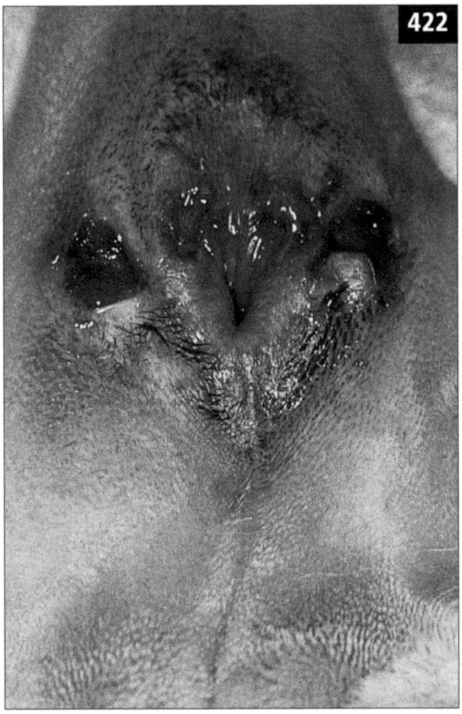

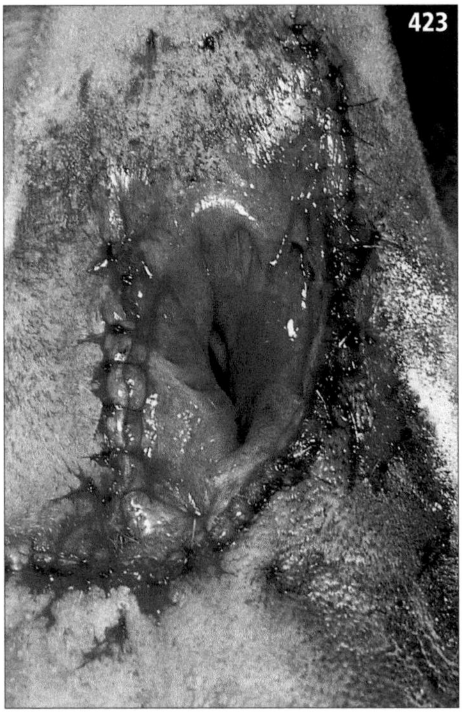

422, 423 Canine anal furunculosis. (**422**) The lesions of anal furunculosis include extensive perianal ulceration and the formation of deep sinus tracts. (**423**) One form of treatment is wide surgical excision of affected tissue and anal sacs, with local reconstruction. (Photographs courtesy B.M.Q. Weaver.)

424

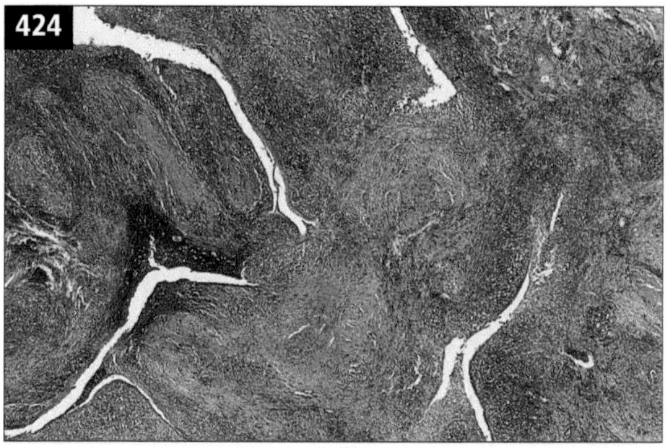

425

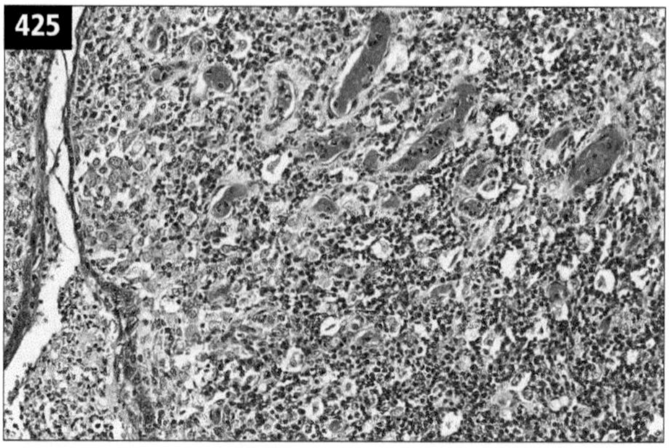

426

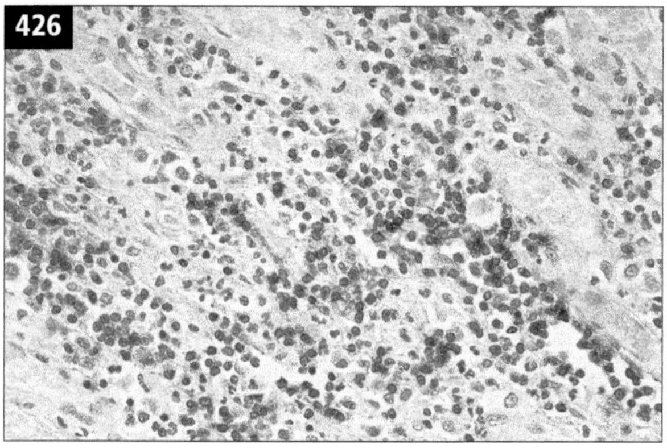

427

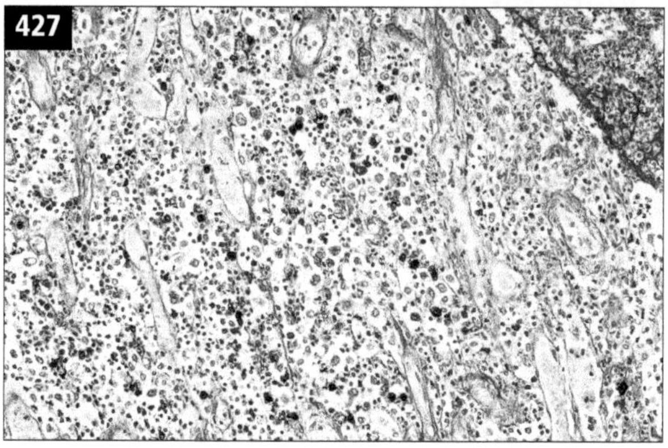

424–427 Canine anal furunculosis. (**424**) Biopsy of perianal tissue from a dog with anal furunculosis. At low power magnification, multiple branching sinus tracts are seen to run through the tissue. There is extensive deposition of granulation tissue between the tracts and intense inflammatory infiltration at the margins of each tract. (**425**) High power magnification of a sinus tract demonstrates that neutrophils and macrophages are associated with the sinus lumen, and that there is an outermost lymphoplasmacytic infiltration. (**426, 427**) Section of tissue from adjacent to a sinus tract demonstrates numerous $CD3^+$ T cells (**426**) and IgA bearing plasma cells (**427**) within the inflammatory infiltrate. (From Day MJ [1993] The immunopathology of anal furunculosis in the dog. *Journal of Small Animal Practice* **34:**381–389, with permission.)

428

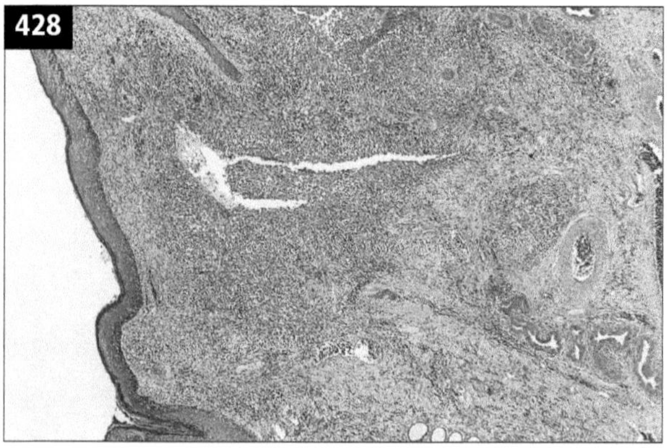

429

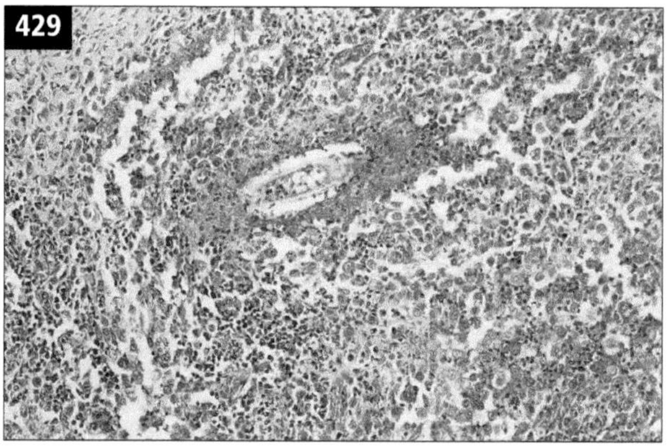

428, 429 Canine anal furunculosis. Low power (**428**) and high power (**429**) views of biopsies of haired perianal skin from dogs with anal furunculosis. In such tissue there is often evidence of folliculitis–furunculosis, which may be a site of initiation of the sinus tracts that characterize the disease. Affected dogs generally have high titred serum antibodies specific for *Staphylococcus intermedius* and these bacteria may be associated with the follicular lesions. Faecal flora may then perpetuate the regional inflammation.

combination with oral prednisolone (tapering from a starting dose of 2mg/kg q24h) and metronidazole (10mg/kg q12h for 2 weeks) and novel protein restriction diet, has also been used. Although such medical therapy has now gained widespread acceptance, it should be noted that when cases are treated by dietary modulation and surgical excision of affected tissue, this also produces an excellent outcome.

The perianal lesions are characterized by infiltration by $CD3^+$ T lymphocytes and plasma cells expressing IgG, IgM and IgA (**424–427**). Affected dogs have normal to elevated serum IgA concentration, elevated serum IgG concentration and high levels of serum antibody specific for *Staphylococcus intermedius*. Expression of cytokine genes and genes encoding PRRs has been examined within lesional tissue biopsies. These studies suggest local activation of Th1 immunity (IL-2 and IFNγ gene expression) and macrophage production of pro-inflammatory cytokines (IL-1, IL-6, TNFα) and matrix metalloproteinases (MMP-9 and MMP-13). Histopathological studies have suggested that staphylococcal folliculitis–furunculosis (**428, 429**) may initiate the perianal disease, and that antigens from staphylococci or faecal flora may drive the lymphoplasmacytic response. There is little evidence to suggest that anal sacculitis underlies anal furunculosis.

IMMUNE-MEDIATED HEPATIC DISEASE

There have been few studies of the hepatic immune system in companion animals. The liver is well-endowed with immune cells distributed throughout the sinusoids and portal areas. The sinusoidal Kupffer cells function as APCs capable of expression of MHC class II and cytokine secretion. Macrophages and dendritic cells are found within the portal triad. A resident population of hepatic T cells is also found within portal areas and the sinusoids and intraepithelial T cells have been described within the feline bile duct epithelium (**430**). Small numbers of B cells and plasma cells may be distributed within the portal areas.

Functional aspects of the canine and feline hepatic immune system can be inferred from studies in other species (**431**). Mesenchymal cells within the space of Disse (Ito cells, stellate cells or hepatic lipocytes) are immunologically active and can secrete a variety of cytokines and chemokines that recruit monocytes and lymphocytes to this site. The liver sinusoidal endothelial cells (LSECs) are arranged with gaps between each cell, are fenestrated, and lack a basement membrane, so there is ready movement of molecules from the sinusoidal blood into the space of Disse. The LSECs can present antigen and express adhesion molecules, which can interact with circulating lymphocytes and dendritic cells, encouraging them

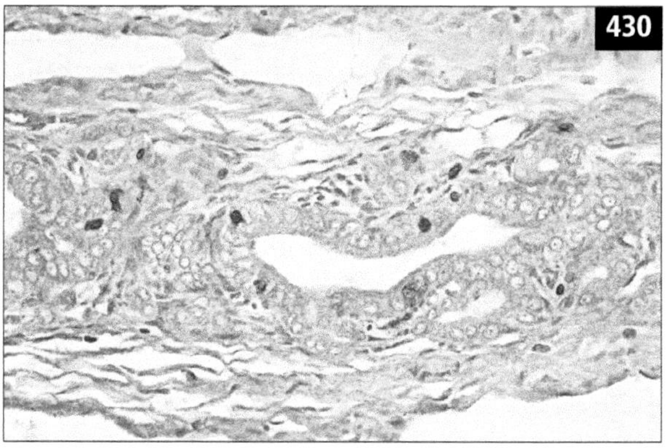

430 Bile duct intraepithelial lymphocytes. Section of portal area from a normal feline liver showing resident $CD3^+$ T lymphocytes within the bile duct epithelium.

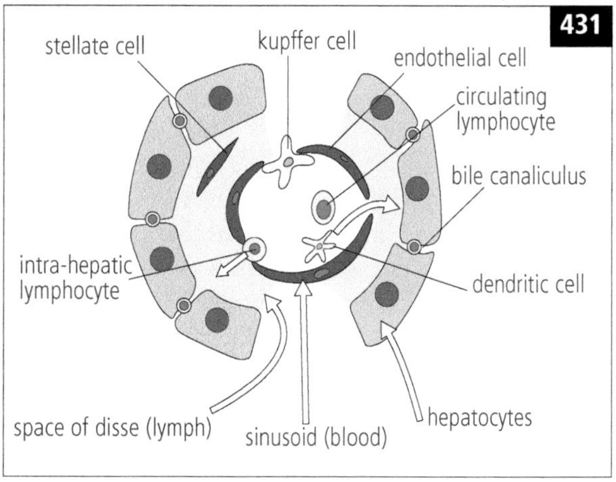

431 Hepatic immune system. A cross-sectional diagram of the major components of the hepatic immune system. A number of key immunological cells (Kupffer cells, lymphocytes and dendritic cells) can migrate from sinusoidal blood into the space of Disse and from there into the portal lymphatic vessels. Recruitment of these populations may be directed by cytokines and chemokines released from mesenchymal cells within the space of Disse (e.g. stellate cells, Ito cells or hepatic lipocytes), and migration is permitted by the fenestrated nature and lack of basement membrane of the liver sinusoidal endothelial cells (LSEC). Immune cell populations are also found within the portal areas. LSEC and bile duct epithelial cells can express MHC class II and thus potentially play a role in local antigen presentation.

to migrate into the space of Disse and from there into the portal lymphatic vessels. Bile duct epithelial cells may also express MHC class II and act as APCs akin to enterocytes (**432**). Bile is IgA-rich in both dogs and cats, but the pathway of IgA secretion into the bile of these species is poorly characterized.

In addition to having the capacity to mount an active immune response, the hepatic immune system is also likely to be able to mediate tolerance (e.g. to food-derived antigens that enter the liver via the portal circulation). The LSECs may present this antigen to hepatic lymphocytes in order to initiate this tolerance response.

CHRONIC HEPATITIS IN THE DOG

Pathogenesis

In man, chronic active hepatitis is a well-defined, primary immune-mediated disease of the liver. It may also occur as part of multisystemic autoimmunity or be secondary to viral infection, drug administration or inborn errors of metabolism. The disease is characterized by the presence of a range of autoantibodies specific for hepatocyte membrane, mitochondrial, cytoplasmic, nuclear and smooth muscle antigens. Histologically there is chronic inflammation of portal tracts, extending through the limiting plate to the periportal parenchyma ('piecemeal necrosis' or 'interface hepatitis') and resulting in the isolation of small groups of hepatocytes and inflammatory cells by fine fibrous septae. T lymphocytes are prominent in the inflammatory infiltrates and are thought to induce hepatocyte apoptosis.

A similar histopathological pattern is recognized in dogs with chronic liver disease. Canine 'chronic hepatitis' (CH) has been defined, although similar hepatic lesions may occur in leptospirosis or adenovirus infection or be related to drug administration (**433**). This type of liver disease is often associated with elevated levels of liver copper, and such copper-associated hepatitis is recognized in a number of breeds including the Dobermann, Bedlington Terrier, West Highland White Terrier, Skye Terrier, Anatolian Shepherd, Dalmatian and Labrador Retriever (**434**). The molecular basis of copper-associated hepatitis has only been defined in the Bedlington Terrier, where there is deletion of exon 2 of the MURR1 (COMMD1) gene involved in the lysosomal storage of copper. Affected Bedlingtons have impairment of biliary copper excretion and progressive lysosomal accumulation

432

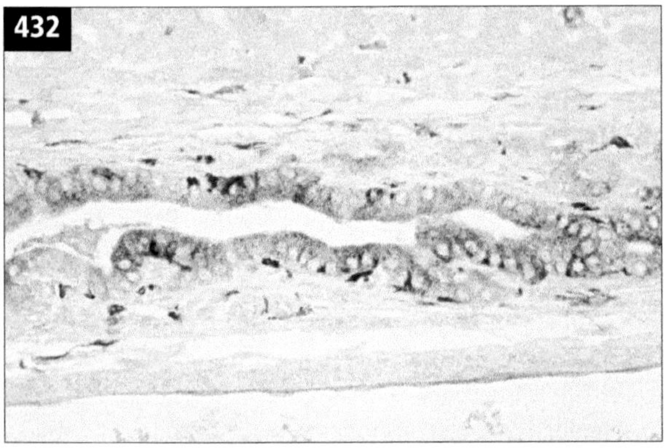

432 Bile duct MHC II expression. Section of portal area from a normal feline liver showing expression of MHC class II by bile duct epithelial cells.

433

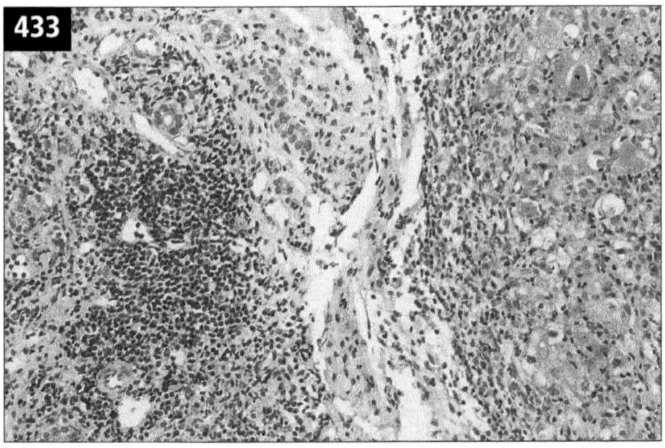

433 Chronic hepatitis. Section of liver from a seven-year-old Labrador Retriever with a two-month history of jaundice and inappetence and reduced hepatic size on ultrasonography. There is extensive portal fibrosis and lymphocytic inflammation, which extends to involve degenerate periportal hepatocytes.

of copper, which becomes apparent histologically from one year of age. MHC associations with the disease in Dobermanns are described in Chapter 3.

Clinical signs

Dogs with CH display a range of clinical signs including depression and weakness, anorexia and weight loss, icterus, polyuria/polydipsia, vomiting and ascites.

Diagnosis

There may be elevated serum alkaline phosphatase and alanine aminotransferase, and hypoalbuminaemia is recorded. Liver biopsy reveals piecemeal necrosis with bile duct proliferation, but there are additional foci of hepatocyte degeneration, inflammation and fibrosis at other levels of the hepatic lobule. Lymphocytes and macrophages dominate the infiltrates, but plasma cells and neutrophils also occur. Although some dogs have serum ANA or antibody to hepatocyte membrane antigens, these are not regarded as being specific disease markers and anti-smooth muscle or anti-mitochondrial antibodies are not found. Peripheral blood mononuclear cell cultures from dogs with chronic hepatitis proliferate in response to liver membrane antigens. Moreover, lesional hepatocytes express membrane and cytoplasmic MHC class II, suggesting that they may be presenting autoantigen to infiltrating T lymphocytes, and class II expression decreases following glucocorticoid therapy. Occasional dogs have had AIHA, hypothyroidism or lymphocytic thyroiditis. Although these findings might suggest that canine CH is a primary autoimmune disease, the observed changes may also reflect immune-mediated liver damage secondary to an unidentified underlying aetiology.

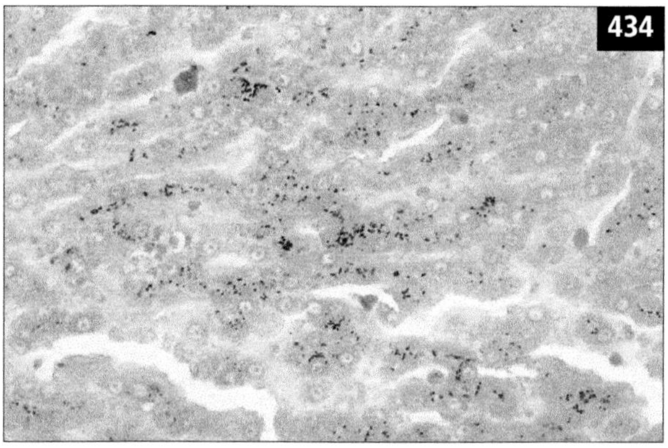

434 Copper toxicosis. Section of liver (stained by rubeanic acid) from a ten-month-old West Highland White Terrier demonstrating accumulation of copper within hepatocytes.

Treatment and prognosis

Supportive therapy with dietary modification, lactulose and antibiotics to control hepatoencephalopathy is usually indicated in the later stages of CH and cirrhosis. Specific treatment aimed at reducing the immune response and consequent fibrosis is based on prednisolone (0.5–2.0 mg/kg p/o q24h). The dosage is less than in other diseases where immunosuppression is attempted because the diseased liver is less able to cope with the catabolic effects of glucocorticoids. Glucocorticoids also modify fibrosis and may halt the deleterious accumulation of α_1-antitrypsin. Immunosuppressive agents (e.g. azathioprine, chlorambucil or cyclophosphamide) can be added to the regime, and colchicine (0.03 mg/kg p/o q24h) may also halt fibrosis. Ursodeoxycholic acid (UDCA, 15 mg/kg p/o q24h) is a hydrophilic bile salt that is of benefit in stimulating bile flow in cholestasis and excluding naturally-occurring, toxic, hydrophobic bile acids. However, it also has some immunomodulatory effect, at least in part through the inhibition of expression of MHC class II.

Hydrophobic bile acids accumulate in cholestasis and perpetuate hepatocyte membrane damage through their detergent action. Oxidative free radicals released in inflammation are also involved in the perpetuation of chronic liver damage, and are the rational basis for the use of anti-oxidants in chronic liver disease. Vitamins C and E, silymarin (milk thistle extract) and s-adenosyl L-methionine (SAMe) have all been reported to be beneficial, although vitamin C is contraindicated if hepatocyte damage is associated with copper accumulation because of an interaction with the copper, reducing it to a more toxic valency.

FELINE INFLAMMATORY LIVER DISEASE

Pathogenesis

The WSAVA Liver Study Group has recently simplified the classification of feline cholangitis, which has a poorly defined aetiopathogenesis that may in part involve immune-mediated mechanisms.

Neutrophilic cholangitis (suppurative or exudative cholangitis/cholangiohepatitis) is characterized by neutrophil-dominated inflammation of portal areas and bile ducts that may extend through the limiting plate to hepatic

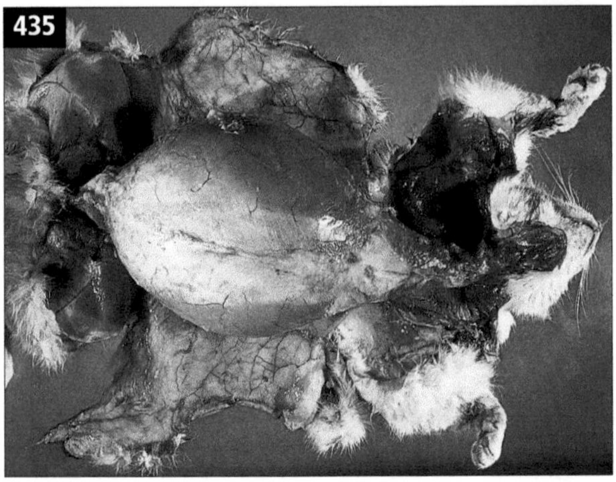

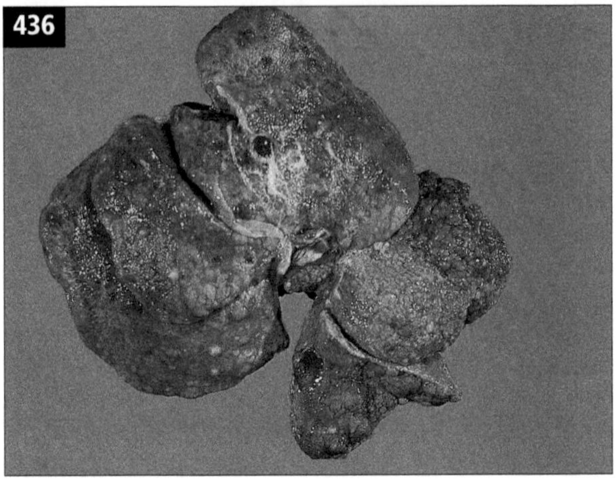

435, 436 Feline progressive lymphocytic cholangitis/cholangiohepatitis. Necropsy examination of an 11-year-old DSH cat with late-stage lymphocytic cholangitis. (**435**) The marked abdominal distension is due to ascites fluid. (**436**) The liver from this cat is firm and tan coloured and has a finely multinodular external appearance.

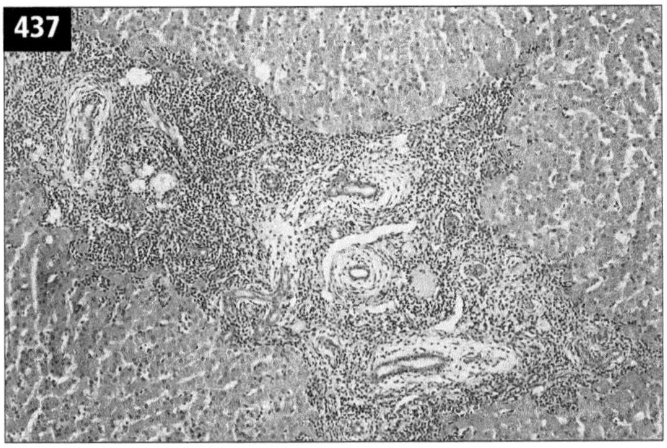

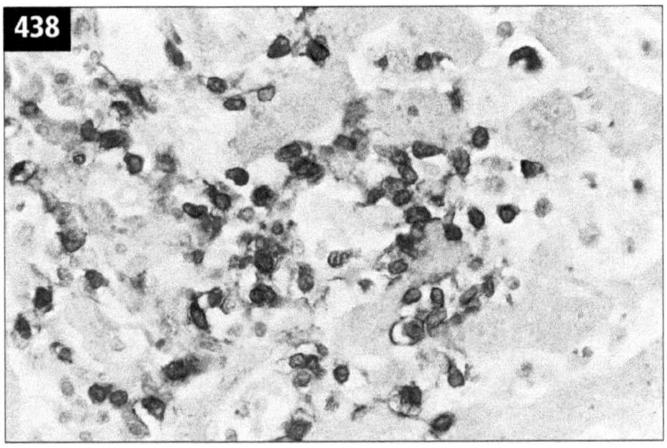

437, 438 Feline progressive lymphocytic cholangitis/cholangiohepatitis. (**437**) Section of liver from a cat with weight loss, dullness, hepatomegaly and jaundice. There is marked lymphocytic infiltration of portal areas. (**438**) The majority of lymphocytes are $CD3^+$ T lymphocytes that infiltrate bile ducts and the periportal parenchyma (shown here).

parenchyma. Cholangiohepatitis may be associated with IBD or pancreatitis, and the proposed pathogenesis involves an ascending bacterial infection of the biliary system. The hepatic damage may be perpetuated by immune-mediated mechanisms following elimination of the bacteria. In the chronic stages of disease (mixed cholangiohepatitis) there may be infiltration of lymphocytes and plasma cells, with fibrosis and bile duct proliferation, and progression to cirrhosis with pseudolobule formation.

The second form of feline portal hepatitis is **lymphocytic cholangitis** (lymphocytic cholangiohepatitis; lymphocytic portal hepatitis; non-suppurative cholangitis) (**435, 436**), which is characterized by an active stage of lymphocytic infiltration of portal areas, with bile duct proliferation (**437, 438**). The infiltrating cells are T lymphocytes that may invade the bile ducts and periportal parenchyma (piecemeal necrosis). There is MHC class II expression by bile duct epithelium. In chronic stages there is progressive portal to portal fibrosis that distorts hepatic architecture. There is no concurrent pancreatic or intestinal disease, and serum autoantibodies (ANA, mitochondria, smooth muscle) were not found in the cases examined.

Clinical signs

The clinical presentation in both forms of cholangitis is similar, with signs including anorexia, weight loss, lethargy and vomiting. Cats with lymphocytic cholangitis may also display polyphagia, ascites and jaundice.

Treatment and prognosis

Neutrophilic cholangiohepatitis is treated with antibiotics chosen, preferably, on the basis of culture/sensitivity testing. In the absence of culture the combination of amoxicillin/metronidazole offers broad-spectrum cover. Immune-mediated inflammation is treated with prednisolone (2–4 mg/kg p/o q24h) in combination with UDCA and/or metronidazole. The response to treatment is often good and the immediate prognosis favourable. However, relapse is common and prolonged treatment is often needed, with a poor long-term prognosis.

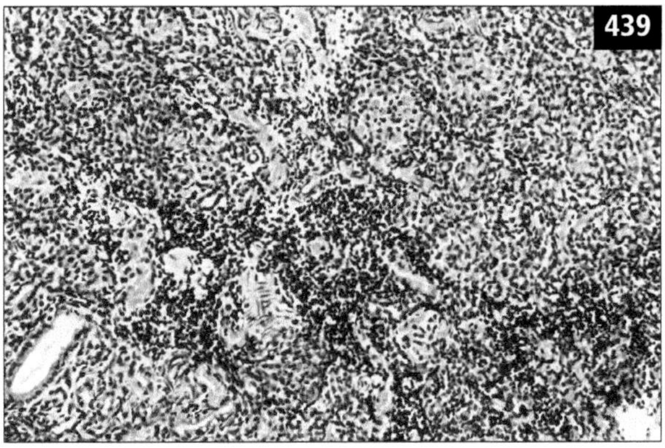

439 Lymphocytic pancreatitis. Section of atrophic pancreas from a one-year-old GSD showing intense lymphocytic infiltration of the exocrine tissue. This immune-mediated process has been described as a cause of exocrine pancreatic insufficiency in this breed.

IMMUNE MEDIATED DISEASE OF THE EXOCRINE PANCREAS

Pathogenesis

Exocrine pancreatic insufficiency (EPI) has been shown to be an inherited condition in GSDs and Rough Collies. Recent histological studies of the pancreas of affected GSDs have revealed the presence of striking lymphocytic infiltration of the exocrine pancreas preceding degenerative changes in exocrine tissue. This lymphocytic pancreatitis is associated with subclinical EPI and a subnormal serum trypsin-like immunoreactivity (TLI). Ultimately this condition may progress to clinical EPI through the development of 'pancreatic acinar atrophy' (PAA) and clinical signs. Immunohistochemical labelling has characterized these infiltrates as predominantly T cell in nature (with similar numbers of $CD4^+$ and $CD8^+$ T cells), and on this basis it has been suggested that this may represent autoimmune destruction of the exocrine pancreas (**439**). Serum autoantibodies that bind exocrine pancreatic tissue may be present at a low titre in some dogs. Endocrine tissue remains unaffected and dogs with PAA rarely develop diabetes mellitus. An autosomal recessive mode of inheritance has not been proven, but recent microsatellite studies have failed to identify a marker gene.

Clinical signs

Affected dogs may display weight loss, polyphagia, soft faeces, poor quality haircoat, borborygmus and flatulence.

Diagnosis

Diagnosis is confirmed by measurement of serum TLI, but false-positive results are reported when assay for faecal elastase is used.

Treatment and prognosis

Therapy is by supplementation of pancreatic enzymes and there has been no clear response to trials of immunosuppression (long-term azathioprine treatment). There is no regeneration of pancreatic tissue, so lifelong supplementation is required.

FURTHER READING

Allenspach K, House A, Smith K *et al.* (2010) Evaluation of mucosal bacteria and histopathology, clinical disease activity and expression of Toll-like receptors in German shepherd dogs with chronic enteropathies. *Veterinary Microbiology* **146**:326–335.

Burgener IA, Konig A, Allenspach K *et al.* (2008) Upregulation of Toll-like receptors in chronic enteropathies in dogs. *Journal of Veterinary Internal Medicine* **22**:553–560.

Dandrieux JR, Bornand VF, Doherr MG *et al.* (2008) Evaluation of lymphocyte apoptosis in dogs with inflammatory bowel disease. *American Journal of Veterinary Research* **69**:1279–1285.

Day MJ (2005) The canine model of dietary hypersensitivity. *Proceedings of the Nutrition Society* **64**:458–464.

Day MJ, Bilzer T, Mansell J *et al.* (2008) Histopathological standards for the diagnosis of gastrointestinal inflammation in endoscopic biopsies from the dog and cat: a report from the World Small Animal Veterinary Association Gastrointestinal Standardization Group. *Journal of Comparative Pathology* **138:**S1–S44.

Garden OA, Pidduck H, Lakhani KH *et al.* (2000) Inheritance of gluten-sensitive enteropathy in Irish Setters. *American Journal of Veterinary Research* **61:**462–468.

German AJ, Hall EJ, Kelly DF *et al.* (2000) An immunohistochemical study of histiocytic ulcerative colitis in Boxer dogs. *Journal of Comparative Pathology* **122:**163–175.

German AJ, Hall EJ, Day MJ (2000) Relative deficiency in IgA production by duodenal explants from German Shepherd Dogs with small intestinal disease. *Veterinary Immunology and Immunopathology* **76:**25–43.

German AJ, Hall EJ, Day MJ (2001) Characterization of immune cell populations within the duodenal mucosa of dogs with enteropathies. *Journal of Veterinary Internal Medicine* **15:**14–25.

German AJ, Hall EJ, Day MJ (2003) Chronic intestinal inflammation and intestinal disease in dogs. *Journal of Veterinary Internal Medicine* **17:**8–20.

German AJ, Day MJ, Ruaux CM *et al.* (2003) Comparison of direct and indirect tests for small intestinal bacterial overgrowth and antibiotic-responsive diarrhea in dogs. *Journal of Veterinary Internal Medicine* **17:**33–43.

Harley R, Helps CR, Harbour DA *et al.* (1999) Analysis of intralesional cytokine mRNA expression in feline chronic gingivostomatitis. *Clinical and Diagnostic Laboratory Immunology* **6:**471–478.

Harley R, Gruffydd-Jones TJ, Day MJ (2003) Salivary and serum immunoglobulin levels in cats with chronic gingivostomatitis. *Veterinary Record* **152:**125–129.

Harley R, Gruffydd-Jones TJ, Day MJ (2011) Immunohistochemical characterization of oral mucosal lesions in cats with chronic gingivostomatitis. *Journal of Comparative Pathology* **144:**239–250

House A, Gregory SP, Catchpole B (2003) Expression of cytokine mRNA in canine anal furunculosis lesions. *Veterinary Record* **153:**354–358.

House AK, Catchpole B, Gregory SP (2007) Matrix metalloproteinase mRNA expression in canine anal furunculosis lesions. *Veterinary Immunology and Immunopathology* **115:**68–75.

Janeczko S, Atwater D, Bogel E *et al.* (2008) The relationship of mucosal bacteria to duodenal histopathology, cytokine mRNA, and clinical disease activity in cats with inflammatory bowel disease. *Veterinary Microbiology* **128:**178–193.

Jergens AE, Schreiner A, Frank DE *et al.* (2003) A scoring index for disease activity in canine inflammatory bowel disease. *Journal of Veterinary Internal Medicine* **17:**291–297.

Jergens AE, Sonea IM, O'Connor AM *et al.* (2009) Intestinal cytokine mRNA expression in canine inflammatory bowel disease: a meta-analysis with critical appraisal. *Comparative Medicine* **59:**153–162.

Jergens AE, Crandell JM, Evans R *et al.* (2010) A clinical index for disease activity in cats with chronic enteropathy. *Journal of Veterinary Internal Medicine* **24:**1027–1033.

Jergens AE, Crandell J, Morrison JA *et al.* (2010) Comparison of oral prednisone and prednisone combined with metronidazole for induction therapy of canine inflammatory bowel disease: a randomized-controlled trial. *Journal of Veterinary Internal Medicine* **24:**269–277.

Littman MP, Dambach DM, Vaden SL *et al.* (2000) Familial protein-losing enteropathy and protein-losing nephropathy in Soft Coated Wheaten Terriers: 222 cases (1983–1997). *Journal of Veterinary Internal Medicine* **14:**68–80.

Lombardi RL, Marino DJ (2008) Long-term evaluation of canine perianal fistula disease treated with exclusive fish and potato diet and surgical excision. *Journal of the American Animal Hospital Association* **44:**302–307.

Luckschander N, Hall JA, Gaschen F *et al.* (2010) Activation of nuclear factor-κB in dogs with chronic enteropathies. *Veterinary Immunology and Immunopathology* **133:**228–236.

Mandingers PJJ, van den Ingh TSGAM, Bode P *et al.* (2004) Association between liver copper concentration and subclinical hepatitis in Doberman Pinschers. *Journal of Veterinary Internal Medicine* **18:**647–650.

Mandigers PJJ, Biourge V, van den Ingh TSGAM *et al.* (2010) A randomized, open-label, positively-controlled field trial of a hydrolyzed protein diet in dogs with chronic small bowel enteropathy. *Journal of Veterinary Internal Medicine* **24**:1350–1357.

Mansfield CS, James FE, Craven M *et al.* (2009) Remission of histiocytic ulcerative colitis in boxer dogs correlates with eradication of invasive intramucosal *Escherichia coli. Journal of Veterinary Internal Medicine* **23**:964–969.

McMahon LA, House AK, Catchpole B *et al.* (2010) Expression of Toll-like receptor 2 in duodenal biopsies from dogs with inflammatory bowel disease is associated with severity of disease. *Veterinary Immunology and Immunopathology* **135**:158–163.

Nguyen Van N, Taglinger K, Helps CR *et al.* (2006) Measurement of cytokine mRNA expression in intestinal biopsies of cats with inflammatory enteropathy using quantitative real-time RT–PCR. *Veterinary Immunology and Immunopathology* **113**:404–414.

Peters IR, Helps CR, Batt RM *et al.* (2003) Quantitative real-time RT–PCR measurement of mRNA encoding α–chain, pIgR and J-chain from canine duodenal mucosa. *Journal of Immunological Methods* **275**:213–222.

Peters IR, Helps CR, Calvert EL *et al.* (2005a) Measurement of messenger RNA encoding the α-chain, polymeric immunoglobulin receptor, and J–chain in duodenal mucosa from dogs with and without chronic diarrhea by use of quantitative real-time reverse transcription polymerase chain reaction assays. *American Journal of Veterinary Research* **66**:11–16.

Peters IR, Helps CR, Calvert EL *et al.* (2005b) Cytokine mRNA quantification in duodenal mucosa from dogs with chronic enteropathies by real-time reverse transcriptase polymerase chain reaction. *Journal of Veterinary Internal Medicine* **19**:644–653.

Simpson KW, Dogan B, Rishniw M *et al.* (2006) Adherent and invasive *Escherichia coli* is associated with granulomatous colitis in Boxer dogs. *Infection and Immunity* **74**:4778–4792.

Spee B, Arends B, van den Ingh TSGAM *et al.* (2006) Copper metabolism and oxidative stress in chronic inflammatory and cholestatic liver diseases in dogs. *Journal of Veterinary Internal Medicine* **20**:1085–1092.

Speeti M, Stahls A, Meri S *et al.* (2003) Upregulation of major histocompatibility complex class II antigens in hepatocytes in Dobermann hepatitis. *Veterinary Immunology and Immunopathology* **96**:1–12.

Stanley BJ, Hauptman JG (2009) Long-term prospective evaluation of topically applied 0.1% Tacrolimus ointment for treatment of perianal sinuses in dogs. *Journal of the American Veterinary Medical Association* **235**:397–404.

Suchodolski JS, Ruaux C, Steiner JM *et al.* (2004) Application of molecular fingerprinting for qualitative assessment of small-intestinal bacterial diversity in dogs. *Journal of Clinical Microbiology* **42**:4702–4708.

Suchodolski JS, Xenoulis PG, Paddock CG *et al.* (2010) Molecular analysis of the bacterial microbiota in duodenal biopsies from dogs with idiopathic inflammatory bowel disease. *Veterinary Microbiology* **142**:394–400.

Tivers MS, Catchpole B, Gregory SP *et al.* (2008) Interleukin-2 and interferon-gamma mRNA expression in canine anal furunculosis lesions and the effect of ciclosporin therapy. *Veterinary Immunology and Immunopathology* **125**:31–36.

Waly NE, Stokes CR, Gruffydd-Jones TJ *et al.* (2004) Immune cell populations in the duodenal mucosa of cats with inflammatory bowel πdisease. *Journal of Veterinary Internal Medicine* **18**:816–825.

Waly NE, Gruffydd-Jones TJ, Stokes CR *et al.* (2005) Immunohistochemical diagnosis of alimentary lymphomas and severe intestinal inflammation in cats. *Journal of Comparative Pathology* **133**:253–260.

Westermarck E, Saari SAM, Wiberg ME (2010) Heritability of exocrine pancreatic insufficiency in German shepherd dogs. *Journal of Veterinary Internal Medicine* **24**:450–452.

Wiberg ME, Saari SAM, Westermarck E (1999) Exocrine pancreatic atrophy in German Shepherd Dogs and Rough–coated Collies: an end result of lymphocytic pancreatitis. *Veterinary Pathology* **36**:530–541.

Wiberg ME, Saari SAM, Westermarck E *et al.* (2000) Cellular and humoral immune responses in atrophic lymphocytic pancreatitis in German Shepherd Dogs and Rough-coated Collies. *Veterinary Immunology and Immunopathology* **76**:103–115.

8 IMMUNE-MEDIATED RESPIRATORY AND CARDIAC DISEASE

Michael J. Day and Cécile Clercx

THE RESPIRATORY TRACT IMMUNE SYSTEM

The normal respiratory tract immune system has recently undergone extensive characterization in the dog and some similar studies have been conducted in the cat. The innate immune system (mucociliary clearance and phagocytic cells) is of particular significance in the respiratory tract (**440**), and relatively high doses of antigen are required to overwhelm these defences and ensure translocation to local lymph nodes for generation of an immune response. The dog has been used as an experimental model for studies of the pulmonary immune response, and instillation of antigens into specific lung lobes is able to generate populations of antigen-specific B lymphocytes that recirculate to sites of antigen deposition, leading to production of specific antibody of the IgG, IgM and IgA classes. Additionally, serum antibody of these classes is also demonstrable. Antigen-specific memory cells are also recruited into the lung after primary immunization, and specific antibody may continue to be produced for several years after antigen exposure. This process may involve continued restimulation by antigen sequestered by pulmonary dendritic cells.

As in other species, the ratio of IgG to IgA alters in secretions from various levels of the canine and feline respiratory tract, with progressively increasing levels of IgG towards the more distal (pulmonary) sites. Intranasal vaccination is an effective means of stimulating local immunity, and antigen-specific IgA can be identified in nasal secretions. Recent studies have examined the cellular component of bronchoalveolar lavage fluid (BALF) from normal dogs and demonstrated the dominance of alveolar macrophages and lymphocytes (both $CD4^+$ and $CD8^+$ with a CD4:CD8 ratio of 3.2 ± 1.9; range 1.7–8.6), with fewer eosinophils, mast cells, epithelial cells and neutrophils.

Immunohistochemical investigations have also characterized the normal immune cell populations of the canine upper and lower respiratory tract. Of note is the fact that organized nasal-associated lymphoid tissue (NALT) or bronchial-associated lymphoid tissue (BALT) was not identified in normal puppies or adult dogs, although the nasopharyngeal tonsil in this species is well developed. IgA^+ plasma cells dominate over IgG^+ or IgM^+ cells at all levels of the respiratory mucosa, but such cells are found in significantly greater number within the nasal mucosa than at lower levels of the respiratory tract (**441**). Adult dogs have a greater number of mucosal plasma cells of all types than are found in the respiratory mucosa of puppies. Similar to the intestinal tract, the respiratory mucosa is rich in IgE expressing mucosal mast cells that are located immediately beneath the epithelial lining (**442**). Mast cells are also found in greater number in the nasal mucosa (compared with lower in the respiratory tract) and are more numerous in the mucosa of puppies than adult dogs. There is a similar distribution for MHC class II expressing APCs, which are enriched in the

440

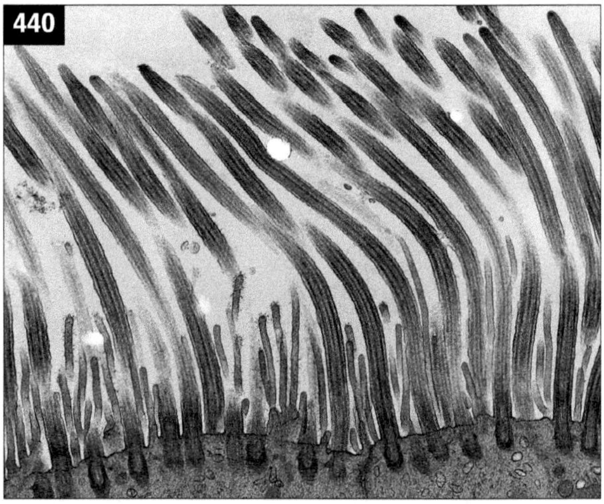

440 Innate immunity of the respiratory tract. Electron micrograph of feline respiratory epithelium showing detail of the cilia that mediate clearance of particulate material from the lower respiratory tract via the 'muco-ciliary escalator'.

nasal mucosa and the mucosa of the younger population. Intriguingly, CD1$^+$ dendritic cells are more numerous in the respiratory mucosa of adult dogs compared with puppies (**443**). Respiratory epithelial cells in the dog rarely express MHC class II, which is a distinct difference when compared with the constitutive expression of this molecule by the intestinal enterocytes (**444**). Scattered T lymphocytes are also distributed throughout the respiratory mucosa and these are a mixed population of CD4$^+$ and CD8$^+$ cells that predominantly express the αβ TCR (**445**). There

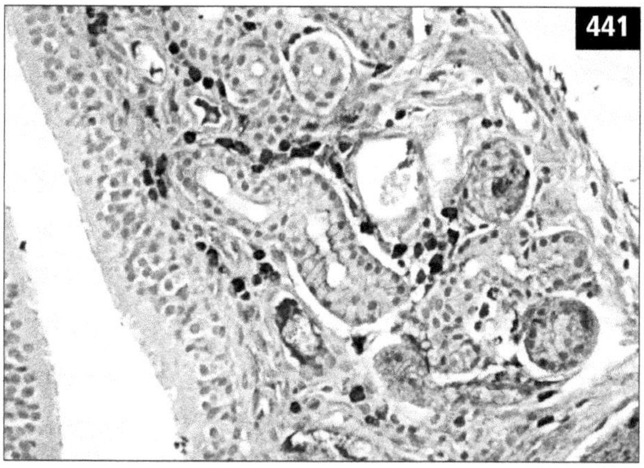

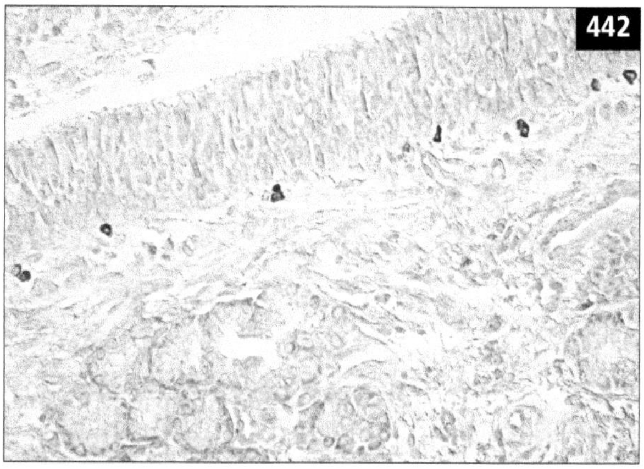

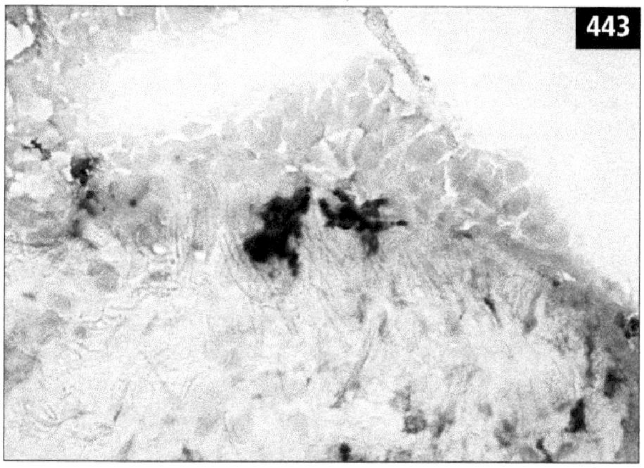

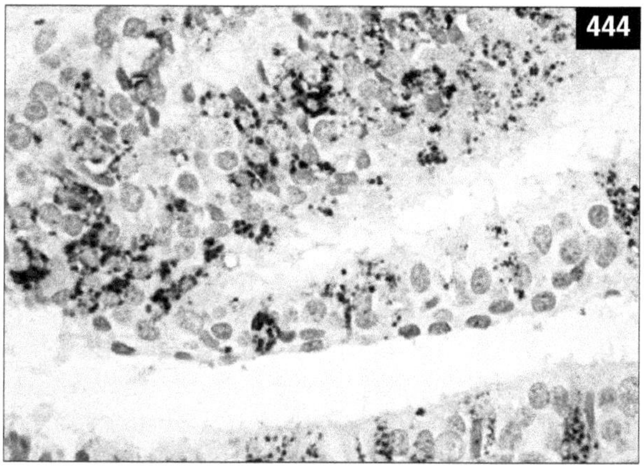

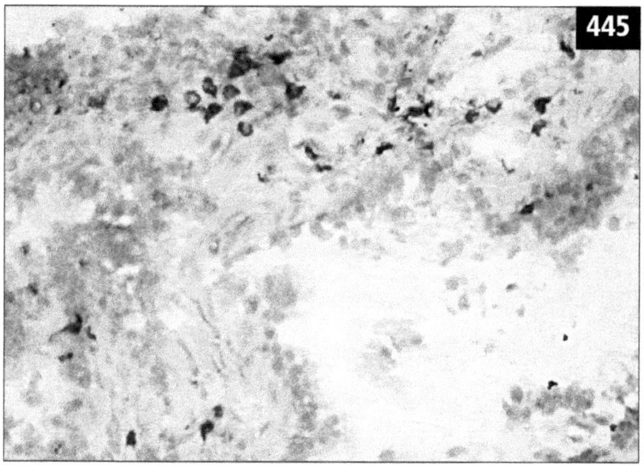

441–445 Normal canine respiratory mucosa. The normal canine respiratory tract is endowed with a range of different immune cell populations that are most concentrated in the mucosa of the nose. (**441**) IgA$^+$ plasma cells are located within the lamina propria of the nasal mucosa and are particularly concentrated around glandular tissue. (**442**) Mast cells are located immediately beneath the epithelial lining in all areas of the respiratory tract. (**443**) CD1$^+$ dendritic cells are located within the lining epithelium and are optimally located for capture of inhaled antigen. (**444**) MHC class II expression is associated with APC populations within the lamina propria and epithelium, and in this section of nasal mucosa there is also expression by epithelial cells. (**445**) A small cluster of T cells expressing the αβ TCR is noted within the pulmonary interstitium. (From Peeters D, Day MJ, Farnir F *et al.* [2005] Distribution of leucocyte subsets in the canine respiratory tract. *Journal of Comparative Pathology* **132**:261–272, with permission).

are more T cells within the respiratory mucosa of adult dogs than of puppies, but at all levels of the respiratory tract there are approximately equal numbers of $CD4^+$ and $CD8^+$ cells. This observation is of note when compared with the dominance of the $CD4^+$ population in normal BALF. The concentration of immune cells within the nasal mucosa likely reflects the greater antigenic exposure that may be predicted at this site, and the fact that adult respiratory mucosa is more richly endowed with immune cells suggests a maturation of the local immune system with increasing age in the dog.

The expression of genes encoding cytokines and chemokines has been examined at different levels of the normal canine respiratory mucosa. Expression of cytokine genes can be detected at all levels from the nose to the lungs, with a dominance of mRNA encoding IL-18 and TGFβ and approximately tenfold less template encoding IL-6, IL-10, IL-12 and TNFα. The least abundant transcripts are those encoding IL-4, IL-5 and IFNγ. The distribution of these cytokine mRNAs is similar at all anatomical levels of the respiratory tract, although at some sites there is greater expression of genes encoding IL-5, IL-18 and TNFα. With respect to chemokines, there is a distinct increase in expression of genes encoding eotaxin-2 and eotaxin-3 (the eosinophil chemotactic molecules) from normal nasal to pulmonary mucosa. Normal puppies and adult dogs express similar amounts of all transcripts at all levels of the respiratory tract. Baseline cytokine and chemokine gene transcription has also been assessed in cats with histologically normal nasal mucosa, and low level transcripts encoding TNFα, IL-12p40, IFNγ, IL-10 and RANTES were described. Canine tracheal epithelial cells have been shown to express genes encoding antimicrobial β-defensins.

IMMUNE-MEDIATED RESPIRATORY DISEASE

The immune-mediated diseases that affect the canine and feline respiratory tract are fundamentally allergic in nature and have a basic type I hypersensitivity pathogenesis, as described in Chapter 3. A number of the primary immunodeficiency disorders described in Chapter 12 present with disease involving the respiratory tract, and lymphoma (see Chapter 13, p. 318) may also involve the respiratory tract.

ALLERGIC RHINITIS

There are sporadic reports of rhinitis of presumptive allergic basis in the dog and cat. Such animals present with oculonasal discharge, sneezing, nose rubbing or head shaking and significant numbers of eosinophils can be demonstrated in nasal exudate or nasal lavage fluid, and infiltrating the nasal mucosa on tissue biopsy (**446, 447**). In the dog, eosinophilic rhinitis may occur concurrently with eosinophilic bronchopneumopathy (described below).

446

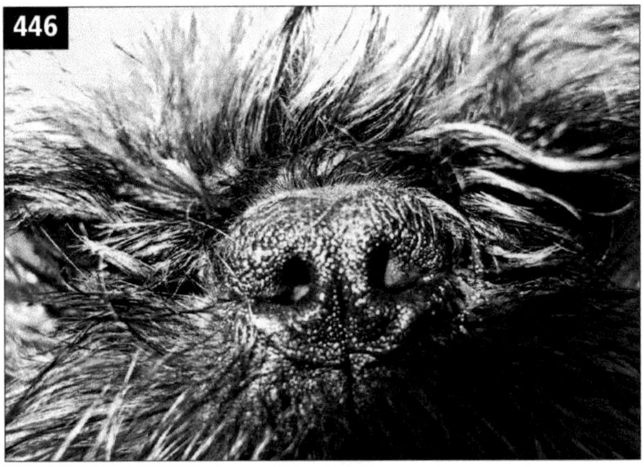

446 Allergic rhinitis. A three-year-old male Belgian Griffon with a two-week history of sneezing and serous nasal discharge. Rhinoscopic examination of the nasal cavity revealed mucosal erythema and eosinophils dominated the cytological preparation in this case.

447

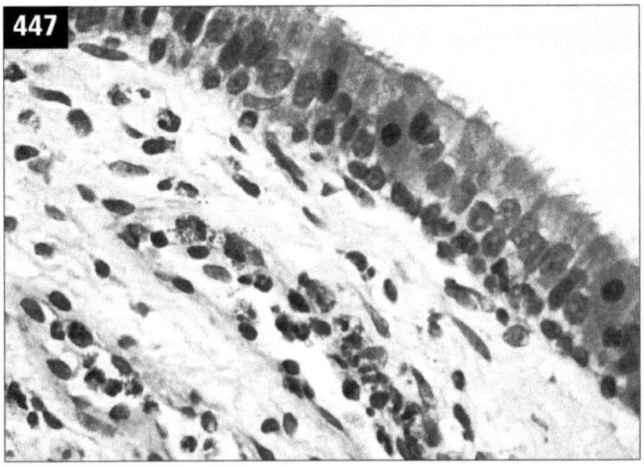

447 Allergic rhinitis. Biopsy of nasal mucosa from a dog with allergic rhinitis. There is oedema of the lamina propria and a prominent cluster of eosinophils within the superficial area of this lamina.

LYMPHOPLASMACYTIC RHINITIS

In some dogs and cats with rhinitis the inflammatory infiltration of the nasal mucosa comprises mixed lymphocytes and plasma cells. In such cases it is generally not possible to find evidence of a microbial aetiology and the disease is often considered to be an idiopathic immune-mediated disorder. Recent studies in dogs and cats have reported the screening of biopsy samples for a range of infectious agents by PCR. In dogs there was no evidence for the presence of canine adenovirus-2, parainfluenza virus-3, *Chlamydophila* or *Bartonella*, although the use of 'universal primers' for bacterial RNA and fungal gene transcription produced positive results in samples from dogs with LPR, nasal aspergillosis and nasal neoplasia. Although it has been suggested that some cases of canine lymphoplasmacytic rhinitis (LPR) may be undiagnosed *Aspergillus* infections, a recent investigation has revealed a distinct immunopathogenesis in these two disorders. In contrast to the Th1-related cytokine mRNA profile in the nasal mucosa of dogs with sino-nasal aspergillosis (see Chapter 2, p. 72), samples from dogs with LPR have a distinct phenotype, with a partial Th2 profile comprising transcription of genes encoding IL-5, IL-8, IL-10, IL-12p19 and p40, IL-18, TNFα, TGFβ and MCP-2 and MCP-3.

In cats with chronic rhinosinusitis (**448**), similar screening of nasal flush or biopsy samples by culture did reveal a greater prevalence of *Mycoplasma* spp. and a range of bacterial (but not fungal) pathogens compared with controls. In this investigation there was no clear association with the presence of FHV-1 DNA (as detected by PCR), but in a separate study there was an association between molecular detection of FHV-1 and up-regulation of cytokine gene expression. This latter result was interpreted to suggest that FHV-1 infection might act as a trigger for secondary immunopathology in this disease.

In a recent retrospective of canine LPR, affected dogs were aged between 1.5 and 14 years and were generally of large breed origin. The nasal discharge was either uni- or bi-lateral and disease had generally been present for longer than six months at the time of referral (**449**). Rhinoscopy and imaging examination (computed tomography) revealed accumulation of fluid and mucus and evidence of turbinate destruction.

ASTHMA-LIKE DISEASE OF THE DOG AND CAT

Asthma is a disease of major importance in human medicine and the mechanisms underlying the various forms of human asthma are the subject of much research. In contrast, spontaneously arising

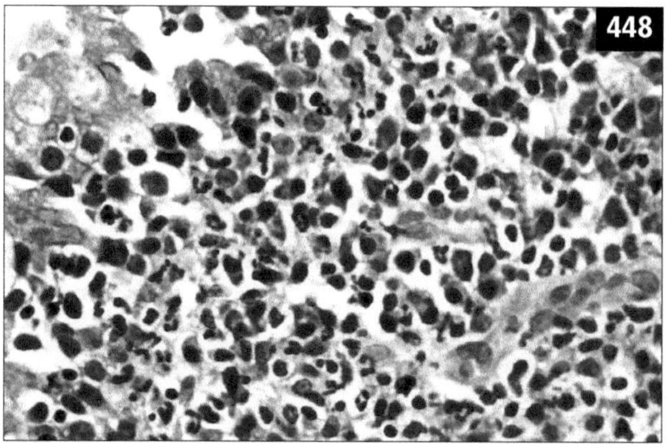

448 Lymphoplasmacytic rhinitis. Biopsy of nasal mucosa from a cat. There is marked infiltration of the lamina propria by lymphocytes and plasma cells. The epithelium is degenerate and superficially there is also a neutrophilic inflammatory response. In the absence of evidence for involvement of feline respiratory viruses, this disorder is often considered to have an idiopathic immune-mediated basis.

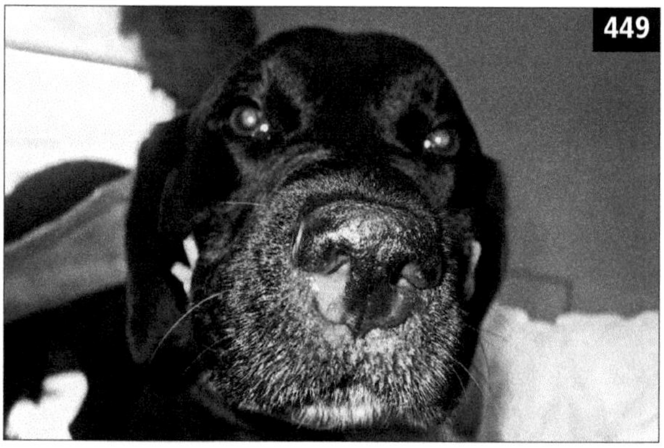

449 Lymphoplasmacytic rhinitis. A seven-year-old male mixed-breed dog with lymphoplasmacytic rhinitis. The dog has been sneezing, with a unilateral serous to mucoid nasal discharge, for the past two months. There is no systemic illness.

allergic lower respiratory disease in the dog and cat is poorly defined and it remains unclear whether these species actually develop an equivalent to human asthma.

Human asthma

The prototype allergic respiratory disease is human asthma. Asthma may have a range of non-immunological causes (e.g. exercise-, anxiety- or drug-induced), where it is defined as intrinsic or non-atopic asthma. In contrast, many cases do have an allergic pathogenesis and these patients are considered to have atopic asthma. This involves a classical type I hypersensitivity response to inhaled aeroallergens, which are generally derived from innocuous environmental agents. As for most immune-mediated diseases, the causation of asthma is multifactorial and there are strong genetic influences. Although human asthma clearly runs within families, strong genetic linkages have proven difficult to identify. Candidate genes that have been examined include those of the major histocompatibility complex (MHC) and the Th2 cytokine gene cluster.

Immunologically, allergic asthma involves sensitization of the affected individual by capture of inhaled allergen by mucosal dendritic cells that process the antigen and present it to antigen-specific lymphocytes within the draining lymphoid tissue of the lung. A classical Th2 immune response is engendered, which results in production of allergen-specific IgE (and probably IgG of

450

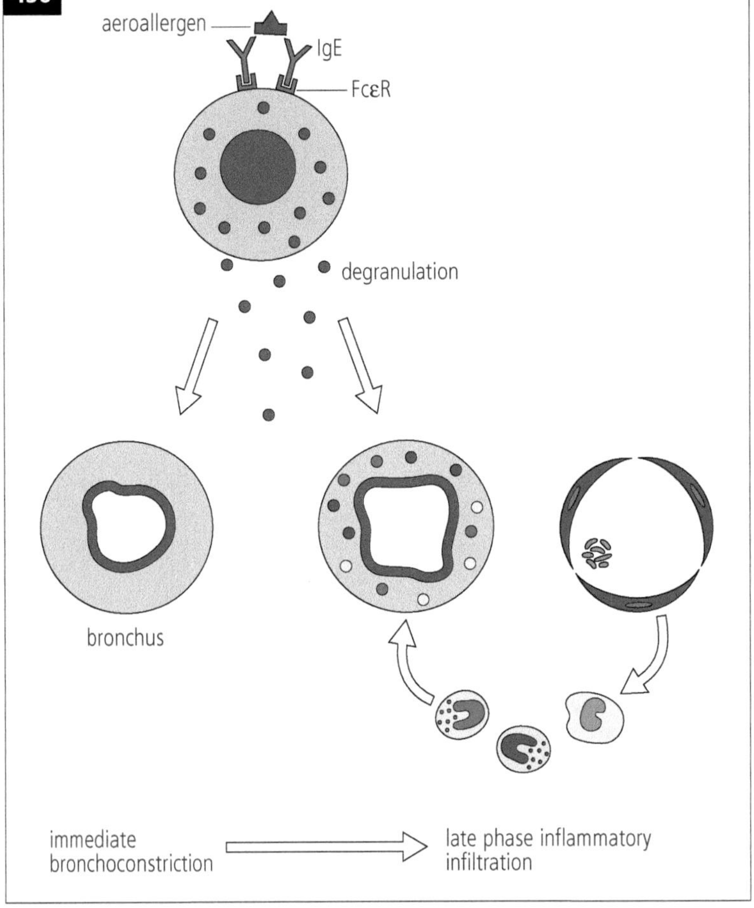

450 Mechanism of asthma. Asthma has a presumptive type I hypersensitivity pathomechanism. Inhaled aeroallergen cross-links IgE bound to mast cell receptors, resulting in mast cell degranulation and local release of inflammatory mediators that cause immediate bronchoconstriction, vasodilation and tissue oedema and infiltration of inflammatory cells including neutrophils, basophils, eosinophils and macrophages. Factors released from these infiltrating cells, and intravascular platelets, perpetuate the response and cause a 'late phase response'.

particular subclasses) that subsequently coats mast cells in the respiratory mucosa. On subsequent exposure to allergen, there is cross-linkage of IgE, with mast cell degranulation leading to immediate (5–60 minutes) bronchoconstriction, vasodilation and late phase (4–24 hours) recruitment of inflammatory cells (e.g. eosinophils, macrophages) to the affected area (**450**). It is now understood that these allergic responses progress such that the nature of the immune regulation changes towards a more cell-mediated (Th1) immunity in chronic phases. The immunological control of the allergic response is mediated by regulatory T cells producing cytokines such as IL-10 or TGFβ.

Experimental models of asthma

The immunology of allergic pulmonary disease has largely been studied in rodent models. It is possible to sensitize mice or guinea pigs of particular strains to standard antigens such as ovalbumin (OVA) (derived from chicken eggs); therefore, when they are challenged by the same antigen (via the respiratory tract), they develop clinical signs and pathology compatible with asthma. The Der p1 allergen of house dust mite has also been used to induce murine experimental asthma in such studies.

Similar experimental studies have been performed in the dog and cat. Beagle dogs sensitized systemically by repeated injection of *Ascaris,* OVA or ragweed antigen develop clinical signs of respiratory disease when challenged by the same allergen via the airways. Physiological studies in these models have confirmed increased airway resistance in challenged dogs. BALF collected from ragweed-sensitized dogs contains a high proportion of eosinophils, and serum allergen-specific IgE and IgG1/IgG4 antibodies are produced. OVA sensitized dogs have been shown to have BALF allergen-specific IgE in the absence of detectable serum levels of the same antibody. The latest of these studies shows that the offspring of ragweed-sensitized dogs show an allergic response to aerosol allergen challenge, whereas offspring of non-sensitized dogs do not.

Experimental sensitization and challenge studies have also been performed in the cat. In one model system, cats were sensitized and challenged with Bermuda grass allergen and shown to mount a serum allergen-specific IgE response that was greatest after aerosol challenge. This was associated with evidence of bronchial hyperreactivity, together with the presence of eosinophils and allergen-specific IgG and IgA in BALF. Analysis of cytokine mRNA production by BALF cells and blood mononuclear cells was determined in this model by quantitative RT-PCR. A Th2 cytokine profile (IL-4, IL-6 and IL-10) was shown. Subcutaneous administration of Th1 enhancing bacterial 'CpG oligonucleotide motifs' prior to sensitization led to reduced production of allergen-specific IgE in sensitized cats. Intranasal and subcutaneous rush immunotherapy has also been shown to be efficacious in this model. Similar studies have been performed with house dust mite, *Ascaris* or OVA as the sensitizing antigen.

Some studies of exercise-induced asthma have also been reported in the dog. Sled dogs working in cold environments have mucus accumulation and neutrophilic inflammation of the lower airways. The extent of these changes is significantly greater than in control dogs that were not exercised for a two-week period before sampling.

Canine allergic bronchitis

The most common cause of canine airway inflammation is infectious tracheobronchitis ('kennel cough') involving pathogens such as *Bordetella bronchiseptica,* adenovirus or parainfluenza virus. This syndrome bears little relationship to asthma.

Dogs with respiratory disease defined as idiopathic 'chronic bronchitis' do bear greater clinical similarity to human asthma. BALF cytology generally shows chronic-active inflammatory change with neutrophils and macrophages, which implies that the disease does not involve type I hypersensitivity. However, BALF of such patients does occasionally show a high proportion of eosinophils, and these dogs might have an allergic component to their respiratory inflammation, although this is not described as 'asthma'.

Eosinophilic bronchopneumopathy

For many years a syndrome has been recognized in the dog that was most often described as 'pulmonary infiltration with eosinophils' (PIE). More recently, the more descriptive name of 'eosinophilic bronchopneumopathy' (EBP) has been applied to this disorder.

451
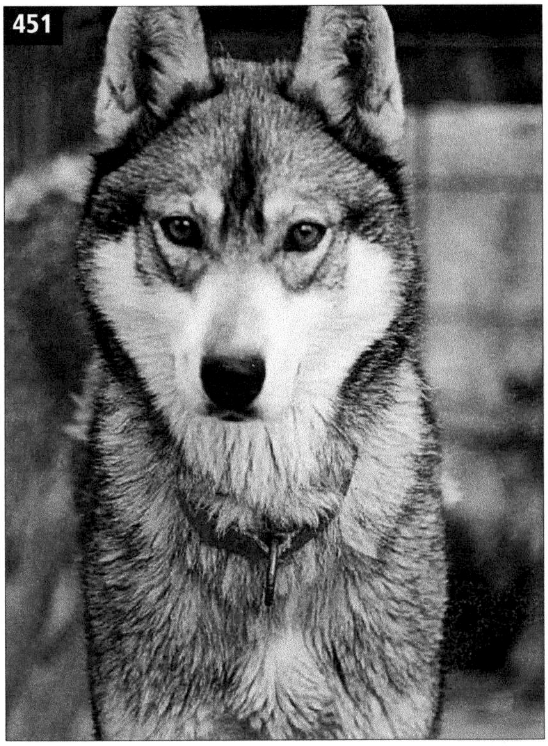

452
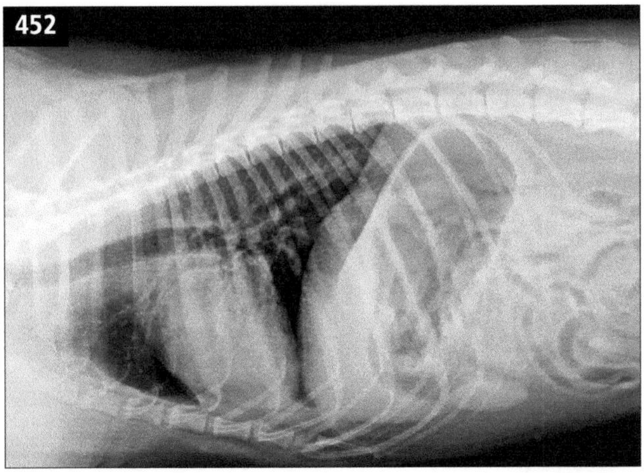

453
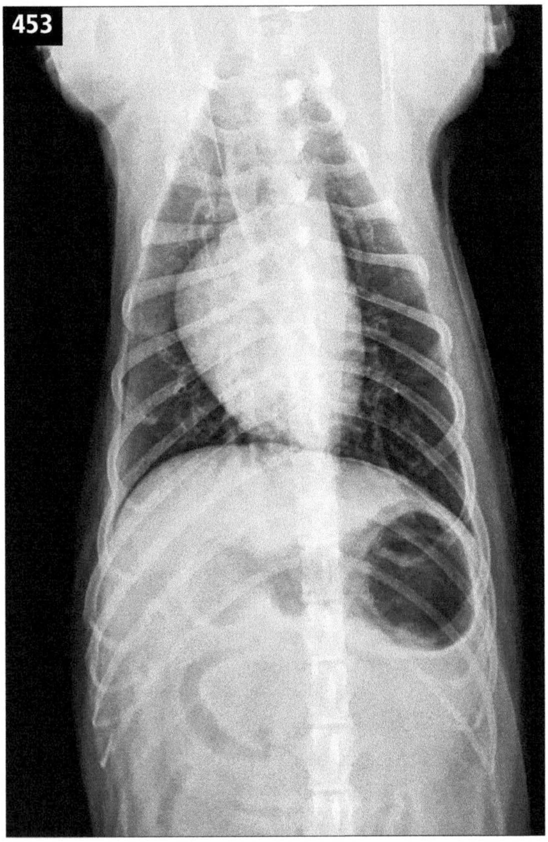

454
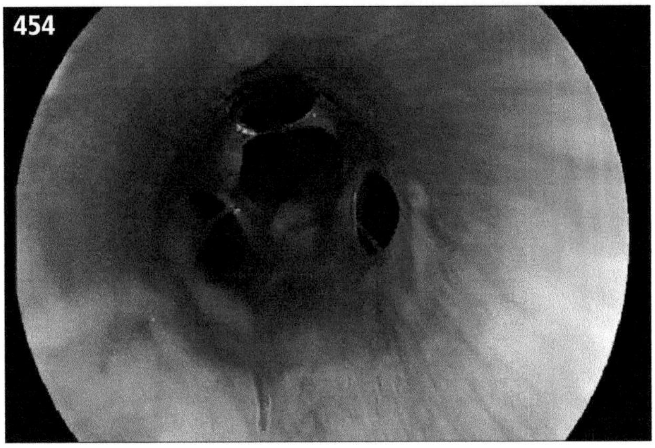

451–454 Eosinophilic bronchopneumopathy. (**451**) A six-year-old Husky dog with EBP. Dogs of this breed are predisposed to this condition. (**452, 453**) Left lateral and dorsoventral thoracic radiographs of a six-year-old mixed-breed dog with EBP, showing a bronchointerstitial pattern and peribronchial cuffing. (**454**) Bronchoscopic examination reveals the presence of characteristic abundant mucoid secretion within the airway.

455
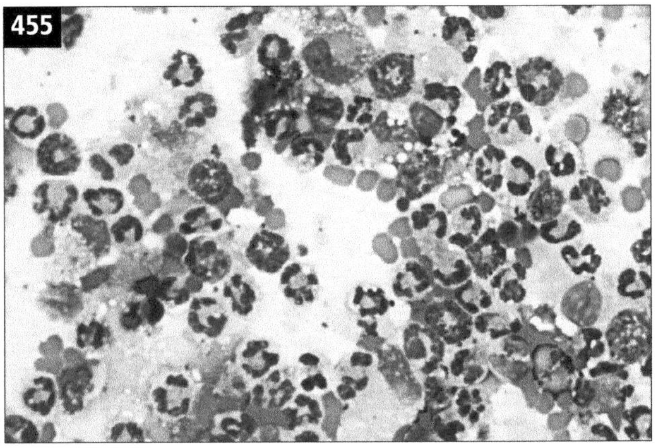

455 Eosinophilic bronchopneumopathy. BALF from a dog with EBP reveals the presence of a mixed inflammatory population with a prominent population of eosinophils.

EBP is not a common disease, but young Husky or Malamute dogs appear predisposed (451). The clinical presentation is of cough, gagging, retching and dyspnoea. The disease can be complicated in some dogs by the presence of concurrent bacterial bronchopneumonia. Up to 50% of affected dogs may also have concurrent eosinophilic rhinitis, and the pathogenesis of this response is presumptively similar to that of the lower respiratory tract.

On radiography, the most common features are a moderate to severe bronchointerstitial pattern (452, 453). Bronchoscopy generally reveals the presence of abundant yellow-green mucoid material, with thickening or polypoid change to the mucosa and occasional partial airway closure during expiration (454).

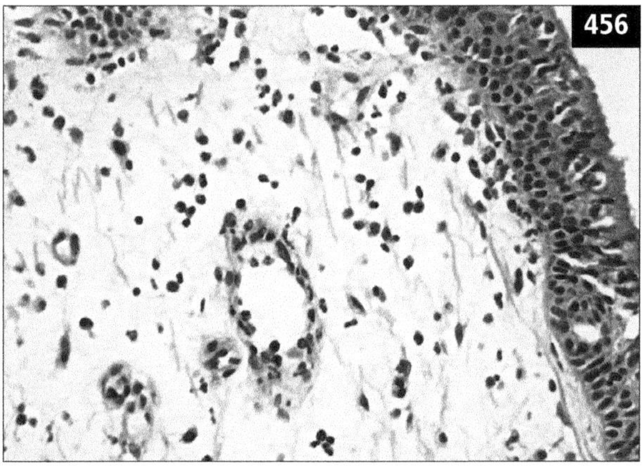

456 Eosinophilic bronchopneumopathy. Bronchial mucosal biopsy from a dog with EBP. There is oedema of the lamina propria and active exocytosis of eosinophils from small capillaries in this sample with early changes.

BALF from dogs with EBP is characterized by a striking eosinophilic component, sometimes with mucus and other chronic inflammatory cells (455). Bronchial mucosal biopsies similarly show a spectrum of change from early eosinophilic infiltration and exocytosis through to late-stage chronic mixed mononuclear inflammation with eosinophils, with tissue destruction and ulceration (456). Similarly, pulmonary biopsies demonstrate the classical intense eosinophil infiltration of alveoli. Approximately 60% of cases have blood eosinophilia.

Immunological studies have shown that there are elevated concentrations of immunoglobulins within the BALF of affected dogs, in particular IgA and IgM, although IgA may be reduced in concentration in the serum. These altered immunoglobulin concentrations revert to normal during therapy with glucocorticoids. The ratio of $CD4^+$ to $CD8^+$ lymphocytes in the BALF is markedly elevated (to 22.6 ± 30.3) compared with normal dogs. This change is caused by a relative increase in the number of $CD4^+$ cells and a concurrent decrease in $CD8^+$ cells. The CD4:CD8 ratio reverts to normal following glucocorticoid therapy. Immunohistochemical labelling of bronchial biopsy material of EBP dogs reveals a number of alterations compared with normal. There is a significant increase in lamina propria APCs (including $CD1^+$ dendritic cells), but not all of these express MHC class II (457). There is also infiltration of plasma cells (expressing predominantly IgA) and T cells, with relatively more $CD4^+$ than $CD8^+$ cells reflecting the change in BALF observed in affected dogs (458).

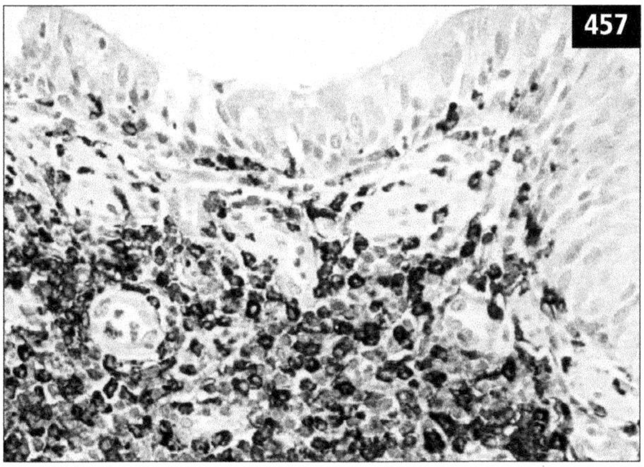

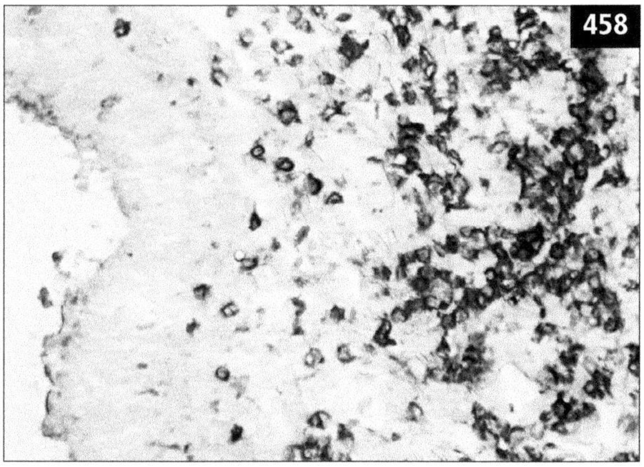

457, 458 Eosinophilic bronchopneumopathy. Biopsies from dogs with EBP labelled to show cells expressing MHC class II (**457**) and CD3 (**458**), indicating infiltration of the bronchial mucosa by APCs and T cells in this disease.

Other studies have investigated cytokine and chemokine mRNA expression in bronchial mucosal biopsies from dogs with EBP. When compared with normal canine bronchial mucosa, EBP dogs have elevation in transcripts encoding eotaxin-2, eotaxin-3 and MCP-3, but a decrease in expression of the inflammatory mediator RANTES. In contrast, there is no alteration in expression of genes encoding a panel of cytokines or those encoding MCP-1, MCP-2 or MCP-4. BALF from dogs with EBP also shows increased expression of the gelatinolytic protease MMP-9 and collagenolytic matrix metalloproteinases MMP-8 and MMP-13, suggesting a role for these molecules in airway destruction and remodelling. Taken together, the range of immunological changes identified in the bronchial mucosa of dogs with EBP adds support to the hypothesis that this is a Th2-mediated allergic disease with similarity to human asthma.

The inciting causes of EBP are poorly defined. Some studies have suggested an association with heartworm, pulmonary parasites or chemicals/drugs. Evidence that EBP might have an allergic basis comes from intradermal testing and the finding of allergen-specific IgE in serum and BALF of dogs with EBP. The currently accepted working hypothesis is that this is an allergic disease (akin to asthma) driven by aeroallergens such as those derived from house dust mites.

Feline asthma

For many years it has been recognized that cats develop a spontaneously arising idiopathic respiratory disease of allergic phenotype, which has been termed 'feline asthma'. Reports of immunological mechanisms underlying this disorder are sparse. Feline asthma should be distinguished from respiratory disease related to

459

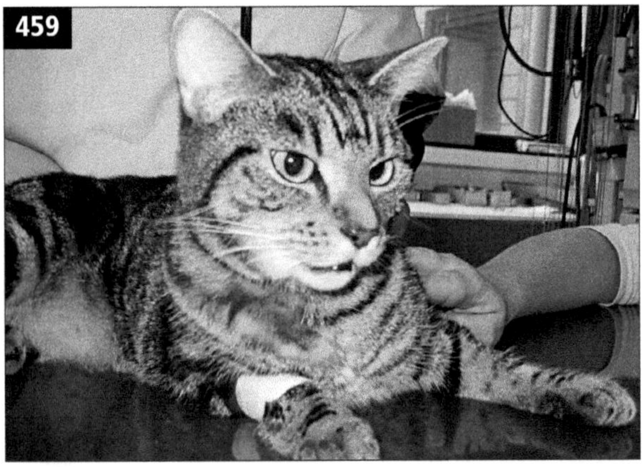

459 Feline asthma. A six-year-old DSH cat, which presented with a history of cough and increasing dyspnoea over a four-month period. Radiography of the chest, bronchoscopy, examination of BALF and bronchial reactivity testing confirmed a diagnosis of feline asthma.

460

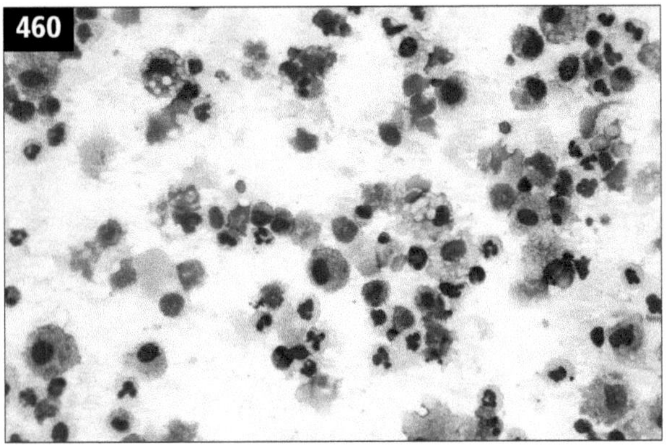

460 Feline asthma. Appearance of BALF cytology from a cat with asthma. There are numerous vacuolated macrophages consistent with a chronic inflammatory reaction, but the high proportion of eosinophils is suggestive of asthma.

461

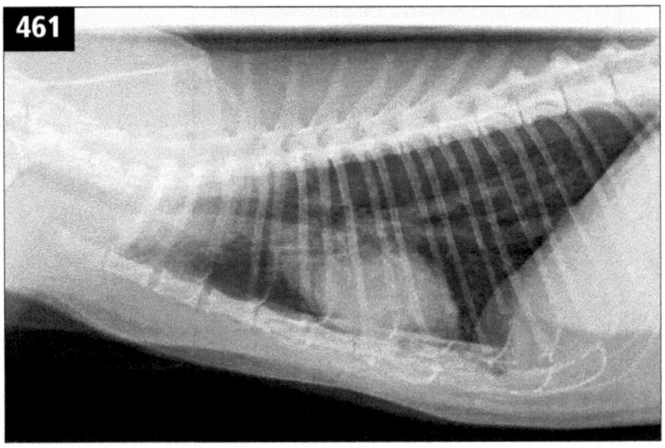

461 Feline asthma. Left lateral thoracic radiograph from the cat described in **459** showing increased bronchial and interstitial pattern in the lungs.

bacterial/mycoplasmal infection, pulmonary parasitism or heartworm infection.

The disease is characterized by recurrent episodes of coughing, wheezing or respiratory distress (**459**). Examination of BALF generally demonstrates a prominent eosinophilic component (**460**). Bronchial biopsies may reveal hyperplasia of glandular tissue, with excess mucus secretion, thickening of airway smooth muscle and eosinophilic infiltration of the mucosa. Measurement of cytokine protein (IL-4, IFNγ, IFNα) or nitric oxide in BALF does not discriminate asthma from chronic bronchitis. Blood eosinophilia is uncommonly present. Radiographically there is evidence of increased bronchial and/or interstitial pattern in the lungs (**461**).

Affected cats may have elevation of total serum IgE concentration and may test positive on intradermal and serological testing. There are reports of clinical improvement following restricted access to allergen or hyposensitization. Human dander has been incriminated as a causative allergen in some individuals.

Treatment of allergic respiratory disease

The spectrum of allergic respiratory diseases in companion animals is generally treated with anti-inflammatory doses of oral glucocorticoids. However, due to the potential side-effects of these drugs, together with the fact that the patients are generally young animals that require lifelong therapy, other therapeutic options have been investigated.

In canine idiopathic eosinophilic broncho-pneumopathy, prednisolone is used initially at a dose of 1 mg/kg q12h and then on alternate days, with progressive tapering of the dose. A maintenance dose of between 0.1 and 1.0 mg/kg every other day is generally achieved. Using this treatment protocol the disease is frequently controlled but rarely cured. In most cases, relapse occurs either directly or within months after drug discontinuation.

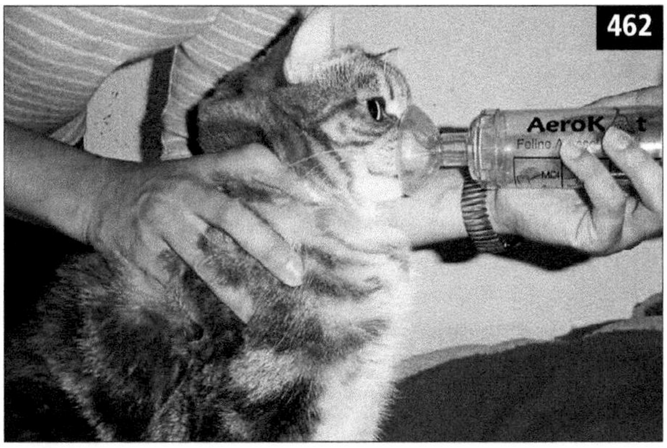

462 Feline asthma. Administration of aerosolized drugs using an adapted metered dose inhaler, spacer and facemask.

Although the most reliable, efficacious and easily administered therapy for feline asthma remains the use of oral prednisolone, there is increasing use of adjunct locally active inhaled glucocorticoid (e.g. fluticasone propionate) or bronchodilators (albuterol sulphate) administered via new delivery systems (metered dose inhalers) adapted for the cat by incorporation of a spacer and a facemask (**462**). Fluticasone propionate is the preferred corticosteroid formulation, as this drug has the greatest potency and longest half-life. Moreover, any fluticasone that is inadvertently swallowed is less likely to be systemically absorbed from the gastrointestinal tract than other formulations. Albuterol is a selective β_2-adrenergic bronchodilator that effects bronchial smooth muscle relaxation. The effects of albuterol are relatively short-lived (under four hours). Several protocols for the treatment of feline asthma, according to the severity of disease, have been described. A standard dosage protocol for the use of fluticasone for cats is 250 μg (one puff into the spacer) q12h. As maximal effect is not expected before three weeks, oral glucocorticoid may be given concurrently with fluticasone at the start of a therapeutic protocol, and tapered over a 2–3-week period. Albuterol may be given, as required, when an animal has evidence of bronchoconstriction and it has an immediate but not prolonged effect, or it can be given once daily before administration of fluticasone. In the Bermuda grass sensitization model of feline asthma, either oral or inhaled glucocorticoid administration led to reduced airway eosinophilia, but had no effect on blood lymphocyte subpopulations or serum and BALF concentrations of allergen-specific IgG and IgA. Only orally administered glucocorticoid was able to reduce the concentration of serum allergen-specific IgE. Spontaneously affected cats rarely show complete cure after a course of therapy and signs may return when therapy is discontinued.

In dogs, similar delivery systems (inhalers with spacer and face mask adapted for this species) have been investigated, but there is a lack of published clinical trials proving their efficacy using either bronchodilators or steroids.

Allergen avoidance is a sensible precaution, but there have been no good clinical studies of the benefits of allergen-specific immunotherapy. In dogs with EBP, ASIT is not efficacious in most cases, but there are anecdotal reports of very good responses. In the Bermuda grass sensitization model of feline asthma, the use of 'rush immunotherapy' (parenteral administration of Bermuda grass antigen in increasing concentration using an abbreviated two-day protocol) has been shown to cause reduced BALF eosinophil numbers, elevated serum antigen-specific IgG, reduced blood lymphocyte response to antigen stimulation, and elevated BALF IFNγ and IL-10 mRNA.

The range of medications used or trialled in human asthma therapy (e.g. antihistamines, leukotriene inhibitors, lipoxygenase inhibitors, mast cell membrane stabilisers, IgE or IL-5 antagonists, ciclosporin, CpG motifs) have not been extensively investigated for use in companion animals, and they may not be appropriate medications for diseases in which classical type I hypersensitivity remains unproven. One study in the feline Bermuda grass allergen sensitization model has shown the benefit of inhaled glucocorticoid, but not a leukotriene antagonist.

One recent experimental study has shown that the induction of antigen-specific oral tolerance in neonatal dogs can prevent allergic ocular and respiratory disease on challenge later in life. Neonatal puppies repeatedly fed OVA failed to develop serum OVA-specific IgE or IgG antibodies after repeated subcutaneous injection of alum-adjuvanted OVA. Moreover, OVA-tolerant dogs developed minimal conjunctival reaction when this antigen was instilled into the eye and, after aerosol challenge with OVA, showed limited bronchoconstriction or inflammation within BALF. Cells from the BALF of tolerant and challenged dogs had significantly higher mRNA encoding the regulatory cytokines IL-10 and TGFβ than controls, suggesting that regulatory cell induction may underlie the observed responses.

IMMUNE-MEDIATED CARDIAC DISEASE

Immune-mediated cardiac disease is probably rare in companion animals, although very few investigations have been performed in this area. The most widely studied entity is canine idiopathic pericardial effusion (IPE), which has been the subject of recent research. This entity arises most frequently in middle-aged, male, large or giant breed dogs. They develop recurrent episodes of accumulation of bloody fluid within the pericardial cavity, which may lead to cardiac tamponade (**463**). The major differential diagnosis is cardiac neoplasia (particularly haemangiosarcoma), but in IPE there is no underlying neoplasia or infectious disease and the pathogenesis is unknown (**464, 465**). Treatment involves pericardiocentesis, but effusion may be recurrent and eventually require pericardiectomy. There are similarities between canine IPE and the pericardial involvement that occurs in some human immune-mediated connective tissue disorders (e.g. scleroderma and SLE), so it has long been proposed that IPE in the dog has an immune-mediated pathogenesis.

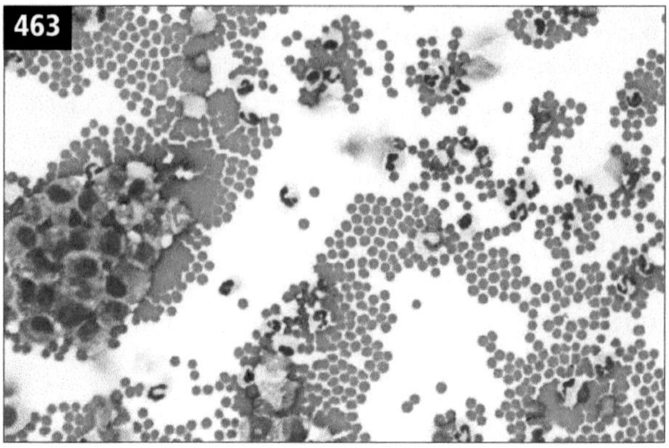

463 Idiopathic pericarditis. Cytological appearance of pericardial fluid from a dog with idiopathic pericarditis. Typically there is a predominance of blood, with numerous vacuolated or haemosiderin-laden macrophages, reactive mesothelia and scattered plasma cells.

Histopathological studies of resected pericardium have revealed extensive pericardial fibrosis, with mononuclear cell inflammatory infiltration that is most prominent at the cardiac surface of the pericardium. The infiltrates have been characterized immunohistochemically as comprising recently emigrated macrophages and IgG or IgA plasma cells, with fewer T lymphocytes and MHC class II expressing APCs. There is no vascular pathology or vascular immune complex deposition. Analysis of the pericardial fluid reveals local concentration of immunoglobulins (IgM and IgA) relative to the blood levels of these proteins. Affected dogs are rarely ANA positive, but flow cytometric studies have revealed alterations in blood lymphocyte populations, specifically a

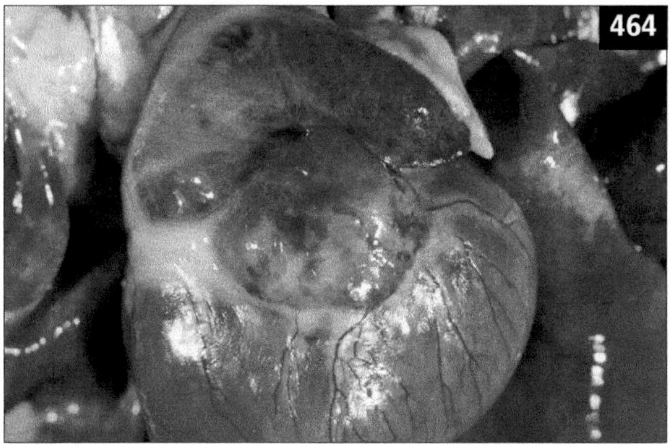
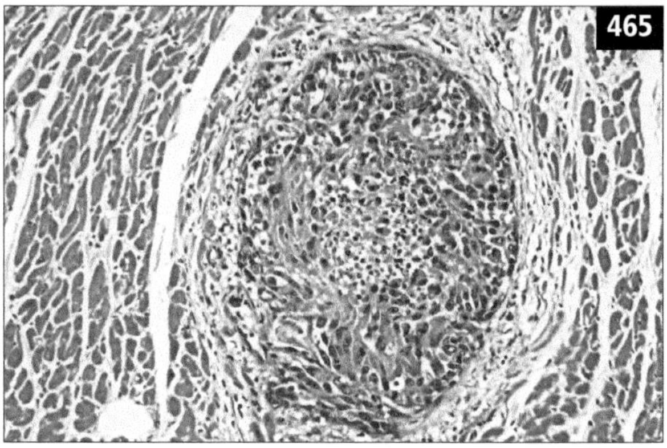

464, 465 Cardiac haemangiosarcoma. The major differential diagnosis for canine idiopathic pericarditis is neoplasia, particularly haemangiosarcoma. Shown is a gross lesion of right atrial haemangiosarcoma (**464**) and an intravascular metastasis within a myocardial vessel (**465**).

reduction in CD4+ T cells, leading to a reduced CD4:CD8 ratio. These findings suggest local and systemic activation of aspects of immunity in IPE, but do not necessarily support a primary, idiopathic immune-mediated pathogenesis for the condition. Molecular studies are required to rule-out the possibility of an infectious aetiology.

Immune-mediated myocardial disease is also poorly documented in companion animals. Lymphocytic myocarditis has been observed in both cats and dogs, but it is more likely to have been triggered by an infectious aetiology. For example, focal lymphocytic myocarditis has been documented in cats experimentally infected with *Bartonella* and so may be a consequence of infection. Some forms of human cardiomyopathy have been suggested to have an immune-mediated component, and compatible anti-mitochondrial autoantibodies have been documented in the serum of English Cocker Spaniels with cardiomyopathy.

Blood lymphocyte subsets have recently been examined in dogs with chronic valvular disease or dilated cardiomyopathy. One investigation revealed reduced CD4+ T cells and CD4:CD8 ratio, but another failed to describe this abnormality. Finally, bacterial valvular endocarditis may give rise to secondary immune-mediated (immune complex) disease such as polyarthritis or glomerulonephritis and particular interest has recently focussed upon canine endocarditis caused by *Bartonella* spp.

FURTHER READING

Barrett EG, Rudolph K, Bowen LE *et al.* (2003) Parental allergic status influences the risk of developing allergic sensitization and an asthmatic-like phenotype in canine offspring. *Immunology* **110**:493–500.

Clercx C, Peeters D, Snaps F *et al.* (2000) Eosinophilic bronchopulmonary disease in dogs: a clinical analysis of 25 cases. *Journal of Veterinary Internal Medicine* **14**:282–291.

Clercx C, Peeters D, German A *et al.* (2002) An immunologic investigation of canine eosinophilic bronchopneumopathy. *Journal of Veterinary Internal Medicine* **16**:229–237.

Day MJ, Martin MWS (2002) Immunohistochemical characterisation of the lesions of canine idiopathic pericarditis. *Journal of Small Animal Practice* **43**:382–387.

Delgado C, Lee-Fowler TM, DeClue AE *et al.* (2010) Feline-specific serum total IgE quantitation in normal, asthmatic and parasitized cats. *Journal of Feline Medicine and Surgery* **12**:991–994.

Erles K, Brownlie J (2010) Expression of β-defensins in the canine respiratory tract and antimicrobial activity against *Bordetella bronchiseptica. Veterinary Immunology and Immunopathology* **135**:12–19.

Guglielmino R, Miniscalco B, Tarducci A *et al.* (2004) Blood lymphocyte subsets in canine idiopathic pericardial effusion. *Veterinary Immunology and Immunopathology* **98**:167–173.

Henderson SM, Bradley K, Day MJ *et al.* (2004) Nasal disease in the cat: a retrospective study of 77 cases. *Journal of Feline Medicine and Surgery* **6**:245–257.

Johnson LR, De Cock HEV, Sykes JE *et al.* (2005) Cytokine gene transcription in feline nasal tissue with histologic evidence of inflammation. *American Journal of Veterinary Research* **66**:996–1001.

Johnson LR, Maggs DJ (2005) Feline herpesvirus type-1 transcription is associated with increased nasal cytokine gene transcription in cats. *Veterinary Microbiology* **108**:225–233.

Kirschvink N, Leemans J, Delvaux F *et al.* (2006) Inhaled fluticasone reduces bronchial responsiveness and airway inflammation in cats with mild chronic bronchitis. *Journal of Feline Medicine and Surgery* **8**:45–54.

Lee-Fowler TM, Cohn LA, DeClue AE *et al.* (2009) Evaluation of subcutaneous versus mucosal (intranasal) allergen-specific rush immunotherapy in experimental feline asthma. *Veterinary Immunology and Immunopathology* **129**:49–56.

Martin MWS, Green MJ, Stafford Johnson MJ *et al.* (2006) Idiopathic pericarditis in dogs: no evidence for an immune-mediated aetiology. *Journal of Small Animal Practice* **47**:387–391.

Michiels L, Day MJ, Snaps F *et al.* (2003) A retrospective study of non-specific rhinitis in 22 cats and the value of nasal cytology and histopathology. *Journal of Feline Medicine and Surgery* **5**:279–285.

Moriello KA, Stepien RL, Henik RA *et al.* (2007) Pilot study: prevalence of positive aeroallergen reactions in 10 cats with small-airway disease without concurrent skin disease. *Veterinary Dermatology* **18**:94–100.

Nafe LA, DeClue AE, Lee-Fowler TM *et al.* (2010) Evaluation of biomarkers in bronchoalveolar lavage fluid for discrimination between asthma and chronic bronchitis in cats. *American Journal of Veterinary Research* **71**:583–591.

Peeters D, Day MJ, Clercx C (2005) Distribution of leucocyte subsets in bronchial mucosa from dogs with eosinophilic bronchopneumopathy. *Journal of Comparative Pathology* **133**:128–135.

Peeters D, Peters IR, Clercx C *et al.* (2006) Real-time RT–PCR quantification of mRNA encoding cytokines, CC chemokines and CCR3 in bronchial biopsies from dogs with eosinophilic bronchopneumopathy. *Veterinary Immunology and Immunopathology* **110**:65–77.

Peeters D, Peters IR, Helps CR *et al.* (2007) Distinct tissue cytokine and chemokine mRNA expression in canine sino-nasal aspergillosis and idiopathic lymphoplasmacytic rhinitis. *Veterinary Immunology and Immunopathology* **117**:95–105.

Reinero CR, Decile KC, Byerly JR *et al.* (2005) Effects of drug treatment on inflammation and hyperreactivity of airways and on immune variables in cats with experimentally induced asthma. *American Journal of Veterinary Research* **66**:1121–1127.

Reinero CR, Byerly JR, Berghaus RD *et al.* (2006) Rush immunotherapy in an experimental model of feline allergic asthma. *Veterinary Immunology and Immunopathology* **110**:141–153.

Stafford Johnson M, Martin M, Binns S *et al.* (2004) A retrospective study of clinical findings, treatment and outcome in 143 dogs with primary pericardial effusion. *Journal of Small Animal Practice* **45**:546–552.

Windsor RC, Johnson LR, Herrgesell EJ *et al.* (2004) Idiopathic lymphoplasmacytic rhinitis in dogs: 37 cases (1997–2002). *Journal of the American Veterinary Medical Association* **224**:1952–1957.

Windsor RC, Johnson LR, Sykes JE *et al.* (2006) Molecular detection of microbes in nasal tissue of dogs with idiopathic lymphoplasmacytic rhinitis. *Journal of Veterinary Internal Medicine* **20**:250–256.

9 IMMUNE-MEDIATED ENDOCRINE DISEASE

Michael J. Day and Susan E. Shaw

INTRODUCTION

The immune and endocrine systems are intrinsically linked by the neuroendocrine immunological loop (see Chapter 1, p. 55), and endocrine tissue and hormones may act as target autoantigens in immune-mediated endocrine disorders. The spectrum of autoimmune endocrine disease is greatest in man, where many clinically significant endocrinopathies are immune mediated (e.g. Hashimoto's thyroiditis, Graves' disease, Addison's disease, type I diabetes mellitus). In contrast, well-defined autoimmune endocrine disease is uncommon in the dog and cat, with the single exception of canine hypothyroidism. This chapter describes those endocrinopathies of dogs and cats for which an immunological basis has been defined, or is proposed.

CANINE HYPOTHYROIDISM

Pathogenesis

Hypothyroidism in the dog is generally attributed to primary thyroid disease (95% of cases) rather than secondary (pituitary) or tertiary (hypothalamic) causes. Histological examination of thyroids from affected dogs reveals one of two changes: either lymphocytic thyroiditis with multifocal infiltration of lymphocytes, plasma cells and macrophages associated with thyroid follicular degeneration (**466**); or non-inflammatory, idiopathic follicular atrophy with an increase in the intervening fibrous or adipose connective tissue matrix (**467**). Although a subject of debate, it is often proposed that follicular atrophy is a late stage of lymphocytic thyroiditis.

Hypothyroidism with thyroid autoantibodies and lymphocytic thyroiditis (infiltration of T lymphocytes and increased expression of MHC class II) has been documented in an inbred cat colony.

The following immunological abnormalities are recognized in dogs with lymphocytic thyroiditis:

- Serum IgG autoantibody specific for thyroglobulin in 50–70% of cases. A recent investigation has reported the fine specificity of such autoantibodies for epitopes within the canine thyroglobulin molecule. Such 'epitope mapping' is crucial for further understanding of autoimmune responses and the development of novel immunotherapeutic approaches.
- Serum autoantibody specific for T3 in 0.2–4.5% of cases, although in one study 38% of hypothyroid sera had anti-T3, and autoantibody specific for T4 (thyroxine) was present in even

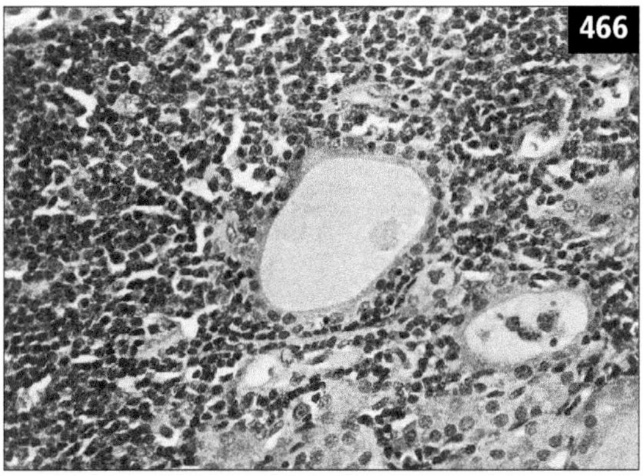

466 Canine lymphocytic thyroiditis. Section of thyroid from a four-year-old Gordon Setter with lymphocytic thyroiditis. There is an intense infiltration of lymphocytes, plasma cells and macrophages, with associated follicular atrophy.

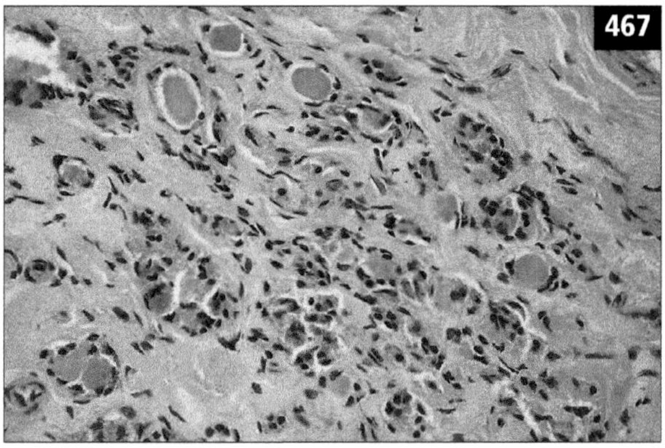

467 Canine idiopathic follicular atrophy. Section of thyroid from a 14-year-old Miniature Poodle with idiopathic follicular atrophy. There is a series of markedly atrophic follicles within a dense fibrous connective tissue matrix, with minimal inflammatory infiltration.

fewer affected dogs. T3 autoantibody may be directed towards an epitope of thyroglobulin that contains T3, and that differs from epitopes that normally elicit autoantibody to thyroglobulin. In a large serosurvey of samples from 287, 948 dogs with clinical signs consistent with hypothyroidism, T3 autoantibody alone was detected in 4.64% and T4 autoantibody alone in 0.63% of samples. Both antibodies were present in 1.03% of samples.

- Serum autoantibody specific for thyroid microsomal antigens has been documented. In a recent study using immunoblotting against purified canine thyroid peroxidase, autoantibodies to this enzyme were demonstrated in 17% of serum samples from hypothyroid dogs that were seropositive for anti-thyroglobulin, anti-T3 or anti-T4. Thyroid peroxidase autoantibodies were not found in the serum of normal dogs or hypothyroid dogs that were seronegative for anti-thyroglobulin, T3 or T4.
- The occasional presence of serum ANA.
- The presence of elevated levels of circulating immune complexes.

In addition, lymphocytic thyroiditis and thyroid autoantibodies have been induced experimentally by administration of thyroglobulin in adjuvant to normal dogs. The immunopathogenesis of lymphocytic thyroiditis involves cytotoxic destruction of thyroid follicular epithelium. Thyroid autoantibodies are thought to be an epiphenomenon rather than have a direct immunopathogenic role (**468**).

Clinical signs

Hypothyroidism is recognized in many breeds, but the disease may have greater prevalence in Golden Retrievers and Dobermanns. Familial hypothyroidism has been reported in the Beagle, Borzoi and Great Dane. MHC gene associations with canine hypothyroidism have been described in Chapter 3. There is no widely accepted gender predisposition and affected dogs are of a wide age range. In the large serosurvey described above, autoantibody-positive dogs were more likely to be of particular breeds (Pointer, English Setter, English Pointer, Skye Terrier, German Wirehaired Pointer, Old English Sheepdog, Boxer, Maltese, Kuvaz and Petit Basset Griffon Vendeen), aged between 2–4

468

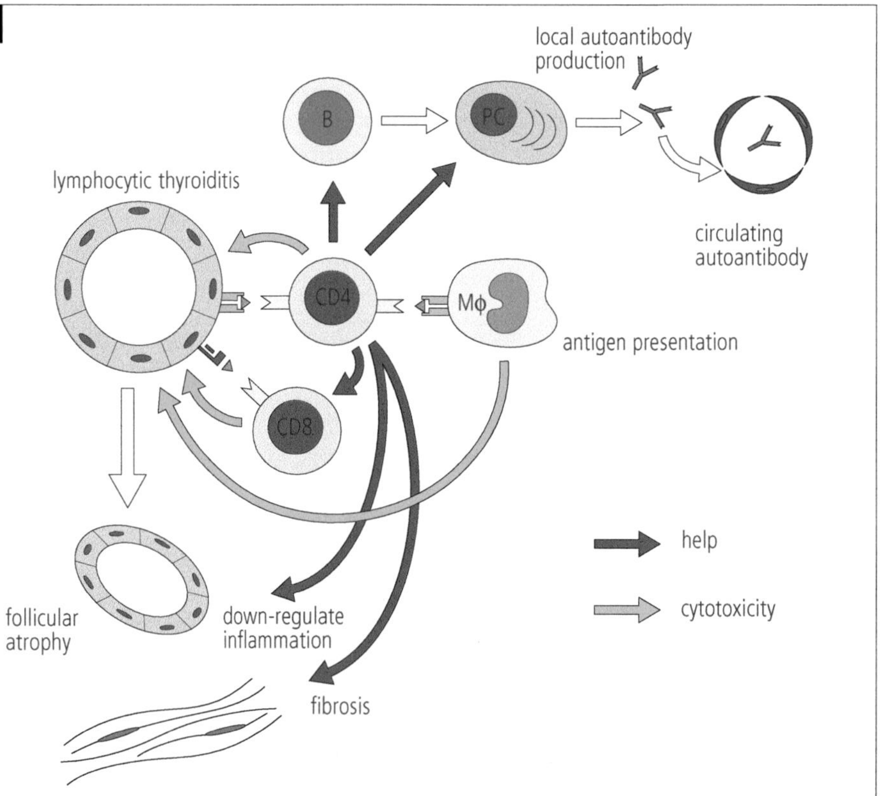

468 Model for the pathogenesis of lymphocytic thyroiditis. In lymphocytic thyroiditis, thyroid follicular epithelial cells present thyroid antigen following up-regulation of MHC class II expression. Infiltrating cytotoxic ($CD8^+$) T lymphocytes recognize autoantigen presented by follicular epithelial cells and infiltrating professional APCs, and mediate cytotoxic destruction of the follicle. Infiltrating $CD4^+$ T cells also provide co-stimulation for differentiation of plasma cells within the thyroid and local synthesis of autoantibody that enters the circulation from this site. Follicular atrophy may be a late stage of lymphocytic thyroiditis, and lymphocyte derived cytokines may initiate deposition of fibrous connective tissue.

years and female. The clinical effects of hypothyroidism are numerous and reflect the generalized role of thyroid hormones on metabolism in many organ systems. Clinical signs include:

- Lethargy, mental dullness.
- Obesity (**469**).
- Endocrine alopecia with hyperpigmentation and/or hyperkeratinization (**470, 471**). Dermal myxoedema (mucinous matrix within the dermis) resulting in 'tragic facial expression' may be seen (**472**). Secondary pyoderma may occur. Atrophic dermatopathy (**473**) is now considered a less common clinical manifestation of hypothyroidism.
- Poor fertility and libido.

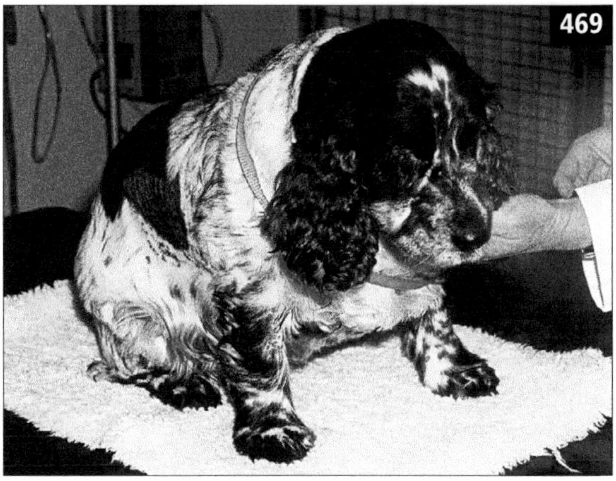

469 Canine hypothyroidism. Hypothyroidism in a seven-year-old neutered female English Cocker Spaniel showing obesity and lethargy. Dermatological manifestations in this case were minimal.

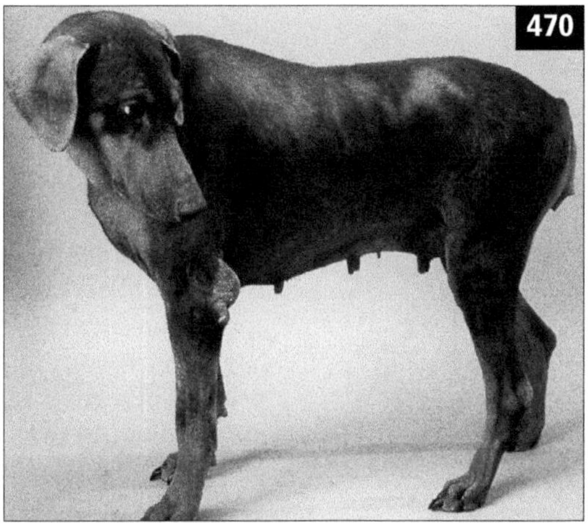

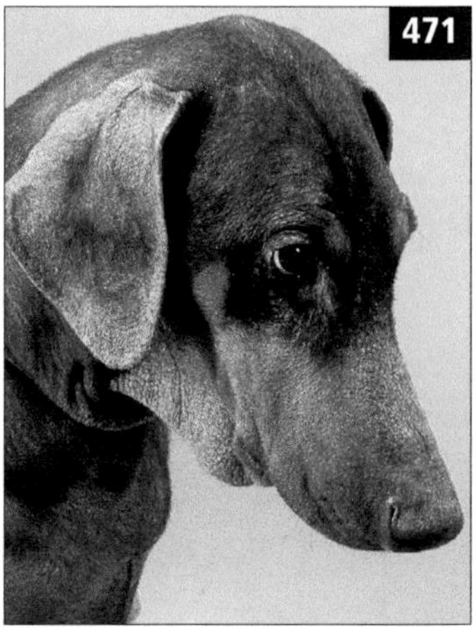

470, 471 Cutaneous changes in canine hypothyroidism. Hypothyroidism in a nine-year-old neutered female Dobermann, illustrating truncal alopecia, scaling and pyoderma. Hair loss over the pinnae is marked and a 'tragic facial expression' is also present. (Photographs courtesy A.J. Shearer.)

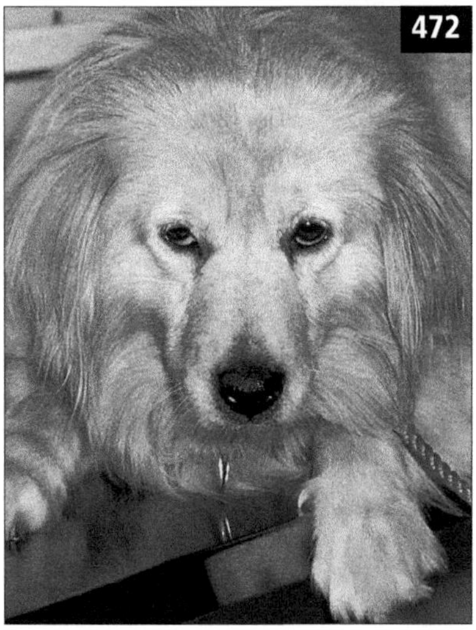

472 Myxoedema in canine hypothyroidism. Myxoedema is an uncommon manifestation of canine hypothyroidism in which there is accumulation of mucopolysaccharide within the dermis. The thickening of facial skin folds gives the classic clinical appearance of a 'tragic facial expression'.

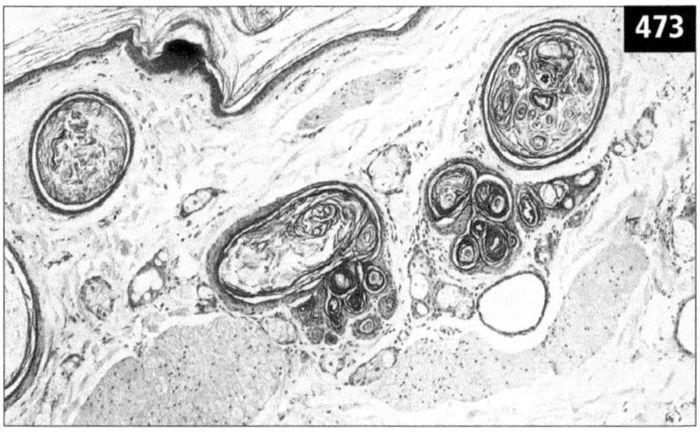

473 Atrophic dermatopathy in canine hypothyroidism. Skin biopsy from a nine-year-old Cairn Terrier with hypothyroidism. The changes of atrophic dermatopathy include epidermal thinning, hyperkeratosis and follicular keratosis, sebaceous gland atrophy and telogen hair follicles. A similar microscopic appearance will be seen with other canine endocrine disease, and hypothyroidism cannot be diagnosed on skin biopsy alone.

- Heat seeking.
- Bradycardia.
- Neuromuscular weakness (hypothyroid myopathy/peripheral neuropathy) with EMG and nerve conduction abnormalities, manifested as stiffness, gait abnormalities or lameness; or vestibular, facial or laryngeal nerve dysfunction.
- Corneal lipidosis.

Lymphocytic thyroiditis may occur concurrently with other autoimmune diseases, or as part of multisystemic autoimmune disease (see Chapter 14, p. 356).

Diagnosis

Screening tests for canine hypothyroidism include:

- Haematological examination, which may reveal mild, normocytic, normochromic anaemia.
- Serum biochemistry, which may reveal hypercholesterolaemia in approximately 66% of cases.
- Assessment of total serum T3 or T4. These are an inaccurate means of diagnosis, as euthyroid dogs with non-thyroidal illness may have reduced levels of these hormones ('euthyroid sick syndrome'). Additionally, some drugs (e.g. glucocorticoids, potentiated sulphonamides) affect T3 and T4 concentration and there may be significant variation in normal levels depending on breed, diurnal fluctuation or the concentration of serum binding proteins. The presence of serum T3 autoantibody may falsely elevate or lower (depending on the test used) serum concentration of T3 in some cases, but the prevalence of such autoantibodies is very low. Analysis of free (non-protein-bound) serum T4 has little advantage over measurement of total T4. However, a modified equilibrium dialysis assay is now available; this may have greater diagnostic accuracy and is unaffected by T4 autoantibodies.
- Endogenous canine TSH measurement is now routinely available for diagnosis of canine hypothyroidism. A low total or free T4 in combination with a high thyroid stimulating hormone (TSH) is considered diagnostic for the condition, but 18–38% of hypothyroid dogs have normal serum TSH and there may be overlap in serum TSH between hypothyroid dogs and euthyroid dogs with dermatological disease.

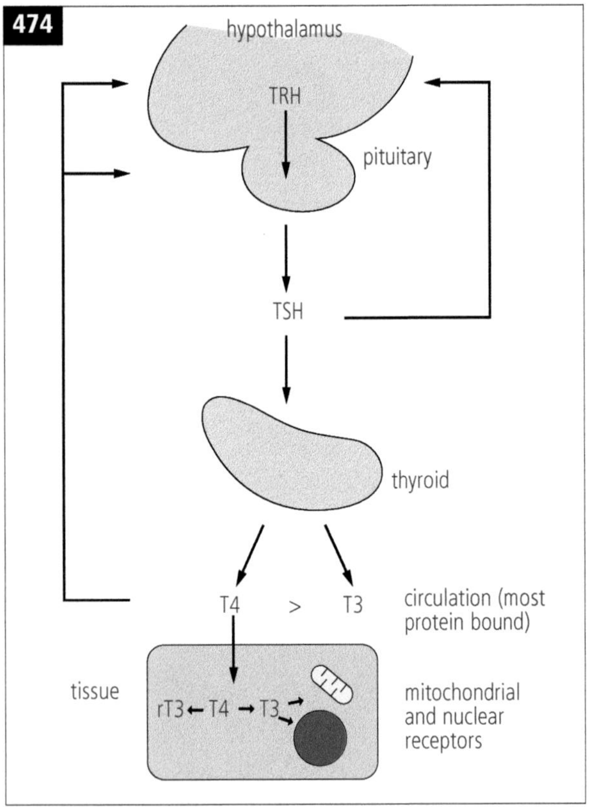

474 The hypothalamic–pituitary–thyroid axis. TRH from the hypothalamus stimulates the release of TSH from the adenohypophysis, which in turn stimulates production of T3 and T4. Negative feedback pathways are in operation at the levels indicated. T4 is present in greater concentration in the circulation and is converted to the active form (T3) within target cells. Some T4 can be converted to the inactive form, reverse T3, as a means of regulation.

In cases where there are borderline changes in thyroid function tests in the face of compatible clinical signs, T4 response to injectable exogenous TSH can be used (**474**). Failure to elevate the level of T4 in a blood sample collected 4–6 hours after intravenous injection or 8–12 hours after intramuscular injection suggests hypothyroidism. However, exogenous TSH is no longer widely available, so alternative diagnostic procedures have been investigated. Stimulation with thyrotropin releasing hormone (TRH) has also been used; however, it is a poor alternative, as TRH fails to stimulate T4 in some euthyroid dogs and the test has a specificity of only 75% for hypothyroidism. Recently, recombinant human TSH has become available and proven to be biologically active in the dog and therefore suitable for performing a TSH response test. However, this product is expensive and sold in a vial size much greater than required for a single canine TSH response test. Aliquots of recombinant human TSH (rHuTSH) may be frozen at –20°C for up to eight weeks without loss of activity.

Another diagnostic approach involves serological confirmation of autoimmunity, usually by ELISA for detection of circulating thyroglobulin autoantibodies (475). This autoantibody will only be found in appreciable titre in 50–70% of hypothyroid dogs, but it may also be found in the serum of euthyroid dogs (10–20%) and in up to 40% of dogs with non-thyroidal endocrine disease (476). The prevalence of such false-positive results may be reduced by selecting an appropriate cut-off value in the ELISA. Moreover, approximately 20% of thyroglobulin autoantibody positive dogs without clinical signs of thyroid disease develop thyroid dysfunction within one year, suggesting that in such cases the presence of autoantibody may be a marker for subclinical disease. Thyroid biopsy may also be undertaken for histological characterization of the thyroid disease.

Treatment and prognosis

The treatment of hypothyroidism is based on oral administration of synthetic levothyroxine sodium (0.01–0.02 mg/kg daily in 2 divided doses). Gradual introduction of therapy is recommended in animals with a decreased ability to metabolize thyroid hormones (e.g. cardiac cases, diabetic animals). In successfully treated hypothyroid dogs, weight loss, improved demeanour, hair regrowth and normalization of hair texture should occur in 1–2 months. When clinical response has been achieved, a single daily dose of levothyroxine is sufficient. The dose regime should be reassessed after four weeks of initial therapy, because metabolic changes may be induced by correction of the hypothyroid state. At this time, 'pre- and post-pill' serum T4 concentrations may be monitored. When once daily dosing with levothyroxine is being used, serum T4 should be at maximum concentration (and within normal range) 6–8 hours after administration.

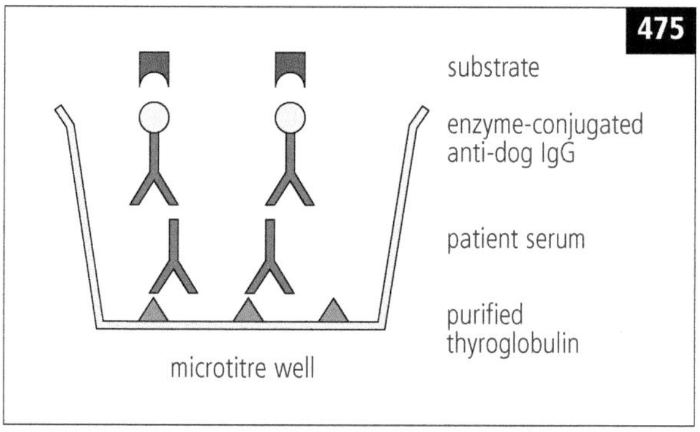

475 ELISA for detection of thyroglobulin autoantibody. The wells of microtitre plates are coated with purified canine thyroglobulin, washed and incubated with appropriate dilutions of patient serum. Binding of thyroglobulin autoantibody is demonstrated by subsequent addition of an enzyme-conjugated antiserum specific for canine IgG and the appropriate enzyme substrate.

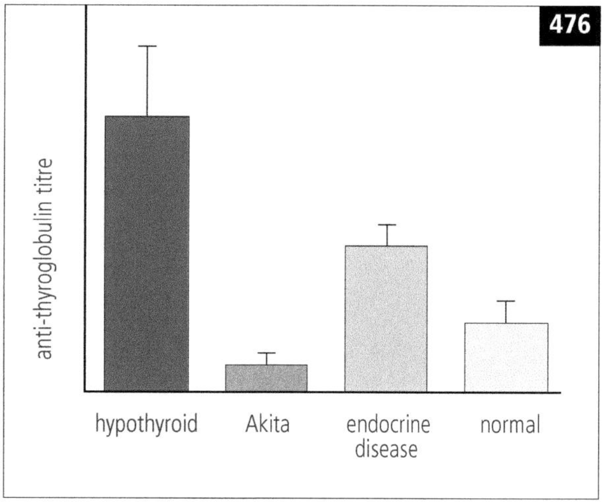

476 Survey of thyroglobulin autoantibodies in the dog. Sera from several groups of dogs were tested by ELISA for the presence of thyroglobulin autoantibody. Titres were greatest in dogs with hypothyroidism confirmed by TSH response testing, but autoantibodies were also occasionally detected in the sera of clinically normal dogs and dogs with other (non-thyroidal) endocrine disease. A survey of samples from Japanese Akitas revealed no significant level of autoantibodies. Dogs of this breed in the USA are reported as susceptible to hypothyroidism, but this survey was conducted in the UK and all dogs made an adequate response to TSH stimulation.

FELINE HYPERTHYROIDISM

The pathogenesis of feline hyperthyroidism involves excessive production of thyroid hormones by hyperplastic or neoplastic (thyroid follicular cell adenoma) thyroid tissue (477–479). Some affected cats may have serum ANA and thyroid-specific antibody, and in some cases there is lymphocytic infiltration of thyroid tissue. The significance of these changes in the pathogenesis of the disease is questionable. Hyperthyroid cats do not have circulating thyroid stimulating antibodies analogous to those of Graves' disease in man. Coincidentally, medical treatment of hyperthyroid cats with the drugs carbimazole or methimazole may lead to the induction of a range of immune-mediated side-effects including IMHA and serum antinuclear antibody.

LYMPHOCYTIC PARATHYROIDITIS

Primary idiopathic hypoparathyroidism in the dog may be associated with lymphocyte and plasma cell infiltration of the parathyroid gland, with fibrosis and loss of chief cells (480). Occasional cases with

477

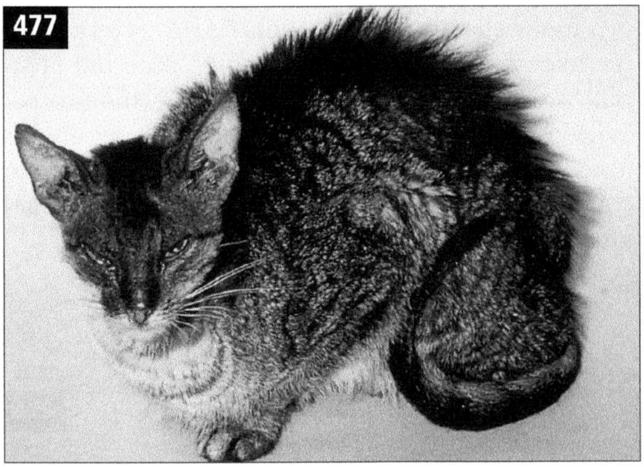

478

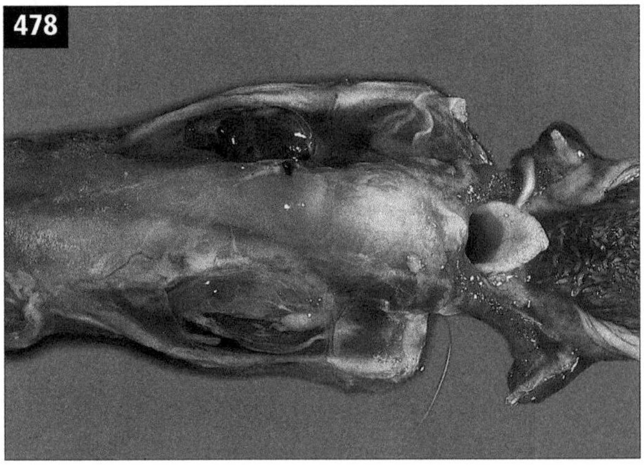

479

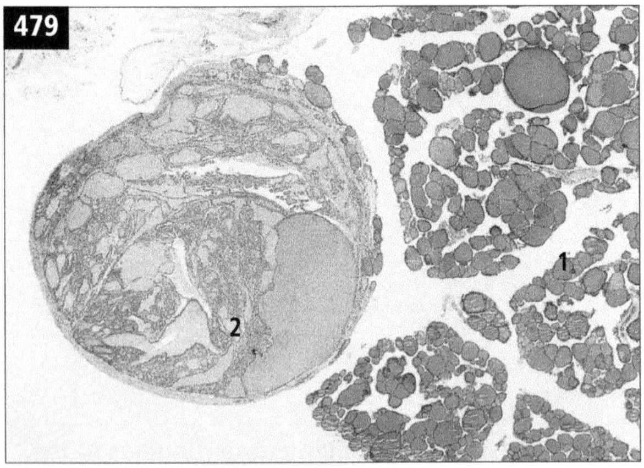

477–479 Feline hyperthyroidism. (**477**) An 11-year-old neutered male DSH cat with hyperthyroidism showing weight loss (despite polyphagia), unkempt coat and excessive claw growth. (**478**) Thyroid glands from a 19-year-old cat with no clinical evidence of hyperthyroidism. There is unilateral, well-circumscribed enlargement of the left thyroid gland. (**479**) Adenomatous hyperplasia of the thyroid of an 11-year-old DSH cat. The section shows the distinction between normal (1) and hyperplastic (2) thyroid tissue.

480

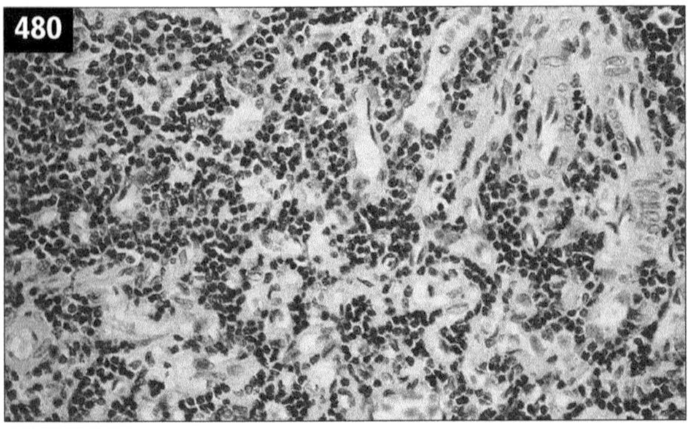

480 Canine lymphocytic parathyroiditis. Section of parathyroid gland from a dog with hypoparathyroidism. There is an intense lymphocytic infiltration of the gland, with reduction in the numbers of chief cells.

similar pathology are reported in the cat. The infiltrating cells have not been phenotyped and there is no documented serum autoantibody.

DIABETES MELLITUS

Human type I diabetes mellitus (juvenile diabetes) is a well-defined autoimmune disease characterized by:

- Macrophage and lymphocyte infiltration of the islets of Langerhans (insulitis) with loss of β cells.
- A strong genetic association with particular MHC allotypes.
- Familial inheritance.
- Serum autoantibodies specific for a range of antigens (e.g. β cell membrane and cytoplasmic components, particularly glutamic acid decarboxylase or GAD_{65}). Autoantibody is present in pre-diabetic sera and may provide an early diagnostic indicator.

Similar serological studies have been performed in dogs with diabetes mellitus. Antibodies specific for β cell cytoplasm have been demonstrated in the serum of diabetic dogs by indirect immunofluorescence using substrate sections of normal pancreas; however, pre-incubation of such sera with insulin abolished this labelling, suggesting that the antibodies were specific for exogenously administered insulin. In a later study, antibodies specific for non-cytoplasmic, β cell-membrane antigens were identified by indirect immunofluorescence in serum from approximately 50% of diabetic dogs before the initiation of insulin therapy. Moreover, it has been possible to distinguish between insulin autoantibody (by assessing reactivity to porcine insulin, which is identical to canine) and antibody specific for heterologous (bovine) insulin, and to examine the specificity of these antibodies for subcomponents of the insulin molecule by ELISA. Using these tests, the presence of insulin autoantibodies in pre-treatment canine diabetic sera has been confirmed. Recombinant canine GAD_{65} has also been produced and used to detect canine autoantibody specific for this molecule, and similar studies have been performed with the C-terminal region of the canine tyrosine phosphatase-like protein IA-2.

On the basis of such serological studies it is suggested that primary canine insulin deficiency diabetes mellitus has an immune-mediated pathogenesis equivalent to the latent autoimmune diabetes of adults (LADA) form of type I diabetes. However, a weakness in this argument is that lymphocytic insulitis is rarely documented in canine diabetes. Instead, canine primary diabetes mellitus appears to be a heterogenous disease that may also arise secondary to pancreatitis (**481**) or congenital β cell hypoplasia.

By contrast, canine insulin resistance diabetes occurs following antagonism of insulin function by other hormones in situations such as dioestrous or gestation, other concurrent endocrinopathy (e.g. hyperadrenocorticism, acromegaly) or iatrogenic administration of glucocorticoids or progestagens. There is little evidence for a canine equivalent to human type II (obesity-related) diabetes.

It is most likely that the observed autoantibodies in diabetic dogs do not have a role in disease pathogenesis, but may be an epiphenomenon, perhaps secondary to β cell damage during pancreatitis. Diabetes mellitus rarely occurs in dogs with other immune-mediated diseases. Some

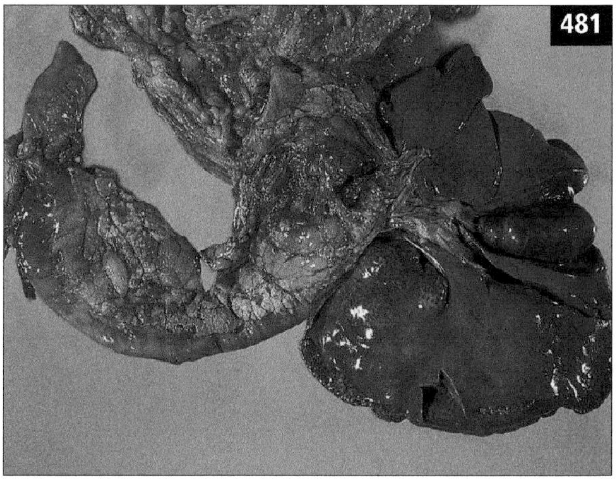

481 Canine diabetes mellitus. The majority of cases of diabetes mellitus in the dog are secondary to underlying factors such as pre-existing acute pancreatic necrosis or chronic pancreatitis. In this necropsy specimen from a six-year-old crossbred dog with acute pancreatitis, there is extensive fat necrosis and omental adhesion within the anterior abdomen largely mediated by local release of pancreatic enzymes. The acute necrosis destroys both exocrine and endocrine pancreas, resulting in diabetes mellitus.

diabetic dogs have also had clinical and serological evidence of hypothyroidism or pancreatic acinar atrophy (see Chapter 7, p. 225), and a single case of a dog with concurrent diabetes mellitus with antibodies specific for β cells, and presumptive AIHA, has been reported.

Breed susceptibilities to diabetes mellitus include the Miniature Schnauzer, Bichon Frise, Miniature Poodle, Samoyed, Tibetan Terrier and Cairn Terrier. The genetic association with DLA haplotypes is described in Chapter 3 and associations with polymorphisms in genes encoding insulin, various cytokines and CTLA-4 are described.

In the cat, diabetes mellitus is also primarily a secondary disease arising due to insulin resistance (e.g. hyperadrenocorticism, progestagen administration) (482). In some cases, β cell-derived amyloid may be deposited within the islets of Langerhans, resulting in loss of islet cells (483). There are also occasional reports of primary lymphocytic insulitis in diabetic cats, where the disease may have a presumptive immune-mediated basis. The lymphocytic infiltrate in one case was predominantly of T cells (484). One recent study has examined the presence of antibodies specific for β cells and insulin in newly diagnosed and insulin treated diabetic cats (with clinically normal and non-diabetes disease controls). Antibodies were only found in a small proportion of insulin treated cats, suggesting that in contrast to the dog, there is little evidence for an immune-mediated pathogenesis for feline diabetes.

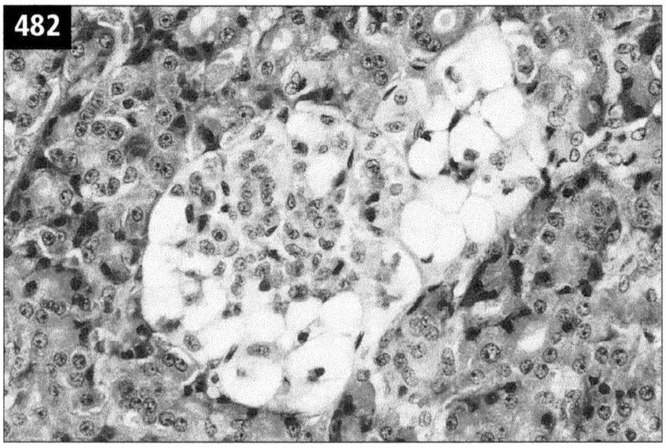

482 Feline insulin-resistant diabetes. Islet cell vacuolation in a six-year-old Burmese cat with hyperadrenocorticism (functional adrenal adenoma) and non-insulin-dependent diabetes mellitus (IDDM).

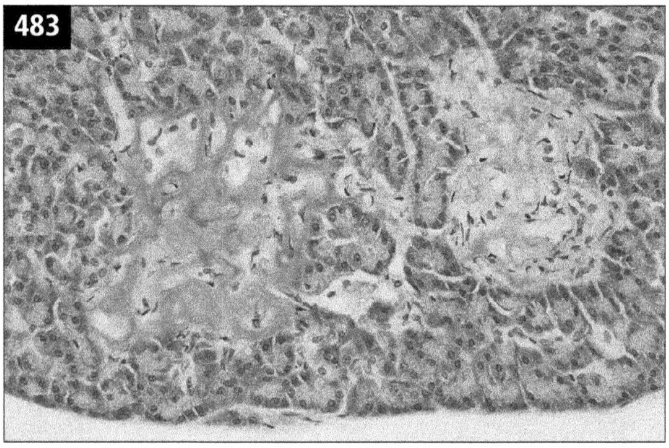

483 Feline islet amyloidosis. Section of pancreas (stained by Congo red) from an 11-year-old DSH cat with diabetes, demonstrating diffuse deposition of amyloid within the islets of Langerhans, with associated loss of islet cells. This islet-amyloid polypeptide is derived from pancreatic β cells, is co-secreted with insulin and may antagonize insulin function, resulting in non-IDDM that may progress to IDDM.

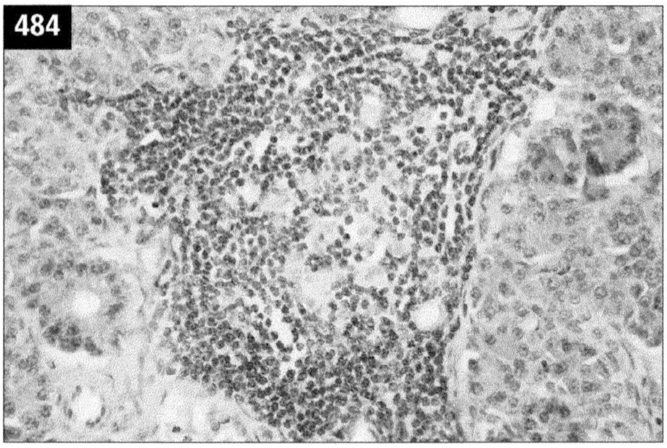

484 Insulitis in feline pancreas. Section of pancreas from a 12-year-old Siamese cat with diabetes in which there is lymphocytic infiltration of most islets of Langerhans, with loss of islet cells.

HYPOADRENOCORTICISM

Hypoadrenocorticism (Addison's-like disease) is most frequently documented in the dog. It occurs when there is significant compromise of adrenal cortical function, resulting in inadequate levels of glucocorticoid and/or mineralocorticoid hormones (**485**) (*Table 17*). A consistent female gender bias has been reported and the majority of affected dogs are of mixed breed. Although a range of underlying causes may result in hypoadrenocorticism (e.g. administration of o,p'DDD, sudden withdrawal from glucocorticoid therapy, destructive adrenal pathology) (**486**), the most commonly reported cause is primary, idiopathic, bilateral adrenal cortical atrophy.

In man, Addison's disease most often has an autoimmune basis as defined by:

- Serum autoantibodies specific for adrenal cortex cells and a series of enzymes involved in steroid metabolism (P450 cytochrome enzymes).
- Lymphocytic infiltration of the adrenal cortex.
- A genetic association with particular MHC types and an inherited basis.
- Association with other autoimmune endocrine diseases and non-endocrine diseases, as part of autoimmune polyglandular syndrome type 1 or 2 (e.g. hypothyroidism, Graves' disease, type I diabetes mellitus, pernicious anaemia, vitiligo).

It has recently been suggested that many cases of canine Addison's-like disease may also have an

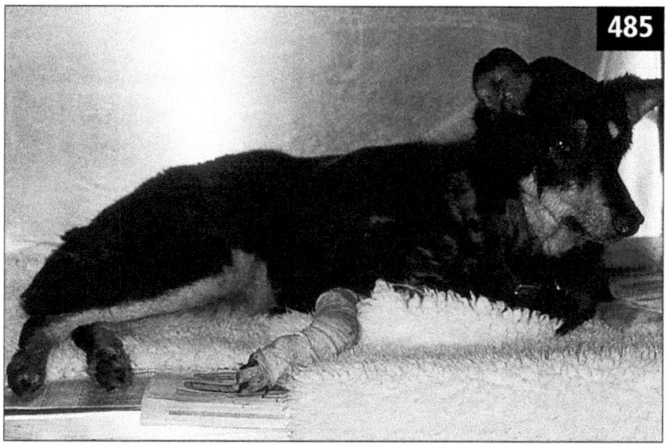

485 Canine hypoadrenocorticism. An 11-year-old female Collie-cross with weight loss, depression, episodic vomiting and diarrhoea, and weakness characteristic of hypoadrenocorticism.

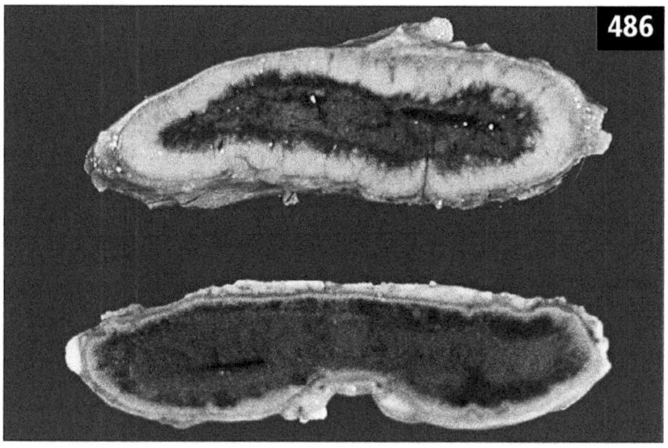

486 Reduced adrenal cortical tissue. Sagittal sections of adrenal gland from a normal dog, and a dog treated for hyperadrenocorticism with o,p'DDD (Lysodren) demonstrating marked reduction in the thickness of the adrenal cortex.

Table 17: Clinical signs of hypoadrenocorticism.
The features noted on clinical examination of dogs with hypoadrenocorticism are compared for two large studies of 111 (Study A) and 42 (Study B) affected dogs, respectively. The percentage of each population demonstrating the listed abnormality is given. Some parameters were not recorded (NR) in either study. (Study A: Feldman EC, Nelson RW (1996) Hypoadrenocorticism (Addison's disease). In *Canine and Feline Endocrinology and Reproduction* (2nd edn). (eds Feldman EC, Nelson RW) WB Saunders, Philadelphia, p. 274; Study B: Melian C, Peterson ME (1996) Diagnosis and treatment of naturally occurring hypoadrenocorticism in 42 dogs. *Journal of Small Animal Practice* **37**:268–275.)

Clinical abnormality	Study A (n = 111)	Study B (n = 42)
Depression	87	88
Thinness	82	NR
Weakness	56	62
Dehydration	35	36
Bradycardia	28	17
Weak femoral pulses	22	14
Melaena/haematochezia	22	17
Collapse	12	43
Abdominal pain	9	21
Hypothermia	NR	43
Reduced capillary refill time	NR	17

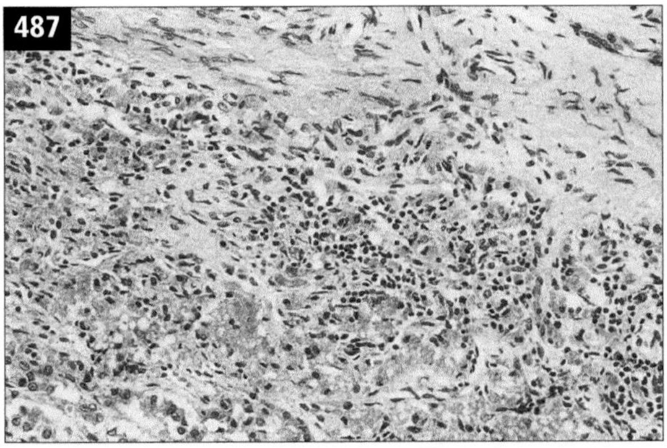

487 Lymphocytic infiltration of adrenal cortex. In this section of adrenal gland from a six-year-old Labrador Retriever with hypoadrenocorticism there is marked reduction in normal cortical tissue, with a prominent connective tissue capsule and adrenal medulla. Within the atrophic cortex is an infiltrate of lymphocytes. This histopathological appearance is consistent with findings in human hypoadrenocorticism and is supportive of an autoimmune pathogenesis for this form of canine Addison's disease.

autoimmune basis. Lymphoplasmacytic infiltration and fibrosis of adrenal cortex may be observed (487), and serum autoantibodies able to bind cortical cells on indirect immunofluorescence have been identified. DLA associations with Adisson's disease are described in Chapter 3.

POLYENDOCRINE DISEASE

A single case of polyendocrine disease with similarity to human polyglandular syndrome type 2 has been described in a middle-aged, female Weimaraner with hypothyroidism and subsequent hypoadrenocorticism. Serum autoantibodies specific for thyroid and adrenal tissue were identified by indirect immunofluorescence, but tissue was not examined microscopically.

FURTHER READING

Catchpole B, Ristic JM, Fleeman LM *et al.* (2005) Canine diabetes mellitus: can old dogs teach us new tricks? *Diabetologia* **48**:1948–1956.

Catchpole B, Kennedy LJ, Davison LJ *et al.* (2008) Canine diabetes mellitus: from phenotype to genotype. *Journal of Small Animal Practice* **49**:4–10.

Davison LJ, Ristic JME, Herrtage ME *et al.* (2003) Anti-insulin antibodies in dogs with naturally occurring diabetes mellitus. *Veterinary Immunology and Immunopathology* **91**:53–60.

Diaz Espineira MM, Mol JA, Peeters ME *et al.* (2007) Assessment of thyroid function in dogs with low plasma thyroxine concentration. *Journal of Veterinary Internal Medicine* **21**:25–32.

Hoenig M, Reusch C, Peterson ME (2000) Beta cell and insulin antibodies in treated and untreated diabetic cats. *Veterinary Immunology and Immunopathology* **77**:93–102.

Lee J-Y, Uzuka Y, Tanabe S *et al.* (2004) Tryptic peptides of canine thyroglobulin reactive with sera of patients with canine hypothyroidism caused by autoimmune thyroiditis. *Veterinary Immunology and Immunopathology* **101**:271–276.

Nachreiner RF, Refsal KR, Graham PA *et al.* (2002) Prevalence of serum thyroid hormone autoantibodies in dogs with clinical signs of hypothyroidism. *Journal of the American Veterinary Medical Association* **222**:466–471.

Rossmeisl JH, Duncan RB, Inzana KD *et al.* (2009) Longitudinal study of the effects of chronic hypothyroidism on skeletal muscle in dogs. *American Journal of Veterinary Research* **70**:879–889.

Short AD, Catchpole B, Kennedy LJ *et al.* (2009) T cell cytokine gene polymorphisms in canine diabetes mellitus. *Veterinary Immunology and Immunopathology* **128**:137–146.

Short AD, Saleh NM, Catchpole B *et al.* (2010) CTLA4 promoter polymorphisms are associated with canine diabetes mellitus. *Tissue Antigens* **75**:242–252.

Skopek E, Patzl M, Nachreiner RF (2006) Detection of autoantibodies against thyroid peroxidase in serum samples of hypothyroid dogs. *American Journal of Veterinary Research* **67**:809–814.

10 IMMUNE-MEDIATED RENAL AND REPRODUCTIVE DISEASE

Michael J. Day and Andrew Mackin

INTRODUCTION

This chapter describes the major immune-mediated renal and reproductive diseases of dogs and cats. The best defined example of the former is immune complex glomerulonephritis (ICGN), which is a relatively common and clinically significant disease of the dog and cat. In contrast, true autoimmune glomerulonephropathy is rarely documented, and the role of the immune system in other diseases such as chronic interstitial nephritis is poorly characterized. Reproductive immunology of the dog and cat is also an area about which relatively little is known compared with other species. Of greatest clinical relevance is the fact that a proportion of cases of infertility in male dogs may have an immune-mediated pathogenesis.

IMMUNE COMPLEX GLOMERULONEPHRITIS

Pathogenesis

The formation of circulating immune complexes (CICs) in situations of moderate antigen excess, and the factors which contribute to their deposition in tissue, have been discussed in Chapter 2. One site that favours immune complex deposition is the renal glomerulus, which is a region of both high blood pressure and ultrafiltration. CICs form in a wide range of infectious, inflammatory, neoplastic or immune-mediated diseases, and may be detected by the assays described in Chapter 5. In many cases the antigenic component of the immune complexes is not identified, but microbial antigens (e.g. bacterial, FIP virus, FeLV, *Leishmania*) are likely to be common, and tissue (e.g. nuclear) antigens may be significant in autoimmune diseases. Elevated concentrations of circulating immune complexes have been demonstrated in dogs with protein losing nephropathy and histopathological evidence of glomerulonephritis. Drugs may also be associated with the development of glomerulonephritis via a type III mechanism, and glomerulonephritis has been documented in Dobermanns treated with sulphonamides and in a dog treated with the immunomodulatory agent *Propionibacterium acnes* (Immunoregulin) for cutaneous melanoma.

CICs may lodge within the glomerulus at different levels, depending largely on their size and charge (**488**). Following immune complex

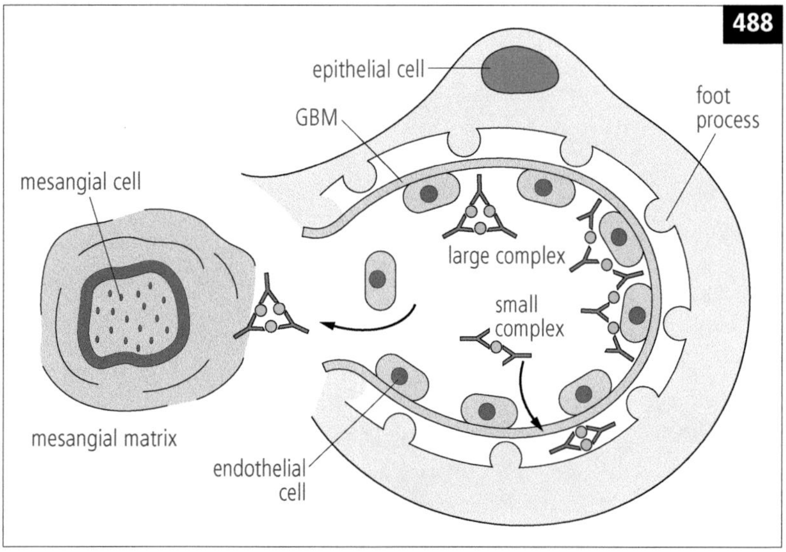

488 Immune complex deposition within the glomerulus. The deposition of CICs within the renal glomerulus depends upon numerous factors, including the size and charge of the complex. Large complexes may be taken into the mesangium or deposit on the endothelial side of the GBM. Small complexes may pass through the GBM and be deposited on the epithelial side of the GBM.

deposition, complement may be activated and the sequence of events that characterizes type III hypersensitivity will be initiated. Primary glomerulitis results in secondary tubular damage and eventual loss of the entire nephron (glomerulonephritis), with interstitial fibrosis and glomerulosclerosis. Alternatively, complexes may be eliminated and the glomerular changes and clinical disease resolve.

An alternative mechanism for ICGN is that immune complexes are formed locally rather than exiting preformed from the circulation. In this instance, circulating antigen of optimum charge would deposit within the glomerulus (subepithelial) and subsequently bind circulating low avidity antibody (489). Experimental data have suggested that this mechanism has a role in canine *Dirofilaria*

489

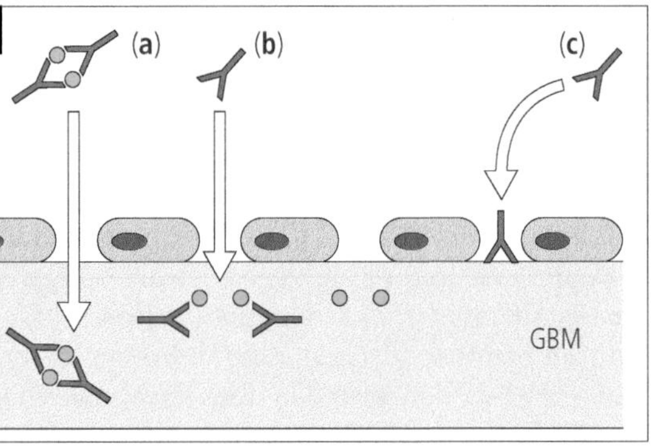

489 Mechanisms of immune-mediated glomerular disease. (**a**) Immune-mediated glomerulonephritis is generally assumed to involve deposition of preformed immune complexes from the circulation at various sites within the GBM or mesangium (see **488**). (**b**) Alternatively, circulating antigen may be deposited initially, and subsequently bind circulating antibody to form an immune complex *in situ*. (**c**) True autoimmune glomerulopathy involves binding of an autoantibody with specificity for epitopes of the GBM, but this form of immune-mediated renal disease is rare in dogs and cats.

490

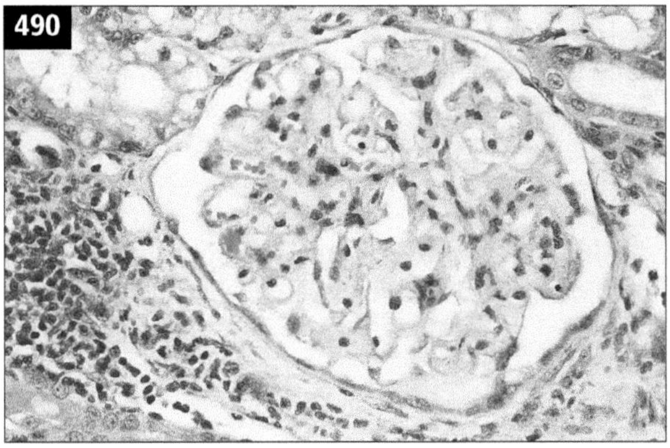

491

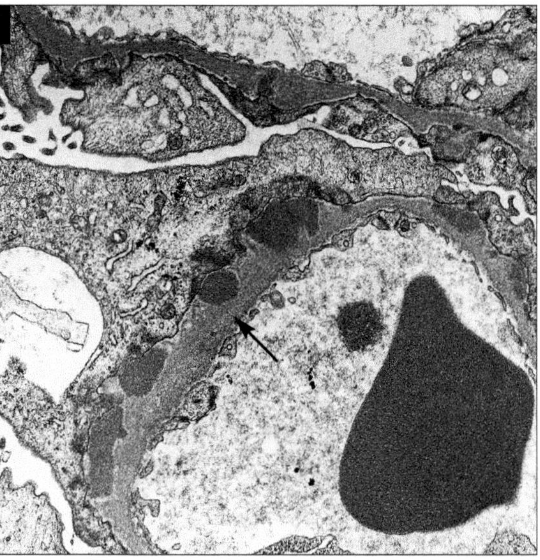

492

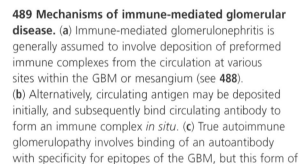

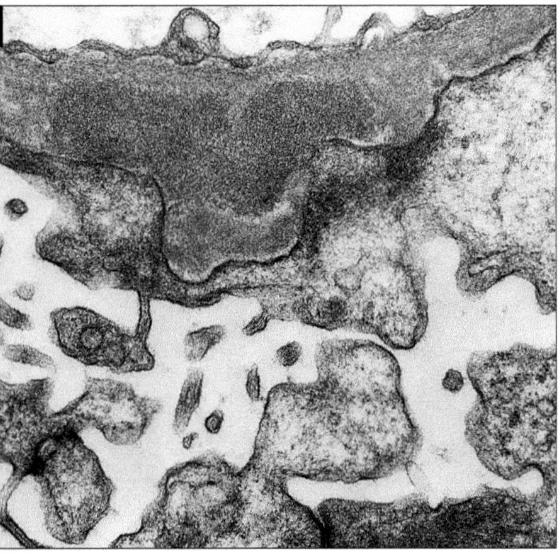

490–492 Membranous glomerulonephritis. (**490**) Section of kidney from a five-year-old DLH cat with ascites and subcutaneous oedema. There is enlargement of the glomerular tuft, with thickening of capillary basement membrane and a focal, mixed mononuclear infiltration of the interstitium. (**491**) Electron micrograph of kidney from a two-year-old DSH cat with ventral oedema, weight loss, proteinuria and hypoproteinaemia due to membranous glomerulonephritis. There are prominent electron-dense deposits on the epithelial side of the basement membrane (arrowed), with fusion of overlying foot processes. (**492**) Higher power detail of similar immune complex deposited within the glomerulus of a two-year-old DLH cat with ascites, ventral oedema, hypoalbuminaemia, proteinuria and elevated blood urea nitrogen. (Electron micrographs **491** and **492** courtesy V.M. Lucke.)

immitis-induced glomerulonephritis. The relative role of CIC deposition or *in situ* immune complex formation is an area of debate; in some situations both mechanisms may be involved. There is also a line of thought suggesting that immune complex deposition or formation is not the primary cause of glomerular damage in glomerulonephritis, but is secondary to damage by other agents.

ICGN may appear microscopically as one of several different morphological variants, depending on the site of complex deposition, although it is possible for more than one glomerular lesion to be present within the same kidney. All forms of ICGN have been documented in dogs with leishmaniosis.

In diffuse **membranous glomerulonephritis,** immune complexes lodge on the epithelial side of the glomerular basement membrane (GBM), resulting in basement membrane thickening but no cellular proliferation or inflammatory infiltration (490–492).

In **membranoproliferative glomerulonephritis,** immune complexes deposit in the mesangium and on either/both endothelial and epithelial sides of the GBM. There is thickening of the GBM in parallel with mesangial, epithelial or endothelial proliferation (493–495).

Mesangioproliferative glomerulonephritis is relatively uncommon and is characterized by increased glomerular cellularity and axial accumulation of mesangial matrix, and is the result of deposition of large immune complexes in the mesangium.

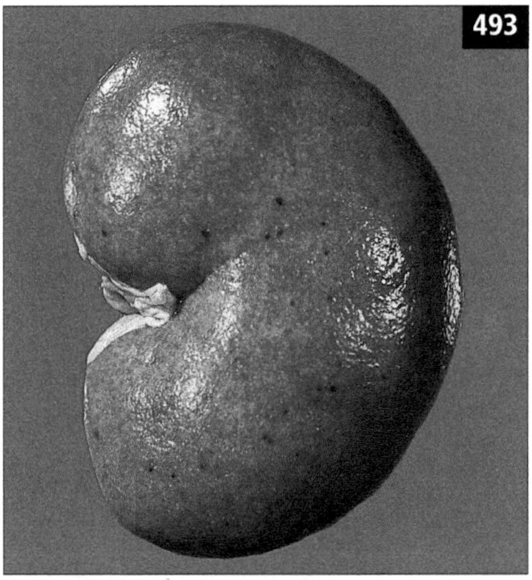

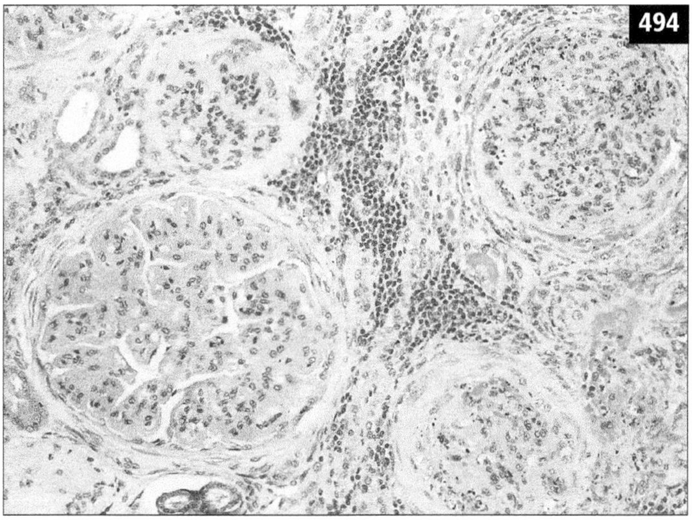

493–495 Membranoproliferative glomerulonephritis. (**493**) Gross necropsy appearance of a kidney from a seven-year-old female Springer Spaniel with chronic renal failure. The kidney has normal overall size and shape, but the surface is flecked with pinpoint white foci and occasional microhaemorrhages are present. (**494**) Section from the same kidney demonstrates glomerular enlargement, increased mesangium and glomerular and interstitial inflammation. (**495**) Section stained by methenamine silver demonstrates enlargement of glomeruli, exaggerated tuft formation (hypercellularity) and 'spike' formation on the GBM.

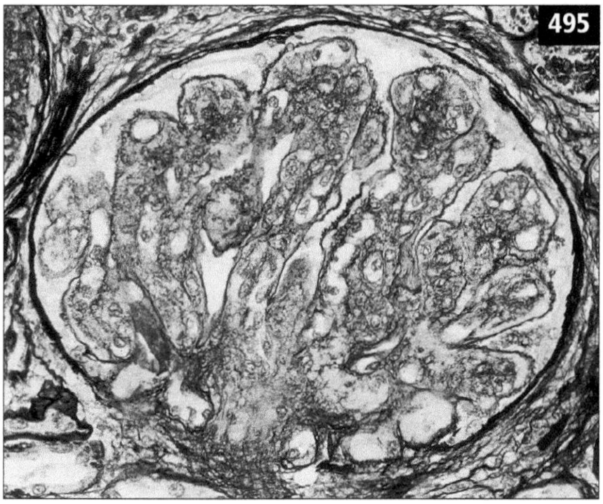

Clinical signs

The end result of advanced ICGN is complete loss of glomerular and tubular function. When more than 75% of functional nephrons have been lost, affected animals will show clinical signs typical of chronic renal failure (**496–499**):

- Loss of tubular concentrating ability, manifest as polyuria, polydipsia and gradual reduction in urine specific gravity towards isosthenuria (1.008–1.014). However, in acute, severe renal failure, oliguria or even anuria may be observed.
- Loss of glomerular ability to excrete solute, leading to azotaemia (elevated blood urea and creatinine) and eventual uraemia (the group of clinical signs and laboratory findings typically associated with advanced renal failure, including anorexia, weight loss, malaise, dehydration, vomiting and oral ulceration, and azotaemia, hyperphosphataemia and anaemia).

However, although active glomerulonephritis will typically progress to renal failure, earlier disease often manifests solely as a protein-losing nephropathy, an indicator of selective loss of one particular glomerular function. In the healthy animal the glomerulus acts as a charge- and size-selective filter, which enables excretion of solutes such as urea while retaining larger molecules (including most proteins) within the circulation. The first major glomerular abnormality associated with glomerulonephritis is loss of this filter function, leading to selective loss of plasma proteins such as albumin. The initial manifestation of protein-losing nephropathy is proteinuria. However, advanced disease can lead to development of the nephrotic syndrome that consists of:

- Proteinuria.
- Hypoproteinaemia (specifically hypoalbuminaemia).
- Hypercholesterolaemia.
- Loss of plasma oncotic pressure leading to ascites, pleural effusion and oedema (although oedema is relatively uncommon in dogs and cats) (**500**).

496

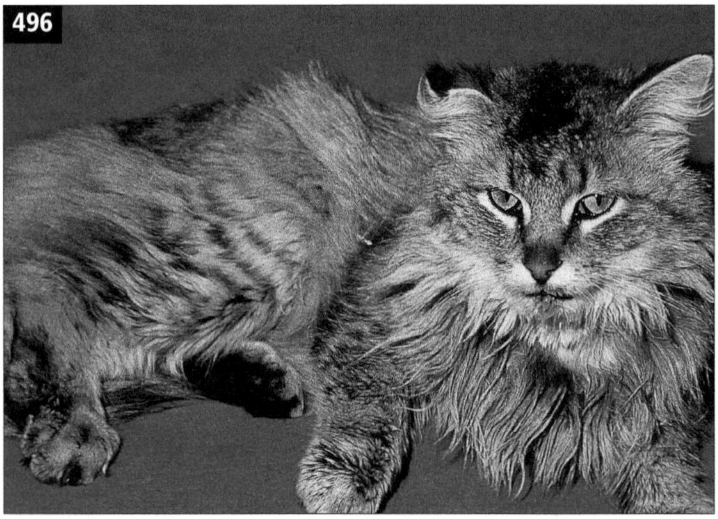

497

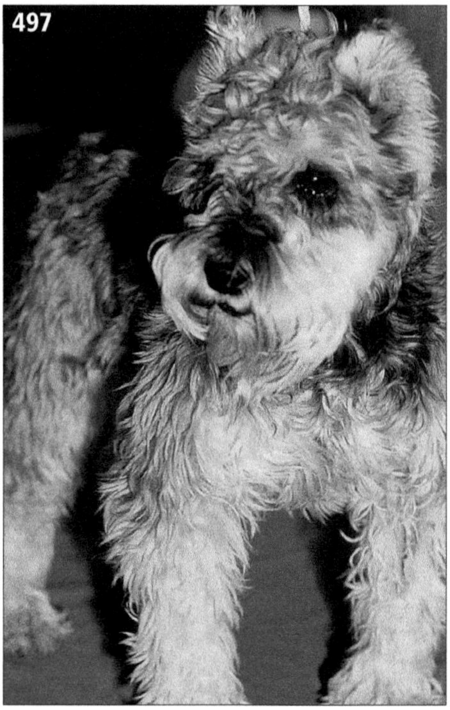

496, 497 Chronic renal disease: clinical presentation. (**496**) Older cat with end-stage renal disease secondary to glomerulonephritis, showing the typical clinical signs of weight loss, anorexia, vomiting, polydipsia and polyuria. Blood analysis revealed mild non-regenerative anaemia, moderate hyperphosphataemia and marked azotaemia. The cat also had hypertrophic cardiomyopathy secondary to hypertension caused by the renal disease. (**497**) Middle-aged Miniature Schnauzer with glomerulonephritis. Although this particular patient had marked proteinuria, mild hypoalbuminaemia and some degree of weight loss, the owners did not present the animal for examination until the renal disease was advanced enough for tubular dysfunction to cause noticeable polydipsia and polyuria.

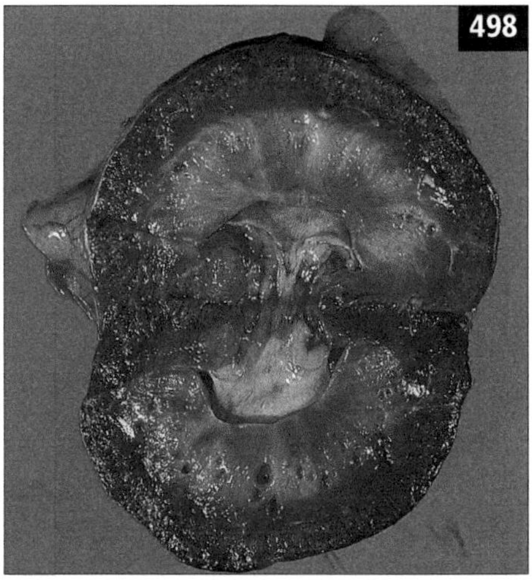

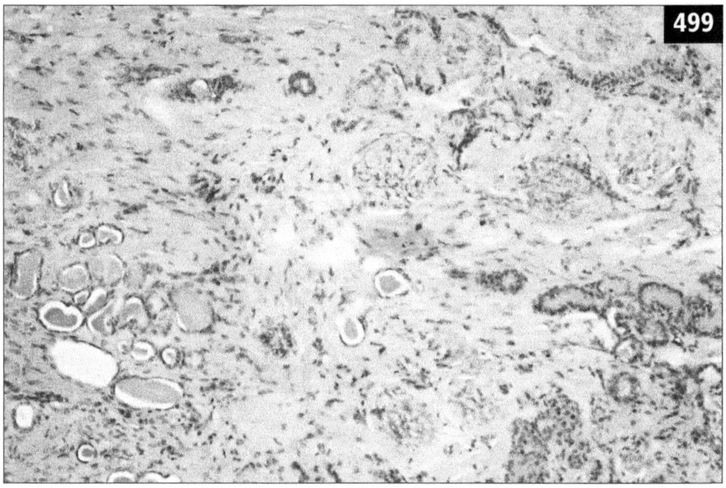

498, 499 End-stage renal disease. (**498**) Sagitally sectioned kidney from a seven-year-old Airedale with vomiting, polyuria/polydypsia and elevated BUN. The kidney is reduced in size, with an irregular, pitted surface and small cystic areas. The microscopic appearance is of diffuse chronic interstitial nephritis. (**499**) Section of kidney from a seven-year-old Dobermann that had progressive renal failure over a two-year period. At necropsy there was gross scarring of both kidneys. Normal renal structure is replaced by extensive areas of fibrosis. Tubular degeneration and regeneration and glomerular sclerosis and calcification are apparent.

500 Nephrotic syndrome. Ascites and some degree of ventral peripheral oedema in a cat with nephrotic syndrome caused by glomerulonephritis. Although the classical features of nephrotic syndrome include ascites and oedema, these particular manifestations are in fact very uncommon in the dog and cat. (Photograph courtesy D. Foster.)

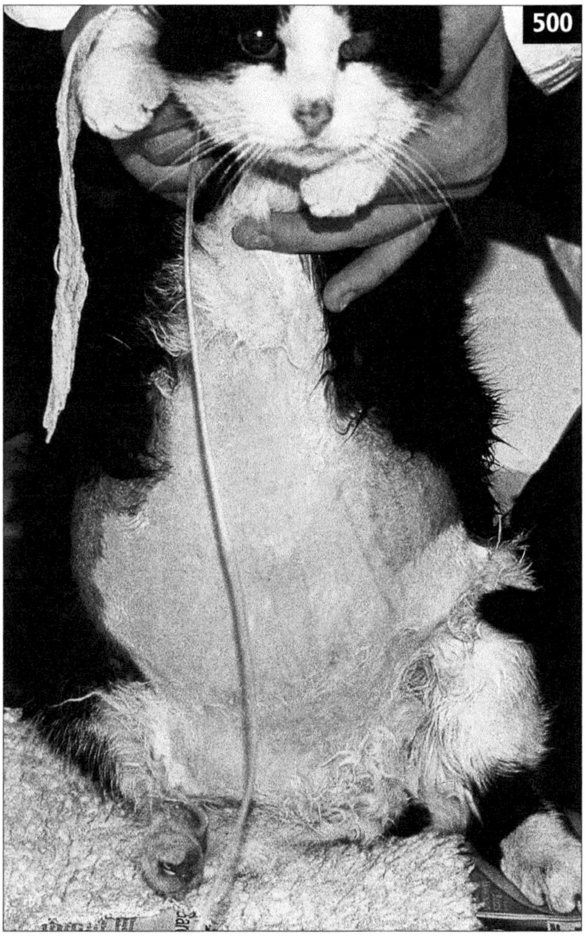

Potential complications of glomerulonephritis, besides nephrotic syndrome and renal failure, include hypertension (with retinal haemorrhage or detachment) and thromboembolic disease (particularly pulmonary thromboembolism). The latter complication is generally attributed to loss of antithrombin III by glomerular leakage.

Diagnosis

In animals suspected of having ICGN, appropriate diagnostic measures should be taken to identify any primary underlying cause (e.g. infection, neoplasia, autoimmunity, drug administration). Antemortem diagnosis of ICGN involves progression through a series of laboratory diagnostic measures (501):

501

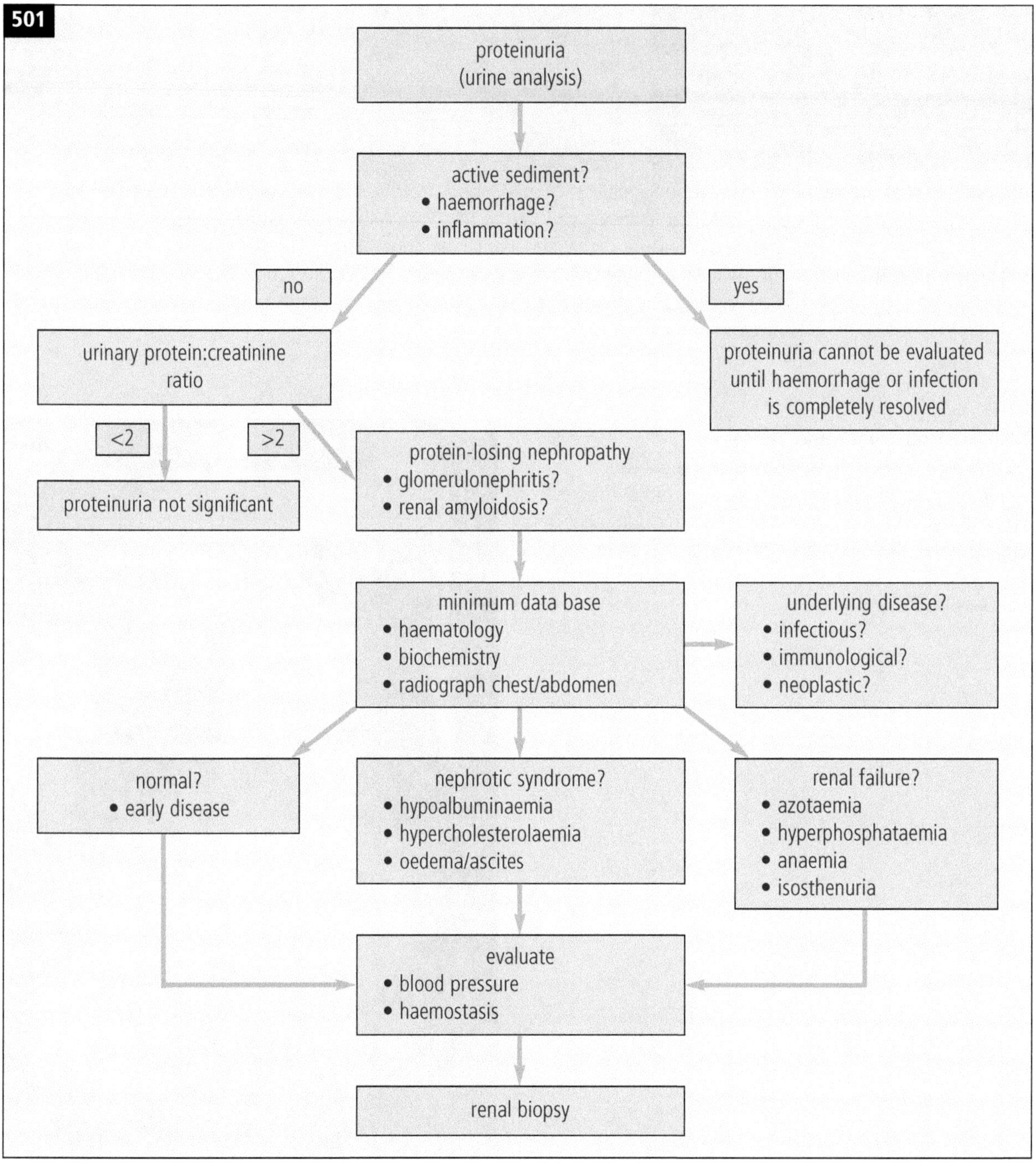

501 Diagnostic approach to proteinuria.

- Urinalysis. Excessive urinary protein loss is the hallmark of ICGN and can be the only detectable abnormality in early cases. Urinary dipstick detection of protein in the absence of urinary tract infection or haemorrhage (i.e. in animals with a normal urinary sediment) should prompt more accurate quantification of protein loss by measurement of the urinary protein:creatinine ratio. A ratio greater than two, in the presence of normal urinary sediment, strongly suggests protein-losing nephropathy. As ICGN progresses to renal failure, urine specific gravity will also steadily decline.
- Serum biochemistry in more advanced cases may reveal evidence of nephrotic syndrome (hypoproteinaemia, hypoalbuminaemia and hypercholesterolaemia) and eventual renal failure (azotaemia, hyperphosphataemia).
- Haematology may reveal a non-regenerative anaemia associated with chronic renal failure in advanced cases. Antithrombin III activity may be reduced in dogs with protein-losing nephropathy.

In dogs and cats the only common causes of protein-losing nephropathy are ICGN and amyloidosis, of which glomerulonephritis is the more prevalent entity. However, in order to confirm a diagnosis of ICGN, and to rule-out amyloidosis, renal biopsy is necessary. Renal biopsy is usually performed by ultrasound-guided percutaneous needle biopsy. The early lesions of glomerulonephritis are often unremarkable on haematoxylin and eosin staining. GBM thickening may be appreciated more readily with the use of periodic acid-Schiff (PAS) or PAS-methenamine silver staining. Whenever feasible, blood pressure and haemostatic parameters should be assessed prior to renal biopsy.

Immunohistochemistry

The definitive diagnostic procedure for demonstrating glomerular immune complexes is immunohistochemical examination of biopsy tissue (see Chapter 5, p. 153). A panel of antisera specific for IgG, IgM, IgA and complement C3 should be used. Such complexes will generally have an irregular, granular appearance associated with the GBM, or they may be identified within the mesangium (502, 503). The Ig most often identified is IgG, but

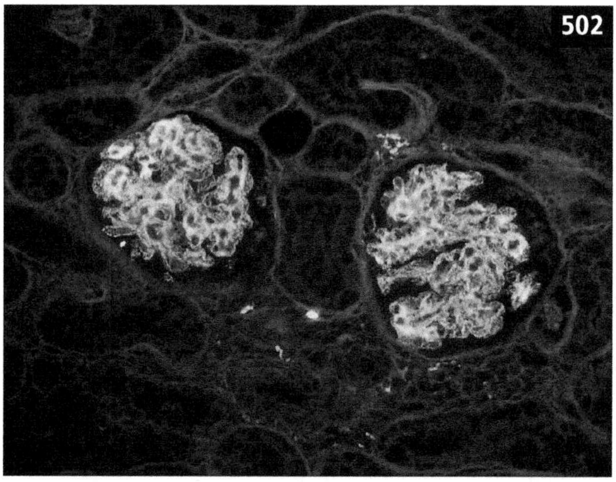

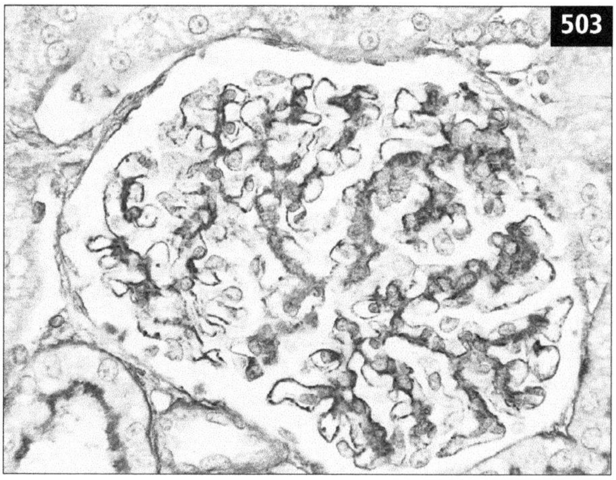

502, 503 Demonstration of glomerular immune complex deposition. The presence and composition of immune complexes may be demonstrated by immunohistochemistry. (**502**) Section of kidney from a three-year-old DSH cat with membranous glomerulonephritis. Labelling with a fluorescein-linked antiserum specific for feline IgG demonstrates granular deposition of immune complex along the basement membrane on UV microscopy. (**503**) Section of kidney from a one-year-old DSH cat with membranous glomerulonephritis labelled by the indirect immunoperoxidase method using an antiserum specific for feline IgG. (From Day MJ (1996) Diagnostic assessment of the feline immune system. Part II. *Feline Practice* **24**:14–25, with permission.) There is multifocal labelling of the glomerular basement membrane.

IgM and IgA may also be present. In one study, positive labelling for IgM and IgA was infrequently associated with electron-dense deposits on electron microscopy, suggesting that this labelling represented non-specific trapping of these Igs in damaged mesangium and GBM. In contrast, the few reports of canine IgA nephropathy involve deposition of IgA associated with mesangioproliferative or membranoproliferative disease. Positive glomerular immunofluorescence may also be demonstrated in the kidneys of many randomly selected dogs that do not have clinical renal disease. In the cat it has been suggested that the presence of IgG alone (with or without C3) is correlated with a favourable long-term prognosis, whereas the addition of IgM and IgA is associated with renal failure.

The absence of demonstrable immunoreactants does not necessarily rule out an immunological pathogenesis, and it may reflect an inappropriate biopsy site or the presence of advanced renal lesions with glomerulosclerosis and reabsorption of immune complex. It is not routinely possible to identify the antigenic component of the immune complexes by immunohistochemistry.

Electron microscopy

Electron microscopy can be used to localize immune complexes to the endothelial (subendothelial) or epithelial (subepithelial) side of the GBM. There may be fusion of the epithelial foot processes over the affected GBM. Subepithelial complexes may be separated by ‘spikes’ of GBM and may eventually be surrounded by, and incorporated into, the GBM. Thus, subepithelial complexes may with time become intramembranous and the presence of intramembranous deposits, in addition to subepithelial deposits, in cats with glomerulonephritis is associated with a poorer clinical prognosis. In membranoproliferative glomerulonephritis the thickening of the GBM may be attributed to infiltration of the membrane by mesangial processes or matrix.

Adjunct tests

The concentration of CICs (see Chapter 5, p. 146) and serum complement components (see Chapter 12, p. 295) may be assessed in ICGN. Reduced levels of complement (C3 or C4) may suggest complement consumption in immune complex removal or a genetic deficiency of specific complement components, which may lead to failure to adequately clear immune complexes. However, one recent study failed to demonstrate reduced serum concentrations of C3 in dogs with protein-losing nephropathy using a sensitive ELISA. Animals with ICGN may also have serum ANA, particularly if underlying autoimmune disease (e.g. SLE) is present, but there is no apparent association between ANA titre and severity of renal disease.

Treatment

Treatment of the disease process that triggered the development of ICGN is the primary consideration, and glomerulonephritis is unlikely to resolve unless the underlying disease is eliminated. However, even when an underlying disease can be identified and eliminated, glomerulonephritis will often progress unless immunosuppressive and anti-inflammatory therapy is instituted.

Immunosuppressive therapy

In theory, oral prednisone or prednisolone alone, at an immunosuppressive dose rate, would be expected to be an effective treatment for ICGN. Indeed, the sporadic individual case of ICGN in dogs and cats does improve, sometimes dramatically, following commencement of glucocorticoid therapy. Unfortunately, many other patients either fail to improve or actually deteriorate after commencing glucocorticoid therapy. Many of the common side-effects of steroid therapy, such as volume retention, increased catabolism and susceptibility to infection, are poorly tolerated in animals with nephrotic syndrome and/or renal failure. Furthermore, by reducing removal of CICs by the mononuclear phagocytic system, glucocorticoids can potentially lead to an increase in deposition of immune complexes at the glomerulus. For these reasons, if glucocorticoids are used at all in patients with ICGN, initial response to therapy should be carefully monitored for potential side-effects and progression of renal disease.

Other immunosuppressive agents have not as yet been shown to be effective for treating ICGN in dogs and cats, although benefits may be seen in the individual patient:

- Azathioprine (dogs only) at a daily oral dose of 2 mg/kg.
- Cyclophosphamide at a dose of either 2 mg/kg or 50 mg/m^2 orally every second day or for 3–4 consecutive days in each week.
- Ciclosporin (dogs only) at a daily oral dose of 5 mg/kg.

Anti-inflammatory therapy

Prostaglandins such as thromboxane, released from platelets activated at the site of immune complex deposition, have a significant role in perpetuating the inflammatory processes that exacerbate glomerular damage in ICGN. Antiplatelet agents such as aspirin and dipyridamole, as well as more specific thromboxane synthetase inhibitors, may therefore delay or reverse the progression of ICGN. Trial therapy with very low (antiplatelet) doses of aspirin (0.5 mg/kg q24h or q12h) is therefore indicated in patients with confirmed ICGN. In contrast, aspirin at standard doses (10–25 mg/kg q12–q8h) is potentially nephrotoxic.

Dietary supplementation with omega-3 fatty acids may also potentially alleviate glomerulonephritis by decreasing the production of harmful prostaglandins such as thromboxane and concurrently increasing the production of prostaglandins, which inhibit platelet function and have a beneficial effect on renal haemodynamics.

Adjunctive therapy

The recommended dietary therapy for patients with ICGN includes sodium restriction to minimize hypertension, volume expansion and susceptibility to oedema, and phosphate restriction in those animals with overt renal failure. Dietary protein should be of a high biological value and modestly restricted, since the feeding of a high protein diet to patients with protein-losing nephropathy (although understandably tempting in those patients with low serum albumin levels) merely increases the magnitude of proteinuria and may actually worsen hypoalbuminaemia.

Ascites and oedema that fails to respond to dietary sodium restriction alone may resolve with strict cage rest and diuretics. Renal haemodynamics, particularly in hypertensive patients, may be improved by the careful use of angiotensin converting enzyme (ACE) inhibitors such as captopril, enalapril and benazepril. Although anticoagulant drugs such as warfarin and heparin may be of some benefit in preventing pulmonary thromboembolism, most clinicians prefer to rely solely on the anti-platelet effects of low doses of aspirin.

Prognosis

Unfortunately, most dogs and cats with ICGN progress to develop severe nephrotic syndrome or terminal renal failure. Descriptions of successful treatment of glomerulonephritis are limited to sporadic case reports. The poor prognosis associated with ICGN probably reflects the fact that proteinuria is usually asymptomatic until glomerulonephritis progresses to nephrotic syndrome or renal failure, so a diagnosis is often only established late in the disease process. Furthermore, it is often not possible to identify and eliminate the underlying cause of the ICGN.

GLOMERULAR BASEMENT MEMBRANE AUTOIMMUNITY

Autoimmune glomerulonephritis occurs when autoantibody binds to epitopes of the GBM, initiating an immunopathological sequence similar to that in ICGN. In this case, immunohistochemistry demonstrates linear deposition of immunoglobulin or complement along the GBM, with initial absence of electron dense deposits on electron microscopy. However, with time, granular immune complexes form and the pattern of immunohistochemical labelling changes. This condition is rarely described in the dog, but it can be induced experimentally in this species.

CHRONIC INTERSTITIAL NEPHRITIS

Chronic interstitial nephritis is one form of tubulointerstitial disease. It is caused by a range of specific agents (microbial, toxic, chemical, drug) in addition to putative immunological mechanisms. The disease is characterized by progressive interstitial inflammation (predominantly lympho-

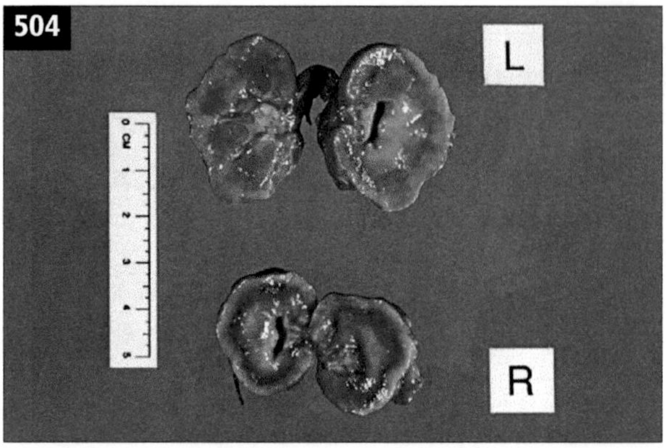

504 Interstitial nephritis. Kidneys from a cat with histological evidence of severe chronic interstitial nephritis. The kidneys are reduced in size and have an irregular cortical outline, with reduction in width of the cortex.

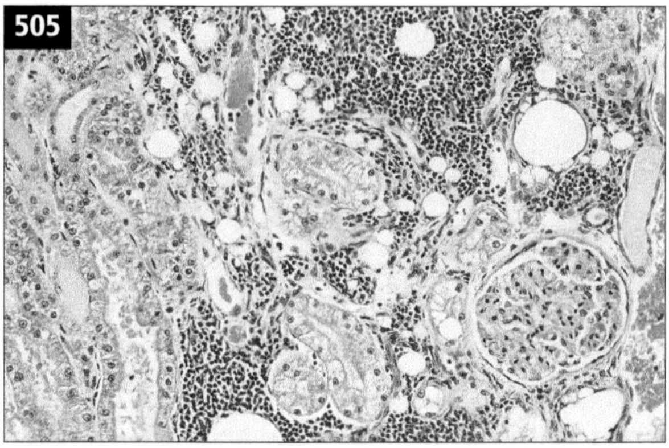

505 Interstitial nephritis. Section of kidney taken at necropsy from a five-year-old Siamese cat with neurological disease. Both kidneys have multiple foci of interstitial lymphoplasmacytic infiltration. Subclinical interstitial nephritis is a common postmortem finding in middle-aged to older cats.

plasmacytic) and fibrosis, with tubular atrophy and degeneration, leading to secondary glomerular injury (504, 505). The clinical features will therefore be associated with failure of tubular, rather than glomerular, function, but in end-stage disease there will be renal failure and uraemia.

In humans and in experimental models, both tubular basement membrane autoantibody-induced and immune complex-induced tubulointerstitial disease is described. Tubular basement membrane autoantibody has been described in a dog with tubulointerstitial nephritis, but production of this antibody may have been secondary to pre-existing renal pathology.

One study has demonstrated expression of MHC class II by tubular epithelial cells, peritubular vascular endothelium, interstitial dendritic cells and infiltrating mononuclear cells in dogs with tubulointerstitial nephritis. Glomeruli were not positively labelled. It was hypothesized that tubular absorption of cytokines (e.g. IFNγ) and immunogenic peptides in these dogs may have induced class II expression by tubular epithelia.

REPRODUCTIVE IMMUNOLOGY

There is a relative paucity of knowledge of the role of the immune system in reproductive disorders of the dog and cat. Infertility in male dogs may have a wide range of causes, but it has been postulated that dogs with spermatogenic arrest or poor semen quality may occasionally have underlying autoimmunity directed at spermatozoa. Such autoantibody may also be generated following testicular damage, with breakdown of the blood-testis barrier and exposure of previously sequestered spermatic antigens to the immune system. The nature of such antigens is poorly defined. Anti-sperm antibodies may also potentially be generated in females and be a cause of infertility. Anti-sperm antibodies have been experimentally induced in dogs following immunization with sperm antigen in adjuvant, and may be detected in the serum (506, 507).

The infertility and testicular atrophy that occurs in dogs chronically infected with *Brucella canis* may have an immunological basis. Evidence for this hypothesis was obtained in an experimental study that demonstrated:

- Serum and seminal fluid antibodies able to agglutinate sperm, with high titred antibodies contained in the IgA-rich fraction of seminal plasma.
- Seminal plasma cytophilic factors that could mediate adherence of sperm to isolated splenic macrophages.
- Positive DTH response on intradermal inoculation of testicular antigen.
- Lymphoplasmacytic infiltration of atrophic testes, with correlation between the strength of the intradermal response and degree of testicular atrophy.

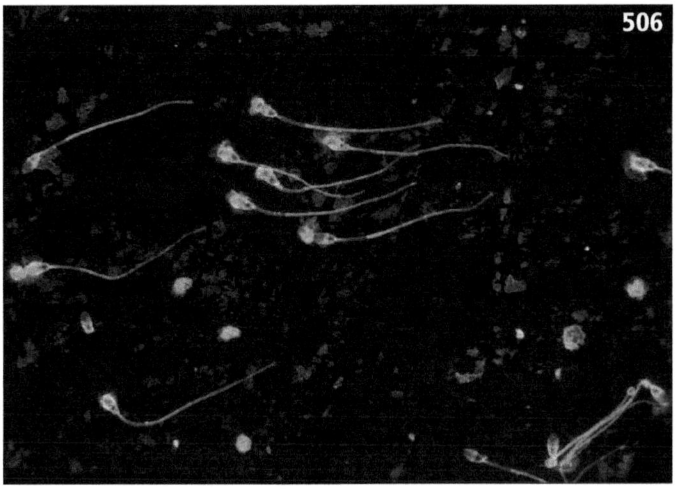

506 Detection of anti-sperm antibodies by indirect immunofluorescence. Fixed smears are made of normal canine sperm that are incubated with serial dilutions of serum from the infertile patient. Binding of antibody to different regions of the spermatozoa (head, midpiece or tail) is visualized by the use of a fluorescein-conjugated secondary antibody. In this example, using equine sperm with serum from a stallion with subnormal fertility, there is immunofluorescence of the head and tail but no staining of the mid-piece. (From Day MJ [1996] Detection of equine anti-sperm antibodies by indirect immunofluorescence and the tube-slide agglutination test. *Equine Veterinary Journal* **28:**494–496, with permission.)

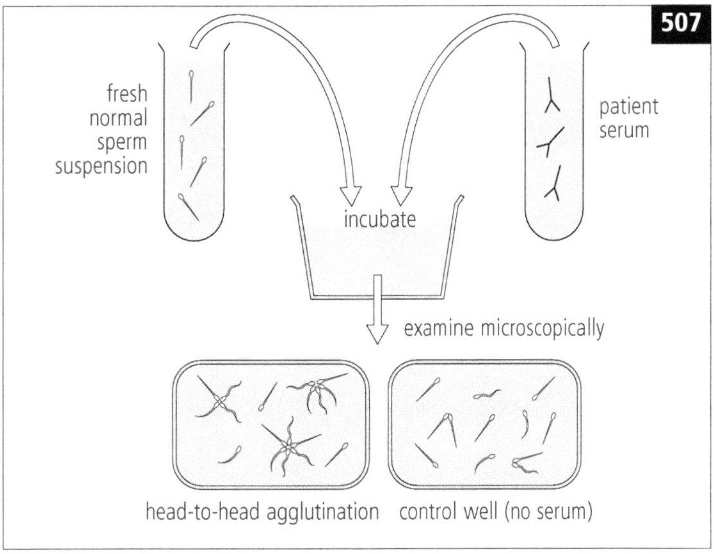

507 Demonstration of anti-sperm antibody by agglutination. In this assay a fresh preparation of washed, normal canine sperm is made and counted. Specific numbers of viable sperm are incubated in microtitre wells with serial dilutions of serum from the infertile dog, and examined microscopically after the period of incubation. The proportion of clumped (agglutinated) sperm is determined by counting and compared with control wells containing no serum. The number of sperm per clump and the orientation of the agglutinated sperm (e.g. head to head, tail to tail) can also be assessed.

In a study of a large inbred Beagle colony, an association was recorded between lymphocytic thyroiditis (see Chapter 9, p. 241) and interstitial lymphocytic orchitis, resulting in testicular atrophy and subnormal fertility. Such an association is also documented in murine models of multisystemic autoimmunity and would suggest an immune-mediated pathogenesis for the testicular disease.

A recent study has examined the immune response in experimentally-induced prostatic hyperplasia in castrated dogs given androgen and/or oestrogen. Hyperplasia was followed by a pronounced mononuclear cell infiltration, dominated by T lymphocytes and including macrophages and B cells forming inflammatory lymphoid follicles. The nature of this response would not be inconsistent with a form of autoimmunity occurring subsequent to prostatic hyperplasia.

FURTHER READING

Acierno MJ, Labato MA, Stern LC *et al.* (2006) Serum concentrations of the third component of complement in healthy dogs and dogs with protein-losing nephropathy. *American Journal of Veterinary Research* **67**:1105–1109.

Aresu L, D'Angelo A, Zanatta R *et al.* (2007) Canine necrotizing encephalitis associated with anti-glomerular basement membrane glomerulonephritis. *Journal of Comparative Pathology* **136**:279–282.

Grauer GF (2005) Canine glomerulonephritis: new thoughts on proteinuria and treatment. *Journal of Small Animal Practice* **46**:469–478.

Mahapokai W, van den Ingh TSGAM, van Mil F *et al.* (2001) Immune response in hormonally-induced prostatic hyperplasia in the dog. *Veterinary Immunology and Immunopathology* **78**:297–303.

Roudebush P, Polzin DJ, Adams LG *et al.* (2010) An evidence-based review of therapies for canine chronic kidney disease. *Journal of Small Animal Practice* **51**:244-252.

Zatelli A, Borgarelli M, Santilli R *et al.* (2004) Glomerular lesions in dogs infected with *Leishmania* organisms. *American Journal of Veterinary Research* **64**:558–561.

11 IMMUNE-MEDIATED OCULAR DISEASE

Michael J. Day and Sheila Crispin

OCULAR IMMUNITY

The ocular immune system has both innate and acquired components. Physical factors, including the blink response, third eyelid and tear film, are a significant means of defence from microbes, chemicals or aeroallergens. The tear film comprises an inner mucin layer produced primarily by the conjunctival goblet cells, and also transmembrane mucin derived from epithelial cells. The middle aqueous layer is secreted by the lacrimal and accessory lacrimal glands as well as the nictitans glands, and there is also an outer oily layer produced mainly by the meibomian glands of the eyelids. Tears contain Ig produced by plasma cells within the lacrimal tissue. In the dog the dominant Ig in tears is IgA (1.0 ± 0.7 mg/ml), with less IgG (0.6 ± 0.6 mg/ml) and very small quantities of IgM (0.02 ± 0.00 mg/ml). Aggregates of lymphocytes and plasma cells are a normal feature of the subepithelial connective tissue of the bulbar conjunctiva and the inner aspect of the third eyelid, and interepithelial lymphocytes are also recognized. This conjunctiva-associated lymphoid tissue (CALT) is poorly characterized in the dog and cat. The normal structure of the eye is reviewed in (508).

The eye is referred to as an 'immunologically privileged site' and is characterized by:

- A paucity of resident lymphocytes and APCs; however, MHC class II-positive Langerhans cells may be found at the periphery of the corneal epithelium and may migrate to the central epithelium under the direction of epithelially-derived cytokines (e.g. IL-1). A sparse population of APCs is also found within the trabecular meshwork of the filtration angle, and class II expression may be induced on uveal vascular endothelium.
- No lymphatic drainage other than conjunctival.
- The 'blood–eye barrier' (blood–aqueous and blood–retinal barriers).

Whilst these features may suggest that the ocular structures are remote from the systemic immune system ('sequestered antigens'), this is not the case, as inoculation of antigen into the anterior chamber can induce a systemic immune response and ocular autoimmunity is well documented. However, at this

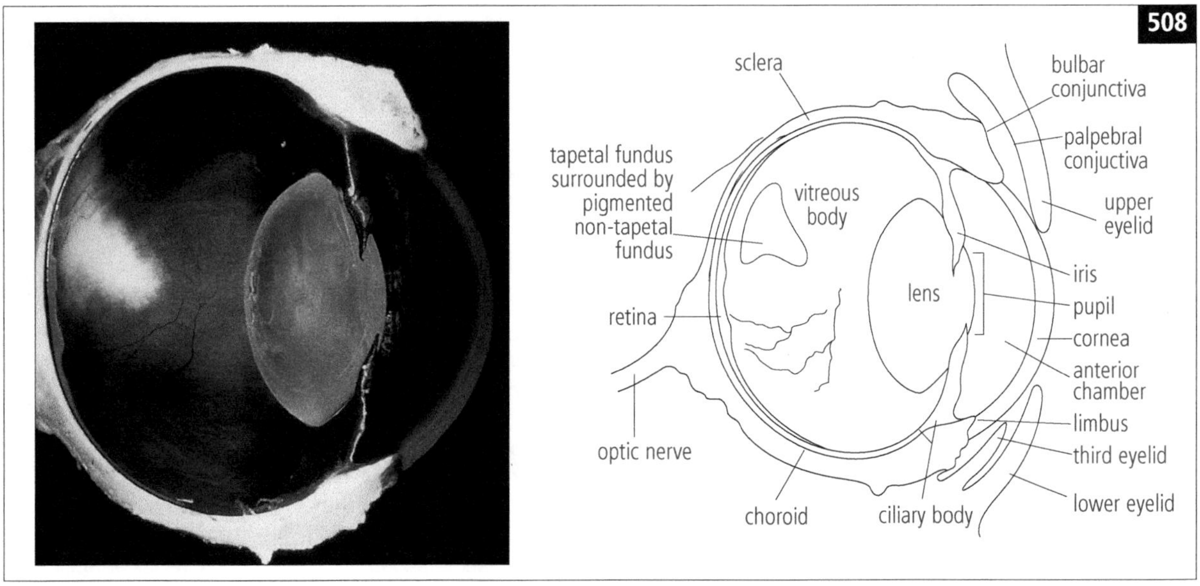

508 Normal ocular anatomy. Diagrammatic representation of the eye and associated structures. (Photograph courtesy J.R.B. Mould.)

privileged site, experimentally allografted cells may escape immunological recognition (within the anterior chamber) and skin grafts bearing the same alloantigens are not rejected. Similarly, corneal grafts are not rejected by individuals presensitized to graft alloantigens; therefore, corneal transplantation is the most successful form of transplant surgery.

An unusual component of the ocular immune system is 'anterior chamber-associated immune deviation' (ACAID), whereby there is a unique systemic immune reactivity following administration of antigen to the anterior chamber. Following inoculation by this route, soluble antigens are processed locally by poorly defined, but presumably unconventional, mechanisms that may be under the control of intraocular cytokines such as TGFβ. Normal aqueous humour contains high levels of TGFβ and neutralization of this cytokine by monoclonal antibodies can prevent the induction of ACAID. Processed antigen then translocates to the spleen via the bloodstream and ACAID does not develop in the absence of the spleen. Here there is induction of an immune response that specifically favours humoral immunity, with inhibition of the DTH response consistent with preferential activation of Th2 lymphocytes or induction of IL-10 secreting regulatory T cells. An alternative form of ACAID occurs when cell-associated antigens are placed into the anterior chamber and $CD4^+$ and $CD8^+$ cytotoxic populations are activated. These recirculate to the inoculated eye (entering via the uveal tract) but fail functionally to differentiate. These cells may be suppressed by local TGFβ or be induced to secrete this cytokine themselves. Alternatively, these cells may express Fas, which interacts with Fas ligand on anterior chamber parenchymal cells to induce deletion by apoptosis. Expression of Fas ligand is widespread in the eye, including the cornea, iris, ciliary body and retina. The expression of this molecule is thought to create a protective barrier, which encircles the eye and protects these structures from the effects of inflammatory cells (expressing Fas) that enter the eye and are induced to undergo apoptosis on engagement of the Fas-Fas ligand molecules. Compromise of this ocular expression of Fas ligand may lead to sight-threatening ocular inflammation and may be one mechanism underlying the initiation of some of the diseases described in this chapter.

The overall effect of these complex and specialized immunological mechanisms is to prevent deleterious intraocular inflammation that may affect sight, but this also renders the eye susceptible to pathogens that require local expression of inflammatory mediators for elimination. This chapter describes the immune-mediated diseases of the cornea, uveal tract and episclera/sclera and retina.

IMMUNE-MEDIATED CONJUNCTIVAL DISEASE

ALLERGIC CONJUNCTIVITIS

Pathogenesis

Allergic conjunctivitis occurs in dogs and cats as a localized conjunctival reaction or in conjunction with cutaneous hypersensitivity (see Chapter 5, p. 126). The initiating allergens are rarely identified, but the absence of other causative agents and response to therapy often underlies diagnosis.

Clinical signs

In dogs (509) and cats (510) the clinical features include bilateral conjunctival hyperaemia, swelling (chemosis), pruritus (rubbing and pawing at the eyes) and serous ocular discharge. There may be

509

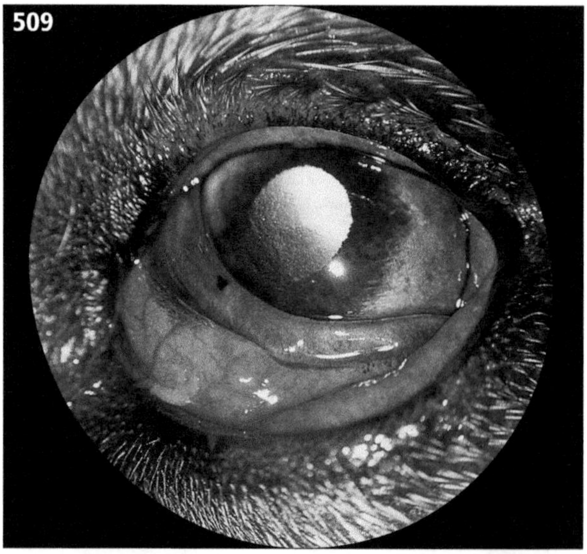

509 Allergic conjunctivitis. Labrador Retriever with atopy and allergic conjunctivitis. There is conjunctival hyperaemia and chemosis, together with a seromucoid discharge.

inflammation of the eyelid margins (marginal blepharitis) and cornea (keratitis), and secondary (often staphylococcal) infection may occur. In chronic cases there may be lymphoid hyperplasia, with the formation of grossly visible follicles (follicular conjunctivitis) (**511**), and cytological examination of these lesions demonstrates a mixed population of lymphocytes and plasma cells (**512**).

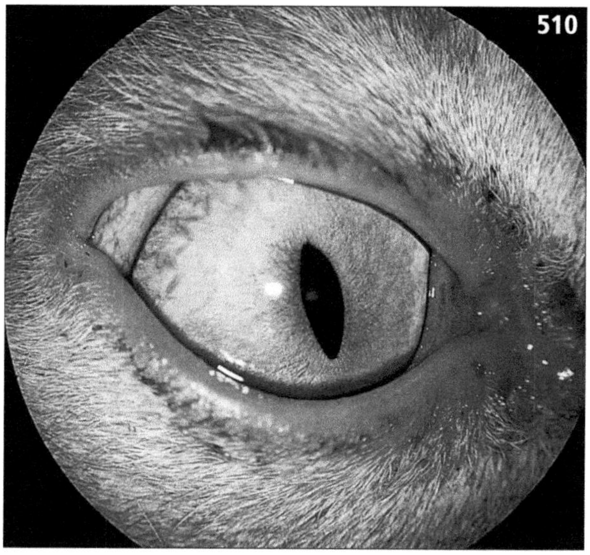

510 Allergic conjunctivitis. Devon Rex cat with allergic conjunctivitis and blepharitis associated with the use of topical tetracycline.

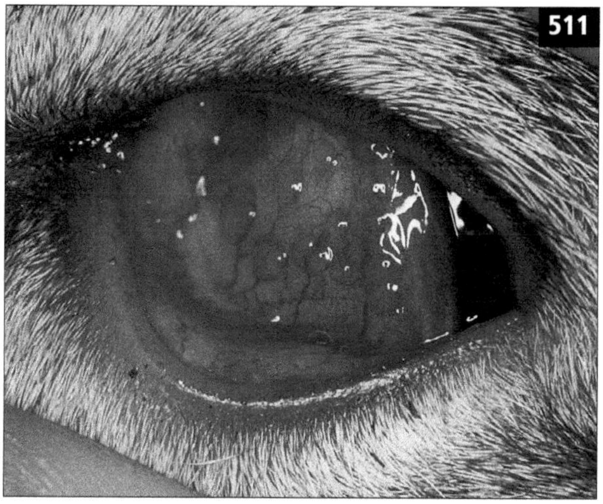

511 Follicular conjunctivitis. DSH cat with follicular conjunctivitis. Note the follicles on the palpebral conjunctiva and the conjunctiva of the third eyelid.

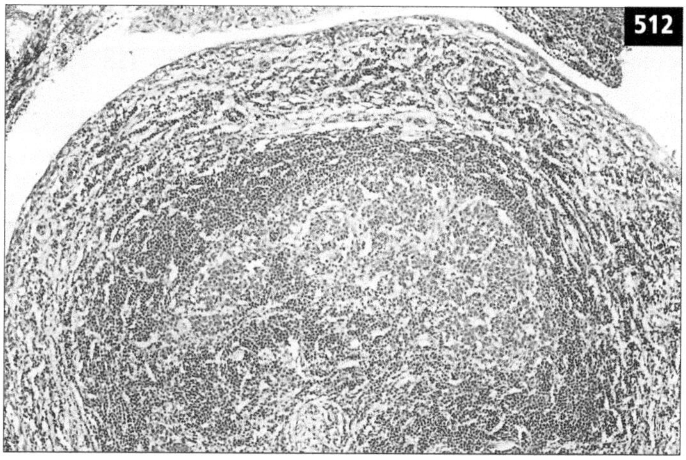

512 Follicular conjunctivitis. Conjunctival biopsy from a Labrador Retriever with a four-week history of conjunctivitis characterized by the presence of scattered white spots over the conjunctiva and inner surface of the third eyelid. Microscopically, these comprise hyperplastic lymphoid follicles surrounded by numerous plasma cells.

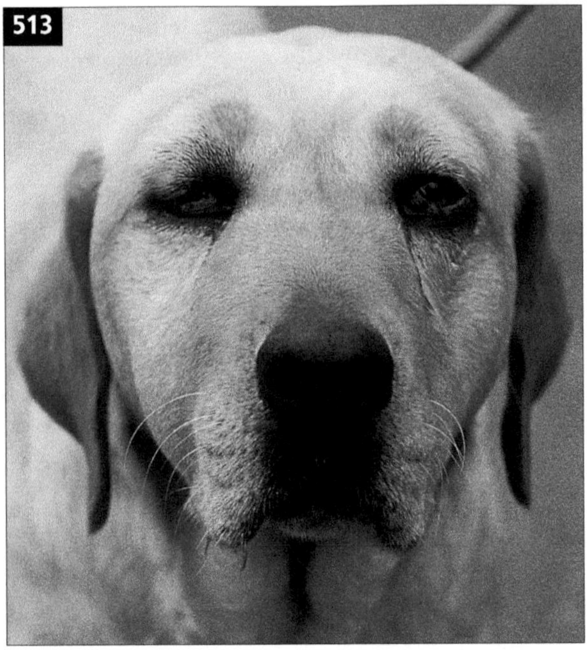

513 Allergic conjunctivitis. Labrador Retriever with allergic conjunctivitis and facial oedema, the result of a bee sting a few hours previously.

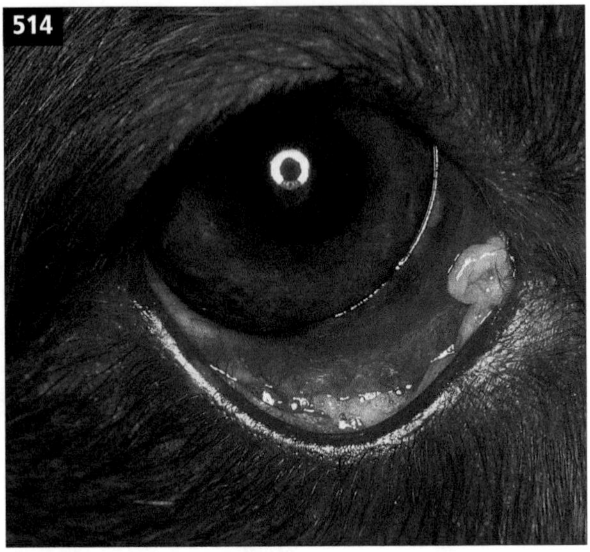

514 Allergic conjunctivitis. English Springer Spaniel with chronic conjunctivitis. The dog had received a great variety of topical treatments to no effect. The conjunctivitis was actually associated with systemic immune-mediated disease.

Diagnosis

The history and clinical appearance may be diagnostic (**513**), but it is often unhelpful, particularly in chronic cases (**514**). Conjunctival scrapes to identify the cell types that are present may be taken with a sterile Kimura spatula, a cytological brush or the blunt end of a disposable scalpel blade. Conjunctival swabs for culture are required if bacterial or viral infection is likely to be present. Conjunctival biopsy demonstrates:

- Epithelial and goblet cell hyperplasia, squamous metaplasia or ulceration.
- Eosinophil infiltration of subepithelial connective tissue and epithelium with few mast cells.
- Lymphoplasmacytic infiltration may follow in chronic lesions.

Treatment and prognosis

Successful management depends on identifying and removing the offending agents, but allergic conjunctivitis is difficult to cure if the allergens cannot be identified. Palliative treatment consists of topical vasoconstrictors or sodium cromoglycate, which inhibits mast cell degranulation. Topical glucocorticoids (betamethasone, fluorometholone and prednisolone) are reserved for more serious cases. The prognosis is guarded if the cause of the allergy cannot be identified or if the patient cannot undergo allergen-specific immunotherapy (see Chapter 5, p. 133).

CANINE NICTITANS PLASMACYTIC CONJUNCTIVITIS

Pathogenesis

Nictitans plasmacytic conjunctivitis (plasmoma) is a chronic, putatively immune-mediated inflammatory disease of the anterior surface of the third eyelid. The condition often occurs in conjunction with chronic superficial keratitis/keratoconjunctivitis (CSK/CSKC). Both diseases are recognized most frequently in GSDs, which may also have ulceration of the medial canthus of both eyelids (medial canthus erosion syndrome).

Clinical signs

The lesions appear as raised, pinpoint nodules that coalesce and result in thickening and inflammation of the anterior surface of the third eyelid (**515**). The histological appearance is of a subepithelial infiltration of large numbers of plasma cells and aggregates of $CD3^+$ T lymphocytes (**516**).

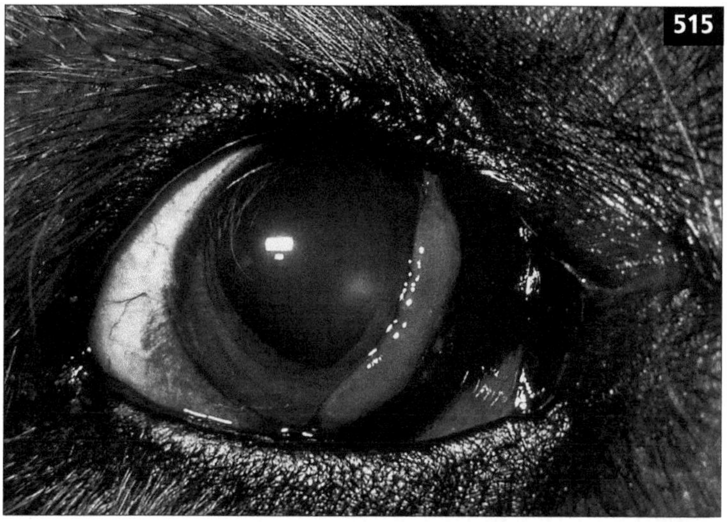

515 Canine nictitans plasmacytic conjunctivitis. GSD with nictitans plasmacytic conjunctivitis. Note the thickening of, and loss of pigment from, the leading edge of the third eyelid.

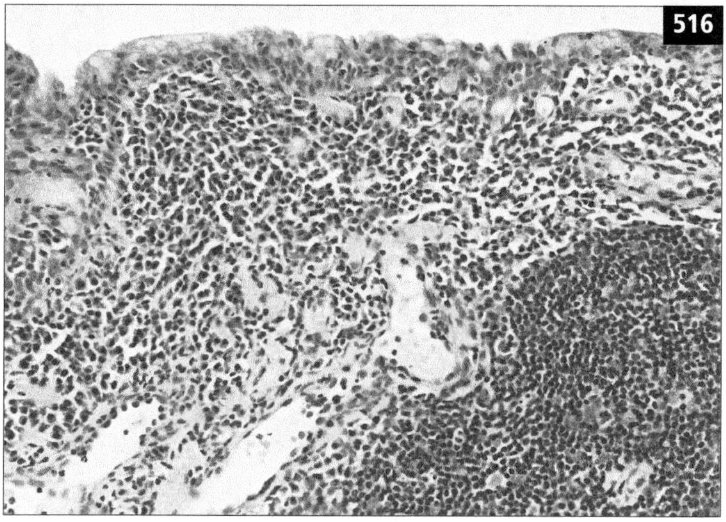

516 Histology of canine nictitans plasmacytic conjunctivitis. Biopsy from the anterior surface of the third eyelid of a three-year-old GSD with a six-month history of recurrent nictitans plasmacytic conjunctivitis. There is a marked infiltrate of plasma cells beneath the mucosal epithelium and an aggregate of small lymphocytes is prominent.

Treatment and prognosis

The disease is responsive to topical ophthalmic ciclosporin applied every 12 hours for at least six weeks. Reduction in the number of plasma cells (but not T cells) is observed in post-treatment biopsies. Lifelong treatment may be needed at the lowest rate of application that prevents recurrence, as the condition recurs when treatment is stopped. Therefore, prognosis for complete cure is guarded.

LIGNEOUS CONJUNCTIVITIS

Pathogenesis

The proposed pathogenesis of ligneous conjunctivitis involves conjunctival vascular injury with excessive permeability and accumulation of mixed albumin, Ig and fibrin that coagulates to form a hyaline deposit. Human patients have absent or very low levels of plasminogen and the underlying cause of ligneous conjunctivitis is now recognized as the presence of one of several different mutations in the gene encoding plasminogen. Plasminogen deficiency has been described in one dog with this disease.

Clinical signs

Ligneous conjunctivitis is occasionally described in dogs (predominantly Dobermanns) and is characterized by thickened and firm palpebral conjunctivae and third eyelids, with formation of an adherent fibrinous membrane (membranous conjunctivitis), and secondary corneal oedema and neovascularization (517–520). In many cases the conjunctival lesion is part of multisystemic disease involving similar changes in the oral mucosa, with urinary or upper respiratory infection.

Diagnosis

No microbial cause is identified and affected dogs are negative for serum ANA. The histological appearance of affected conjunctiva includes:

- Epithelial ulceration and fibrinocellular crusting.

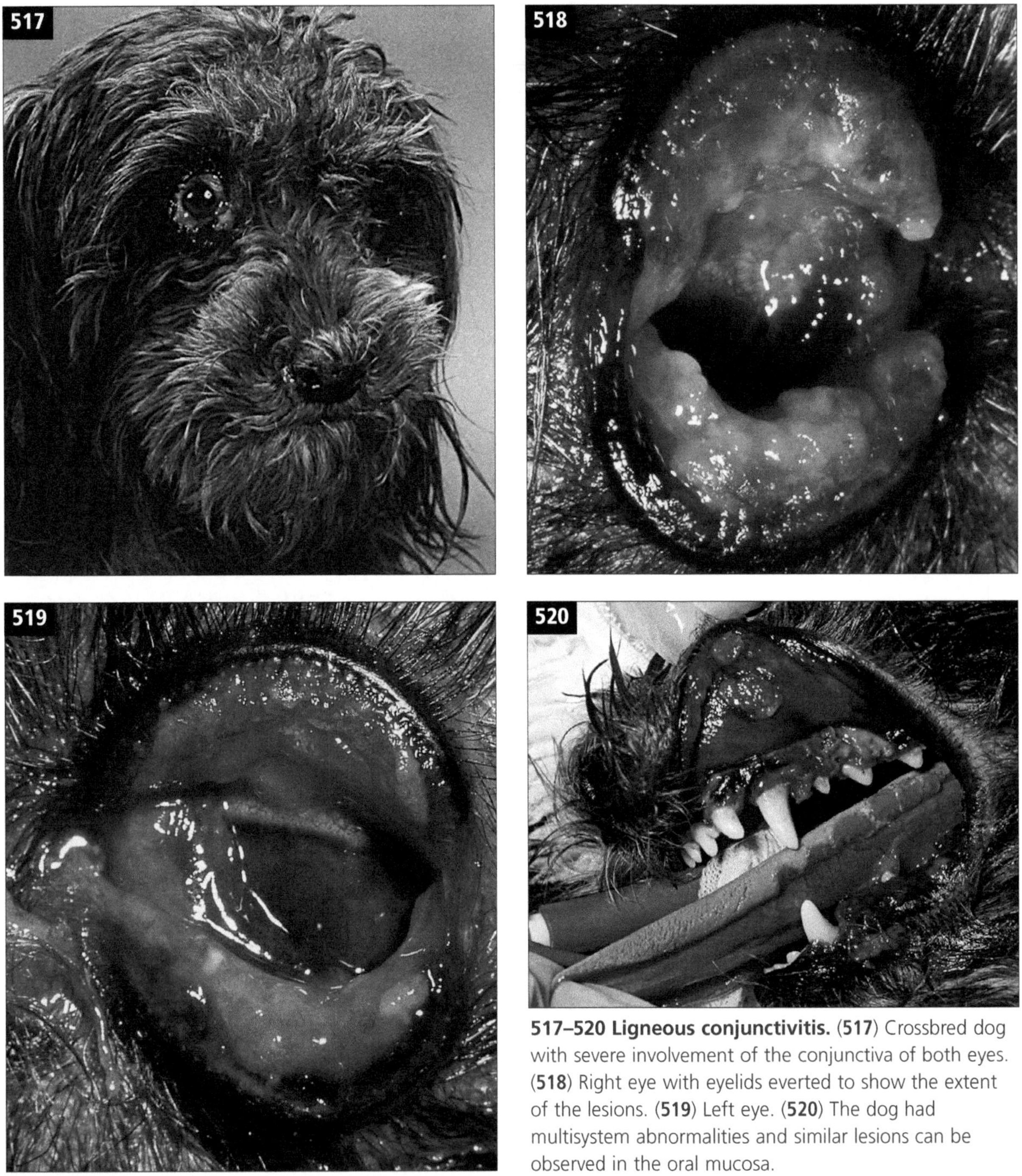

517–520 Ligneous conjunctivitis. (**517**) Crossbred dog with severe involvement of the conjunctiva of both eyes. (**518**) Right eye with eyelids everted to show the extent of the lesions. (**519**) Left eye. (**520**) The dog had multisystem abnormalities and similar lesions can be observed in the oral mucosa.

- Neutrophil infiltration of the superficial mucosa.
- Deposition of thick, hyaline, eosinophilic material within the mucosa. This has a fibrillary appearance on electron microscopy but does not stain for amyloid or Ig.
- A lymphoplasmacytic perivascular infiltration of the mucosa, with an infiltrate of macrophages, lymphocytes ($CD3^+$) and plasma cells (IgG and IgA) at the deep margin of the hyaline deposit.

Treatment and prognosis

Treatment is generally unsatisfactory, with poor response to both topical and systemic approaches. Success is often gauged in terms of remission of clinical signs rather than cure. A suggested regime includes topical use of an antibiotic–glucocorticoid preparation and ciclosporin ointment, and systemic treatment with prednisolone and azathioprine. If there is a satisfactory response, the dose of azathioprine can be reduced to a maintenance level and all other drugs gradually withdrawn over several weeks. The fibrinous membranes may be surgically removed, but they can recur. The prognosis is extremely guarded when there are associated multisystem abnormalities.

Therapy with topical fresh frozen plasma, plasmin or plasminogen has been used to effect in the management of the condition in man.

AUTOIMMUNE CONJUNCTIVITIS

The conjunctiva may be involved in the autoimmune skin diseases described in Chapter 5 (**521, 522**).

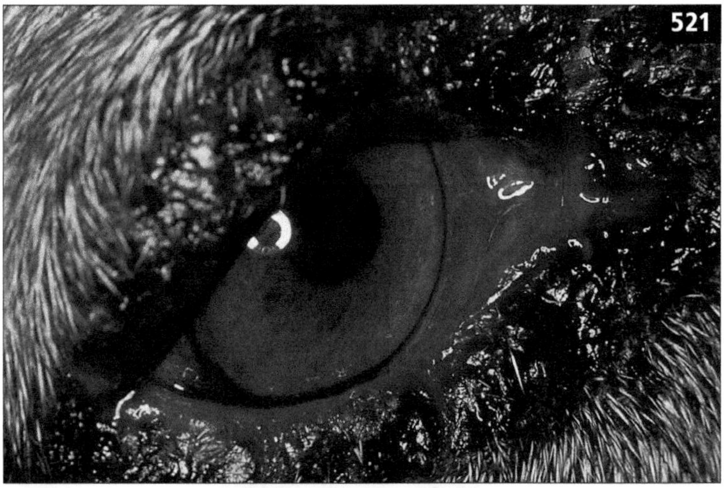

521 Autoimmune conjunctivitis. Conjunctival involvement in pemphigus foliaceus in a GSD.

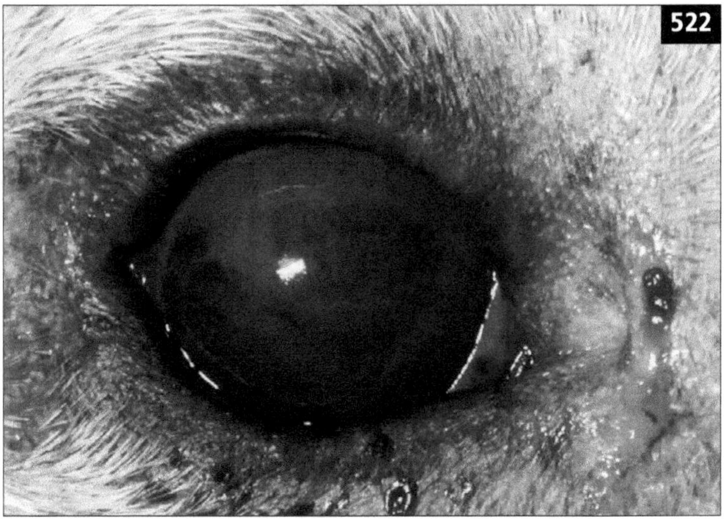

522 Erythema multiformae. Complex tear film disorder with secondary vascular and pigmentary keratitis in a Labrador Retriever with erythema multiforme.

IMMUNE-MEDIATED DISEASES OF THE CORNEA

Corneal inflammation (keratitis) may have a variety of causes, but in each case the lesions have a similar progression, involving:

- Corneal oedema.
- Leukocyte infiltration from tears and limbic vessels.
- Corneal stromal vascularization and fibrosis, with epithelial metaplasia and pigmentation.
- Keratomalacia may be a rare feature of some immune-mediated types of keratitis (**523**).

Keratitis may primarily involve the cornea or it may occur by extension of inflammation of the conjunctiva or uveal tract.

CHRONIC SUPERFICIAL KERATITIS/ KERATOCONJUNCTIVITIS

Pathogenesis

CSK/CSKC (pannus keratitis, Uberreiter's syndrome) is a chronic, usually bilateral, non-ulcerative, proliferative stromal keratitis that has greatest prevalence in middle-aged GSDs. A DLA risk haplotype (DLA DRBI*01501/ DQAI*00601/DQBI*00301) is defined in this breed. The inflammatory infiltrates include $CD4^+$ (and fewer $CD8^+$) T lymphocytes, which secrete IFNγ, plasma cells and macrophages. There is hyperplasia and pigmentation of the corneal epithelium and the epithelial cells express MHC class II. Most cases have diffuse deposition of IgG in the superficial stroma of the limbal conjunctiva, and a few dogs have IgG deposition within the superficial corneal stroma or along the corneal epithelial basement membrane. An immune-mediated pathogenesis is proposed, involving an autoimmune response towards corneal antigens that may be modified by factors such as ultraviolet (UV) light or viral infection.

Clinical signs

The clinical appearance of CSK/CSKC is characteristic. The presentation is of corneal opacity due to superficial stromal inflammation, vascularization and fibrosis extending from the limbus. The deep corneal stroma is unaffected. The earliest lesions are usually observed in the lower lateral (inferotemporal) conjunctiva in the region of the limbus and adjacent cornea. With time these may extend to involve the whole cornea (**524, 525**). Associated pigment migration is common in breeds with a pigmented perilimbal region (**526**). There is slight discomfort and mild epiphora may be present.

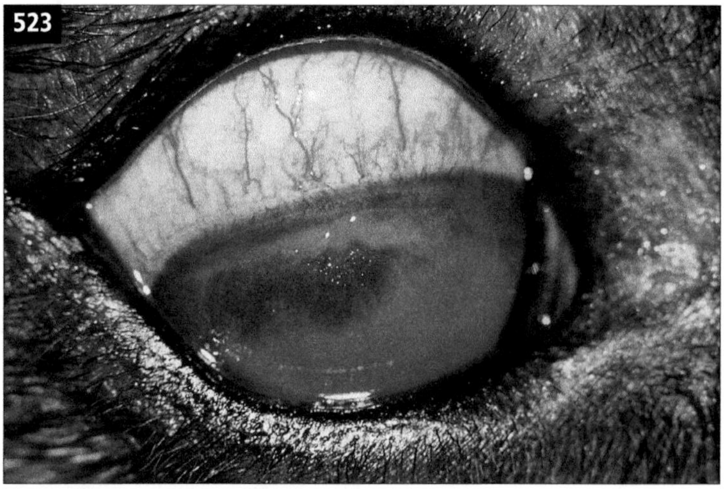

523 Immune-mediated keratitis. Limbal keratomalacia in a GSD that had been treated for bacterial keratitis (*Pseudomonas aeruginosa* isolated) a few weeks earlier.

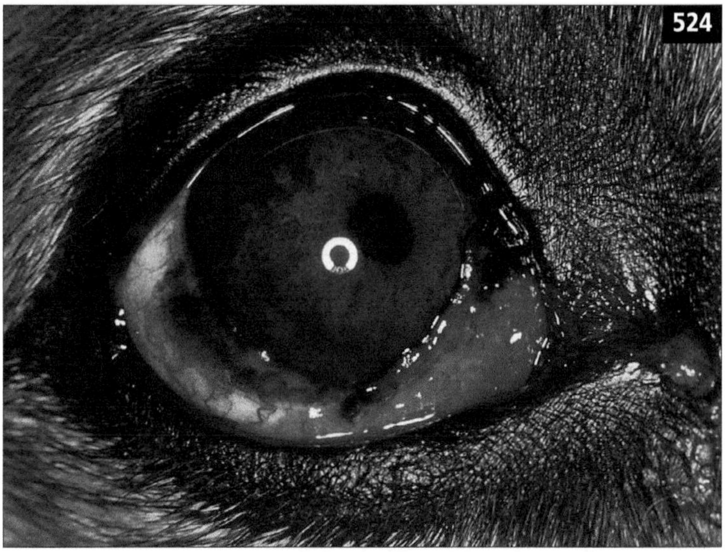

524 Chronic superficial keratoconjunctivitis. Early involvement in a GSD. Note the subtle changes inferotemporally at the limbus and the more obvious involvement of the third eyelid.

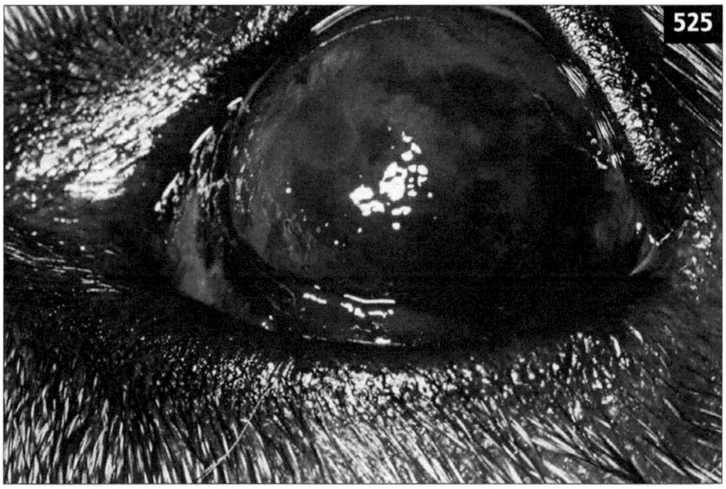

525 Chronic superficial keratoconjunctivitis. Almost the entire cornea is involved in this GSD.

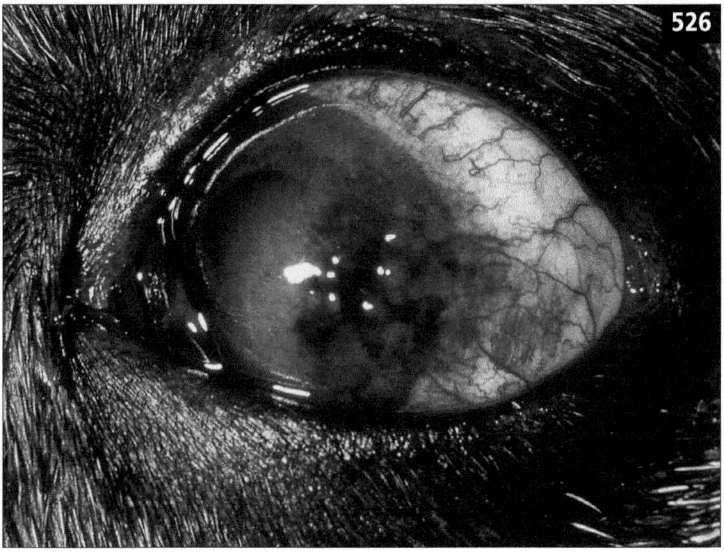

526 Chronic superficial keratoconjunctivitis. Another GSD with more extensive inferotemporal corneal involvement. In addition to the characteristic fibrovascular infiltration, there is associated pigment migration.

Treatment and prognosis

Topical ciclosporin applied every 12 hours is the treatment of choice and has all but replaced the use of topical glucocorticoids, radiotherapy or surgery. In a small proportion of cases it may be possible to withdraw treatment once the eyes are of normal appearance, but in most cases (particularly in at-risk breeds such as the GSD), treatment is required for life, as the condition recurs as soon as treatment is stopped. The prognosis is reasonable as long as treatment does not lapse, but CSK/CSKC is more difficult to control when predisposing factors such as UV light and altitude cannot be avoided. As with nictitans plasmacytic conjunctivitis, long-term treatment should be at the lowest rate of application that serves to prevent recurrence.

KERATOCONJUNCTIVITIS SICCA

Pathogenesis

Keratoconjunctivitis sicca (KCS; desiccation keratitis) is most frequently documented in the dog, and generally follows destruction of the lacrimal and often also the nictitans glands, with failure to produce adequate aqueous tears. KCS may be secondary to periorbital (lacrimal) trauma, drug reactions (particularly sulphonamides) or acute lacrimal inflammation; however, the most common cause is lymphocytic infiltration of the lacrimal gland, with subsequent atrophy and fibrosis. This is presumed to be a primary autoimmune event based on the following evidence:

- The lesions are analogous to the ocular component of the human autoimmune disease, Sjögren's syndrome. Although rarely documented in companion animals, two cases of canine Sjögren's syndrome have been described. In these dogs there was KCS in conjunction with xerostomia, vaginal dryness, lymphocytic thyroiditis and serum autoantibodies. This collection of findings also characterizes the human disease. These dogs were part of an experimental colony that was bred to develop SLE, therefore it was likely that they had a genetic predisposition to the development of autoimmunity. Although considered rare, it has been suggested that canine Sjögren's syndrome may be underdiagnosed and that a proportion of dogs with KCS may have subclinical histopathological changes in salivary tissue. One study of 50 dogs with KCS identified ten patients with a degree of xerostomia.
  A single cat with Sjögren's syndrome has been documented in the literature.
- The lesions may be reversed by immunosuppressive therapy.
- Affected dogs have hypergammaglobulinaemia, and serum autoantibodies (rheumatoid factor, ANA, anti-lacrimal antibody) may be found.
- KCS may occur as part of multisystem autoimmune disease (e.g. SLE) or concurrently with hypothyroidism, RA, diabetes mellitus, CH or autoimmune skin disease.
- Immunohistochemical characterization of the gland of the third eyelid of dogs with KCS revealed infiltration of T lymphocytes with $CD8^+$ cells dominating over $CD4^+$ lymphocytes. The number of $CD8^+$ cells decreased with treatment. These infiltrating lymphocytes have reduced expression of markers of apoptosis, but glandular epithelial cells have elevated marker expression as a likely consequence of their cytotoxic destruction. In contrast, dogs with KCS have no abnormality in the response of peripheral blood lymphocytes to mitogen, and have normal blood lymphocyte counts and a normal blood CD4:CD8 ratio (2.4–2.8:1).

Clinical signs

Breed predisposition for the English Bulldog, Lhasa Apso, Shih Tzu and West Highland White Terrier (527) is recognized and the clinical features (528) include:

- Mucoid to mucopurulent ocular discharge.
- Conjunctivitis.
- Superficial keratitis and, in chronic severe cases, extreme dryness (xerosis).
- Blepharitis.
- Secondary bacterial infection.

The corneal changes include:

- Epithelial hyperplasia, pigmentation and keratinization; ulceration is sometimes a feature, especially in acute cases.
- Stromal vascularization and fibrosis.
- Superficial stromal inflammation.

Diagnosis

Diagnosis is based on the breed predisposition and characteristic ocular signs. Affected dogs usually present with mild blepharospasm and pain,

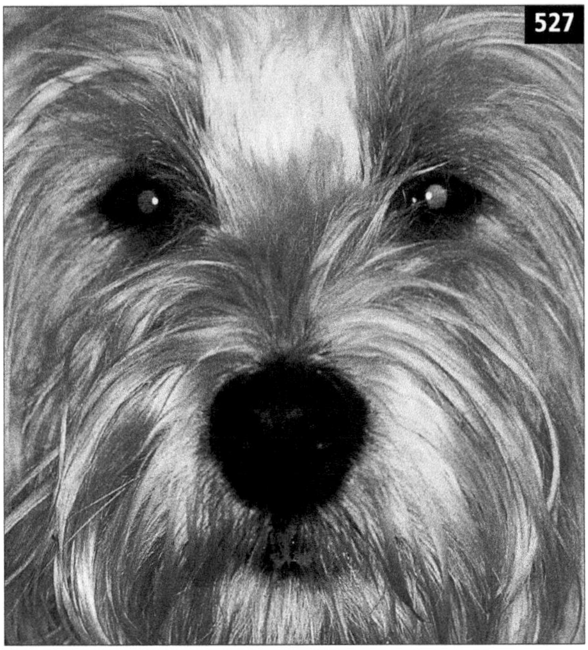

527 Keratoconjunctivitis sicca. West Highland White Terrier with early KCS. Note that the eyes look relatively normal from a distance, although mild ocular discomfort was present. Schirmer I tear testing gave readings of 0 and 3 mm per minute in the right and left eyes, respectively.

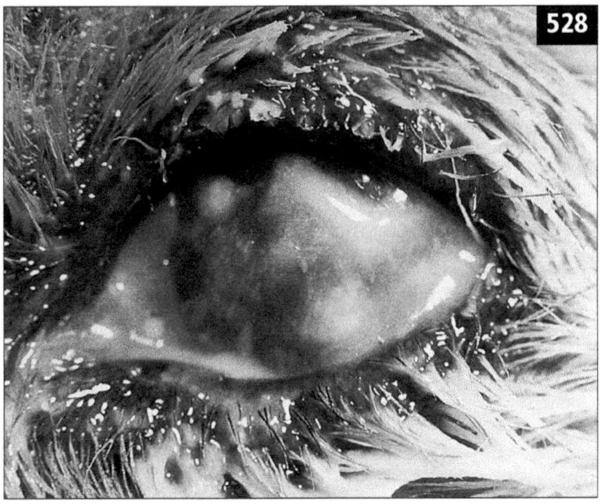

528 Keratoconjunctivitis sicca. West Highland White Terrier with more chronic KCS. Note the profuse mucopurulant discharge, dull cornea and mild conjunctivitis.

although more severe pain will be present when ulcerative keratitis occurs. KCS may start unilaterally, but it becomes bilateral with time. A Schirmer I tear test is used to confirm the diagnosis. Both eyes should be tested. In normal dogs, values in excess of 10 mm per minute (20 ± 5 mm) are expected, but in affected dogs 0–5 mm per minute is usual.

Treatment and prognosis

The treatment of choice for KCS of autoimmune origin is topical ciclosporin every 12 hours. Treatment will be required for life. Newer topical drugs such as the macrolide lactone tacrolimus are also being evaluated. Early management may require careful removal of excessive ocular discharge and, in cases with abnormal mucin production, acetylcysteine 3–4 times daily may be beneficial initially. Judicious short-term use of topical glucocorticoids can be a useful adjunct to initial therapy, provided that corneal ulceration is not present. Tear replacement therapy with a new generation carbomer (polyacrylic acid) preparation may be helpful until tear production has improved as a result of the ciclosporin therapy. Alternative strategies (surgical transplantation of the parotid duct) should only be considered if there is no response to a six-week trial of ciclosporin. The prognosis is reasonably good in cases that respond to ciclosporin, provided that the ciclosporin therapy is maintained.

FELINE EOSINOPHILIC KERATOCONJUNCTIVITIS (FELINE PROLIFERATIVE KERATOCONJUNCTIVITIS)

Pathogenesis

This condition is characterized by uni- or bilateral, proliferative, superficial stromal keratoconjunctivitis of unknown aetiology (**529**).

Clinical signs

The clinical signs include ocular discomfort, mild blepharospasm and a low-grade ocular discharge. Tear production may be increased as a result of ocular discomfort, although occasionally it is reduced. The palpebral and bulbar conjunctivae are often reddened and oedematous and, rarely, are swollen enough to obscure the cornea. There may be focal conjunctival papillae (raised projections of mixed epithelia, stroma and inflammatory cells).

Corneal infiltration and vascularization are key features of the condition. Usually, the dorsolateral (superotemporal) or inferotemporal quadrants of the cornea are affected, but the whole cornea becomes involved as the condition progresses. Corneal oedema and minute erosions may be present. The characteristic feature of proliferative keratoconjunctivitis is a superficial, creamy white, plaque-like material, which is described as of 'cottage cheese' appearance. There is no clear relationship to the mucocutaneous eosinophilic lesions of the cat (see Chapter 5, p. 141), but there may be other concurrent hypersensitivity disease (e.g. upper respiratory tract allergy; see Chapter 8, p. 230).

Diagnosis

The diagnostic approach may include cytological examination of corneal scrapings, which will demonstrate numerous eosinophils but only occasional mast cells (**530**). On biopsy the stromal inflammation consists of macrophages, plasma cells, eosinophils and mast cells, with superficial stromal vascularization and fibroplasia (**531**).

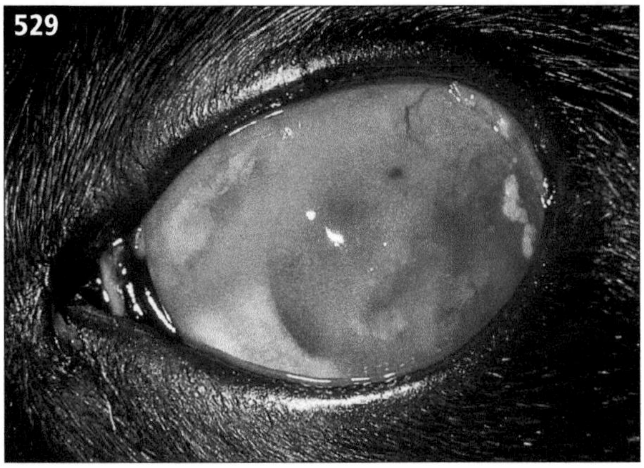

529 Feline eosinophilic keratoconjunctivitis. DSH cat with extensive corneal infiltration, which is densest temporally. Note the characteristic white material, which is present in and on the superficial cornea and on the palpebral conjunctiva of the upper eyelid.

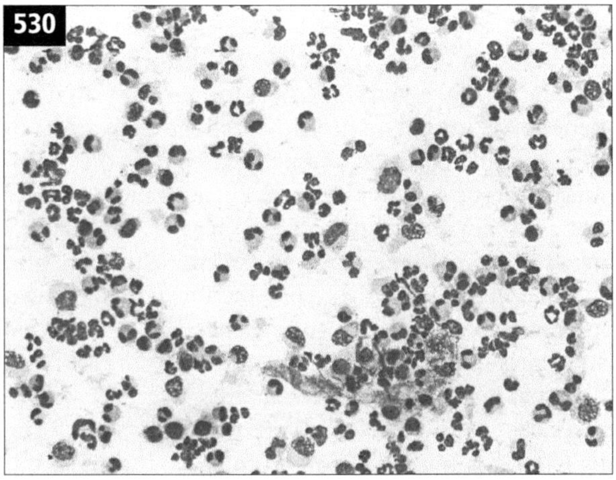

530 Feline eosinophilic keratitis. Corneal scraping from an 18-month-old Maine Coon cat with progressive corneal inflammation over a six-month period. The cytological preparation contains numerous eosinophils, with fewer neutrophils, macrophages and lymphocytes.

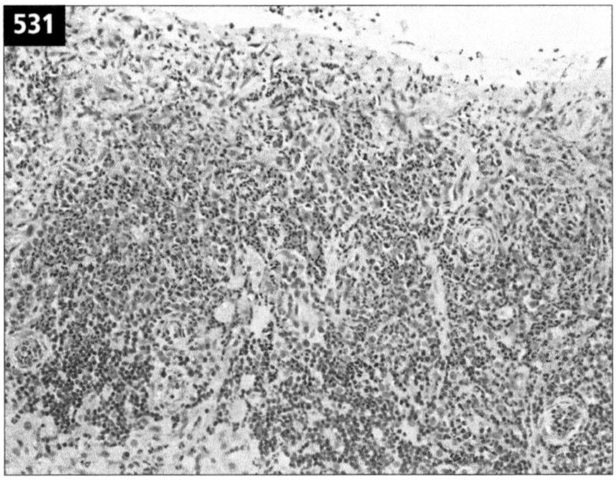

531 Feline eosinophilic keratoconjunctivitis. Conjunctival biopsy from a nine-year-old Burmese cat with eosinophilic conjunctivitis. There is surface ulceration and an intense eosinophil infiltration of conjunctiva, with deep lymphoplasmacytic aggregates.

Treatment and prognosis

Response to treatment and, by inference, the prognosis will be adversely affected by concurrent problems such as infection with feline herpesvirus, FeLV or FIV. In the absence of complicating factors, the disease responds to topical glucocorticoid therapy and also to glucocorticoids or megestrol acetate (a progestogen with immunosuppressive activity) given orally as a short-term course of treatment. As megestrol acetate can induce diabetes mellitus, it should not be a first line treatment. Topical ciclosporin appears less effective than other treatments in the early stages, but may be useful for long-term therapy. Lesions will recur in a proportion of cases when treatment is stopped. A suggested treatment regime might include initial induction of localized immunosuppression with topical glucocorticoids, followed by maintenance with topical ciclosporin if the lesions recur.

IMMUNE-MEDIATED DISEASES OF THE UVEA

Most forms of uveitis in the dog and cat reflect local immunopathology as part of systemic disease (**532, 533**). The classical example occurs in canine adenovirus (CAV) 1 infection (or use of vaccines incorporating CAV1), where there is formation of viral immune complex in the uvea, with neutrophil infiltration and secondary corneal endothelial damage and oedema ('blue eye') (**534**). In the cat,

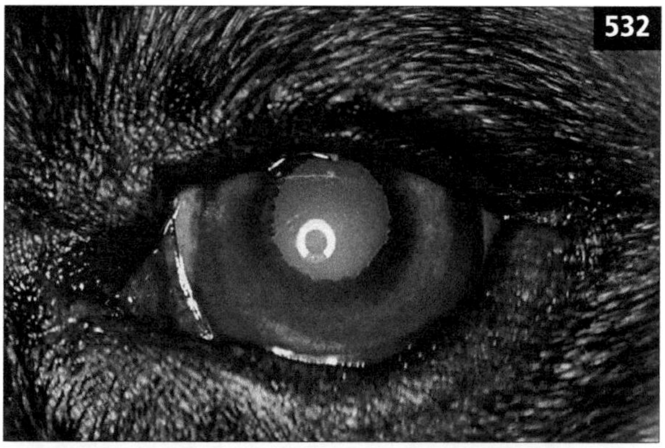

532 Canine uveitis. Keratouveitis in a Boxer with leishmaniosis.

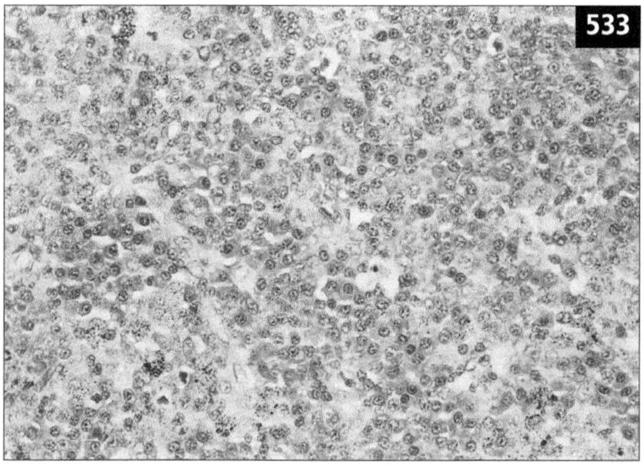

533 Canine uveitis. Ciliary body from a four-year-old Boxer with cutaneous and ocular leishmaniosis. This is a granulomatous uveitis with large numbers of plasma cells. Amastigotes were identified within the cytoplasm of some macrophages.

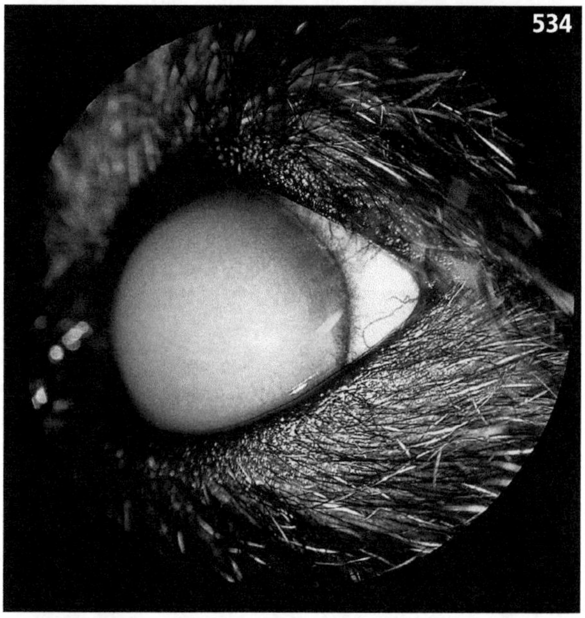

534 Immune-mediated uveitis. Crossbred dog with corneal oedema (blue eye) associated with canine viral hepatitis.

uveitis is generally associated with viral infection (535–539) (FIV, FIP, FeLV), toxoplasmosis, bartonellosis or mycosis. However, lymphoplasmacytic uveitis does occur in the dog and cat in the absence of identified causative agents or conclusive serological evidence of infection, and such cases are often attributed to primary immune-mediated (autoimmune) disease. Defined ocular antigens (rhodopsin,

535

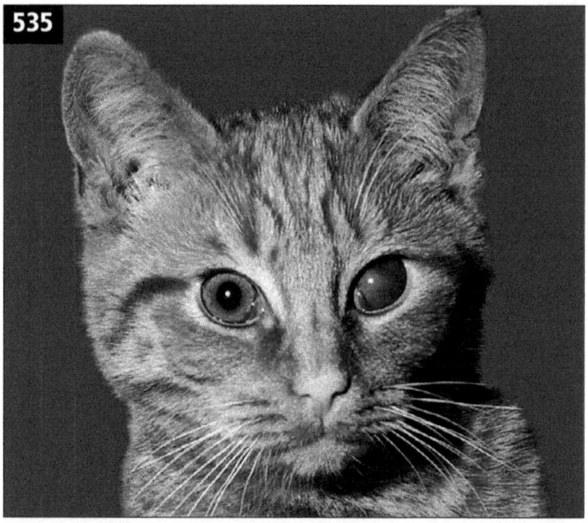

536

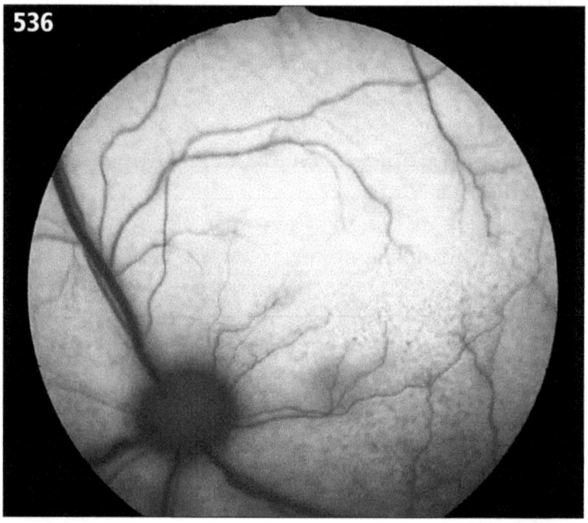

537

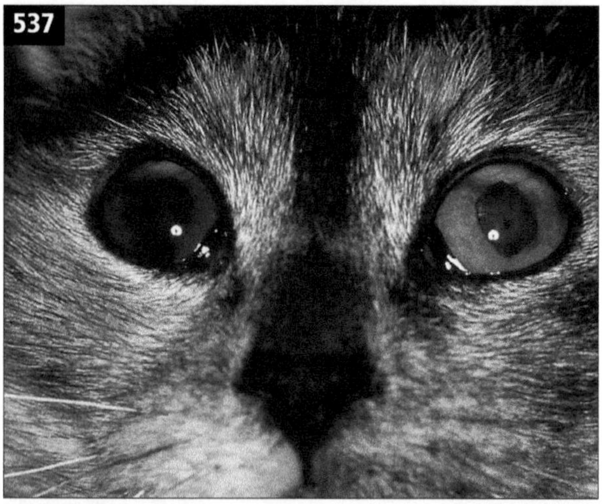

538

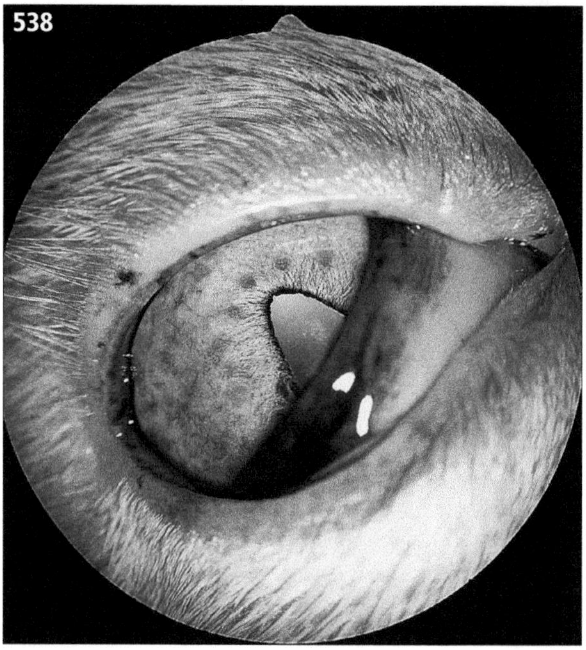

539

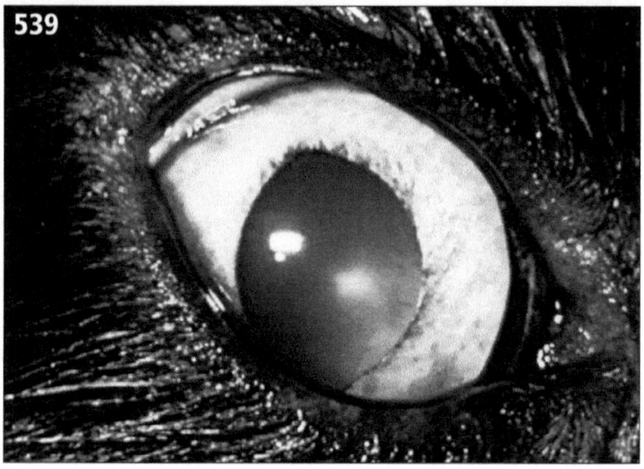

535–539 Feline uveitis. Uveitis in the cat is generally associated with an infectious agent. (**535**) In this cat the ocular disease is secondary to FIP virus infection. (**536**) Extensive vasculitis and perivascular oedema of the retinal vessels in a young cat with FIP infection. (**537, 538**) Uveitis secondary to FeLV (**537**) and FIV (**538**) virus infections. (**539**) Anterior and intermediate uveitis in a cat with concurrent FIV infection and toxoplasmosis.

retinal S antigen, interphotoreceptor-binding protein) may induce CD4+ T cell-mediated autoimmune uveoretinitis in experimental rodent models.

IMMUNE-MEDIATED UVEITIS

Clinical signs

Immune-mediated uveitis most commonly presents acutely in the dog and chronically in the cat. Acute uveitis is usually an intensely painful condition, with associated blepharospasm, lacrimation and genuine photophobia. There may be visual impairment or blindness. The salient ocular features include ciliary injection, varying degrees of corneal oedema, aqueous flare, a miotic pupil that responds sluggishly to different lighting conditions, and a swollen iris with loss of fine detail (540). If it is possible to examine the posterior segment, choroiditis and optic neuritis may be present. The intraocular pressure is low in initial stages.

Chronic uveitis is not usually painful. The eye is not necessarily reddened and the cornea may be clear except for keratic precipitates on the ventral posterior surface. Aqueous flare may be present or absent. The pupil is likely to be irregular if posterior synechiae have formed and the iris may be slightly darker with prominent vessels (rubeosis iridis) and nodules. Inflammatory deposits may be present on the anterior and posterior lens capsule, and hyphaema may be present (541). Posterior segment changes include chorioretinitis, chorioretinal degeneration, retinal detachment, optic neuritis and optic atrophy. The intraocular pressure may be normal or lowered, or increased if secondary glaucoma has occurred. In cats a slightly higher incidence of both glaucoma and secondary lens luxation has been associated with primary, idiopathic lymphoplasmacytic uveitis. It is not usually possible to determine the cause of uveitis from the ocular presentation.

Treatment and prognosis

Immune-mediated uveitis responds poorly to treatment and has a guarded prognosis. Anterior uveitis requires topical treatment with glucocorticoids (prednisolone acetate) and a mydriatic cycloplegic (1% atropine). Topical NSAIDs may be used in conjunction with topical glucocorticoids. Intermediate and posterior uveitis requires systemic treatment with corticosteroids, and panuveitis requires both topical and systemic corticosteroids as well as topical atropine. Combinations of anti-inflammatory and immunosuppressive drugs (see dermatouveitis below) have not been evaluated scientifically for these conditions.

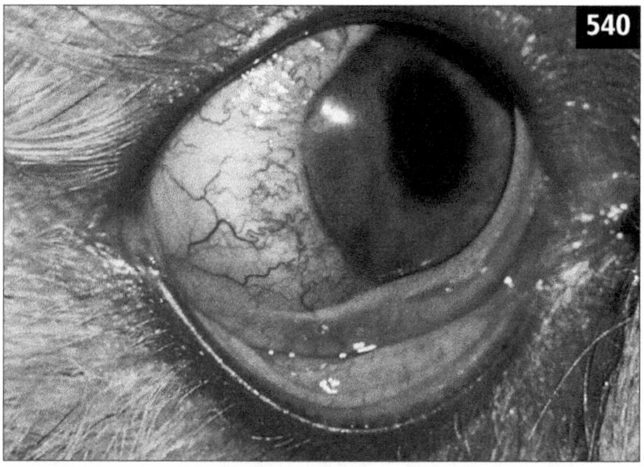

540 Immune-mediated uveitis. Crossbred dog with acute uveitis as a sequela to IBD. Both eyes were affected and the intraocular pressure was 7 mm Hg in the eye illustrated. Note the perilimbal hyperaemia, aqueous flare, keratic precipitates on the posterior surface of the cornea, iris swelling and loss of iris detail. The pupillary light response was poor and the pupil was moderately constricted and of irregular outline. There was also posterior segment inflammation. The uveitis had been present in this eye for at least two days and the eye was very painful.

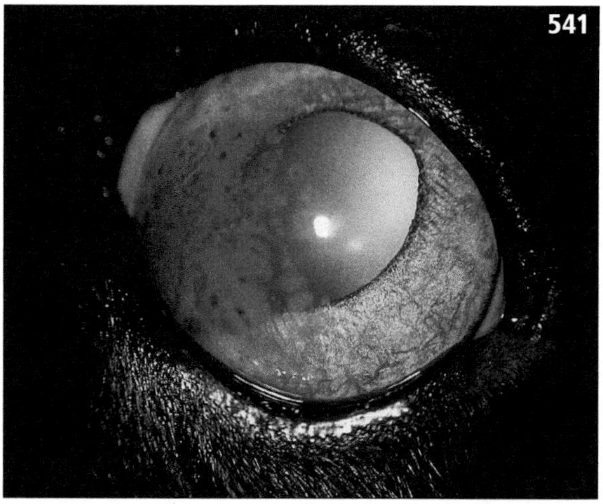

541 Immune-mediated uveitis. DSH cat with bilateral idiopathic lymphoplasmacytic uveitis. Note the keratic precipitates on the posterior cornea and the obvious blood vessels on the surface of the iris. The eye was not painful and the intraocular pressure was 14 mm Hg. Secondary lens luxation was present in the other eye.

CANINE DERMATOUVEITIS

Pathogenesis

Dermatouveitis (canine granulomatous uveitis, Vogt-Koyanagi-Harada-like syndrome [VKH], uveodermatological syndrome) is most commonly recognized in the Japanese Akita, Siberian Husky, Samoyed, Chow Chow, Golden Retriever, Old English Sheepdog, Shetland Sheepdog, St. Bernard, Irish Setter and Australian Setter. The proposed pathogenesis is an autoimmune reaction to melanin-containing cells. Japanese Akitas have a greater risk for the development of dermatouveitis if they carry the MHC class II allele DLA-DQA1*00201.

A recent immunohistochemical study of the ocular and cutaneous lesions in affected Japanese Akita dogs has suggested that these might have distinct immunopathogenesis. The intraocular infiltrates were dominated by B lymphocytes and macrophages displaying minimal MHC class II expression (542), whereas the cutaneous lesions comprised a dominant T lymphocyte infiltrate with strong class II expression by local APCs and keratinocytes (543, 544). These features are consistent with a Th2-regulated immune response within the eye and a Th1-dominated response within affected skin.

Clinical signs

The clinical presentation (545) is of a combination of depigmentation of skin (eyelids, nose, lips, footpads, scrotum, anus) and bilateral uveitis. This combination of uveitis with characteristic skin lesions in susceptible breeds is unlikely to be confused with other ocular problems. The ocular lesions consist of an acute and painful panuveitis of

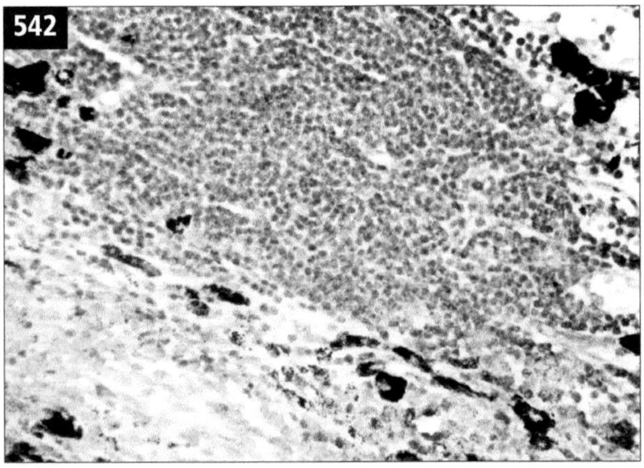

542 Canine dermatouveitis. Immunohistochemical labelling for expression of CD3 within a lymphoid aggregate within the retina of the dog in **545**. Very few of the cells are positively labelled. Immunolabelling of a serial section confirmed that these were B lymphocytes that expressed the CD79a molecule. B cells and non-MHC class II expressing macrophages dominate the intraocular lesions of dermatouveitis.

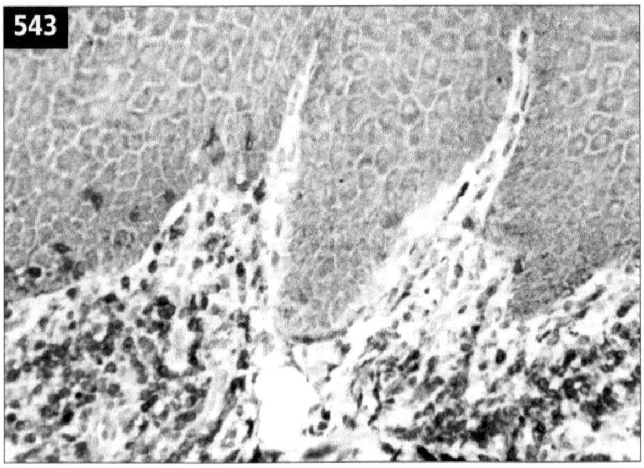

543 Canine dermatouveitis. Immunohistochemical labelling of lesional skin from an Japanese Akita with dermatouveitis demonstrates infiltration of $CD3^+$ T lymphocytes into the dermis and epidermis.

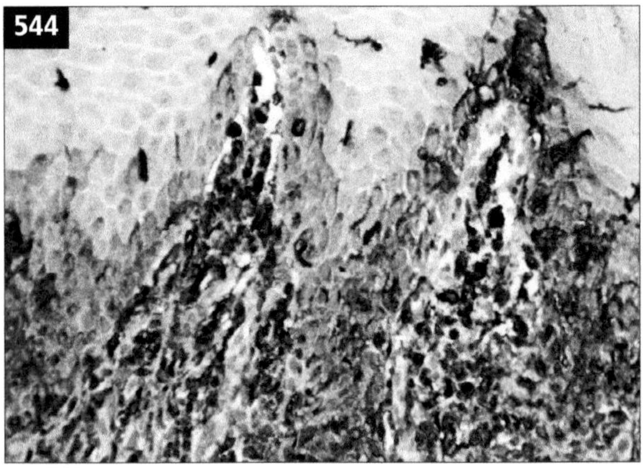

544 Canine dermatouveitis. Immunohistochemical labelling of a serial section of skin from the dog in **545** demonstrates strong expression of MHC class II by infiltrating dermal APCs, epidermal Langerhans cells and basal keratinocytes.

both eyes that may present as loss of visual acuity or even blindness. The lesions are as described above for anterior uveitis and there is often evidence of previous inflammatory episodes (546). Posterior segment changes include chorioretinitis, pigmentary disturbance, serous retinal detachment and optic neuritis (547).

Diagnosis

Histologically there is destructive granulomatous endophthalmitis, with abundant melanin granules, which may involve the choroid and pigmented retinal epithelium and lead to retinal detachment (548). Anti-retinal antibodies have been demonstrated in one dog using a substrate of

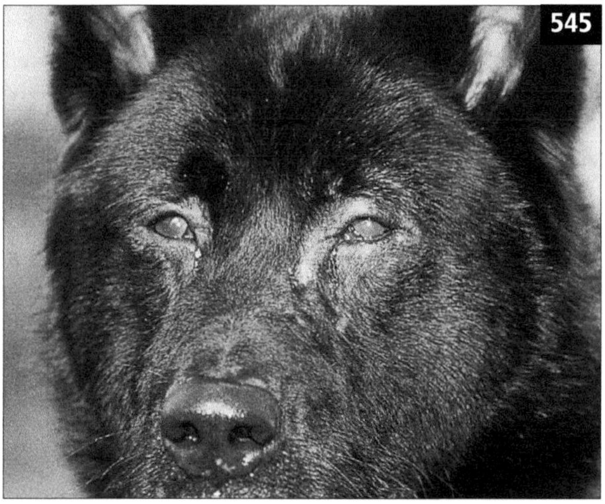

545 Canine dermatouveitis. Japanese Akita with dermatouveitis. Both eyes are affected and there is obvious pain and photophobia. Note also the periocular hair loss and depigmentation and whitening of hair in the muzzle region of this young dog.

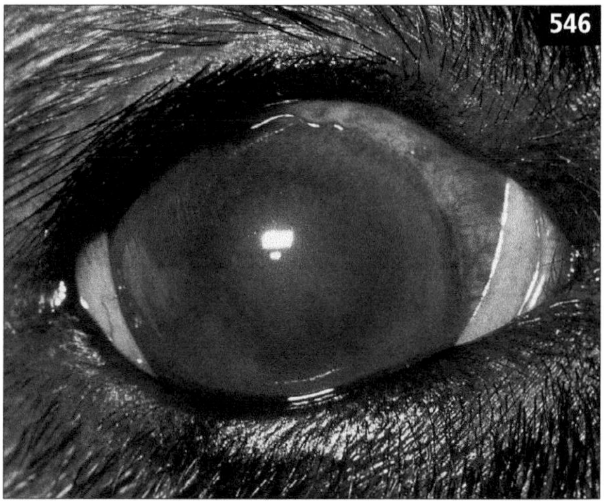

546 Canine dermatouveitis. Japanese Akita with acute recurrent panuveitis associated with dermatouveitis. Note the peripheral corneal vascularization and a discrete focal haemorrhage on the anterior lens capsule. The irregular, partially fixed pupil is indicative of previous inflammatory episodes.

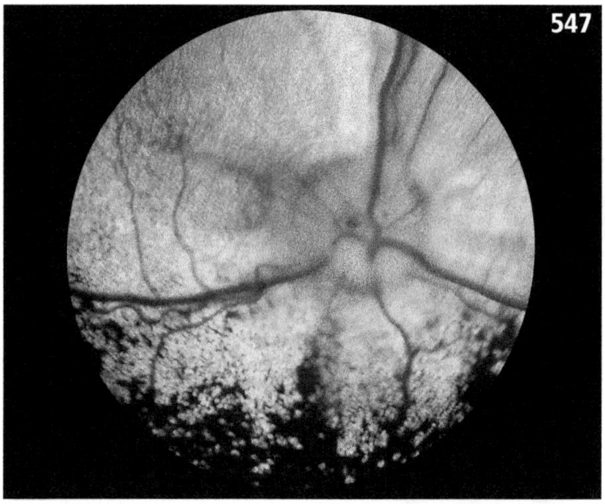

547 Canine dermatouveitis. Japanese Akita with acute recurrent uveitis associated with dermatouveitis. Note that optic neuritis is present. There is also peripapillary serous detachment of the retina and subtle changes in pigmentation are also apparent in the upper part of the illustration.

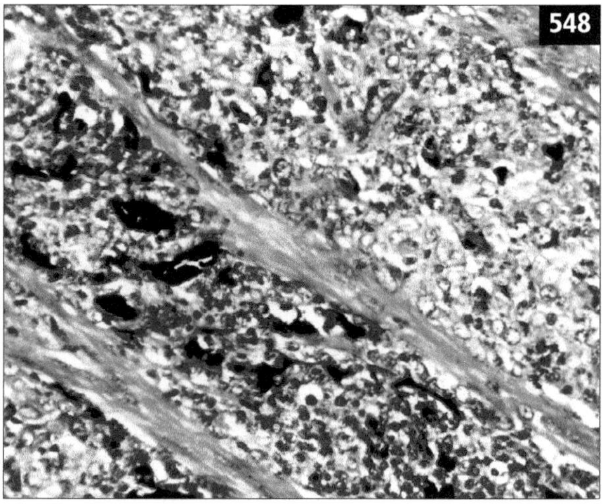

548 Canine dermatouveitis. Granulomatous infiltration of the ciliary body in an Japanese Akita with dermatouveitis.

bovine retinal extract by ELISA, but such antibodies have been demonstrated in dogs with a range of ocular diseases and are likely to be secondary to retinal degeneration rather than a primary cause of disease. Target autoantigens are proposed in human VKH patients to be melanocyte-associated antigens such as Melan-A, MART-1 and tyrosinase. The cutaneous lesions are characterized by infiltration of superficial dermis by macrophages, lymphocytes and plasma cells, but there is only a mild interface reaction. The dermal macrophages contain melanin and there may be reduced pigmentation of epidermis with fewer epidermal melanocytes.

Treatment and prognosis

The management of canine dermatouveitis is not simple and at best the prognosis is guarded. Topical ocular treatment consists of glucocorticoid (prednisolone acetate applied 5 times daily initially, with a reducing regime when the eye has 'quietened'). In severe cases a topical NSAID (e.g. ketorolac trometamol) can be used as an adjunct to topical glucocorticoid. In addition, a mydriatic cycloplegic (1% atropine) is applied as often as necessary to overcome the intense miosis that is part of the acute presentation. Systemic treatment with a glucocorticoid (usually prednisolone) and an immunosuppressant (usually azathioprine) is also necessary, and the combination is safer, with fewer side-effects, than either drug used alone. Both topical and systemic treatment are continued until there is remission (including the return of normal pigmentation), and then the amount and frequency of treatment is gradually reduced. Sudden cessation of treatment may be accompanied by severe recrudescence of inflammation. Even with excellent management the condition is typified by episodic relapses, and permanent blindness or painful secondary glaucoma may occur.

LENS-INDUCED UVEITIS

Two forms of lens-induced uveitis are documented in the dog. The first is associated with leakage of lens protein through the intact capsule of a resorbing cataract (phacolytic uveitis) (**549**). Normal individuals become tolerant to lens protein by continual release of small quantities, but phacolytic uveitis may involve breaking of tolerance and an autoimmune response to these antigens, manifest as mild, lymphoplasmacytic uveitis, and this can be managed medically with topical anti-inflammatories if required.

The second form occurs subsequent to rupture of the lens capsule (phacoclastic uveitis) and is associated with severe inflammation, fibroplasia and, sometimes, endophthalmitis (**550–552**). Small puncture wounds in the lens capsule may seal and such cases can be managed medically, but when there is extensive or sustained release of lens contents, surgical intervention to remove the antigenic protein, usually by phacoemulsification, should be undertaken without delay.

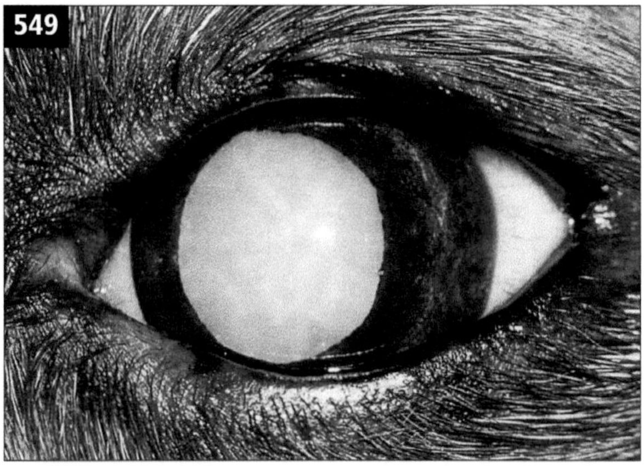

549 Phacolytic uveitis. Phacolytic uveitis associated with resorption of cataract in a diabetic Border Collie. Note the darkening of the iris, the different densities within the lens and the folding of the lens capsule.

IMMUNE-MEDIATED DISEASES OF THE CANINE RETINA

Immune-mediated retinal disease in the dog is a rare occurrence and generally attributed to a defined underlying causation. The induction of anti-retinal antibodies in diseases such as dermatouveitis is discussed above. One further example of this phenomenon occurs in toxacariasis, where the inflammatory reaction to migrating larvae is thought to trigger release of autoantigens and production of retinal autoantibodies (553).

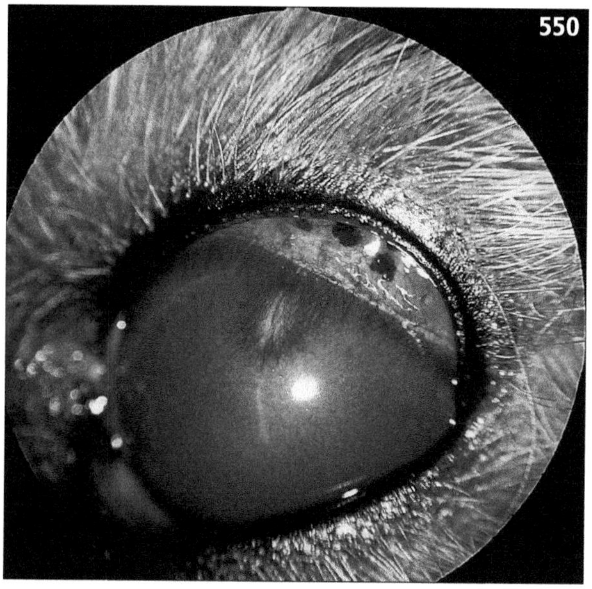

550 Phacoclastic uveitis. Phacoclastic uveitis and secondary glaucoma associated with traumatic rupture of the lens following penetrating injury in a West Highland White Terrier. The white area at 12 o'clock marks the site of original corneal penetration.

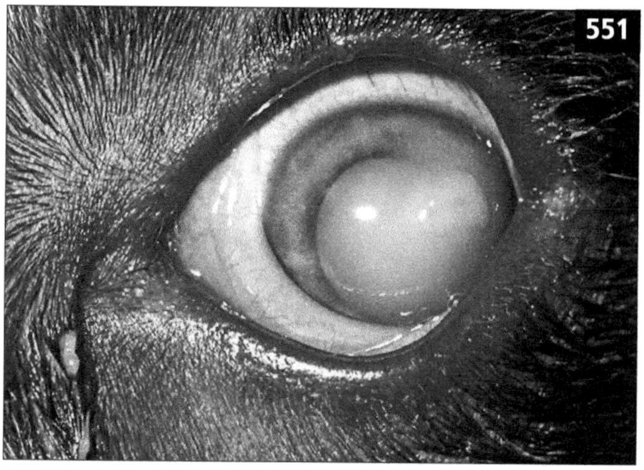

551 Phacoclastic uveitis. Full thickness corneal injury and lens penetration in a puppy as a result of a cat claw injury. There is uptake of fluorescein at site of corneal penetration.

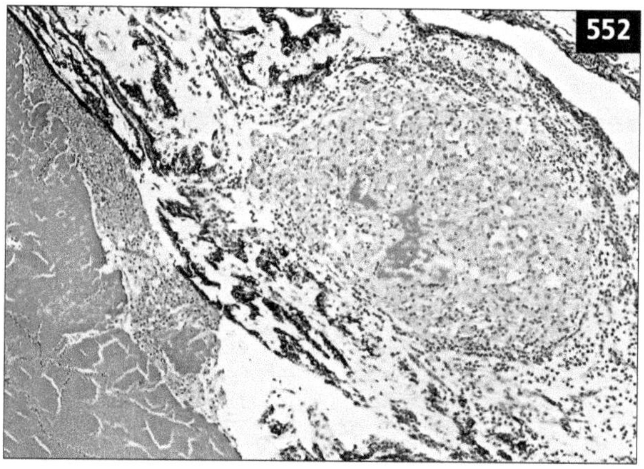

552 Phacoclastic uveitis. Eye from a one-year-old rabbit with rupture of the lens capsule and associated pyogranulomatous inflammation that has extended to the ciliary body and cornea. This presentation may be a consequence of *in utero* infection with the microsporidian parasite *Encephalitozoon cuniculi,* which causes capsular rupture later in life.

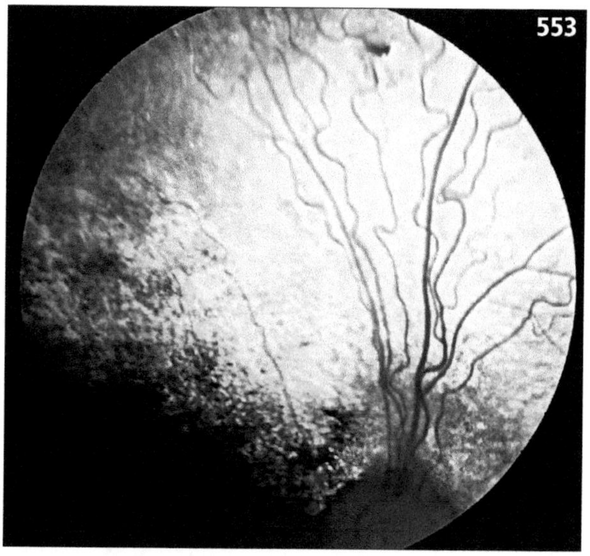

553 Immune-mediated chorioretinitis. Extensive damage is apparent as a result of previous chorioretinitis and optic neuritis. This dog had a heavy infestation of *Toxocara canis* and the severe ocular inflammation followed worming; retinal autoantigens are thought to play a role in this type of inflammatory response.

IMMUNE-MEDIATED DISEASES OF THE CANINE SCLERA AND EPISCLERA

DIFFUSE EPISCLERITIS

Pathogenesis

Diffuse episcleritis (and associated conjunctivitis or keratitis) is characterized by vascular congestion and oedema, with inflammation and thickening of the episcleral/conjunctival tissue (554). These changes are often bilateral and acute in onset, and they may be recurrent. The disease may be immune-mediated, as there is episcleral vasculitis with deposition of immunoreactants in the vascular wall and a lymphoplasmacytic infiltration.

Clinical signs

Diffuse episcleritis presents as mild to marked, acute episodic reddening of episcleral and conjunctival vessels. Peripheral corneal oedema and infiltration by lipid is common to both episcleritis and scleritis, and the level of corneal involvement helps determine whether the inflammation is episcleral or scleral.

Diagnosis

Examination of the 'white' of the eye will aid assessment of the level of inflammation, and daylight and red-free (green) light are better for this than artificial light. A directly acting sympathomimetic (e.g. 10% phenylephrine) will vasoconstrict superficial conjunctival and episcleral vessels and make it easier to differentiate scleral inflammation.

Treatment and prognosis

The condition is episodic and not painful, so treatment is not always necessary. However, topical corticosteroids may be used. If there is associated lipid deposition, it is important to perform lipid and lipoprotein analysis (preferably during an inflammatory episode) to distinguish reactive hyperaemia due to high circulating lipid.

NODULAR EPISCLERITIS

Clinical signs

Nodular episcleritis (episclerokeratitis, nodular fasciitis, fibrous histiocytoma, inflammatory pseudotumour) presents as single or multiple firm, nodular swellings below the bulbar conjunctiva or just posterior to the limbus. The accurate classification of this disease is difficult, as is evident from the multiplicity of descriptive names, and terms such as fibrous histiocytoma, which imply malignancy, are best avoided. Nodular episcleritis (555) differs from nodular episclerokeratitis (556) only in terms of the corneal involvement. Histologically the lesion comprises a non-encapsulated mixture of spindle and mononuclear cells (557). There is minimal collagenous stroma, but reticulin fibres are readily demonstrated.

Diagnosis

Diagnosis is usually based on clinical appearance, histopathology of the lesions and response to treatment.

554

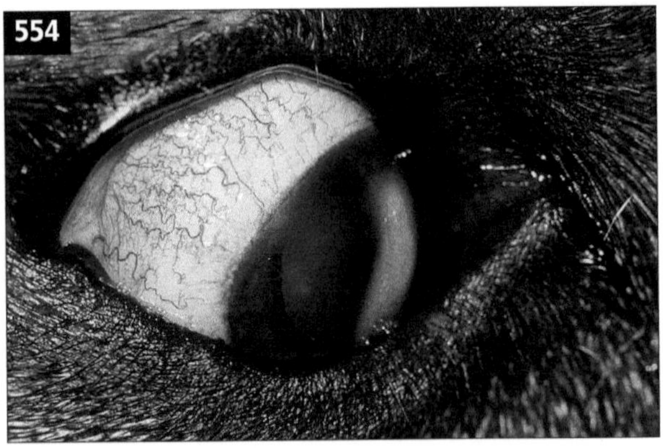

554 Canine diffuse episcleritis. Great Dane with diffuse episcleritis and a linear streak of corneal lipid deposition in an area of cornea subject to mild mechanical trauma from a sebaceous adenoma of the lower eyelid. The dog was hyperlipoproteinaemic.

555

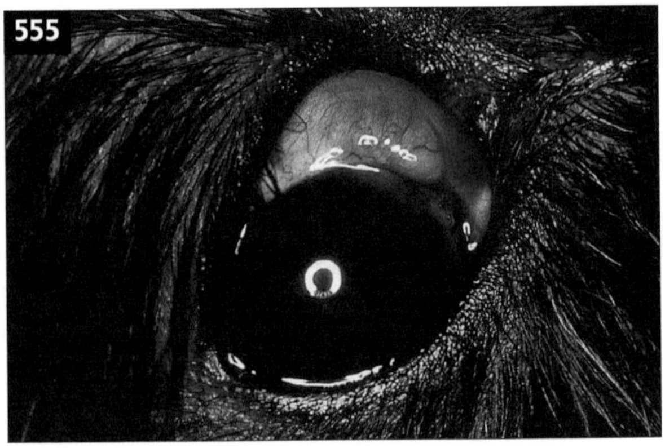

555 Canine nodular episcleritis. Cairn Terrier with a large episcleral nodule and a very faint rim of peripheral oedema in the adjacent cornea.

Treatment and prognosis

Long-term topical glucocorticoids are the medical treatment of choice and may be combined with excisional biopsy. Other topical agents (e.g. ciclosporin) require evaluation. The use of systemic cytotoxic drugs (e.g. azathioprine) is debatable for what is, in essence, a benign, slowly growing inflammatory lesion.

DIFFUSE AND NODULAR SCLERITIS

Pathogenesis

The aetiology of these disorders is unknown, but they are considered immune-mediated. Most cases are organ specific, but the possibility of coexisting connective tissue disease should be considered and assessment of serum RF and ANA may be useful.

Clinical signs

Primary scleral inflammation may have a diffuse (rare) or nodular (more common) presentation. The scleral thickening observed in diffuse scleritis may be sufficient to cause proptosis. The change may be uni- or bilateral and may involve the conjunctiva or episclera.

Diagnosis

Diagnosis is based on the clinical appearance of dark red, almost purple, scleral injection. Topical phenylephrine will blanch overlying superficial vessels for easier identification of the affected area (558, 559). Low-grade uveitis is present in some

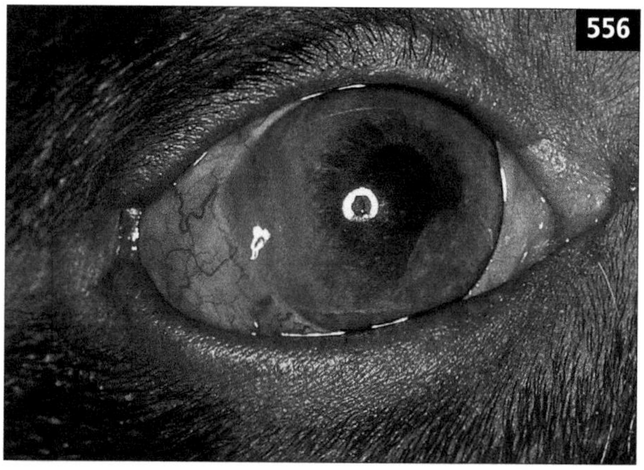

556 Canine nodular episclerokeratitis. English Springer Spaniel with nodular episclerokeratitis. Note that the nodule has infiltrated the cornea.

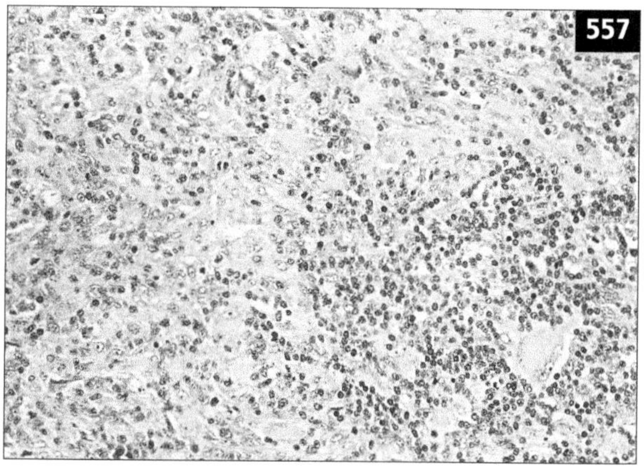

557 Canine nodular episcleritis. Enucleated eye from a six-year-old Manchester Terrier with a focal episcleral nodule present for three months. The nodule is composed of a background stroma of collagen and fibroblasts, with a mixed mononuclear inflammatory population including occasional multinucleate giant cells.

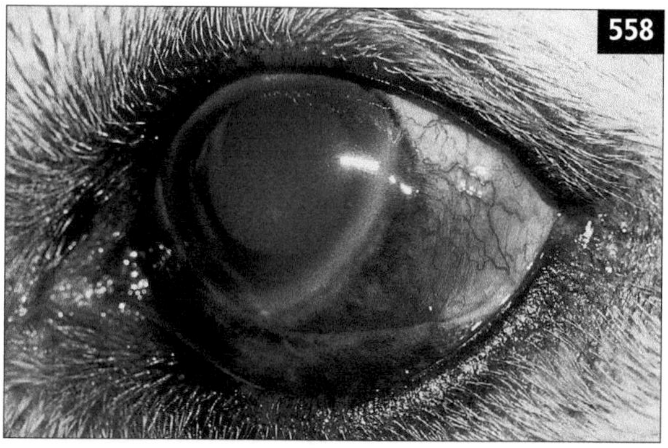

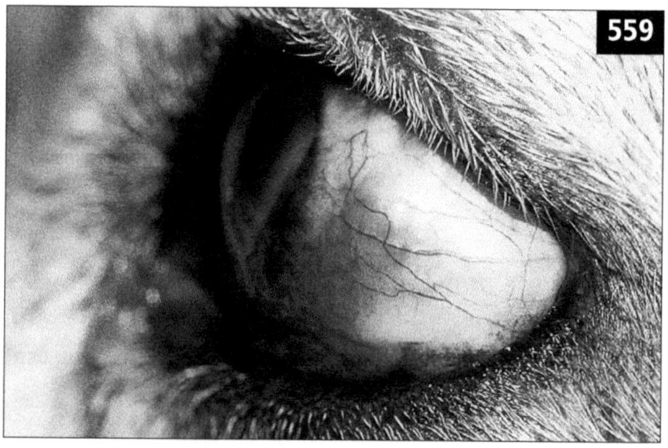

558, 559 Canine nodular scleritis. (**558**) Labrador Retriever with nodular scleritis; low-grade uveitis with fine keratic precipitates is also present. (**559**) The same dog after 10% phenylephrine has been applied to the eye to blanch the superficial vessels in order to demonstrate the nodule more clearly.

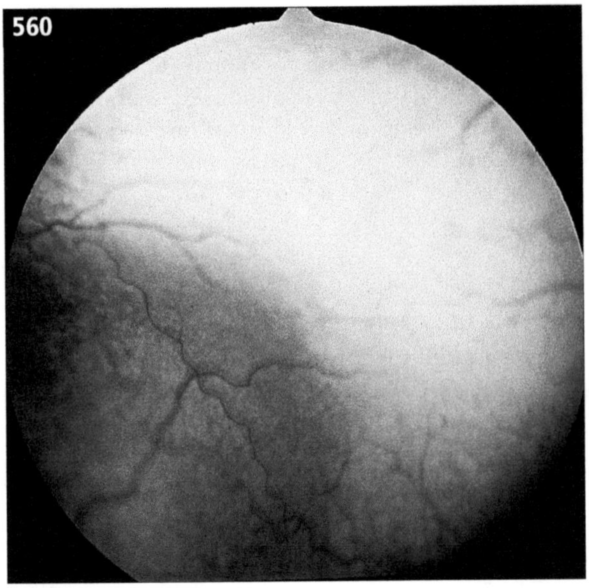

560 Canine nodular scleritis. German Shorthaired Pointer with nodular scleritis. A nodule is clearly visible on ophthalmoscopic examination as a fawn elevation between 6 o'clock and 9 o'clock.

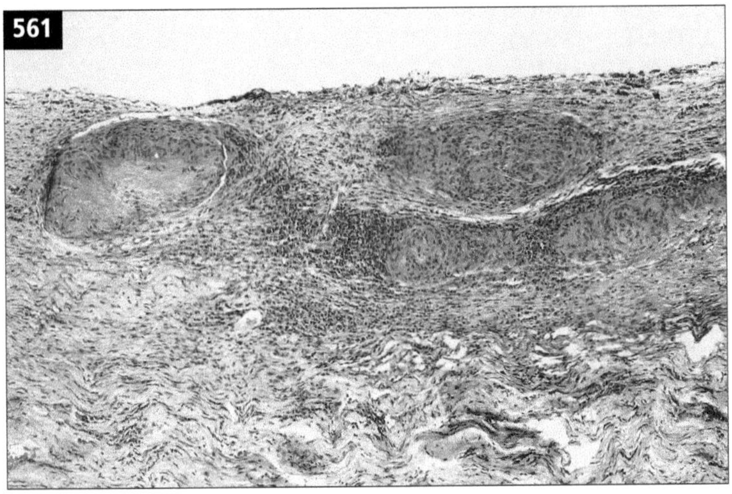

561 Canine necrotizing scleritis. Section of sclera with diffuse, mixed mononuclear to granulomatous inflammation, focal collagen degeneration and vasculitis. Immunohistochemical examination of this lesion revealed a dominant $CD3^{+}$ T cell infiltrate and evidence of IgG deposition within affected vascular walls.

cases and fundus changes (**560**) may be observed following mydriasis, with or without scleral depression to extend the field of view. Diagnostic imaging (ultrasonography and magnetic resonance imaging [MRI]) can demonstrate the extent of inflammation and aid in monitoring the efficacy of treatment.

Treatment and prognosis
Treatment is as described for dermatouveitis and the prognosis is guarded, especially with bilateral involvement.

NECROTIZING SCLERITIS
Pathogenesis
Necrotizing scleritis is very rare and may be a severe manifestation of scleritis or an organ-specific, immune-mediated vasculitis arising in the anterior sclera. There are coalescing scleral granulomas with central remnants of denatured collagen, with or without eosinophils; alternatively, a diffuse granulomatous reaction may be observed (**561**). Rarely, similar lesions arise in the skin of affected dogs, suggesting that the disease may present as a systemic immune complex disorder affecting scleral and dermal vessels (**562**). Immunohistochemical studies have demonstrated deposition of IgG within the vascular walls and an inflammatory infiltration of $CD3^{+}$ T lymphocytes, MHC class II expressing

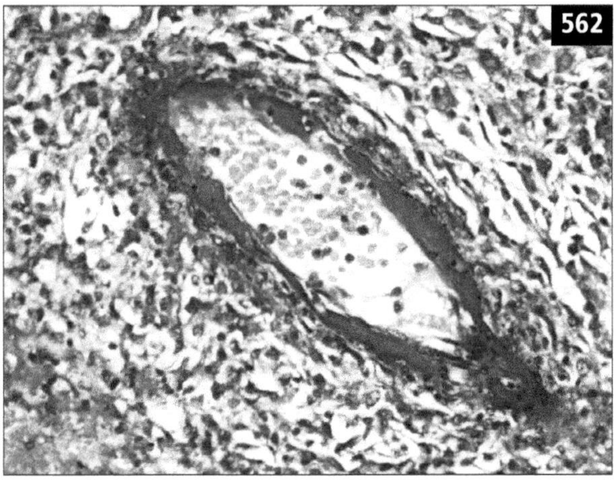

562 Canine necrotizing scleritis. Section of sclera stained by Martius scarlet blue to demonstrate fibrin (red) within the wall of an inflamed scleral vessel. There is an intense granulomatous inflammatory infiltrate surrounding the vessel.

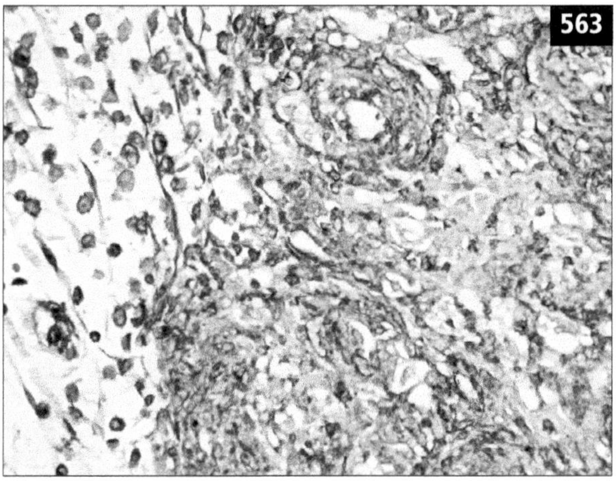

563 Canine necrotizing scleritis. Section of sclera from the dog in **554** labelled immunohistochemically to show marked expression of MHC class II by infiltrating macrophages.

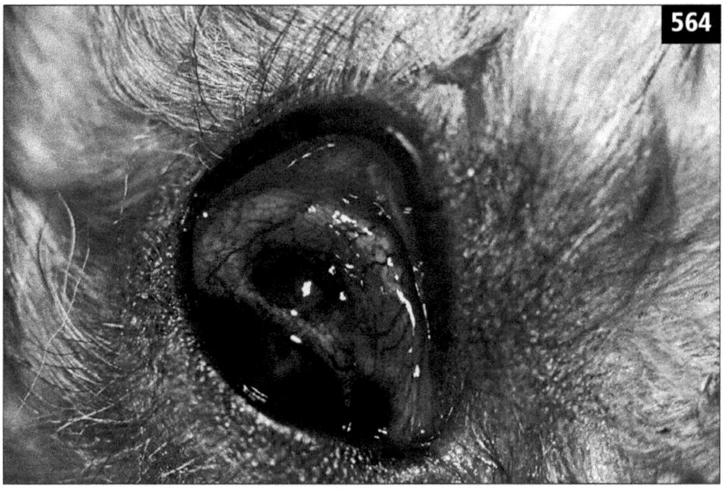

564 Canine necrotizing scleritis. Scleromalacia perforans is a rare complication of necrotizing scleritis.

macrophages and IgG plasma cells (563). The immunopathology appears identical in both ocular and cutaneous lesions.

Clinical signs

The lesions may spread circumferentially around the sclera and involve the uvea and retina.

Diagnosis

Diagnosis is based on clinical appearance, imaging examination and histopathology. Biopsy is not always easy due to the potential for scleromalacia perforans (564), and the biopsy site may require the postoperative support of a cartilage-containing graft or donor sclera.

Treatment and prognosis

Prognosis is poor due to likely complications (scleromalacia perforans), and the eye may be lost. Treatment, if attempted, must be aggressive and hospitalization is required. An initial intravenous bolus of glucocorticoid may be required and subsequent systemic glucocorticoid therapy is usually combined with azathioprine or cyclophosphamide and, possibly, ciclosporin. Ocular glucocorticoid therapy should be applied topically, not by the subconjunctival route, because of the risk of scleromalacia perforans.

FURTHER READING

Angles JM, Famula TR, Pedersen NC (2005) Uveodermatologic (VKH-like) syndrome in American Akita dogs is associated with an increased frequency of DQA*00201. *Tissue Antigens* **66**:656–665.

Breaux CB, Sandmeyer LS, Grahn BH (2007) Immunohistochemical investigation of canine episcleritis. *Veterinary Ophthalmology* **10**:168–172.

Carter J, SM Crispin, DJ Gould *et al.* (2005) An immunohistochemical study of uveodermatologic syndrome in two Japanese Akita dogs. *Veterinary Ophthalmology* **8**:17–24.

Carvalho ARR, Naranjo C, Leiva M *et al.* (2009) Canine normal corneal epithelium bears a large population of CD45-positive cells. *Veterinary Journal* **179**:437–442.

Davidson MG (2000) Toxoplasmosis. *Veterinary Clinics of North America: Small Animal Practice* **30**:1051–1062.

Day MJ, Mould JRB, Carter WJ (2008) An immunohistochemical study of canine necrotizing scleritis. *Veterinary Ophthalmology.* **11**:11–17.

Donaldson D, Day MJ (2000) Epitheliotrophic lymphoma (mycosis fungoides) presenting as blepharoconjunctivitis in an Irish Setter. *Journal of Small Animal Practice* **41**:317–320.

Gilger BC, Rose PD, Davidson MG *et al.* (1999) Low-dose oral administration of interferon-alpha for the treatment of immune-mediated keratoconjunctivitis sicca in dogs. *Journal of Interferon and Cytokine Research* **19**:901–905.

Izci C, Celik I, Alkan F *et al.* (2002) Histologic characteristics and local cellular immunity of the gland of the third eyelid after topical ophthalmic administration of 2% cyclosporine for treatment of dogs with keratoconjunctivitis sicca. *American Journal of Veterinary Research* **63**:688–694.

Jokinen P, Rusanen EM, Kennedy LJ *et al.* (2011) MHC class II risk haplotype associated with canine chronic superficial keratitis in German shepherd dogs. *Veterinary Immunology and Immunopathology* **140**:37–41.

Massa KL, Gilger BC, Miller TL *et al.* (2002) Causes of uveitis in dogs: 102 cases (1989–2000). *Veterinary Ophthalmology* **5**:93–98.

Sanchez RF, Innocent G, Mould J *et al.* (2007) Canine keratoconjunctivitis sicca: disease trends in a review of 229 cases. *Journal of Small Animal Practice* **48**:211–217.

Spiess AK, Sapienza JS, Mayordomo A (2009) Treatment of proliferative feline eosinophilic keratitis with topical 1.5% cyclosporine: 35 cases. *Veterinary Ophthalmology* **12**:132–137.

Torres M-D, Leiva M, Tabar M-D *et al.* (2009) Ligneous conjunctivitis in a plasminogen-deficient dog: clinical management and 2-year follow-up. *Veterinary Ophthalmology* **12**:248–253.

van der Woert A (2001) Management of intraocular inflammatory disease. *Clinical Techniques in Small Animal Practice* **16**:58–61.

Williams DL, Pierce V, Mellor P *et al.* (2007) Reduced tear production in three canine endocrinopathies. *Journal of Small Animal Practice* **48**:252–256.

12 IMMUNODEFICIENCY DISEASE

Michael J. Day

INTRODUCTION

Immunodeficiency disease may be primary or secondary in nature. Primary immunodeficiency is a congenital, inherited defect of one or more components of the immune system. Such disorders are uncommon in dogs and rare in cats. In contrast, defective immune function secondary to infectious, neoplastic, metabolic or chronic inflammatory diseases, or to administration of drugs, often occurs in these species.

SECONDARY IMMUNODEFICIENCY

The range of secondary immunodeficiencies recorded in dogs and cats is broad. Selected examples are discussed below.

Physiological

Immunological parameters vary with the age, breed and sex of an animal. Numerous recent studies have now examined the age-related changes that occur in the canine and feline immune systems. In common with humans, in older dogs and cats there are alterations in the balance of circulating lymphocytes (reduced $CD4^+$ T cells and $CD21^+$ B cells, with elevated $CD8^+$ T cells and thus reduced CD4:CD8 ratio), reduction in blood lymphocyte mitogen-driven proliferative responses, and elevations in the serum concentration of IgG and IgA. Mitogen responsiveness is also influenced by the season (maximal in spring to summer) and time of day of sample collection, and there is similar diurnal variation in the concentration of serum IgA in the dog. The serological response to vaccine antigens does not appear to diminish with age, and innate immune function (e.g. NK cell activity, neutrophil phagocytosis) is also relatively stable with ageing.

Dietary factors, particularly protein, mineral and vitamin intake, have major effects on immune function and there has been much recent focus by pet food manufacturers on developing diets that are able to optimize immune system function or even counteract the effects of ageing. Approaches such as alteration of the n3:n6 polyunsaturated fatty acid balance or incorporation of anti-oxidants such as vitamin E or betacarotene have been shown to have some effect on age-related decline in immune function.

Hormonal effects on immune function are not well characterized in dogs and cats, but in man the concept of the neuroendocrine immunological loop has been widely studied (see Chapter 1, p. 55). One clear example of this phenomenon is the observation that pregnancy in women is associated with transient remission from autoimmune diseases such as RA. In similar fashion, mobilization of latent *Toxocara canis* in the pregnant bitch may be permitted by such immunosuppression.

Drug therapy

Many drugs have pronounced effects on the immune system and such treatment should be withdrawn for several weeks before performing *in vitro* immunological studies. For example, glucocorticoids have wide ranging effects on granulocyte, monocyte and lymphocyte function, and ciclosporin has potent suppressive effects on lymphocyte proliferation.

Chronic disease

Animals with chronic disease may have secondary reduction of immunological function. Dogs with demodicosis often have depressed lymphocyte proliferation, with decreased IL-2 production and IL-2 receptor expression by the stimulated cells. Early studies suggested that this was related to a suppressive factor in autologous serum, which was also able to decrease the chemotactic migration of normal dog neutrophils. This serum factor may be associated with concurrent bacterial pyoderma, and immune complexes of antibody and staphylococcal antigen have similar suppressive function. Despite these systemic abnormalities, there is active mononuclear infiltration of the cutaneous lesions of demodicosis (565, 566). Serum factors that suppress lymphocyte proliferative responses have been identified in a range of other diseases including immunoproliferative small intestinal disease of the Basenji.

Dogs with deep pyoderma, or nasal or disseminated aspergillosis, may have secondary depression of lymphocyte proliferation or neutrophil function. Similarly, dogs with anal furunculosis may have depressed mitogen-induced lymphocyte proliferation, which returns to normal after recovery from disease. Neutrophils from dogs with diabetes mellitus have decreased ability to adhere to nylon wool, and this defect may contribute to development of secondary infection in this disease. Reduced lymphocyte function is also documented in bitches with pyometra.

A range of viral infections induces secondary immunological abnormalities. CDV, canine parvovirus, feline parvovirus and FeLV infections may cause depletion of lymphoid tissue (567) and suppress lymphocyte proliferative responses. A reduced CD4:CD8 ratio has been documented in FeLV-infected cats.

Feline immunodeficiency virus

The most striking example of secondary immunodeficiency in dogs and cats is the profound immunological imbalance that occurs in FIV infection. FIV is a T lymphotropic lentivirus that can infect $CD4^+$ and $CD8^+$ T cells, $SmIg^+$ cells, monocytes and macrophages, follicular dendritic

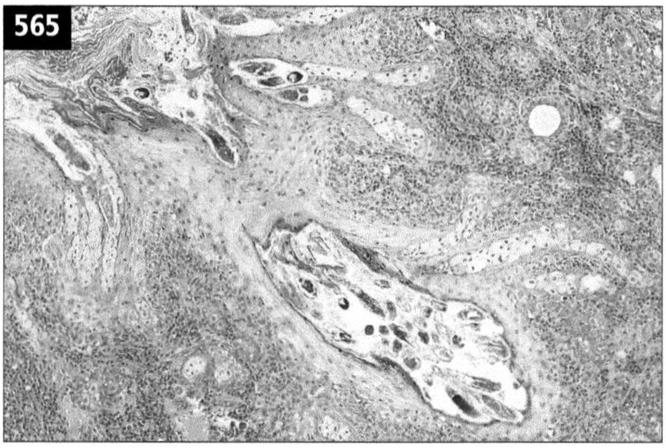

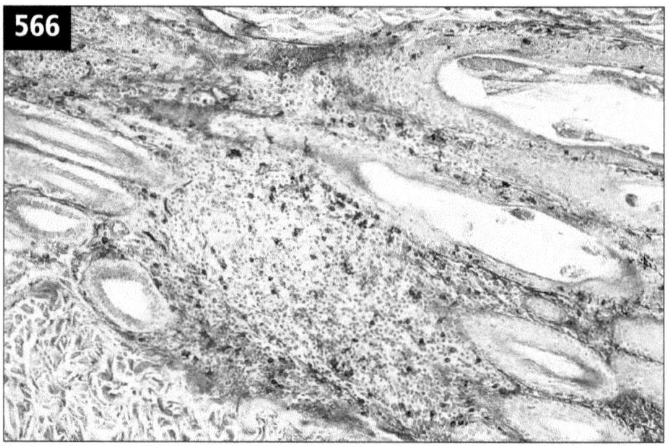

565, 566 Canine demodicosis. The local cutaneous immune response in canine demodicosis comprises a vigorous infiltration of T cells ($CD4^+$ and $CD8^+$), MHC class II expressing macrophages and dendritic cells, and plasma cells of the IgG, IgM and IgA classes. (**546**) Section of skin from a dog with demodicosis demonstrating numerous mites within the upper follicular lumen. (**547**) IgM-bearing plasma cells within the perifollicular infiltrate in a dog with demodicosis.

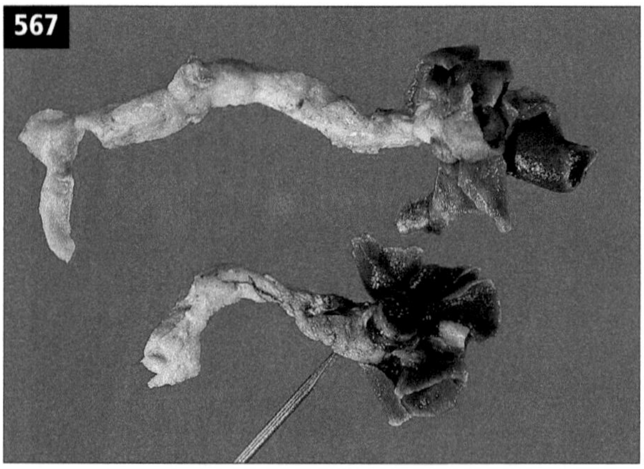

567 Thymic hypoplasia. Thoracic contents from a poorly grown, two-week-old Siamese kitten (upper specimen) and an unrelated kitten of similar age (lower specimen). The thymus is clearly visible in the lower specimen, but not apparent in the upper one (position indicated by metal probe). Microscopic examination of the adipose tissue in this area revealed remnants of depleted thymic lobules. This gross appearance would most commonly be attributed to *in utero* infection by FIE virus, but in this kitten there was no other histological evidence of viral infection, suggesting primary thymic hypoplasia. (From Day MJ [1997] A review of thymic pathology in 30 cats and 36 dogs. *Journal of Small Animal Practice* **38:**393–403, with permission.)

cells and astrocytes (**568**). The primary viral receptor is now known to be CD134 (OX40), which is a member of the TNF receptor superfamily of molecules. CD134 interacts with FIV gp95 and viral infection of the cell also involves an interaction with the chemokine receptor CXCR4. The virus is most likely transmitted via biting, as FIV is readily isolated from saliva. There is also evidence for *in utero*, perinatal or venereal transmission, but this is likely to occur infrequently. Infection has been associated with:

- Chronic disease of multiple systems including gingivostomatitis, respiratory infection, enteritis, dermatitis, weight loss, pyrexia and lymphadenomegaly (**569**).
- Opportunist infection by feline calicivirus, FeLV or feline foamy virus (FeFV; feline syncytium forming virus). Other infections are documented in FIV-positive cats (*Toxoplasma, Mycoplasma, Candida, Cryptococcus, Demodex* or *Mycobacterium*), but no statistically significant associations are recorded.
- Haematological abnormalities including non-regenerative anaemia, leukocytosis or leukopenia.
- Neurological disease including meningitis, meningoencephalitis and choroiditis.
- Lymphoma (mostly B cell) or myeloproliferative disease. This effect is generally attributed to concurrent FeLV infection, but lymphoma also occurs in FeLV-negative, FIV-infected cats. FIV proviral DNA cannot be isolated from lymphoma cells, suggesting an indirect role for FIV.

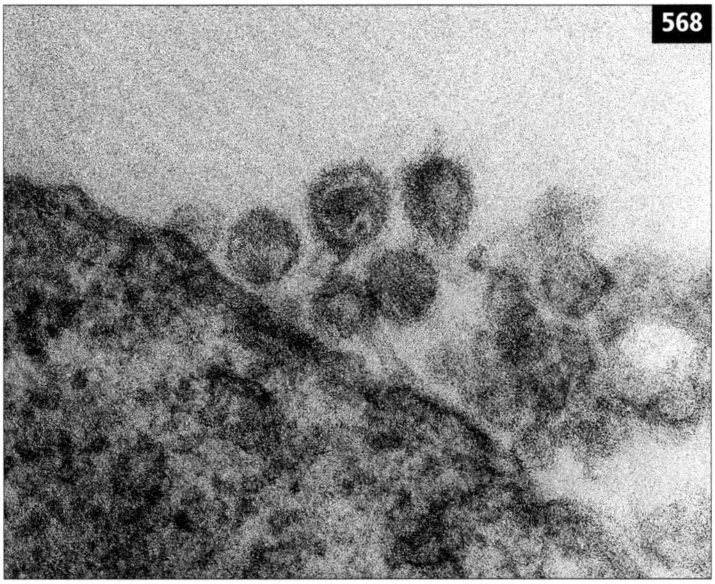

568 FIV. Transmission electron micrograph of FIV particles adjacent to the membrane of an infected lymphocyte.

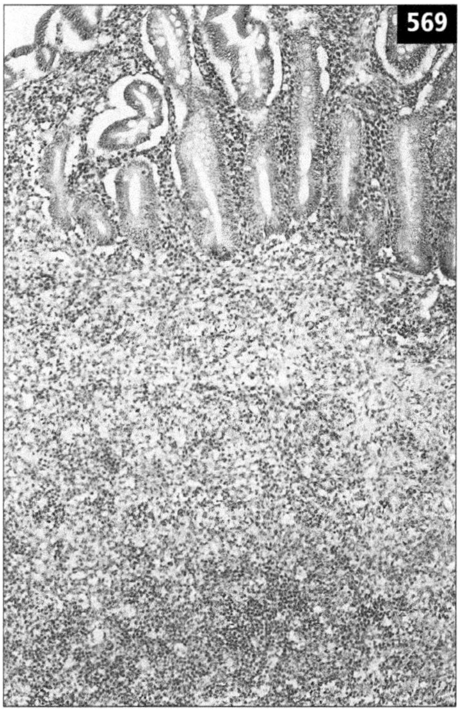

569 FIV infection. Section of colon from a five-year-old DSH cat with FIV infection and clinical signs of weight loss, anorexia, vomiting and pyrexia. There is a granulomatous colitis extending to muscle layers. Intestinal lesions are often documented in cats with FIV infection, but specific aetiological agents are not identified by special stains.

In contrast, many infected cats will remain clinically normal for protracted periods, although they remain a reservoir of infection for other animals.

The clinical course of FIV infection has largely been determined from experimental studies. An acute phase of mild illness (pyrexia, anorexia, lymphadenomegaly, with progressive decline in circulating $CD4^+$ T cells) may persist for some months (stage 1) and is followed by an asymptomatic phase (with continued gradual decline in $CD4^+$ T cells) that may last several years (stage 2). During stage 3 there is recurrence of mild illness, which may respond to symptomatic treatment, but in stages 4 and 5 there is progressive onset of the AIDS-like syndrome described above. Death usually occurs within 12 months of the onset of stage 4–5 disease.

Diagnostic measures include demonstration of virus in blood T cells, amplification of FIV nucleic acid sequence by conventional or real-time PCR, or demonstration of FIV-specific antibody. A range of in-practice test kits based on ELISA or immunochromatography are available, and these may allow concurrent testing for FeLV. Laboratory methodology for antibody testing includes indirect immunofluorescence and western blotting. A positive in-practice test from a clinically ill animal should generally be considered accurate; however, in the case of test-positive cats that are clinically normal, a confirmatory test should be performed by a laboratory. Similarly, an animal with high clinical index of suspicion that tests negative using an in-practice kit should be retested by laboratory-based methodology.

The observed immunological abnormalities in FIV infection may include:

- Progressive decrease in CD4:CD8 ratio. CD8 and B lymphocyte numbers may increase to normalize the total lymphocyte count.
- Depressed response of blood mononuclear cells to mitogens or specific antigens, with reduced IL-2 production on mitogen activation but increased production of IL-1, IL-6 and TNFα.
- Altered macrophage function.
- Abnormal lymphoid tissue (570, 571).
- Polyclonal gammopathy.

570
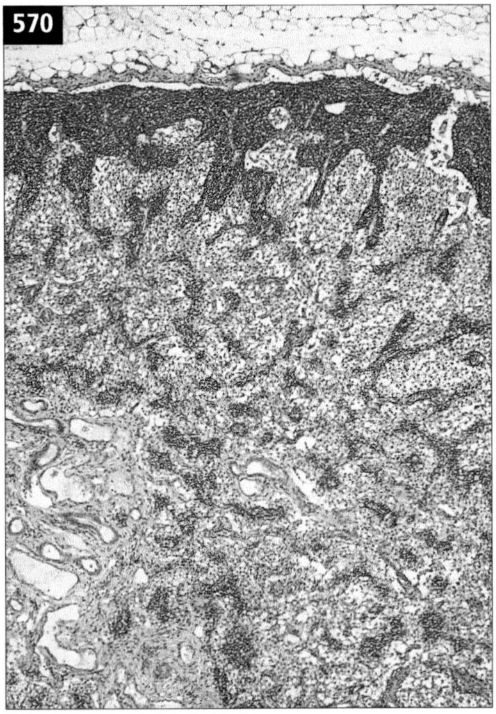

571
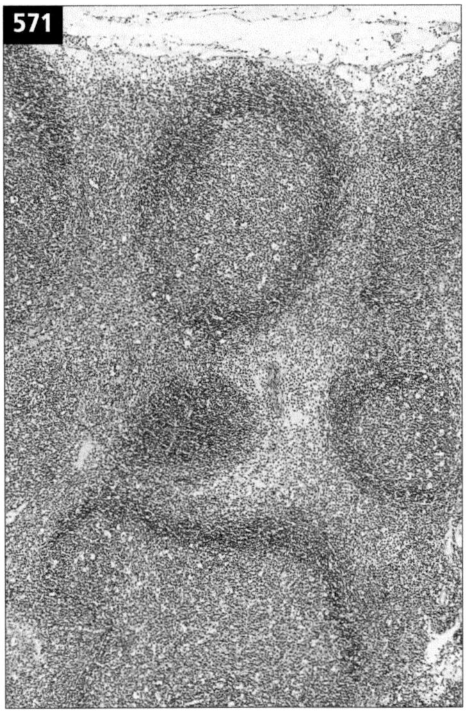

570, 571 Lymph node abnormalities in FIV infection. Sections of lymph node from cats with FIV infection showing examples of the range of histological abnormalities including marked depletion of cortical lymphoid tissue (**570**) and lymphoid hyperplasia with large and irregular follicle formation (**571**).

PRIMARY IMMUNODEFICIENCY

The specific defect in primary immunodeficiency may involve any part of the immune system during any stage of immunological development (572). A defect of an early developmental stage results in life-threatening disease, whereas abnormalities of late development may result in chronic, low-grade disease.

Primary immunodeficiency disease may be suspected where there is:

- Chronic, recurrent infection in young, littermate animals.
- Infection at multiple sites.
- Failure to respond to standard antimicrobial therapy.
- Infection with unusual microorganisms (e.g. environmental saphrophytes).
- Persistent leukocytosis or hypergammaglobulinaemia.
- Persistent leukopenia or hypogammaglobulinaemia.
- Failure to respond to vaccination.
- Concurrent autoimmunity, allergy or immune system neoplasia.
- An absence of possible causes of secondary immunodeficiency.

Although numerous primary immunodeficiency states have been documented in the dog, in reality their immunological and molecular basis is poorly understood. For this reason, many canine immunodeficiency states should only be considered as 'putative' immunodeficiencies until such time as the molecular pathogenesis is defined. This is the case for only three canine immunodeficiency diseases (cyclic haematopoiesis, canine leukocyte adhesion deficiency and severe combined immunodeficiency), which are described below.

Diagnosis of immunodeficiency

The aim of diagnosis is to localize the immunological defect to one or more components of the immune system. Optimally, the affected animal should be subject to a full panel of tests of cell-mediated and humoral immune function in

572

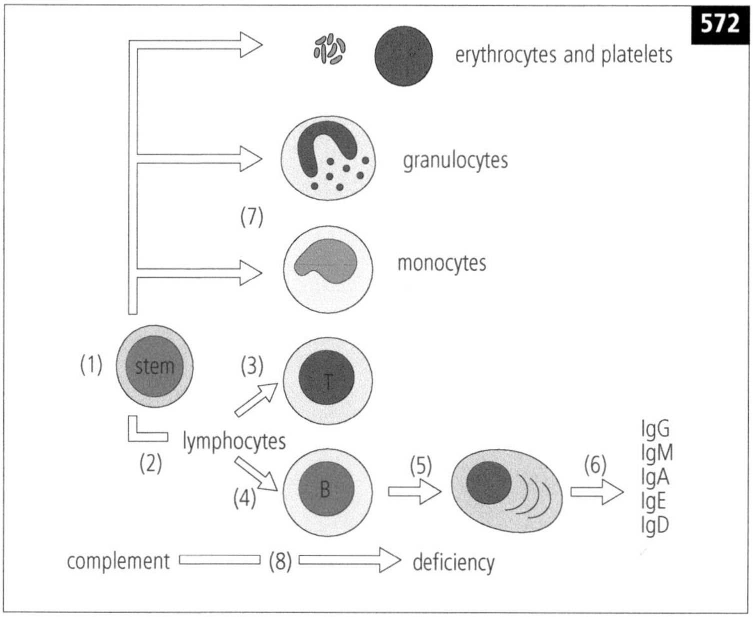

572 Primary immunodeficiency disease. This diagram summarizes the development of haemopoietic and lymphoid cells and the possible points at which developmental abnormality may give rise to primary immunodeficiency disease. These include (1) failure of differentiation of the pluripotent stem cell; (2) failure of differentiation of the committed stem cell; (3) failure of T cell development; (4) failure of B cell development; (5) blockade of B cell differentiation into plasma cells; (6) failure to produce selected class(es) of immunoglobulin; (7) failure to produce functional neutrophils or macrophages; or (8) failure to produce one or more complement components.

order to establish where the defect may lie. In reality, such tests are not readily available other than by arrangement with a specialist or research laboratory. The diagnostic approach may include:

- Haematology profile.
- Bone marrow biopsy.
- Lymph node biopsy.
- Serum protein analysis (**573, 574**).
- Characterization of infectious agents by serology or culture.
- Full necropsy of any dead littermates.
- Quantification of serum Igs (see below).
- Assessment of the antibody response to vaccine antigens.
- Complement function testing (see below).
- Determination of complement component concentration (see below).
- Peripheral blood lymphocyte phenotyping and calculation of the CD4:CD8 ratio (see below).
- Assessment of the ability of blood lymphocytes to respond to mitogens or specific antigens (see below).

573

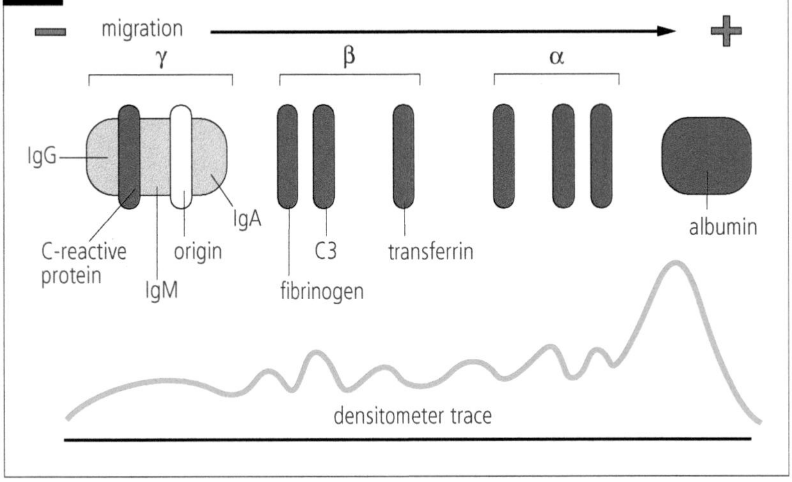

574

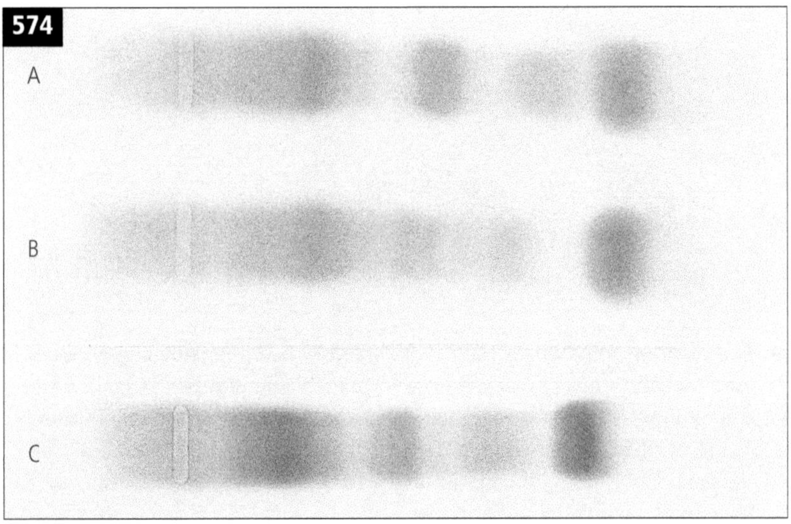

573, 574 Serum protein electrophoresis. (**573**) Serum proteins are electrophoretically separated in an agarose gel that is then stained for protein and may be subject to densitometric analysis. The test is a useful screen for reduced concentration of gamma globulin. (**574**) Protein electrophoresis of serum from a normal dog (lane B), a Dobermann with discospondylitis (lane A) and a Dobermann with demodicosis (lane C). There is elevation of β globulins in both Dobermanns; the broad-based band in lane C likely reflects polyclonal gammopathy.

- Neutrophil and macrophage function testing (see below).
- Assessment of the DTH response to intradermal injection of mitogen (e.g. PHA) or contact sensitization to DNCB (1-chloro-2, 4-dinitrobenzene).

Any test producing an abnormal result should be repeated on at least two occasions and performed on any available relatives. Function tests should be performed in parallel with samples from age-matched controls.

Quantification of serum immunoglobulins

Determination of the concentration of the major serum immunoglobulins (IgG, IgM and IgA) is the most widely available test of immune function in the dog, but is less accessible for feline samples. The most widely employed methodology is the single radial immunodiffusion test (SRID) (**575, 576**), but

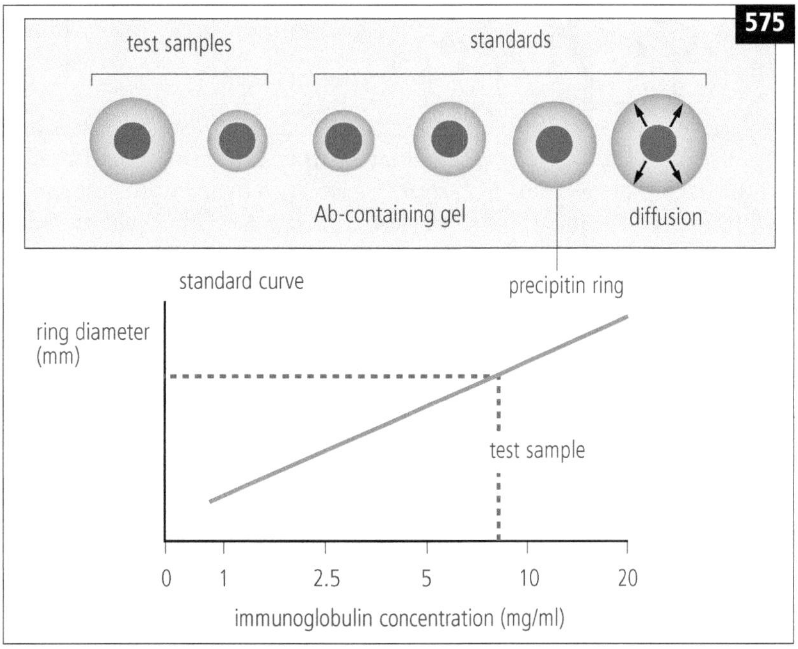

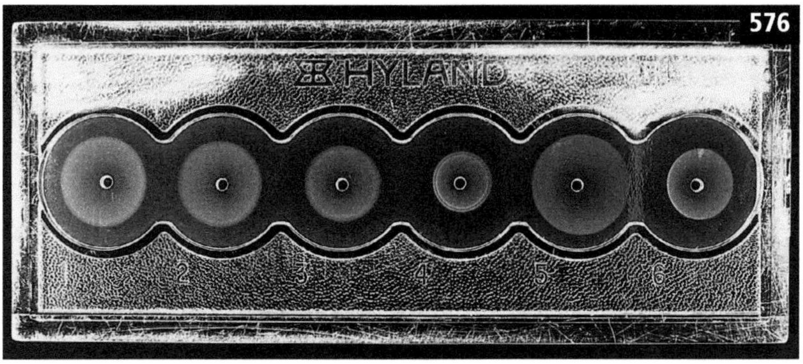

575, 576 Single radial immunodiffusion. (**575**) Antiserum specific for one class of Ig (e.g. anti-IgG) is incorporated into an agarose gel. Samples of test sera are loaded into wells cut into the gel, and a set of Ig standards of known concentrations are loaded to other wells. The gel is incubated for 24 hours and Ig diffuses from the well to form soluble complexes (in antigen excess) with the antibody. These continue to diffuse outwards and bind more antibody until the point of equivalence is reached and the complexes form a ring of precipitation. The ring diameter is proportional to the concentration of Ig, and the Ig concentration in the test samples (mg/ml) can be determined by interpolation from the standard curve. (**576**) The SRID plate shown is a determination of canine serum IgG concentration. The IgG standards are in wells 1–4 and test sera in wells 5 and 6. (From Day MJ [1996] Diagnostic assessment of the feline immune system. Part II. *Feline Practice* **24:**14–25, with permission.)

in a research setting, ELISA is more often used (577, 578). The concentrations of serum Igs in normal dogs and cats are given in *Table 18*.

Complement testing

Testing of complement function (579, 580) is rarely performed, as the assays are technically demanding and serum samples must be frozen to –70°C within two hours of collection due to the lability of complement. The total haemolytic complement assay (CH_{50}) indicates the overall function of the classical and terminal pathways and assesses the ability of complement in patient serum to lyze RBCs sensitized with optimal amounts of anti-RBC antibodies. Complement activity is expressed in terms of CH_{50} units, where a unit is defined as the

577

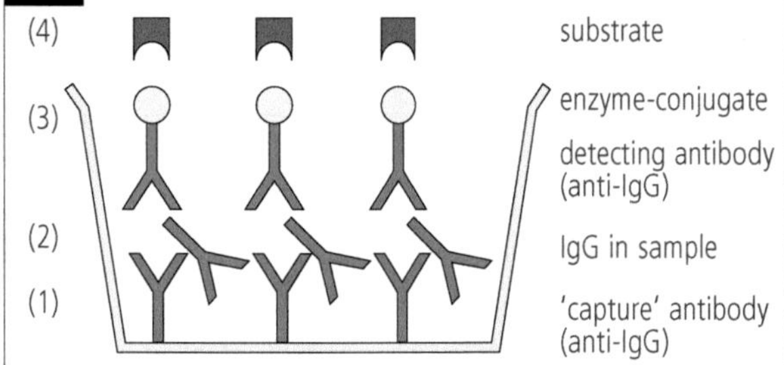

578

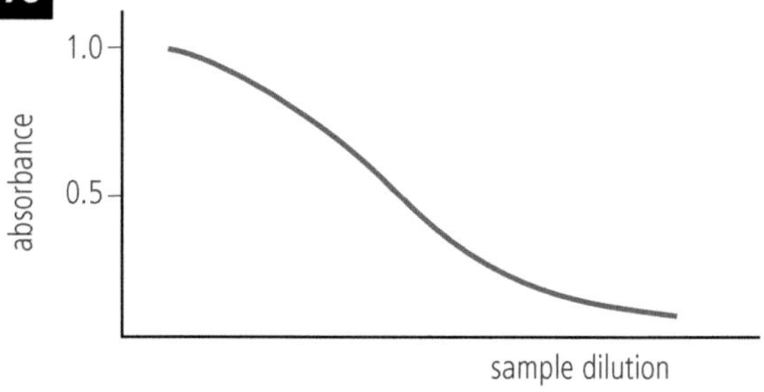

577, 578 Capture ELISA for determination of Ig concentration. In a research setting, Ig concentration is generally measured by capture ELISA. (**577**) Microtitre wells are coated with a capture antibody specific for the Ig to be assayed, and then serial dilutions of the test sample (and standards of known concentration) are added to a series of wells. After incubation and washing, specific binding is detected using a second antibody (or sometimes the same antibody as used in 'capture') that is conjugated to enzyme. The reaction is visualized by addition of substrate and the absorbance is read by an ELISA plate reader. (**578**) Characteristic dilution curve from such an assay demonstrates decreasing absorbance with increasing dilution of the sample. The precise concentration of Ig in the sample may be determined by comparison with a standard curve (often after log transformation of the values). Ig concentration may be determined in serum, tears, saliva, milk, colostrum, duodenal juice, bile or cerebrospinal fluid by this method.

Table 18: Serum Ig in the dog and cat. Numerous studies have defined the range of concentrations of the major serum Igs in the dog and cat. There is variation in the reported normal ranges that likely depends on factors such as geographical location, age, breed and sex of the normal population, and the laboratory methodology employed in the assays (SRID or ELISA). This Table presents a composite of such reports. The bracketed figure represents the full spectrum of concentrations defined as normal in the literature. Interpretation of normal for any case should be based on regional normal data provided by the testing laboratory.

Parameter	Dog	Cat
Serum IgG (mg/ml)	10.0–20.0 (2.5–37.5)	5.0–20.0 (3.9–38.0)
Serum IgM (mg/ml)	1.0–2.0 (0.3–2.7)	0.2–1.5 (0.2–3.6)
Serum IgA (mg/ml)	0.4–1.6 (0.0–3.13)	0.3–2.0 (0.0–6.0)
Serum IgG1 (mg/ml)	8.17 ± 0.95	Not defined
Serum IgG2 (mg/ml)	8.15 ± 3.16	Not defined
Serum IgG3 (mg/ml)	0.36 ± 0.43	Not defined
Serum IgG4 (mg/ml)	0.95 ± 0.45	Not defined
Serum IgE (μg/ml)	1–41	Not defined

quantity of serum complement required to produce 50% lysis of RBCs under standardized conditions of RBC sensitization with antibody. It is expressed as the reciprocal of the serum dilution giving 50% haemolysis. The assay may also be performed using agarose plates that contain the sensitized RBCs. Serum is added to wells cut in the agarose and allowed to diffuse for 20 hours at 4°C. The plates are then incubated at 37°C for 90 minutes to effect haemolysis, which is visualized as a cleared ring surrounding each well, the diameter of which is proportional to the log of the concentration of complement in the serum. The concentration of individual components of the complement

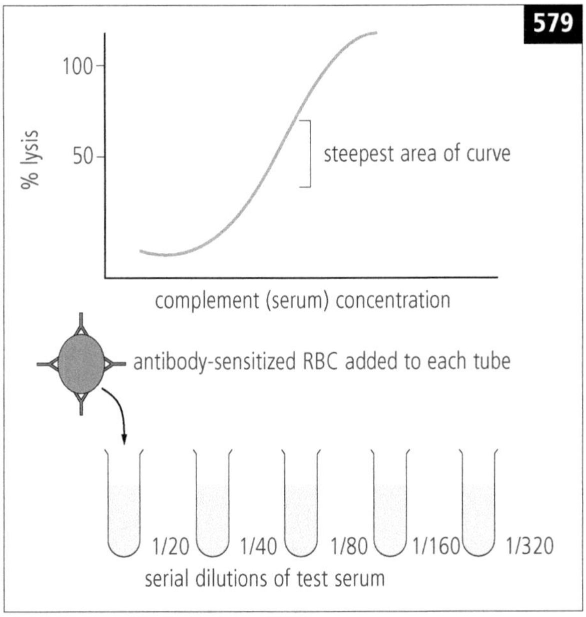

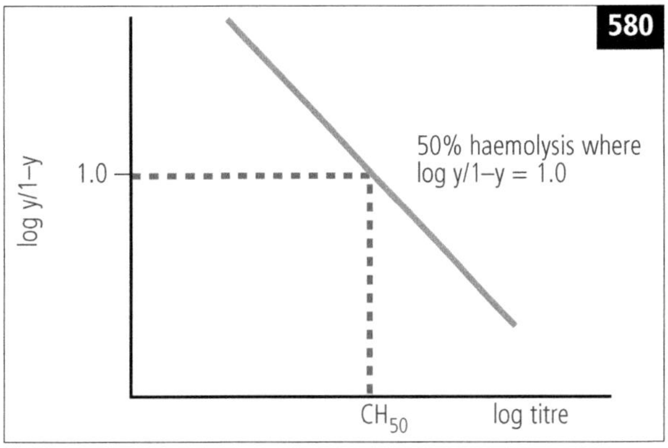

579, 580 CH_{50} assay. (**579**) In the CH_{50} assay, test and reference sera are serially diluted within the range 1/20 to 1/320 and then a standard suspension of erythrocytes optimally sensitized by antibody are added to each dilution. The complement within the serum will be fixed by the antibody and cause lysis of the erythrocytes proportional to the concentration of complement within the particular dilution. The released haemoglobin is measured spectrophotometrically after the period of incubation. Controls for 0% lysis (buffer alone) and 100% lysis (distilled water) of the erythrocytes are included. The assay will produce a sigmoidal curve and the value of 50% lysis is chosen to define the CH_{50} as this point falls within the steepest area of the curve, where lysis is most sensitive to small changes in complement activity. (**580**) The percentage lysis for each serum dilution is calculated using the formula:

$$\% = \frac{\text{OD test} - \text{OD (0\%)}}{\text{OD (100\%)} - \text{OD (0\%)}} \times 100$$

and the value y/1–y is calculated for serum dilutions in which $10\% \leq y \leq 90\%$. This value is then plotted against the titre on a log-log scale, and the titre of the serum that intersects the curve at the value y/1–y = 1.0 is the CH_{50} for that serum.

pathways can be determined using the haemolytic assay described in (**581**).

Peripheral blood lymphocyte phenotyping

The methodology used to determine the percentage (or absolute number) of lymphocytes of particular subsets (most often $CD4^+$, $CD8^+$ T cells and $CD21^+$ B cells) is described in (**582–586**). The most widely used data from such analysis is the ratio of CD4 to CD8 T cells, which for normal dogs is approximately 1.7 and for normal cats 1.9.

Lymphocyte function testing

These assays test the ability of blood lymphocytes to respond to mitogens or specific antigens. Mononuclear cells isolated from blood may be used in *in vitro* functional assays, either as an unfractionated population or as purified

581

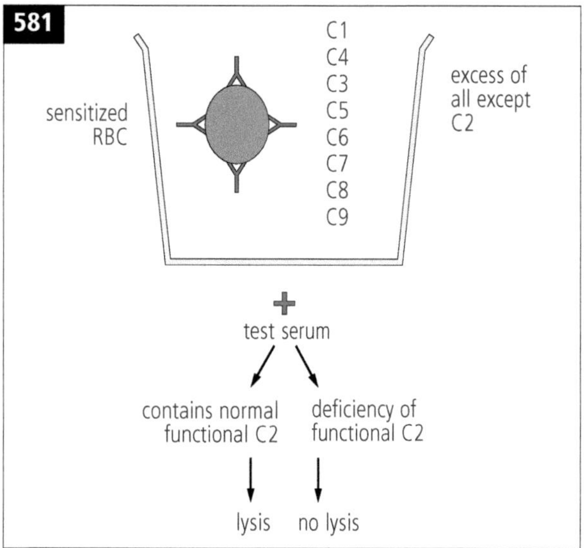

581 Haemolytic titration assay for assessment of individual complement components. In this assay, sensitized RBCs are incubated with an excess of all complement components except the one under assay. The test serum thus provides the component in question, permitting lysis if present in adequate amount. The test has been used to define the activity of C1–C9 in the dog and cat. SRID has also been used to measure the concentration of C3 and C4 in canine serum.

582

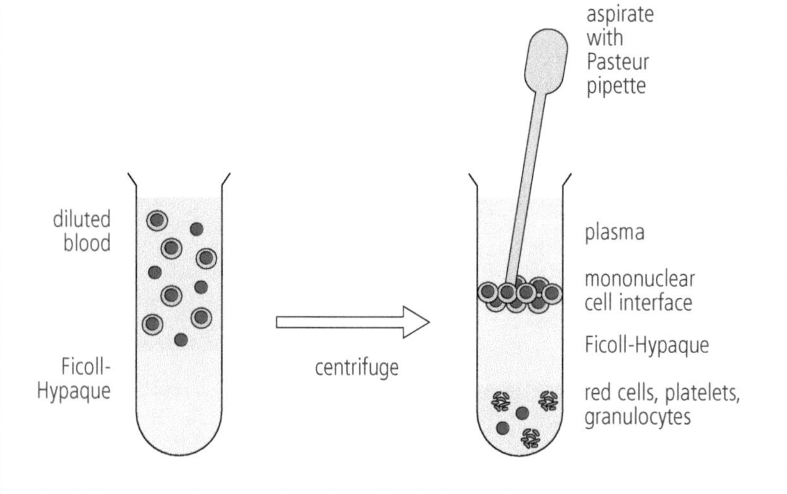

582 Isolation of blood mononuclear cells by density gradient centrifugation. Blood is diluted in tissue culture medium or buffered saline and layered on top of a density gradient solution (most commonly Ficoll-Hypaque of specific gravity 1.077). The tube is centrifuged, during which time the erythrocytes, platelets and granulocytes within the blood sample pass through the Ficoll to pellet at the bottom of the tube. The mononuclear cells (lymphocytes and monocytes) remain at the interface of the medium and the Ficoll and may be carefully aspirated with a Pasteur pipette. The purity and viability of the mononuclear suspension can be assessed by staining with vital dye, and the number of cells are counted in a haemocytometer chamber or with a cell counter. The relative numbers of lymphocyte subsets within the interface can be determined by immunolabelling (**583–586**).

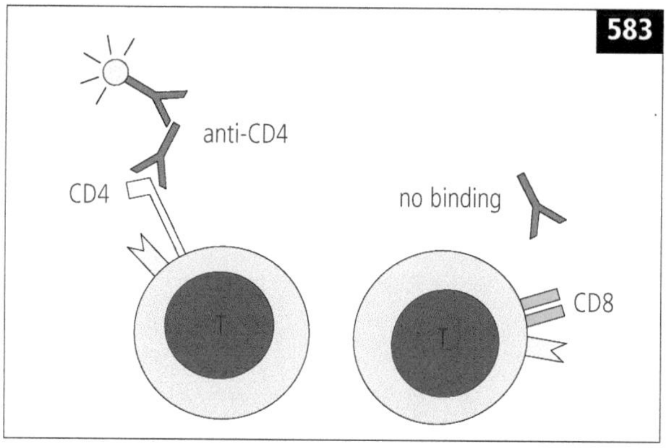

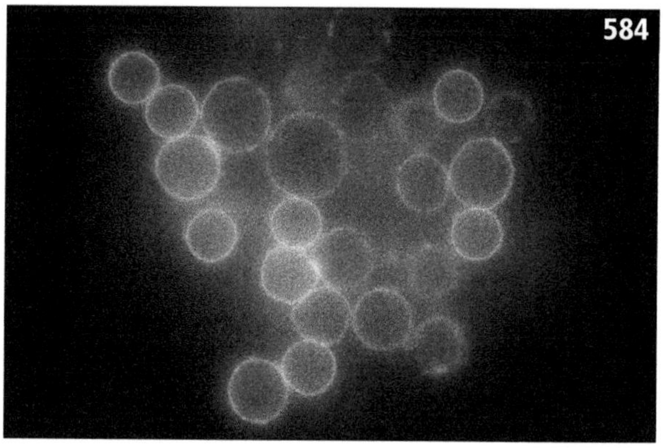

583, 584 Identification of lymphocyte subsets within a mixed population. (583) Monoclonal antibodies have been produced that specifically bind to epitopes on surface molecules unique to individual lymphocyte subpopulations (e.g. CD4 or CD8). The binding of these monoclonal antibodies (usually mouse or rat origin) can be detected using a second antibody (anti-mouse or rat), conjugated to fluorescein, that will produce apple-green rim fluorescence of the cell under UV light. Fab'$_2$ fragments of the second antibody are generally used in order to avoid non-specific binding of this antibody to Fc receptors on the surface of the lymphocytes. (**584**) In this preparation of canine blood mononuclear cells, T lymphocytes within the sample have been identified with a rabbit antiserum specific for all T cells (pan-T cell marker) and a secondary anti-rabbit reagent conjugated to fluorescein.

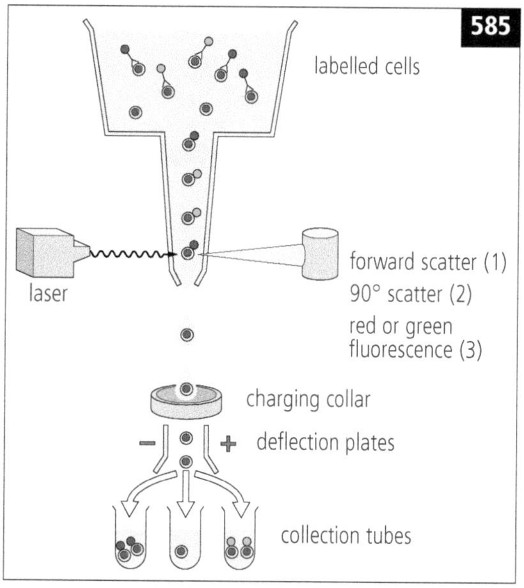

585, 586 Fluorescence-activated cell sorter. (585) The technique of flow cytometry has revolutionized the study of lymphocyte subsets. Lymphocyte subpopulations within a mixture can be enumerated using a flow cytometer (FACScan) or sorted into purified viable populations using a FACS. Two subsets within a mixture can be differentially labelled using monoclonal antibodies and secondary antibodies conjugated to different fluorochromes (e.g. fluorescein or phycoerythrin) that produce green or red fluorescence under UV light. The suspension of labelled cells is taken up into a vibrating flow chamber from which the cells exit individually encased in a sheath of buffer fluid. Each cell in the sample then passes a spot on which is focused an 'interrogating' laser beam; the cell emits a pulse of light that is captured by a series of photosensors. These detect (1) the forward angle light scatter as a measure of cell size; (2) the 90° light scatter as a measure of cell granularity; and (3) the emitted fluorescent light (green or red). In sample analyses, 10,000 cells are assessed for these parameters. The cell stream is then subject to vibration to cause it to break into droplets, and each droplet is given a charge dependent on the type of cell that it contains. The droplets (and thus cells) may be separated by passing the stream between a pair of electrostatic deflection plates, and the purified populations (usually 99% pure) are collected into different tubes. (**586**) In this example of 'two colour' labelling, peripheral blood lymphocytes from a dog have been labelled with monoclonal antibodies specific for CD4 (directly conjugated to phycoerythrin) and CD8 (directly conjugated to fluorescein). The two non-overlapping subsets are depicted in this 'contour plot' and the unlabelled cells are found in the lower left quadrant. (Data from Moore PF, Rossitto PV, Danilenko DM *et al.* [1992] Monoclonal antibodies specific for canine CD4 and CD8 define functional lymphocyte T subsets and high density expression of CD4 by canine neutrophils. *Tissue Antigens* **40**:75–85.)

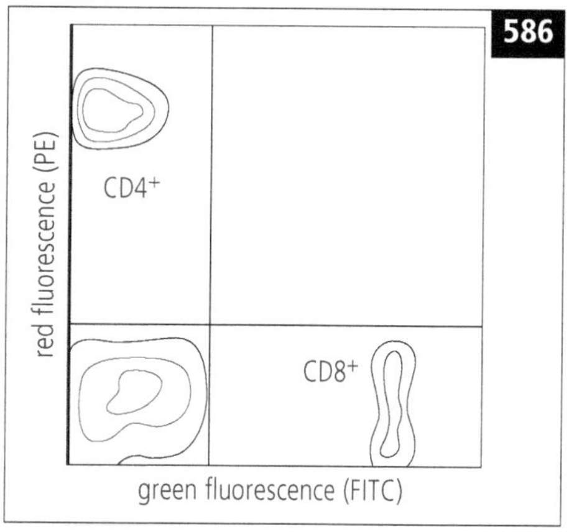

T ($CD4^+$ or $CD8^+$) or B cell populations obtained by depleting unwanted cell types or selecting those that are required. The most commonly performed test of lymphocyte function involves assessing response to stimulation by mitogens (587). Mitogens are substances (often plant derived) that non-specifically stimulate multiple clones of lymphocytes by binding to surface carbohydrate molecules. Some mitogens preferentially activate T lymphocytes (e.g. concanavalin A [ConA], phytohaemagglutinin [PHA]), whereas others primarily effect B cells (e.g. pokeweed mitogen, bacterial lipopolysaccharide).

587

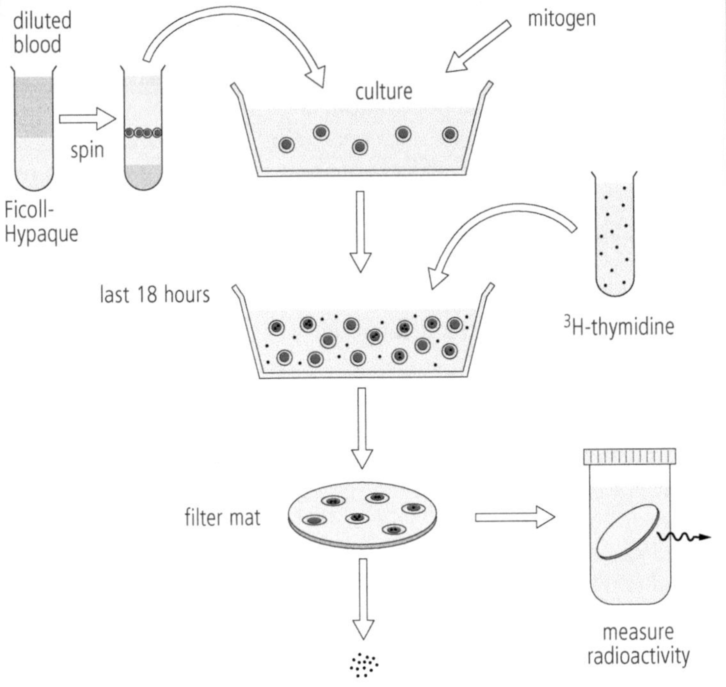

587 Lymphocyte stimulation test. Peripheral blood mononuclear cells (including lymphocytes) are obtained by density gradient centrifugation (see **582**) and co-cultured with mitogen in the wells of microtitration plates for a 48–72 hour period. Unstimulated control cultures are also established. During the last 18 hours of culture, the wells are 'pulsed' with ^{3}H-thymidine, which is incorporated into the DNA of dividing cells. The cells are then harvested onto a glass fibre filter disc and the amount of incorporated radioactivity measured by placing the disc in scintillation fluid into a beta counter. The results of the assay may be given as counts per minute (cpm) of incorporated radioactivity, or as a stimulation index (SI) that gives the ratio of cpm in stimulated to unstimulated cultures. Alternative, non-radioactive methods of determining lymphocyte proliferation have also been utilized.

588

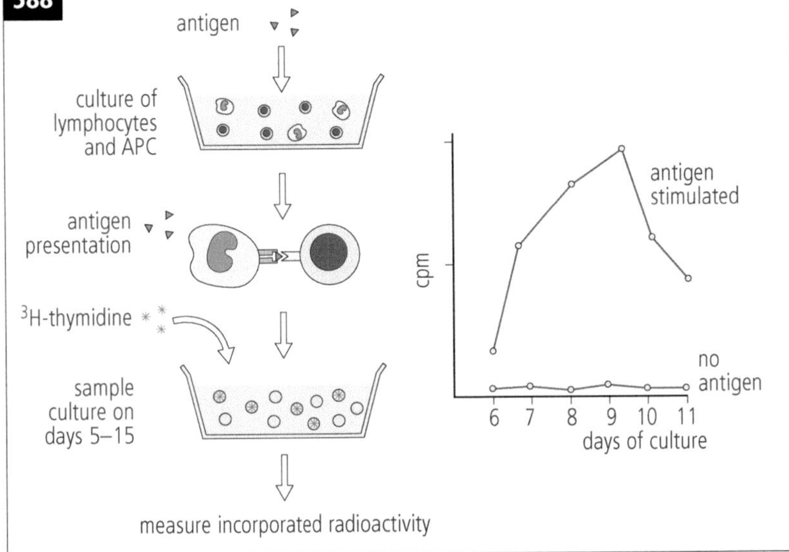

588 Antigen specific lymphocyte proliferation assay. Mononuclear cells (including lymphocytes and monocytes as APCs) are cultured in a large tissue culture well in the presence of specific antigen that is processed and presented to cause lymphocyte proliferation. Small aliquots of the cultured cells can be serially withdrawn on days 5 to 15 of culture and pulsed with ^{3}H-thymidine, and the kinetics of the proliferative response demonstrated. In a 'primary' cell culture, the mononuclear cells are exposed to a previously unseen foreign antigen (e.g. keyhole limpet haemocyanin) and give maximal response on day 9 of culture. Following primary culture, lymphocytes can be provided with fresh medium, fresh APCs and antigen and restimulated *in vitro* to demonstrate a 'secondary' (memory) response to antigen that peaks at an earlier time point (e.g. day 6).

Antigen-specific lymphocyte stimulation assays involve *in vitro* processing of antigen and selective activation of antigen-specific clones through the T cell receptor (**588**). Alternative means of assessing activation of cultured lymphocytes involve phenotypic analysis (e.g. for expression of activation markers such as the IL-2 receptor) after culture, or quantification of cytokines released into the tissue culture medium by the activated cells. Cytokines can be measured by ELISA or bioassay (**589**). Alternatively, cells can be collected from culture after stimulation and cytokine-specific mRNA detected by RT-PCR (see Chapter 1, p. 40). Primers have been designed to enable determination of mRNA encoding most dog and cat cytokines, and very recently a set of monoclonal antibodies has become available commercially that allows detection of key canine and feline cytokine proteins by capture ELISA or a commercial microbead-based multiplex assay. Measurement of cytokine protein is always the preferred methodology, as there is not necessarily a correlation between the presence of mRNA and secretion of the protein product. In the case of B lymphocytes, *in vitro* stimulation may lead to the release of Ig into the culture medium, which may be detected by ELISA. The function of cytotoxic lymphocytes or NK cells can also be assessed *in vitro* (**590**).

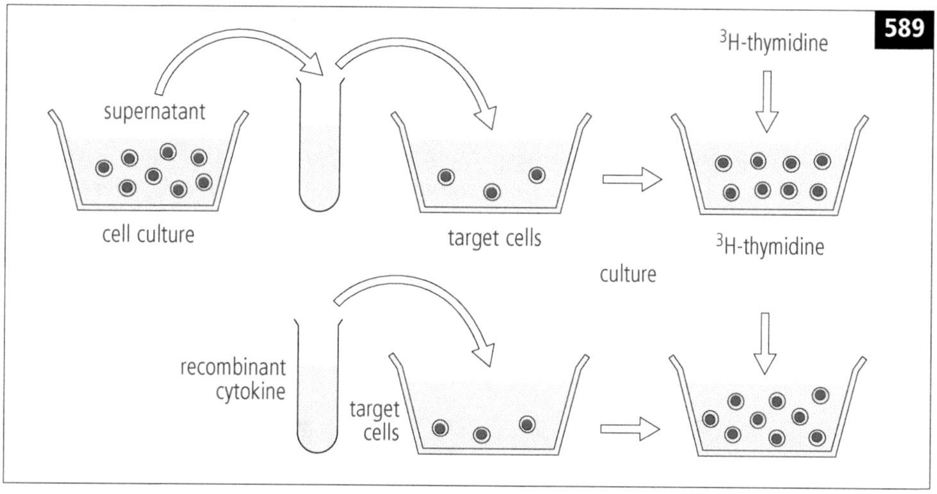

589 Bioassay for measurement of cytokine production. Lymphocytes are stimulated by antigen or mitogen in culture and release cytokine to the culture medium during proliferation. An aliquot of this supernatant (containing cytokine) is added to a culture of a cell line that is dependent on a specific cytokine (e.g. IL-2) for growth. A control culture is stimulated by a source of recombinant cytokine of known quantity. If the cytokine of interest is produced by the original cell culture, the supernatant fluid will support the growth of the indicator cell line and the relative activity can be calculated in comparison to that of the recombinant standard. Cytokines such as IL-1, IL-2, IL-6, TNF and IFNγ have been measured using bioassay.

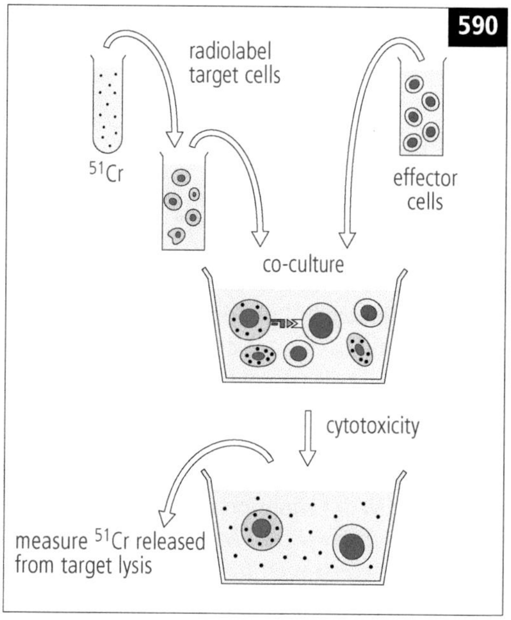

590 Cytotoxicity assay. Target cells are radiolabelled by incubation with ^{51}Cr and then co-cultured with effector cells (cytotoxic lymphocytes or NK cells) at different target:effector ratios. During culture there is MHC-restricted target cell killing. The radiolabelled chromium released from lysed target cells is then measured. Target cell lines may be virally infected, histoincompatible or tumour cells.

Neutrophil and macrophage function testing

The major functions of neutrophils (adhesion, chemotaxis, phagocytosis, intracellular killing) can be assessed *in vitro*. Neutrophils are readily isolated from blood by density gradient centrifugation. Isolated neutrophils can migrate along chemotactic gradients established by chemicals, serum, cytokines, complement components or inflammatory mediators. The most common means of assessing chemotaxis involves use of the 'Boyden chamber', where neutrophils are placed into one side of a chamber separated from the chemotactic substance by a millipore filter through which the agent diffuses. Neutrophils that migrate towards the agent are trapped within the filter, which may be stained and examined microscopically. In the 'under-agarose assay', neutrophils placed into one well of an agarose gel migrate beneath the gel towards chemoattractant placed in a second well. The creation of suction blisters in canine skin to examine *in vivo* chemotaxis of neutrophils in response to autologous serum has been reported.

Assessment of neutrophil phagocytosis (**591**, **592**) and neutrophil killing of organisms such as *Staphylococcus* can be made *in vitro* (**593**). The respiratory burst of neutrophils following phagocytosis can be assessed using the nitroblue tetrazolium (NBT) test. This involves reduction of the colourless dye NBT to dark blue formazan, which can be assessed spectrophotometrically. Alternatively, in the chemiluminescence assay the light released during the oxidative burst is measured by a chemiluminometer. Blood monocytes become adherent macrophages during *in vitro* culture and the ability of these cells to phagocytose and kill may be assessed.

Immunoglobulin deficiency

Immunoglobulin deficiency may arise due to failure to ingest adequate colostrum, delayed onset of endogenous Ig production (transient hypogammaglobulinaemia) or a primary genetic deficiency resulting in failure to synthesize adequate concentrations of one or more classes of Ig. Immunoglobulin deficiency is the most common form of immunodeficiency recognized in man and animals. The clinical signs of primary immunodeficiency disease (e.g. infection) generally do not become manifest until there is degradation of maternal Ig by 12–15 weeks of age (**594**), but neonates that fail to ingest adequate colostrum may be susceptible to infection earlier in neonatal life. Individual pups within a litter with delayed onset of endogenous Ig production (transient hypogammaglobulinaemia) have been reported to develop recurrent upper respiratory tract infection until six months of age.

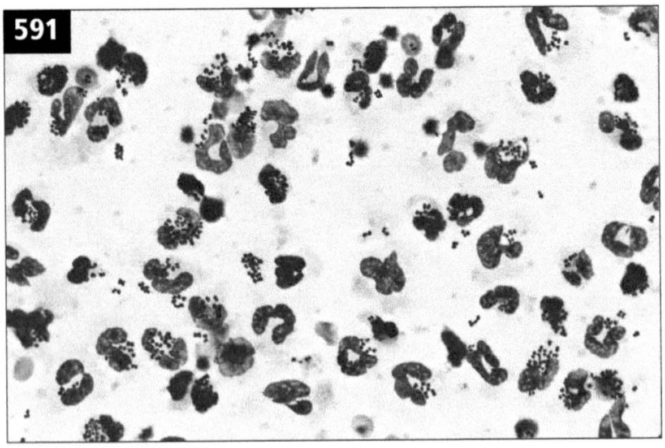

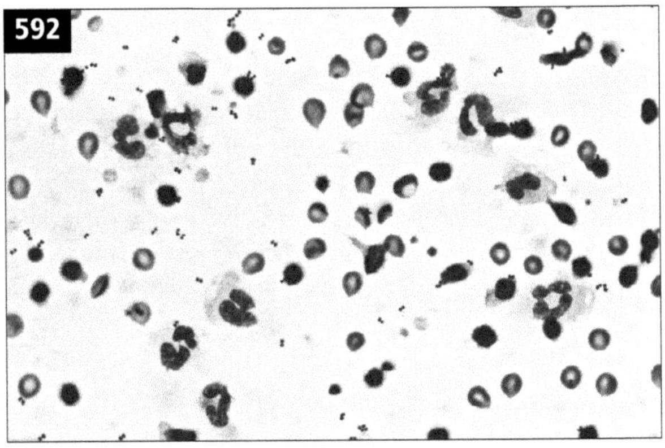

591, 592 Neutrophil phagocytosis assay. Neutrophils were isolated from the blood of a normal dog and incubated with suspensions of staphylococci that had been previously opsonized by canine serum (**591**) or not opsonized (**592**). After a ten-minute period the reaction was stopped and cytocentrifuge samples were prepared from each tube. In **591** the neutrophils have phagocytosed large numbers of opsonized staphylococci, with numerous organisms within the cytoplasm of most cells. In contrast, in **592** relatively few unopsonized staphylococci have been phagocytosed. (From Day MJ, Mackin A, Littlewood J [2000] *Manual of Canine and Feline Haematology and Transfusion Medicine*. BSAVA, Gloucester, with permission.) Other particulate substances may be used in this assay (yeast, latex beads) and autologous serum should be used in parallel with normal serum to detect any deficiency in opsonins. These assays have also been adapted for the flow cytometer by incorporating the use of fluorescently-labelled targets.

Failure of passive transfer

The nature of canine and feline placentation is such that newborn pups and kittens are born with only approximately 5–10% of adult levels of serum immunoglobulin, as these molecules are unable to cross the endotheliochorial barrier. In one study, newborn kittens lacked serum IgG and IgA, but had low concentrations of IgM. Therefore, as with other domestic animal species, there is an obligate requirement to take in colostrum within the first 24 hours of birth in order to provide passively acquired immunity until endogenous production of Ig commences. Uptake of maternal immunoglobulin is permitted by modifications to the neonatal intestine, in particular expression of a specific receptor molecule (FcγRn), which binds the

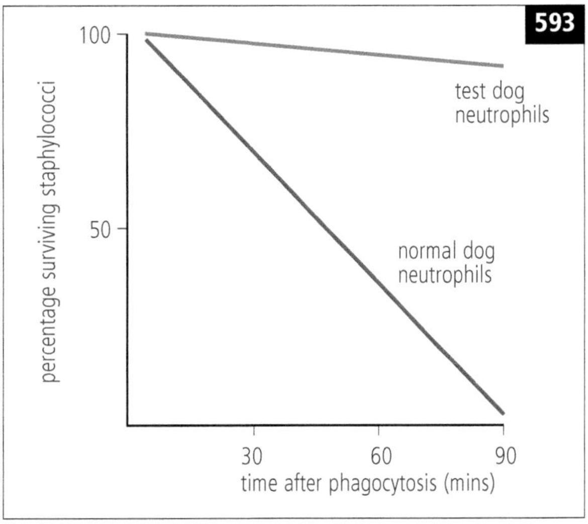

593 Neutrophil killing assay. A suspension of opsonized staphylococci was incubated with normal dog neutrophils and neutrophils from a dog with suspected neutrophil killing abnormality. Neutrophils were incubated with a defined number of opsonized organisms and, after phagocytosis had occurred (ten minutes), extracellular staphylococci were lyzed by addition of specific enzyme. At various time points thereafter (0, 30, 60 and 90 minutes), intracellular staphylococci were liberated by osmotic lysis of the neutrophils and serial dilutions of the viable intracellular bacteria were plated onto agar; colonies were enumerated after incubation of the plate. The number of viable intracellular organisms at each time point is a fraction of the original number of organisms, and this data enables construction of a curve of the kinetics of intracellular killing. Over a 90 minute time course, phagocytosed staphylococci were progressively killed by the normal dog neutrophils, but neutrophils from the test dog were unable to kill the phagocytosed organisms.

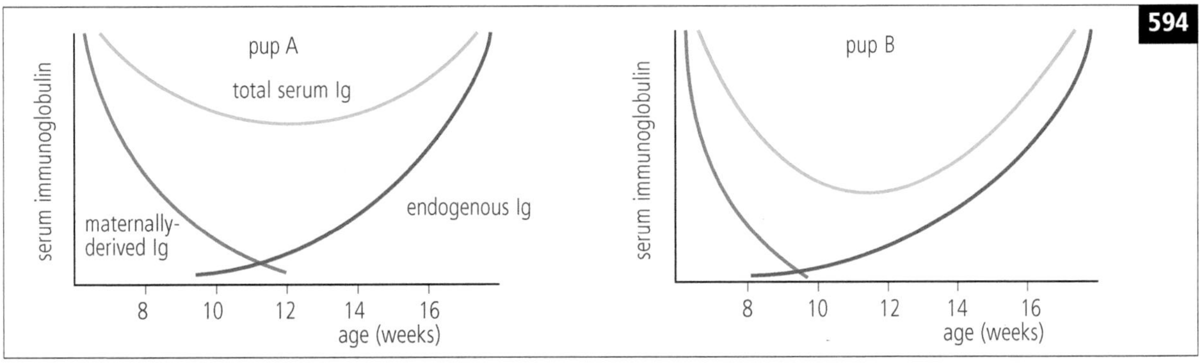

594 Serum Ig in neonatal animals. Serum Ig levels in neonatal dogs and cats are affected by the transfer of maternally-derived (colostral) immunity. The presence of maternal Ig prevents endogenous production by neonatal B cells (and effective vaccination with most currently licensed products) until such time as it has been degraded. The mechanisms underlying this suppression likely involve antigen neutralization by maternal Ig and cross-linkage of B cell SmIg with antigen and maternal Ig bound to the FcR. Individual neonates may take in different amounts of colostral Ig. In the example shown, pup A has greater maternally-derived Ig than pup B and it may be expected to have a relatively delayed onset of endogenous Ig production. Primary, congenital immunodeficiency diseases are generally not clinically apparent until there is loss of maternal protection.

Fc portion of maternal Ig, resulting in transport across the epithelial barrier and absorption into the circulation. The concentrations of IgG, IgM and IgA in canine and feline colostrum and milk are given in *Table 19*. Failure of a newborn pup or kitten to ingest sufficient colostrum will leave that individual with insufficient immune defences in early life. Although well documented in equine and production animal medicine, this phenomenon has been poorly documented in dogs and cats. Failure of passive transfer might arise via a number of possible mechanisms, such as competition for colostrum with stronger littermates, premature birth or lactation, or poor mothering ability. Lack of colostral Ig uptake may be confirmed by measuring serum immunoglobulins after the first 24 hours of life, and such testing is routinely performed in equine stud medicine. Ig replacement in colostrum deprived animals is discussed below (Therapy for immunodeficiency disease, p. 313).

IgA deficiency

Canine selective IgA deficiency is recognized when the serum IgA concentration is below 0.2–0.4 mg/ml, depending on the definition of normal range for a particular study. IgA deficiency was documented in two Shar Peis with respiratory infection (2/2) and conjunctivitis, demodicosis, ringworm infection and pruritic dermatitis responding to dietary restriction (1/2). In a subsequent survey, the majority of clinically normal dogs of this breed were also shown to have subnormal IgA concentration. A second form of immunodeficiency is also recognized in the Shar Pei. Affected dogs have recurrent infection of the skin and the respiratory and gastrointestinal

Table 19: Immunoglobulin concentrations in canine and feline serum, colostrum and milk. This Table presents a composite of published data concerning Ig concentration in these secretions relative to concentrations in serum. The canine values for colostrum and milk are recorded as a percentage of mean serum concentration of that Ig, whereas the feline values are absolute (mg/ml). The day of sampling for milk values is also noted. Both canine and feline colostrum are enriched for IgG and IgA but contain little IgM. Canine milk is dominated by IgA, whereas the feline equivalent contains predominantly IgG. (Canine data from Heddle RJ, Rowley D (1975) Dog immunoglobulins. I. Immunochemical characterization of dog serum, parotid saliva, colostrum, milk and small bowel fluid. *Immunology* **29:**185–195; feline data from Claus MA, Levy JK, MacDonald K *et al.* (2006) Immunoglobulin concentrations in feline colostrum and milk, and the requirement of colostrum for passive transfer of immunity to neonatal kittens. *Journal of Feline Medicine and Surgery* **8:**184–191 and Casal ML, Jezyk PF, Giger U (1996) Transfer of colostral antibodies from queens to their kittens. *American Journal of Veterinary Research* **57:**1653–1658.)

	Dog	**Cat**
Serum IgG (mg/ml)	5.2–17.3 (mean 9.8)	15.0 ± 5.4
Serum IgM (mg/ml)	0.7–2.7 (mean 1.7)	3.7 to 6.4
Serum IgA (mg/ml)	0.2–1.2 (mean 0.5)	1.9 ± 1.4
Colostral IgG	15.68 (160% of mean serum)	62.0 ± 23.8
Colostral IgM	0.23 (14% of mean serum)	0.4–2.0
Colostral IgA	2.5 (500% of mean serum)	14.3 ± 11.6
Milk IgG	0.098 (1% of mean serum; days 25–50)	5.3 ± 7.3 (day 7) 2.0 ± 1.3 (day 42)
Milk IgM	0.15 (9% of mean serum; days 25–50)	
Milk IgA	1.35 (270% of mean serum; days 25–50)	2.9 ± 2.3 (day 7 and 42)

tracts and a susceptibility to development of a range of tumours. There is deficiency of one or more immunoglobulin classes (mostly IgM) in addition to impaired T cell response to mitogens, suggesting a combined immunodeficiency.

IgA deficiency was reported in a colony of Beagles in association with chronic respiratory and cutaneous infection. Affected dogs sometimes had serum RF and they were unable to generate IgA plasma cells following stimulation of lymphocytes with pokeweed mitogen. A colony of English Cocker Spaniels with various autoimmune diseases and serum autoantibodies was also affected by IgA deficiency (see Chapter 14, p. 367).

Young Irish Wolfhounds with chronic rhinitis and/or bronchopneumonia are recognized throughout the world, and one recent international investigation has shown pedigree relationships between affected dogs in several countries. In the absence of evidence for a defect in function of the cilia lining the respiratory mucosa (ciliary dyskinesia), it has been proposed that affected dogs may have an underlying primary immunodeficiency disorder. Indeed, studies of affected dogs have shown selective reduction in serum IgA concentration (595–597), but there appears to be no defect in the concentration of mucosal IgA measured in bronchoalveolar lavage fluid. The blood CD4:CD8 ratio in these patients was normal, but within BALF there was an elevated ratio consistent with CD4 T cell responsiveness in the affected mucosa.

The most complex putative defect of IgA and mucosal immunity occurs in the GSD, a breed that is uniquely predisposed to a range of immune-mediated infectious or inflammatory diseases involving the skin or mucosal surfaces,

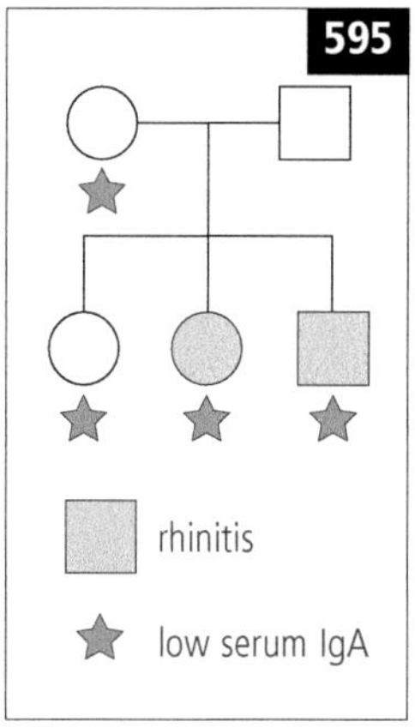

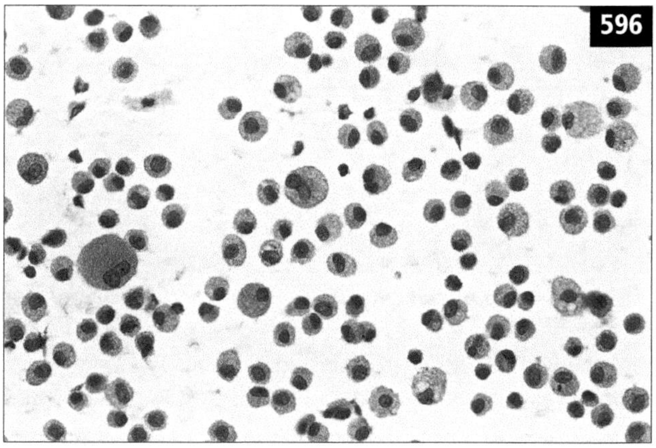

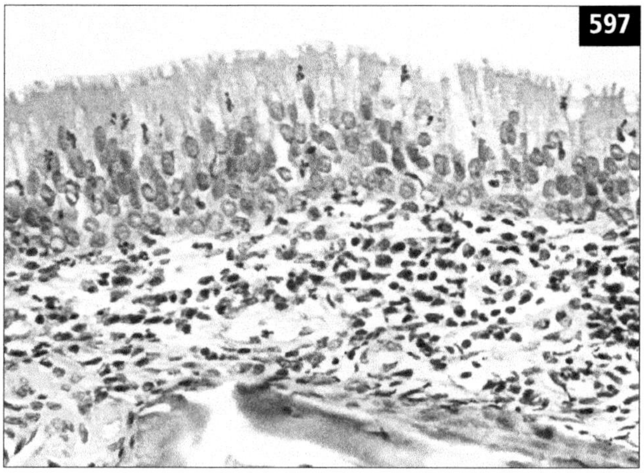

595–597 IgA deficiency in Irish Wolfhounds with chronic rhinitis and/or bronchopneumonia. (**595**) A family of Irish Wolfhounds in which two 13-week-old littermate animals presented with chronic rhinitis that progressed to pneumonia. Each affected animal had normal serum IgG and IgM concentrations, but reduced serum IgA. The clinically normal littermate animal and the dam of the litter also had selective reduction in serum IgA. (**596**) Bronchiolar-alveolar lavage fluid from an affected pup demonstrating large numbers of vacuolated macrophages and some large multinucleate cells indicative of chronic inflammation. (From Day MJ [1998] Mechanisms of immune-mediated diseases in small animals. *In Practice* **20**:75–86, with permission.) (**597**) Section of nasal mucosa from an Irish Wolfhound with chronic, recurrent rhinitis. There is an inflammatory infiltration of the lamina propria, with exocytosis of neutrophils through the overlying epithelium.

including ARD, IBD, anal furunculosis (see Chapter 7, p. 219), deep pyoderma (598–600), monocytic ehrlichiosis and disseminated aspergillosis. Disseminated aspergillosis provides a good example of an infectious disease of GSDs for which an underlying immunodeficiency would in part explain the breed predisposition to the infection. The disease is recognized in Australia, the US and Europe, and almost exclusively affects GSDs (601, 602). The causative agent is the

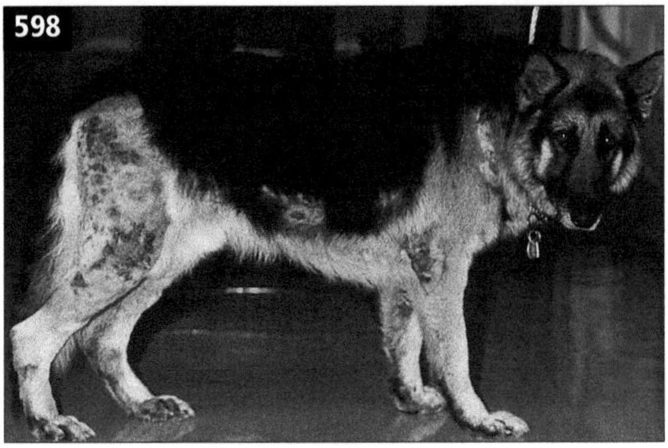

598 Deep pyoderma in GSDs. Clinical presentation of generalized deep pyoderma of GSDs. There are multiple, draining sinus tracts, with a generalized distribution in this dog, but localized forms of the disease occur. The causative agent is *Staphylococcus intermedius*. Some dogs have concurrent anal furunculosis. (Photograph courtesy S.E. Shaw.)

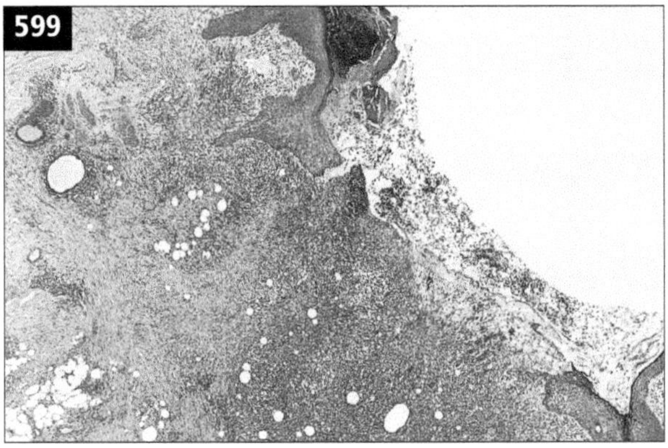

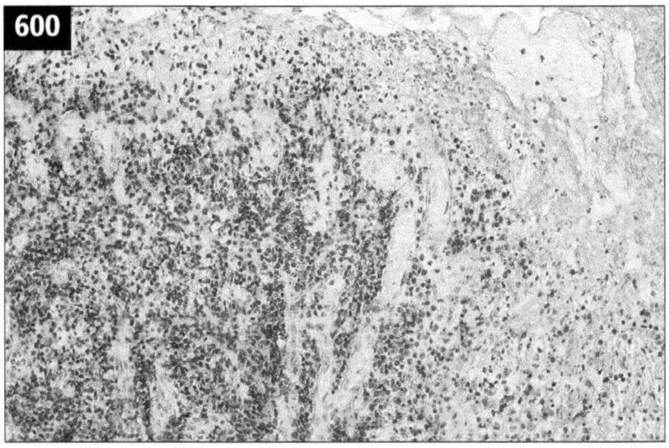

599, 600 Deep pyoderma. (**599**) Histological appearance of a skin biopsy from an English Bull Terrier with deep pyoderma. There is a region of epidermal ulceration overlying an intense lymphoplasmacytic infiltrate that is centred on ruptured hair follicles (furunculosis). (**600**) The lesion contains large numbers of $CD3^+$ T cells (shown here) and plasma cells of the IgG, IgM and IgA classes. In contrast, biopsies from GSDs with deep pyoderma have a relative paucity of T lymphocytes but similar numbers of plasma cells. This may suggest failure of T cell homing to sites of cutaneous inflammation in the GSD. (From Day MJ [1994] An immunopathological study of deep pyoderma in the dog. *Research in Veterinary Science* **56**:18–23, with permission.)

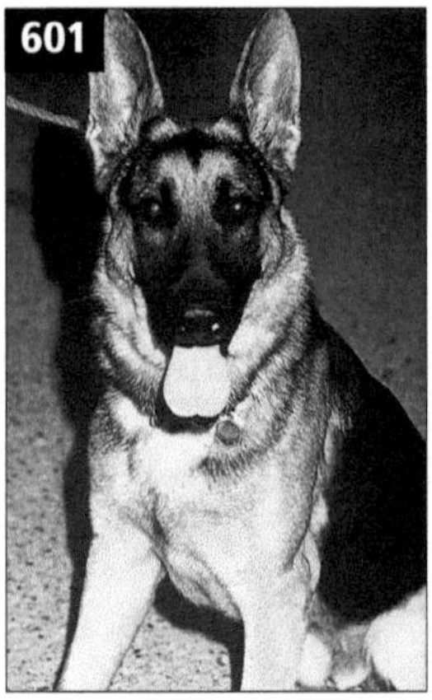

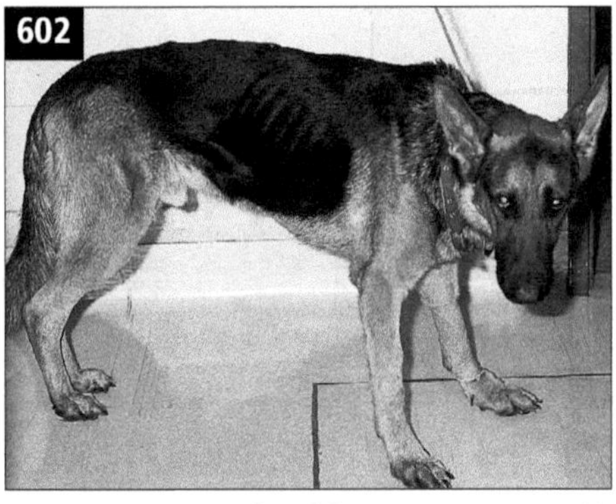

601, 602 Disseminated aspergillosis. (**601**) A two-year-old male GSD at the time of initial presentation with a four-week history of non-specific abdominal pain. *Aspergillus* hyphae were present in the urine and a diagnosis of disseminated aspergillosis was made. (**602**) The same dog eight weeks later showing marked loss of body condition and generalized depression. At necropsy examination there was extensive disseminated *Aspergillus* infection. (Photographs courtesy C.E. Egar; [**602**] from Day MJ, Mackin A, Littlewood J [2000] *Manual of Canine and Feline Haematology and Transfusion Medicine*. BSAVA, Gloucester, with permission.)

environmental saphrophyte *Aspergillus terreus*, although other *Aspergillus* species and other opportunist fungi are occasionally incriminated (603). Affected dogs have systemic fungal granulomata, particularly of vertebrae or long bones, kidney, spleen and lymph nodes (604–607). The disease is progressive and usually fatal, although antifungal agents (e.g. itraconazole) may prolong life and sometimes induce remission. Studies have failed to demonstrate a simple

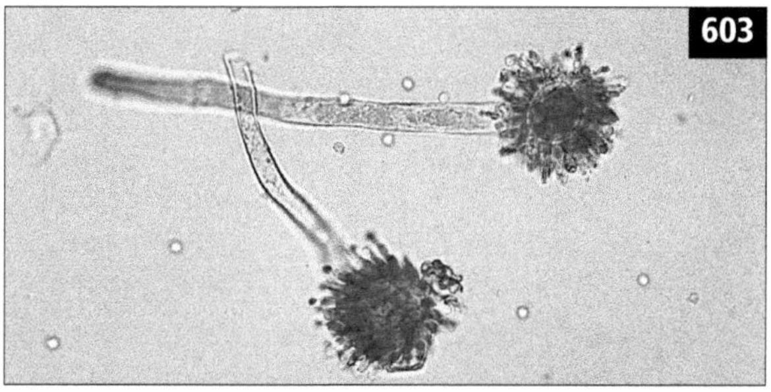

603

603 *Aspergillus terreus*. Wet preparation (lactophenol cotton blue stain) showing the connidial heads of *Aspergillus terreus*, the major causative agent of disseminated aspergillosis in the GSD.

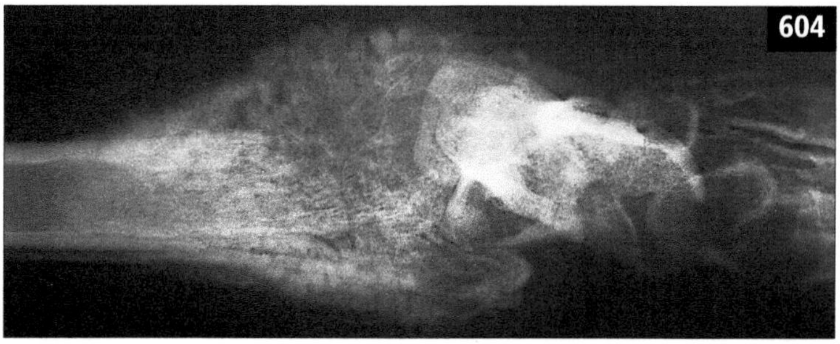

604

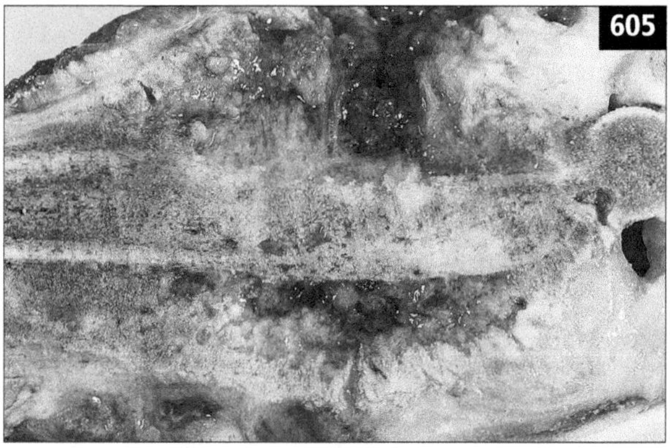

605

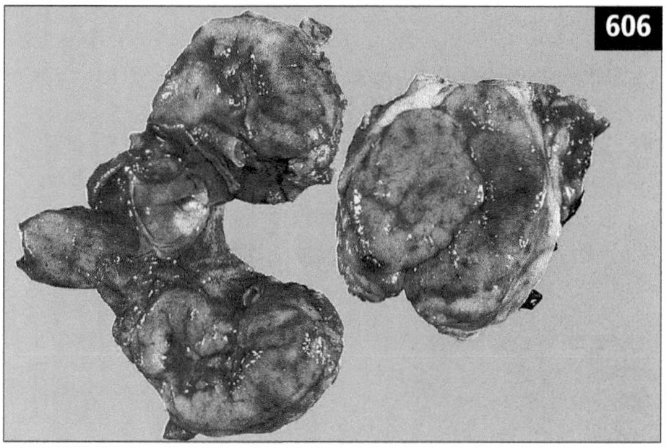

606

604–606 Disseminated aspergillosis. (**604**) Radiographic appearance of the tarsal bones of a GSD with disseminated aspergillosis demonstrating extensive long bone destruction. (Photograph courtesy S.E. Shaw) (**605**) Cross-section of humerus from a dog with disseminated aspergillosis showing osteolysis, new bone formation and extensive soft tissue inflammation. (**606**) Lymph nodes from a dog with disseminated aspergillosis. The nodes are markedly enlarged, with loss of normal corticomedullary distinction on the cut surface. (Photographs courtesy Pathology Unit, Murdoch University.)

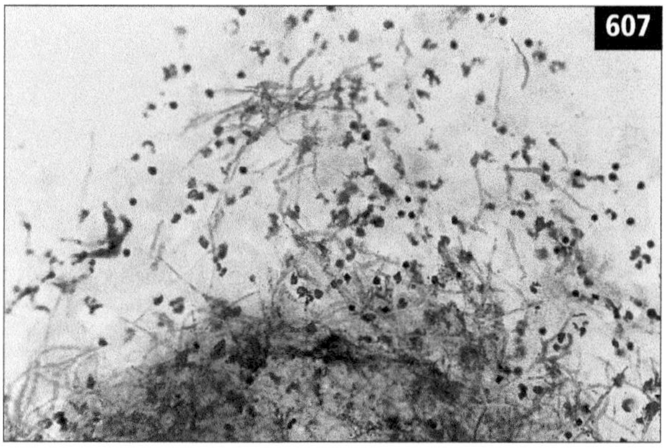

607

607 Disseminated aspergillosis. Fine needle aspirate taken from one of the lymph nodes in **606** ante mortem. There is a large mycelial mat with mixed inflammatory cells. (Photograph courtesy J.N. Mills.)

immunological defect, but it remains a likelihood that abnormal mucosal immunity is a major factor permitting initial penetration of fungal spores.

Evidence for impaired mucosal immunity in GSDs has been acquired over many years and includes:

- Either IgA deficiency or wide variance in serum IgA in normal GSDs. Other studies have not shown abnormality in serum IgA concentration in dogs of this breed.
- Reduced IgA concentration in tears of normal GSDs (described in one study, but not replicated in another).
- Reduced IgA concentration in faeces of GSDs. This is again a contentious observation, as there are conflicting data from different studies. The most recent reports describe some GSDs with consistently low faecal IgA concentration on repeat sampling.
- Increased numbers of $SmIgA^+$ lymphocytes in the blood of GSDs with disseminated aspergillosis.
- 'Inappropriate' usage of IgA in the systemic granulomata of disseminated aspergillosis (**608, 609**).
- No reduction in the numbers of IgA plasma cells in the intestinal mucosa of GSDs with ARD, but reduced concentration of IgA in duodenal juice, suggesting failure to synthesize or secrete IgA (see Chapter 7, p. 209).
- A CD4:CD8 imbalance (increased $CD8^+$ cells) and decreased proportion of $CD21^+$ B cells in GSDs with deep pyoderma.
- Polymorphisms in genes encoding TLRs.

In genetic terms, the GSD is an interesting breed. Evolutionarily it is one of the oldest canine breeds and thus more closely related to the wolf ancestors of this species. GSDs have a relatively heterozygous MHC, but studies with microsatellite markers have suggested that heavy inbreeding may have occurred amongst these dogs. Also of note is the recent observation that all GSDs express a single molecular variant of the IgA heavy chain hinge region compared with the greater heterozygosity found amongst other breeds.

IgG deficiency

Three candidate syndromes characterized fundamentally by IgG deficiency have been described in the dog.

The first of these is the widely recognized syndrome of chronic, recurrent infection in young Weimaraner dogs. In 1980 a colony of Weimaraners was described in which there was growth hormone deficiency, thymic aplasia and failure of blood lymphocytes to respond to T cell mitogens. Affected dogs had a wasting syndrome and were susceptible to infection. This entity has never been reported subsequently and appears unrelated to the disease that currently affects this breed and which was first reported in Australia in 1984 and has since been documented in the US, Europe and the Middle East. These dogs have chronic recurrent infections of multiple body systems, left shift neutrophilia and neutrophil-dominated inflammatory lesions at necropsy (**610**). In the US, affected dogs more often appear

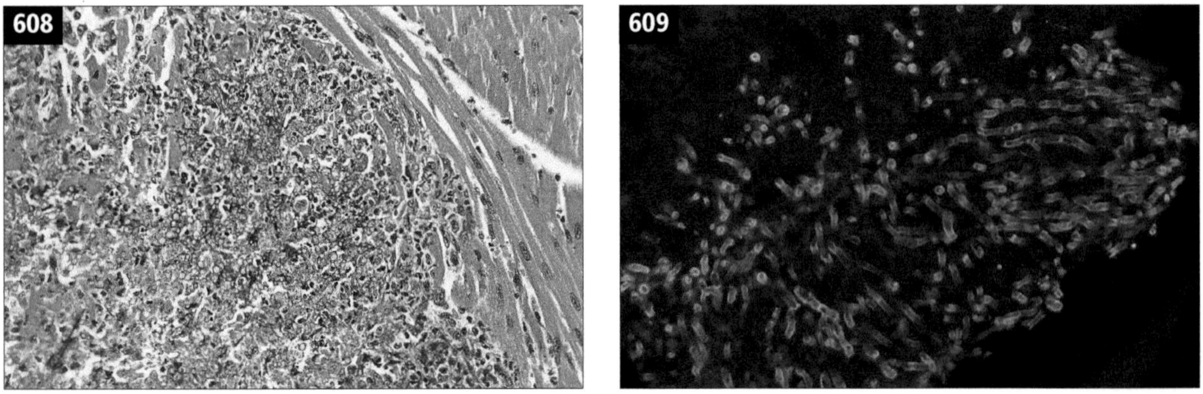

608, 609 Inappropriate IgA usage in disseminated aspergillosis. (**608**) Section of fungal granuloma within the myocardium of a GSD with disseminated aspergillosis. (**609**) Immunofluorescence labelling of this tissue reveals marked deposition of IgA on the surface of the intralesional fungal hyphae, and IgA-bearing plasma cells are often prominent within the inflammatory infiltrates of such systemic lesions. The dominance of IgA in non-mucosal lesions is of note; this class of Ig would normally be expected to be produced in a mucosal immune response.

to present with hypertrophic osteodystrophy (HOD), also known as metaphyseal osteopathy, and the disease is often referred to as 'HOD of the Weimaraner'.

There is some confusion over the nature of the likely immunological defect in these dogs. Initial studies of the Australian cases failed to demonstrate abnormality of neutrophil or lymphocyte function, but subsequent investigations in the US suggested that there was a defect in neutrophil function (chemiluminescence), with normal lymphocyte, monocyte and NK cell function. A single case from Belgium was reported with defective neutrophil phagocytosis but normal chemotaxis. Despite this, the most consistent immunological abnormality in affected dogs is reduced concentration of serum IgG (and sometimes IgM and IgA) (**611**). This low serum IgG concentration cannot be attributed to the presence of serum immune complexes, which are not elevated in affected dogs, and moreover it appears to be a persistent finding when these dogs are serially monitored over time during periods of active disease and remission. Subnormal serum IgG concentration has in fact now become the most accessible means of definitively diagnosing this disease syndrome.

An intriguing aspect of the 'Weimaraner immunodeficiency syndrome' is the apparent role of vaccination as a trigger factor for the clinical disease. In the majority of cases where vaccination history has been studied, the onset of clinical signs is in the weeks following the final injection of the puppy's series of vaccines. In one 'experimental' study, a litter of Weimaraner pups was subdivided into two groups, which received different vaccination regimes. The group of pups that received more frequent administration of multi-component vaccine went on to develop more severe disease than those pups undergoing a less extensive vaccinal protocol.

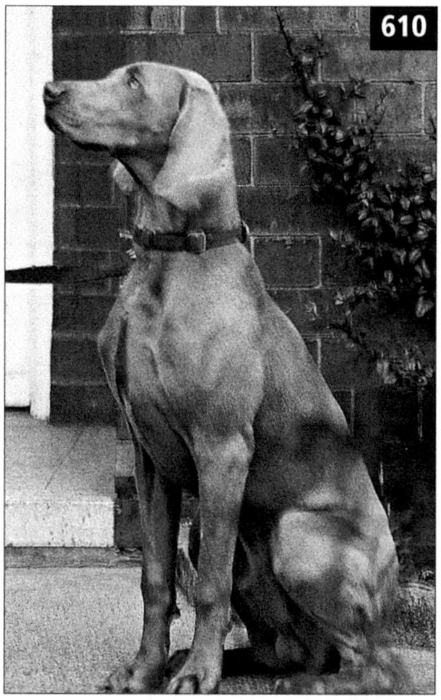

610 Immunodeficiency in Weimaraners. This Weimaraner was first presented at 15 weeks of age (after waning of maternal Ig) with chronic, recurrent infections of the alimentary tract, joints, skin and conjunctivae. There was peripheral lymphadenomegaly and a left shift neutrophilia during episodes of disease that responded to antimicrobial therapy. The dog was monitored over a 230 day period and shown to have consistently reduced serum IgG and IgA concentration. This patient eventually succumbed to repeated infection.

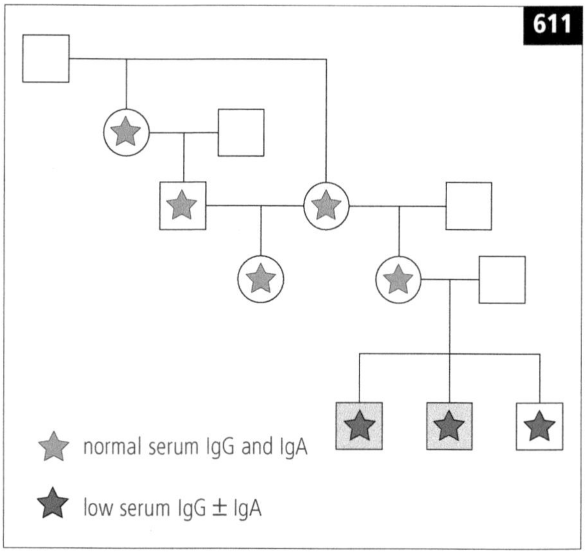

611 Immunodeficiency in Weimaraners. Pedigree of the Weimaraner shown in **610**. The littermates of this animal both had reduced serum IgG and one had concurrent reduction in IgA concentration. One of these littermate dogs died suddenly at 27 weeks of age and the second had pyoderma. Other relatives of this litter (including the dam) had normal serum Ig levels.

Affected dogs may make a clinical response to anti-inflammatory (glucocorticoid or NSAID) and antimicrobial therapy. The clinical outcome of this syndrome is variable. Some animals develop such severe disease that they must be euthanased, others recover but develop chronic recurrent infections, and yet others appear to fully recover and do not undergo disease relapse. The response to therapy, and the possibility of clinical recovery, are not features generally associated with primary immunodeficiency disease.

The second disease entity with a putative underlying IgG deficiency is the recently reported syndrome of *Pneumocystis carinii* pneumonia in young adult Cavalier King Charles Spaniels (CKCSs). This organism is an opportunist pathogen, which is a major cause of infection and disease in human patients with immunodeficiency disease. Affected CKCSs are young adults (mean age 3.5 years) with respiratory signs initiated by the organism. Some dogs have also had cutaneous demodicosis, again suggestive of underlying immunodeficiency. Affected dogs have subnormal serum IgG concentration and often an elevation in serum IgM (which may be a compensatory mechanism), and these findings persist in patients that are serially monitored (**612, 613**). The dogs may respond to appropriate antimicrobial therapy, but disease relapse may occur in subsequent years.

Finally, a litter of Rottweiler pups was described in which several littermates developed multi-systemic inflammatory or infectious disease. These dogs generally had subnormal IgG and/or IgA, together with abnormalities in development of lymphoid tissues (**614**). The basis for this defect has not been defined and other affected litters have not

612

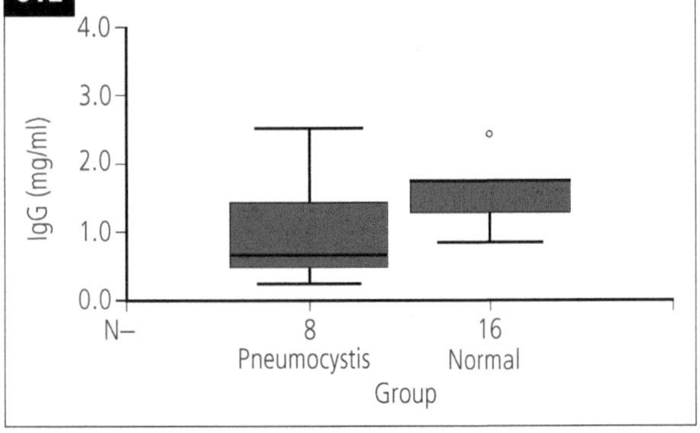

613

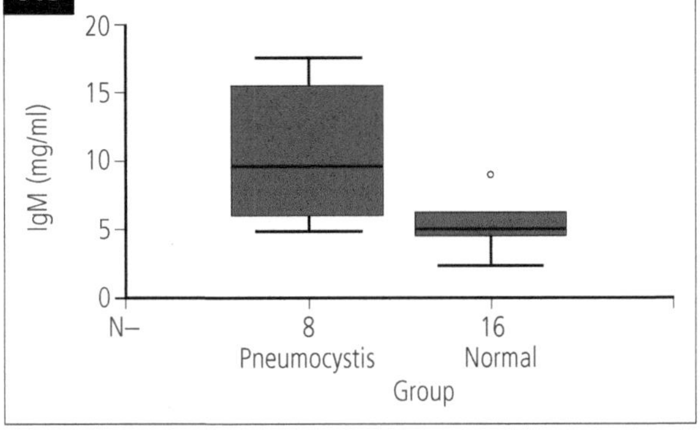

612, 613 Pneumocystis pneumonia in Cavalier King Charles Spaniels. Serum IgG (**612**) and IgM (**613**) concentrations in a group of CKCSs with pneumocystis pneumonia compared with a group of clinically normal CKCS dogs. Affected dogs have subnormal serum IgG concentration and elevation of serum IgM concentration. (Data from Watson PJ, Wootton P, Eastwood J *et al.* [2006] Immunoglobulin deficiency in Cavalier King Charles Spaniels with *Pneumocystis* pneumonia. *Journal of Veterinary Internal Medicine* **20**:523–527.)

614

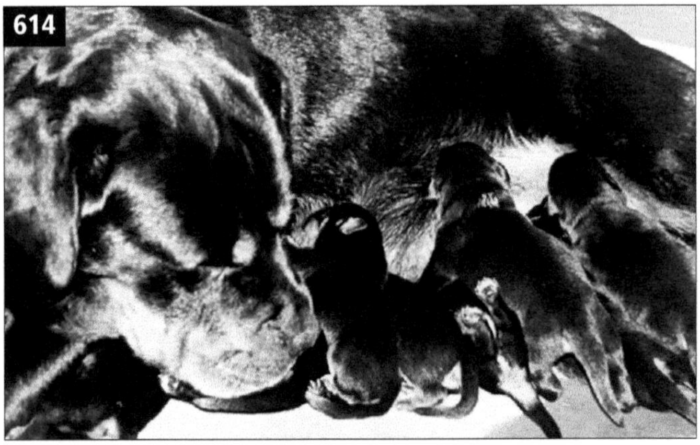

614 Immunodeficiency in Rottweilers. Pups within this litter developed multisystemic inflammatory/infectious disease related to subnormal concentrations of serum IgG and/or IgA. There were also developmental abnormalities in lymphoid tissues of affected pups.

been described, but it is of note that this is a breed that has long been recognised as a 'poor responder' to vaccination and susceptible to parvovirus infection.

Complement deficiency

Some dogs in a colony of Brittanys with hereditary spinal muscular atrophy were reported to have selective deficiency of complement C3. Affected dogs were susceptible to bacterial infection, and two dogs developed renal pathology (ICGN or renal amyloidosis). These dogs had 0.0003% of normal serum C3 and decreased CH_{50}, with normal levels of other classical pathway components except C2, which was lowered in some dogs. The deficiency was not secondary to a serum inhibitor of C3, as the decreased CH_{50} activity was restored by addition of purified C3, and serum from an affected dog mixed with normal dog serum did not alter the level of C3 in the normal sample. Affected dogs had 'C3-like functional activity' at 10% of that of normal dog serum, which may reflect the presence of an altered form of C3 or another protein with limited C3 function. Serum from affected dogs was less effective in chemotactic and opsonization assays and was unable to lyze rabbit RBCs via the alternative pathway. The deficiency was inherited in a non-MHC-linked, autosomal recessive manner and a single base deletion in the C3 gene has been identified.

Cellular immune deficiency

Canine leukocyte adhesion deficiency

In 1975 an Irish Setter with chronic recurrent infection (dermatitis, gingivitis, and osteomyelitis), pyrexia, lymphadenopathy and left-shift neutrophilia was shown to have defective neutrophil bacteriocidal activity (but normal phagocytosis) that was inherited in an autosomal recessive manner. The disease was termed 'canine granulocytopathy syndrome' and neutrophils from affected dogs had reduced glucose oxidation by the hexose monophosphate shunt and increased ability to reduce NBT. In 1987 an Irish Setter-cross with severe bacterial infections and peripheral blood neutrophilia, but lack of tissue pus formation, was described. This animal had an inherited (autosomal recessive) deficiency in expression of the surface integrin molecules CD11b and CD18, manifest as an inability of neutrophils to adhere to various surfaces. There was impaired neutrophil chemotaxis and aggregation, with reduced lymphocyte responsiveness to mitogens. The relationship of this latter condition to canine granulocytopathy syndrome was not definitively established. Twelve Irish Setters with CD11b/CD18 deficiency and recurrent infections were reported from Sweden in 1992, and the disease is also recognized in the UK. The disease has been named 'canine leukocyte adhesion deficiency' (CLAD) and there is an equivalent entity in humans and cattle (BLAD). Although predominantly affecting red Irish Setters, the canine disease has also been documented in red and white Irish Setters. The range of clinical abnormalities in dogs with CLAD has recently been reviewed and includes pyrexia, omphalophlebitis, gingivitis, lymphadenopathy, neutrophilia, metaphyseal osteopathy, cranio-mandibular osteopathy, osteomyelitis, mild interstitial pneumonia and skin wounds.

This syndrome has since become an excellent example of the successful application of molecular diagnosis to a monogenic immunodeficiency in the dog. The precise genetic mutation underlying the disorder was defined and a widely available molecular test able to detect heterozygotes and homozygous carriers was developed. With the cooperation of the Irish Setter breed society in various countries, a programme of testing and controlled breeding has been instigated that may eventually mean that this disease is eliminated from the breed. Indeed, in the relatively isolated population of these dogs in Australia, this disease-free status has almost been achieved. A recent experimental study has reported the use of the CLAD model to study stem cell transplantation, with successful reversal of the signs of disease in the recipient dog (see Chapter 16, p. 411).

Defective neutrophil function in Doberman Pinschers

A series of related Doberman Pinschers with chronic rhinitis and pneumonia was reported a number of years ago, but this syndrome does not appear to have been documented since. Affected dogs had defective neutrophil killing of phagocytosed *Staphylococcus* and decreased ability to reduce NBT and produce superoxide after stimulation. Serum Ig and complement concentrations were normal to elevated, and there was no defect in mitogen-induced lymphocyte proliferation.

Canine cyclic haematopoiesis

Cyclic haematopoiesis (cyclic neutropenia, Grey Collie syndrome) occurs in Collies with poor growth, diluted coat colour and cyclic (every 12 days for approximately three days) neutropenia in addition to neutrophil myeloperoxidase deficiency (**615**). There is also cycling of monocytes, reticulocytes and platelets, but there is no genetic mutation of haemopoietic stem cell factor. The neutropenic episodes are associated with combinations of pyrexia, diarrhoea, conjunctivitis, gingivitis or arthritis. Epistaxis and gingival haemorrhage may occur. Affected dogs have persistently elevated serum CH_{50} that is maximal during periods of neutrophil rebound.

The disease is inherited in an autosomal recessive fashion and, recently, the precise genetic mutation has been defined. This is a mutation in the gene encoding the adaptor protein complex 3 β subunit, the effect of which is to disrupt the intracellular movement of neutrophil elastase. Although humans also suffer from cyclic neutropenia, the genetic mutation is distinct. Again, molecular diagnosis for heterozygote and homozygote dogs is now possible, although this disease is not commonly reported in the wider canine population outside of experimental groups bred to study the equivalent human disease.

Pelger Huët anomaly

This syndrome is documented in several breeds including the American Foxhound, Cocker Spaniel, Boston Terrier and Basenji. There is decreased segmentation of granulocyte nuclei and defective neutrophil chemotaxis is variably described, but there is no abnormality of phagocytosis or intracellular killing. The defects do not predispose to infection and there is no impairment of the antibody response to exogenous antigen or of mitogen-driven lymphocyte proliferation. The anomaly also occurs in cats, where there is additional abnormality of monocytes and megakaryocytes. The disease should be suspected where there is a persistent left shift with normal white cell count in a healthy animal.

Trapped neutrophil syndrome (TNS) of Border collies

TNS is an autosomal recessive disease, widespread in this breed, presenting as neutropenia due to failure to release neutrophils from the bone marrow. Affected dogs may have stunted growth, pyrexia, vomiting, diarrhoea, inappetance, poor coat condition, lameness and joint swelling. A genetic mutation has been identified, but remains unpublished.

Chediak Higashi syndrome

This syndrome is an autosomal recessive trait of blue smoke Persian cats, characterized by abnormal lysosomes and granules within granulocyte cytoplasm. This may be associated with defective neutrophil chemotaxis, degranulation and bactericidal activity, and is accompanied by abnormalities of pigmentation of hair coat and ocular fundus and increased susceptibility to infection. There is an associated bleeding tendency, which may reflect abnormal platelet function.

An hereditary neutrophil granulation abnormality has also been described in Birman cats. This entity is inherited in an autosomal recessive fashion, but the presence of neutrophil cytoplasmic

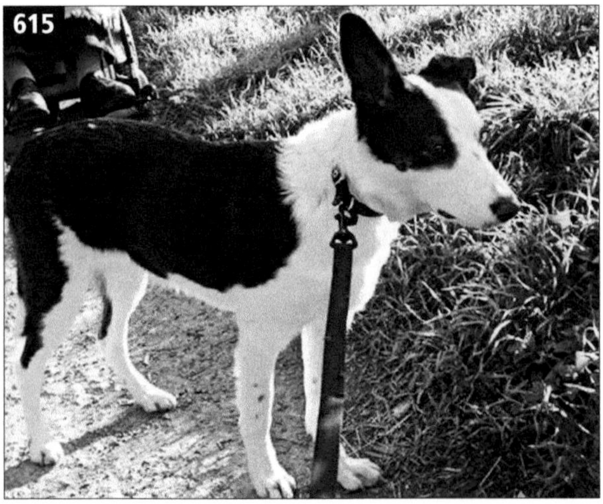

615 Persistent neutropenia. This young Border Collie dog is poorly grown and has repeated episodes of infection and neutropenia. Trapped neutrophil syndrome is suspected.

granules appears to cause no functional abnormality or susceptibility to infectious disease.

Severe combined immunodeficiency

Severe combined immunodeficiency (SCID) has now been described as a recessive trait in Basset Hounds, Cardigan Welsh Corgis and Jack Russell Terriers. In Basset Hounds the disease is X-linked (X-SCID) and affected dogs succumb to bacterial and viral infection after loss of maternal immunity. There is lymphoid hypoplasia and initial T lymphopenia, with normal numbers of circulating B cells. However, older dogs do develop some blood T cells, suggesting limited thymic emigration or extra-thymic expansion of peripheral T cells. Those lymphocytes that circulate do not respond to PHA, ConA or to recombinant IL-2, but IgM synthesis occurs after stimulation by pokeweed mitogen. There is normal serum IgM concentration and low or absent IgG and IgA, suggesting a late-stage defect in B cell maturation, with failure of the Ig class switch. The underlying defect in these dogs is a mutation in the common γ chain of the receptor for IL-2, IL-4, IL-7, IL-9 and IL-15. SCID in the Corgi is not X-linked and involves a distinct mutation in the same cytokine receptor γ chain gene. The disease in the Jack Russell Terrier is a genetic mutation in the DNA protein kinase gene, which means that affected dogs are unable to produce viable T and B cell receptor molecules, with similar marked consequences for immune function of these lymphoid lineages.

Lethal acrodermatitis of Bull Terriers

This syndrome is defined by stunted growth, splayed digits, cutaneous parakeratosis, nail disease, paronychia, footpad hyperkeratosis and skin and respiratory infections (**616, 617**). Affected dogs have subnormal plasma zinc levels, but they do not respond to oral zinc supplementation. There is reduced serum IgA, depletion of T cells from tissues and depressed lymphocyte response to mitogens. Neutrophils have normal ability to phagocytose and kill. The disease is inherited in an autosomal recessive fashion.

Mexican Hairless dogs

Mexican Hairless dogs appear susceptible to perinatal mortality. In one study of dogs of this breed there was impaired antibody and cutaneous DTH responses, with lymphoid depletion of thymus and spleen. There are clear links between hairlessness and immune dysfunction in other species, in particular the inbred laboratory strains of 'nude' rats and mice that are athymic and lack T lymphocytes.

Pneumocystis pneumonia of Miniature Dachshunds

Related young adult Miniature Dachshunds in Australia, New Guinea and South Africa appear predisposed to respiratory disease (hyperpnoea,

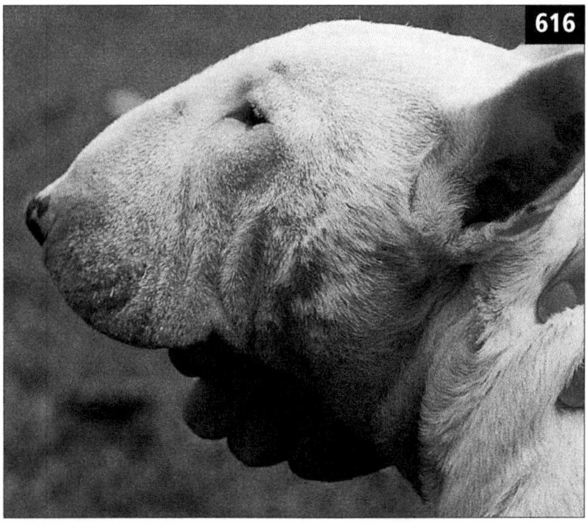

616

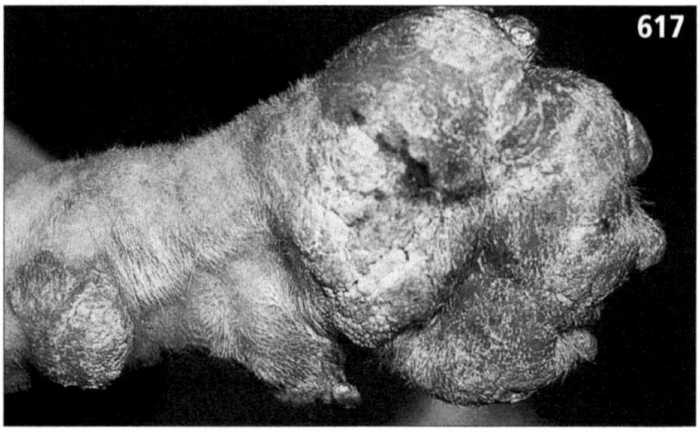

617

616, 617 Lethal acrodermatitis in Bull Terriers. (**596**) Stunted Bull Terrier with lethal acrodermatitis demonstrating submandibular lymphadenopathy. (**597**) There is abnormal keratinization of the footpads, with fissuring, exfoliation and onychodystrophy. (Photographs courtesy S.E. Shaw.)

tachypnoea, exercise intolerance) caused by the opportunist pathogen *Pneumocystis carinii* (**618**). Some dogs also have skin lesions, which may be due to either demodicosis or bacterial pyoderma. Underlying immunodeficiency may explain this breed association. On immunohistochemical evaluation these dogs may have reduced mitogen response of blood lymphocytes, reduced levels of serum IgG, IgM and IgA, and reduced populations of B lymphocytes in lymphoid tissue. As for the syndromes affecting Weimaraners and CKCSs described above, this disease is not a classical immunodeficiency, as affected dogs recover with appropriate antimicrobial treatment.

Disseminated mycobacteriosis in Miniature Schnauzers

An increasing prevalence of systemic infection with *Mycobacterium avium* complex is reported in Miniature Schnauzers in North America, Australia and Europe. These are related young dogs (ten months to three years of age) presenting with non-specific illness and marked lymphadenopathy. On necropsy examination there is extensive granulomatous inflammation throughout the liver, spleen, bone marrow and lymph nodes, with large numbers of acid-fast organisms. The respiratory tract is generally unaffected and it is likely that infection occurs via oral exposure. Limited studies of immune function have suggested a normal CD4:CD8 ratio amongst blood lymphocytes, but an elevation in the proportion of B cells. There are depressed mitogen responses. No clear mode of inheritance is thus far defined, but molecular studies are currently being conducted.

Feline primary immunodeficiency

Primary, congenital immunodeficiency in the cat appears rare relative to the spectrum of disorders that are described in dogs. The Chediak Higashi syndrome and Pelger Huët anomaly are described above. One further example is the single report of Birman kittens born without a thymus or hair coat (thymic aplasia and hypotrichosis). These animals died by 13 weeks of age and had depletion of T cell areas of secondary lymphoid tissue. It was suggested that this disease may be inherited in an autosomal recessive fashion. Sporadic cases of thymic hypoplasia with secondary infection are recorded in kittens (see Chapter 15, p. 370). Finally, it has recently been suggested that the apparent susceptibility of Abyssinian cats to disseminated infection with bacteria of the *Mycobacterium avium-intracellulare* complex might be related to an uncharacterized immunodeficiency.

618

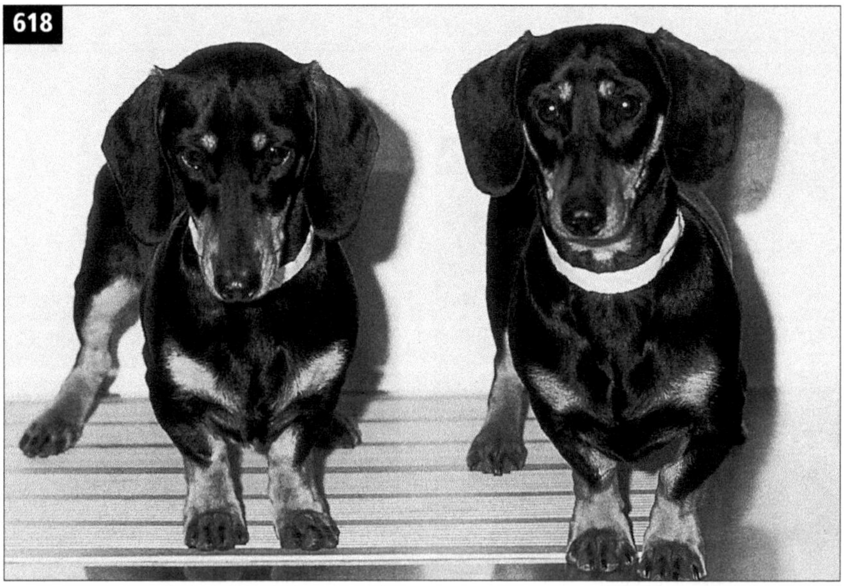

618 *Pneumocystis* pneumonia in Miniature Dachshunds. These two eight-week-old Miniature Dachshund littermates presented with respiratory tract disease attributed to *Pneumocystis carinii.* Both dogs had normal complement CH_{50} and serum C3 and C4 concentrations. One dog had normal lymphocyte response to the mitogen PHA, but consistently reduced serum IgG on three occasions tested. Pedigree analysis revealed that a number of related dogs had died from respiratory disease. (Photograph courtesy W.T. Clark.)

THERAPY FOR IMMUNODEFICIENCY DISEASE

In many of the diseases described above, symptomatic and antimicrobial therapy may induce temporary clinical improvement, but most true primary immunodeficiency disorders are invariably fatal. Immunomodulatory drugs (see Chapter 16, p. 369) have occasionally been used in the therapy of immunodeficiency, but there are no efficacious licensed products that can restore or boost immune function in companion animals.

Ig replacement therapy is standard procedure for many human immunodeficiencies, but there are no reports of its use in dog and cat immunodeficiency disease other than for the management of colostrum-deprived kittens. In this situation commercial milk replacer may be mixed with serum from a well-vaccinated adult cat (50 ml + 50 ml) and fed to animals under 3 days of age. For older kittens serum may be injected subcutaneously or intraperitoneally or plasma may be given i/v. Donor serum should come from a cat of compatible blood type (see Chapter 4, p. 115) that has been screened for infectious disease. As an alternative approach, the use of commercially available lyophilized equine IgG was investigated for the management of colostrum-deprived kittens. The equine IgG was absorbed more efficiently following subcutaneous injection than following oral administration, but the horse IgG had a shorter half life than feline IgG and failed adequately to opsonize bacteria for phagocytosis in an *in vitro* assay.

There is potential for the use of recombinant cytokines in the management of immunodeficiency diseases. Canine granulocyte-colony stimulating factor and canine stem cell factor have been used successfully to treat cyclic haematopoiesis, and bone marrow transplantation has also proven successful in this disease. Immune function has also been successfully restored in X-SCID dogs following bone marrow transplantation and following transplantation of heterologous stem cells into an affected dog that received partial myeloablation (irradiation) and medical immunosuppression after transplantation.

Recently, gene replacement therapy has been successfully applied to the treatment of canine cyclic haematopoiesis and X-SCID in an experimental setting as a model for human disease (see Chapter 16, p. 407). Realistically, such therapies will not (and should not) be used for the treatment of individual dogs. It is far more important to develop valid molecular diagnostic tests and initiate genetic counselling of breeders to enable elimination of such traits from affected breeds.

FURTHER READING

Benson KF, Li F–Q, Person RE *et al.* (2003) Mutations associated with neutropenia in dogs and humans disrupt intracellular transport of neutrophil elastase. *Nature Genetics* **35**:90–96.

Claus MA, Levy JK, MacDonald K *et al.* (2006) Immunoglobulin concentrations in feline colostrum and milk, and the requirement of colostrum for passive transfer of immunity to neonatal kittens. *Journal of Feline Medicine and Surgery* **8**:184–191.

Clercx C, Reichler I, Peeters D *et al.* (2003) Rhinitis/bronchopneumonia syndrome in Irish Wolfhounds. *Journal of Veterinary Internal Medicine* **17**:843–849.

Crawford PC, Hanel RM, Levy JK (2003) Evaluation of treatment of colostrum-deprived kittens with equine IgG. *American Journal of Veterinary Research* **64**:969–975.

Day MJ (1999) Possible immunodeficiency in related Rottweiler dogs. *Journal of Small Animal Practice* **40**:561–568.

Day MJ (2010) Ageing, immunosenescence and inflammageing in the dog and cat. *Journal of Comparative Pathology* **142**:S60–S69.

Foale RD, Herrtage ME, Day MJ (2003) Retrospective study of 25 young Weimaraners with low serum immunoglobulin concentrations and inflammatory disease. *Veterinary Record* **153**:553–558.

Foureman P, Whiteley M, Giger U (2002) Canine leukocyte adhesion deficiency: presence of the Cys36Ser β-2 integrin mutation in an affected US Irish Setter crossbreed dog and in US Irish Red and White Setters. *Journal of Veterinary Internal Medicine* **16**:518–523.

Hall JA, Chinn RM, Vorachek WR *et al.* (2010) Aged beagle dogs have decreased neutrophil phagocytosis and neutrophil-related gene

expression compared to younger dogs. *Veterinary Immunology and Immunopathology* **137**:130–135.
Harus S, Waner T, Aizenberg I *et al.* (2002) Development of hypertrophic osteodystrophy and antibody response in a litter of vaccinated Weimaraner puppies. *Journal of Small Animal Practice* **43**:27–31.
Jobling AJ, Ryan J, Augusteyn RC (2003) The frequency of the canine leukocyte adhesion deficiency (CLAD) allele within the Irish Setter population of Australia. *Australian Veterinary Journal* **81**:763–765.
Kijas JMH, Juneja RK, Gafvert S *et al.* (2000) Detection of the causal mutation for canine leukocyte adhesion deficiency (CLAD) using pyrosequencing. *Animal Genetics* **31**:326–328.
McEwan NA, McNeil PE, Thompson H *et al.* (2000) Diagnostic features, confirmation and disease progression in 28 cases of lethal acrodermatitis of Bull Terriers. *Journal of Small Animal Practice* **41**:501–507.
Perryman LE (2004) Molecular pathology of severe combined immunodeficiency in mice, horses, and dogs. *Veterinary Pathology* **41**:95–100.
Shearman JR, Wilton AN (2007) Elimination of neutrophil elastase and adaptor protein complex 3 subunit genes as the cause of trapped neutrophil syndrome (TNS) in border collies. *Animal Genetics* **38**:188–189.
Suter SE, Gouthro TA, O'Malley T *et al.* (2007) Marking of peripheral T-lymphocytes by retroviral transduction and transplantation of $CD34^+$ cells in a canine X-linked severe combined immunodeficiency model. *Veterinary Immunology and Immunopathology* **117**:183–196.
Trowald–Wigh G, Ekman S, Hansson K *et al.* (2000) Clinical, radiological and pathological features of 12 Irish Setters with canine leukocyte adhesion deficiency. *Journal of Small Animal Practice* **41**:211–217.
Watson PJ, Wotton P, Eastwood J *et al.* (2006) Immunoglobulin deficiency in Cavalier King Charles Spaniels with *Pneumocystis* pneumonia. *Journal of Veterinary Internal Medicine* **20**:523–527.
Yanay O, Barry SC, Katen LJ *et al.* (2003) Treatment of canine cyclic neutropenia by lentivirus-mediated G-CSF delivery. *Blood* **102**:2046–2052.

13 IMMUNE SYSTEM NEOPLASIA

Michael J. Day and Jane M. Dobson

INTRODUCTION

All of the cell types that comprise the immune and haemopoietic systems and their developmental stages have the potential for malignant transformation (**619**). The aetiology of any tumour is multifactorial and there is progression through initiation and latent phases to clinical disease (**620**). Factors involved in the development of haemopoietic and immune system tumours in the dog and cat are poorly understood, with the single exception of tumours induced by FeLV. Predisposing factors in oncogenesis include genetic background, age, sex, diet, environment, immune suppression and stress. There are likely to be genetic influences on the development of such tumours in dogs and cats; for example, lymphoma is recognized in particular breeds of dog (*Table 20*) and within certain canine pedigrees. Recent studies have demonstrated genetic susceptibility to the development of either T or B cell lymphoma within specific ancestral breed groups (e.g. T cell lymphoma in Spitz breeds and dogs of the Shih Tzu group; B cell lymphoma in more recently developed European breeds). Canine lymphoma is a disease of middle-aged to older dogs (80% aged 5–11 years). FeLV-induced lymphoma is more common in younger cats (50% aged less than five years), but also arises in older animals following activation of latent FeLV provirus, although lymphoma is

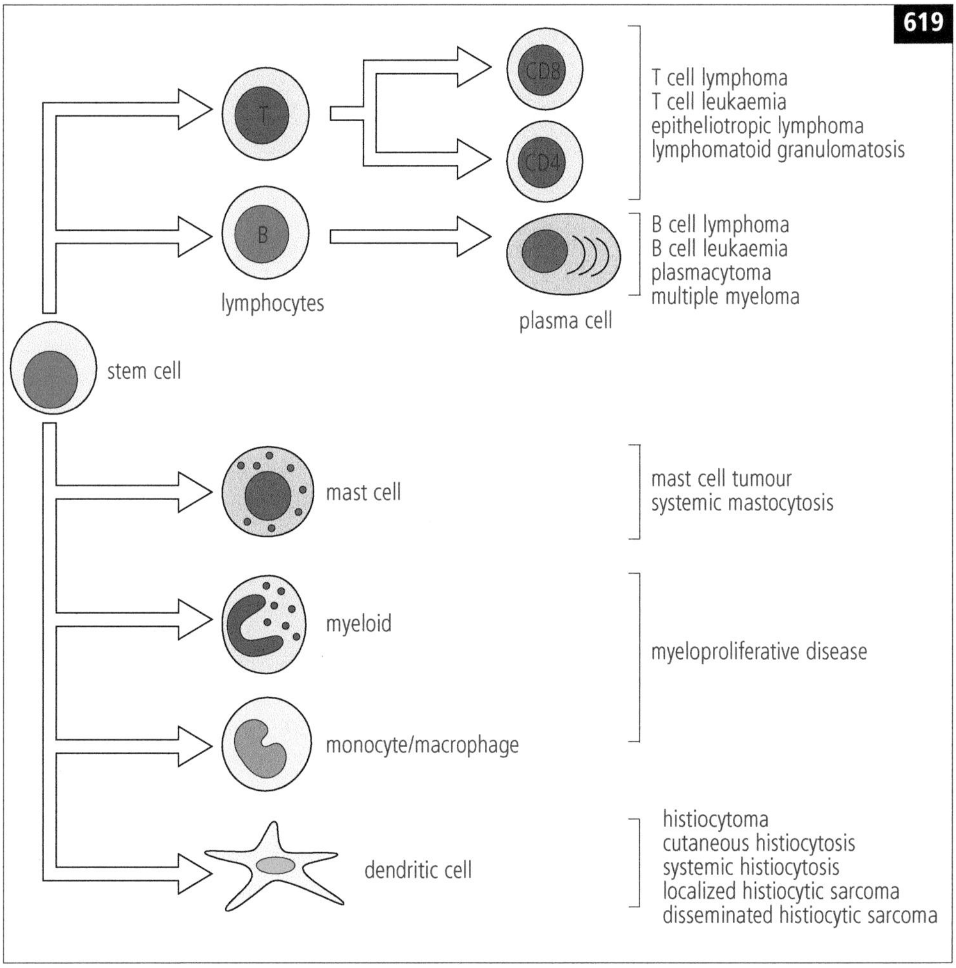

619 Tumours of the immune system. This diagram depicts the developmental stages of lymphoid and haemopoietic cells and lists the major tumours that may arise from each cell type. Cells at different stages of development may become neoplastic and this may be reflected in the anatomical location of the tumour, its histological and cytological appearance, and the range of surface membrane molecules displayed by the transformed cells.

Table 20: Breed prevalence in canine lymphoma. Breed prevalence in three studies of canine lymphoma are presented. Study A, Bristol, UK: Day MJ, Whitbread TJ (1995) Pathological diagnoses in dogs with lymph node enlargement. *Veterinary Record* **136:**72–73; Study B, Cambridge and Glasgow, UK: Dobson JM, Gorman NT (1993) Canine multicentric lymphoma. 1. Clinicopathological presentation of the disease. *Journal of Small Animal Practice* **34:**594–598; Study C, Glasgow, UK: Blackwood L, Sullivan M, Lawson H (1997) Radiographic abnormalities in canine multicentric lymphoma: a review of 84 cases. *Journal of Small Animal Practice* **38:**62–69. The normal population comprises all dogs presented to the Department of Veterinary Medicine, University of Bristol between 1990 and 1994 (n = 3,299). Such breed susceptibility data must be interpreted with care, as in most instances the prevalence of lymphoma in a particular breed correlates with the popularity of that breed in the normal population.

Breed	**Study A (n = 278)**	**Study B (n = 90)**	**Study C (n = 84)**	**Normal population (n = 3,299)**
Crossbred	11.5	27.7	21	11.1
German Shepherd Dog	9.7	5.5	7	7.5
Boxer	7.5	2.2	6	5.5
Labrador Retriever	6.5	11.1	16	7.9
Golden Retriever	6.1	7.7	7	6.2
Collie	3.9			1.0
Dobermann	3.9	6.7	2	3.6
Rottweiler	3.6	4.4	3	1.6
Bull Mastiff	2.9		3	0.3
Yorkshire Terrier	2.5	1.1		2.0
Jack Russell Terrier	2.5		1	2.0
Great Dane	2.1	1.1	2	1.6
English Springer Spaniel	2.1	4.4	1	3.9

NB: Data presented as a percentage of the entire population.

increasingly recognized in FeLV negative cats of all ages. No consistent gender influence has been documented for these tumours in dogs, and canine lymphoma cells do not express oestrogen or progesterone receptors. In contrast, male cats more frequently develop lymphoma, reflecting the horizontal transmission of FeLV.

The best defined initiating factor in feline lymphoma is FeLV, but recent data suggest that FIV may have an indirect, non-FeLV-associated role in the development of feline lymphoma (see Chapter 12, p. 288). Extensive discussion of the molecular biology of FeLV is beyond the scope of this summary, but in brief, FeLV type A proviral DNA recombines with host DNA and incorporates a host oncogene (c-myc). The recombinant FeLV-A virus then includes this host oncogene, which is under the control of the virus and thus permits transformation of host cells that are infected by the recombinant. Less commonly, there may be rearrangement of the host c-myc gene without direct transduction of the gene by FeLV but by integration of FeLV provirus adjacent to the c-myc gene. Recent reviews have suggested that since the advent of FeLV testing and vaccination, the prevalence of FeLV-negative lymphoma (especially the alimentary form) has increased and the mean age of affected cats has thus also increased. FeLV-negative lymphoma is also more prevalent in Australia, which reflects the reported low frequency of this viral infection in that country. In contrast, 50% of cats with spontaneously arising lymphoma in one Australian study were FIV positive, suggesting that this retroviral infection might predispose to development of the tumour. An association between feline gastric lymphoma and *Helicobacter* infection has been proposed.

Despite occasional reports, there is no conclusive evidence for a viral aetiology in canine lymphoma. An association between mineral deposition within canine lymph nodes and the development of lymphoma has been proposed (see Chapter 3, p. 88), and experimental rodents inoculated with mineral species have DNA damage, resulting in lymphomagenesis. Associations between canine lymphoma and exposure to magnetic fields or the

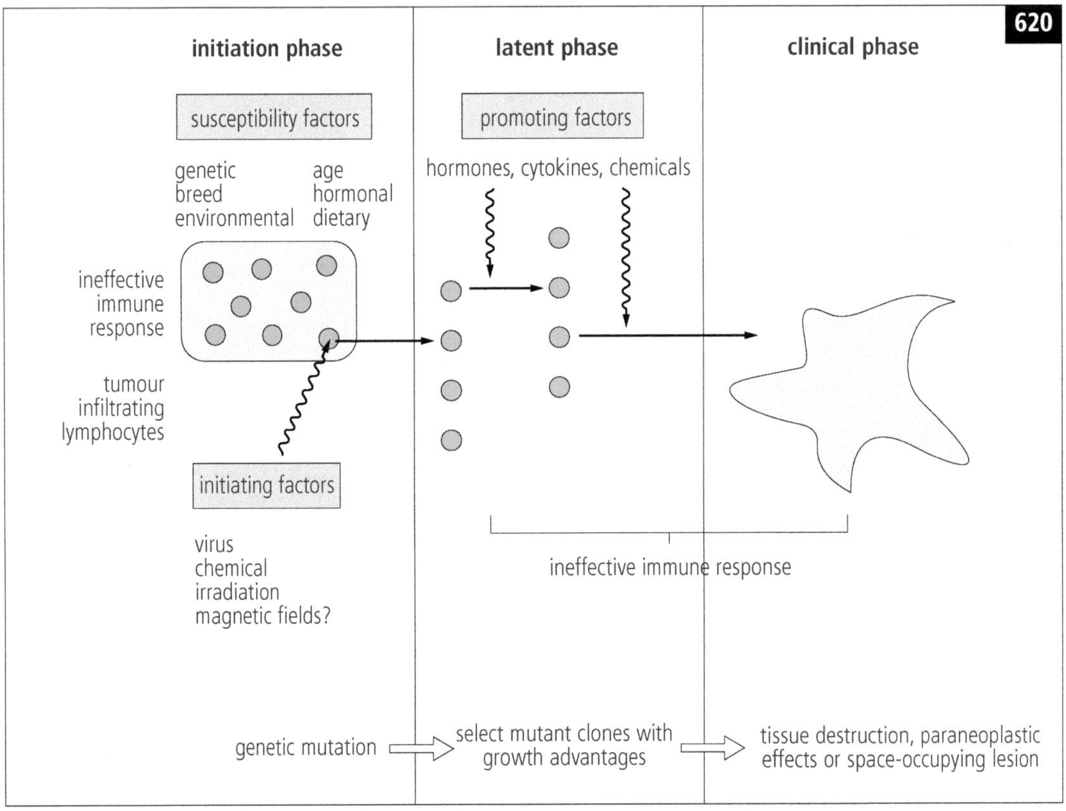

620 Stages in oncogenesis. The development of any tumour proceeds through three stages. An optimum combination of susceptibility factors may permit appropriate initiating factors to induce genetic mutation of a cell within a tissue (**initiation phase**). This cell is transformed and undergoes uncontrolled proliferation, during which time promoting factors act to select those mutant clones that have growth advantages (**latent phase**). During the **clinical phase** of neoplasia the tumour reaches sufficient size to induce clinical signs by tissue destruction, paraneoplastic production of soluble factors or by acting as a space occupying lesion in a confined anatomical space. Current theory proposes that a small population of **cancer stem cells** maintain the tumour by giving rise to **daughter cancer cells** of lesser replicative potential.

herbicide 2,4-dichlorophenoxyacetic acid have been reported. A recent investigation has shown linkage between development of canine lymphoma and residency in industrial areas or the use of paints and solvents within the home environment. These various associations remain largely speculative at this time. Experimental studies have demonstrated that radiation can induce myeloproliferative disease in the dog.

There are a number of stages in oncogenesis (620). Initiating factors trigger uncontrolled growth of the target cell through insertion, deletion or mutation of specific DNA sequences. Neoplastic growth requires inactivation of genes that normally trigger apoptosis (e.g. the p53 gene), and/or inappropriate activation of genes that encode factors that inhibit apoptosis (e.g. bcl-2) or of oncogenes that encode growth factors, growth factor receptors or transducers, or nuclear oncoproteins. Transformation may arise via loss of regulation normally provided by 'tumour suppressor genes' (e.g. p53), and deletion or mutation of the p53 gene is commonly recognized amongst neoplastic cells. The feline p53 gene has been cloned and point mutations recognized in feline lymphoma. FeLV-induced T cell lymphoma-derived cell lines and sections of spontaneously arising feline lymphoma strongly express the bcl-2 protein, although expression is more commonly present in T cell neoplasms compared with B cell neoplasms. The contribution of 'tumour infiltrating lymphocytes' to oncogenesis is now recognized. These Treg cells inappropriately suppress the function of anti-tumour cytotoxic cells and have become a new therpeutic target.

Six essential alterations in cell physiology that collectively dictate malignant growth are:

- Self-sufficiency in growth signals.
- Insensitivity to growth-inhibitory signals.
- Evasion of apoptosis.
- Limitless replicative potential.
- Sustained angiogenesis.
- Tissue invasion and metastasis.

Little is known of the sequence of development of lymphoid or haemopoietic tumours in the dog and cat, but in both species alimentary lymphoma may follow lymphoid hyperactivity in lymphoplasmacytic enteritis. Similarly, myeloproliferative disease may be preceded by myelodysplasia, characterized by clonal instability and resulting in cytopenia, marrow hypercellularity and maturation defects.

LYMPHOMA

Lymphoma may be classified at a variety of levels from gross anatomical distribution to molecular rearrangements in tumour DNA.

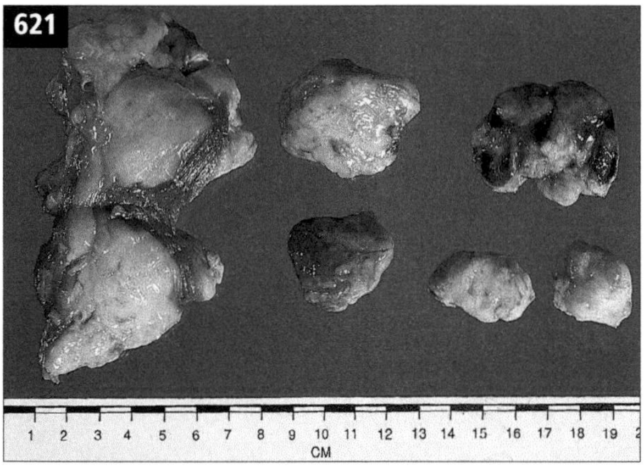

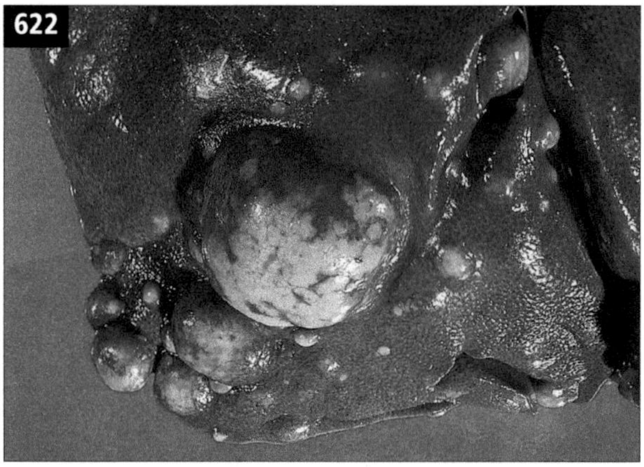

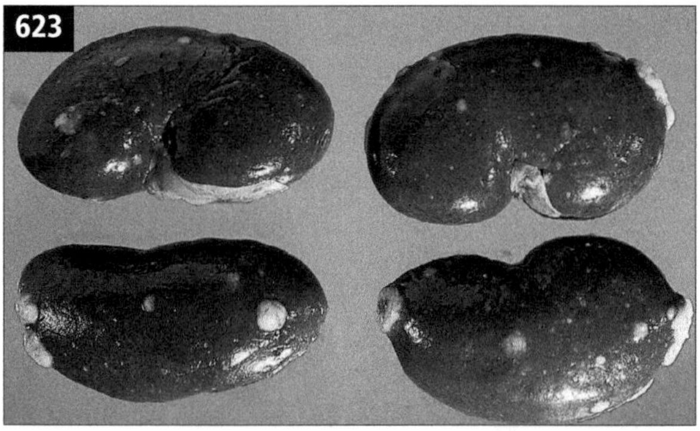

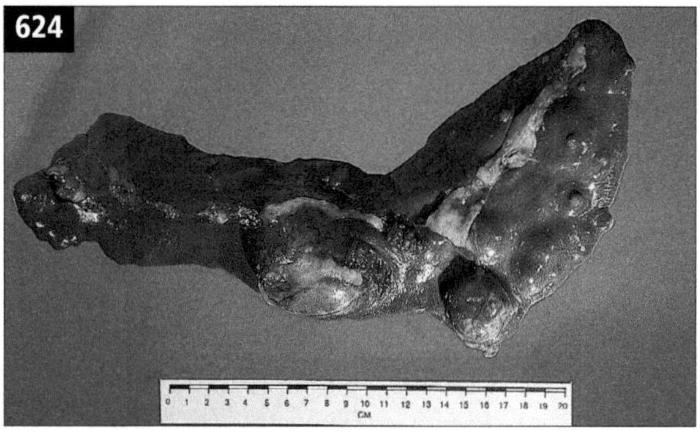

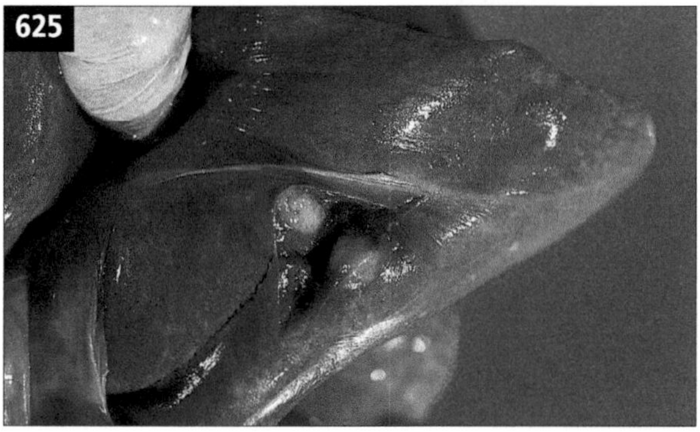

621–625 Canine multicentric lymphoma. Gross necropsy appearance of the lesions of multicentric lymphoma in an eight-year-old male Flat Coated Retriever. (**621**) There is marked enlargement of all the peripheral lymph nodes and the mesenteric and other visceral lymph nodes, with cream nodular masses in the liver (**622**), kidneys (**623**), spleen (**624**) and lung (**625**).

Anatomical distribution

In the dog and cat the anatomical distribution of lymphoma may be:

- **Multicentric** (621–625): involving multiple sites throughout the body, most frequently primarily involving the lymph nodes and then infiltrating organs such as the spleen, liver, kidney, lung, heart, gut and bone marrow. This distribution most likely reflects metastatic spread of a primary neoplasm rather than independent transformation of multiple lymphoid clones at different locations.
- **Thymic** (**mediastinal**) (**626**): restricted to the thymus and regional lymph nodes. A major differential is thymoma (see Chapter 15, p. 370).
- **Alimentary** (**627, 628**): involving any level of the gastrointestinal tract and mesenteric lymph nodes. The liver, kidney or spleen may occasionally be involved.
- **Solitary (extra-nodal)**: uncommon, but appears as a single lesion within the body (e.g. within one kidney) (**629**).

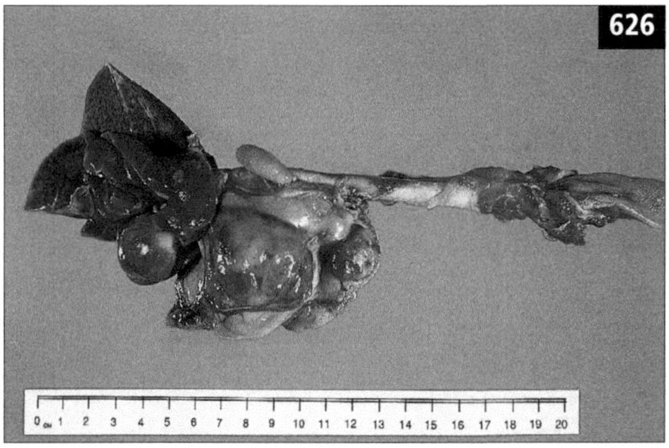

626 Feline thymic lymphoma. Thymic lymphoma experimentally induced in a cat by infection with FeLV. There is a large, cream, multinodular mass within the anterior mediastinum causing caudal displacement of the heart and lungs, and dorsal deviation of the overlying trachea and oesophagus.

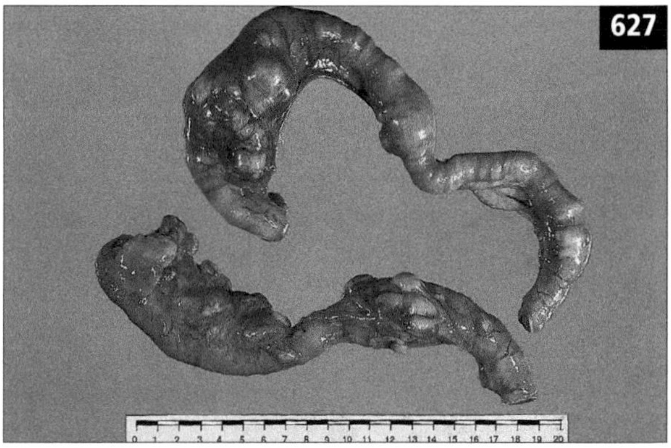

627 Alimentary lymphoma. Portion of small intestine from a six-year-old Welsh Springer Spaniel with a history of vomiting, melaena and haematemesis. At necropsy examination there was gross evidence of alimentary lymphoma. There were multiple, firm, cream nodules along the length of the small intestine. The mesenteric lymph nodes and kidneys of this dog were also affected.

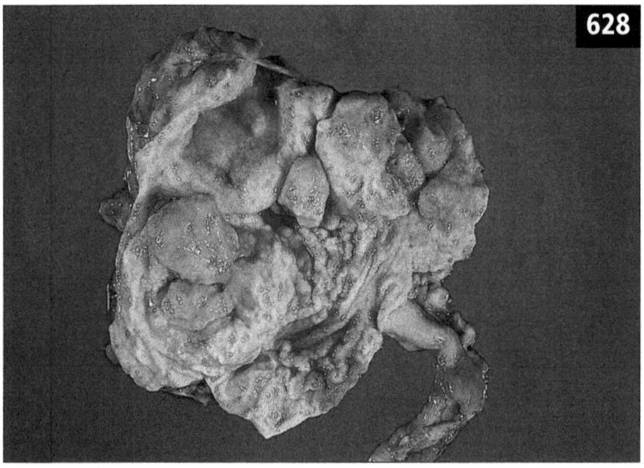

628 Alimentary lymphoma. Stomach from a nine-year-old DSH cat with a six-month history of weight loss, haematemesis and anaemia. Normal gastric mucosa is largely replaced by a series of coalescing, cream nodules. The kidneys of this cat were similarly affected.

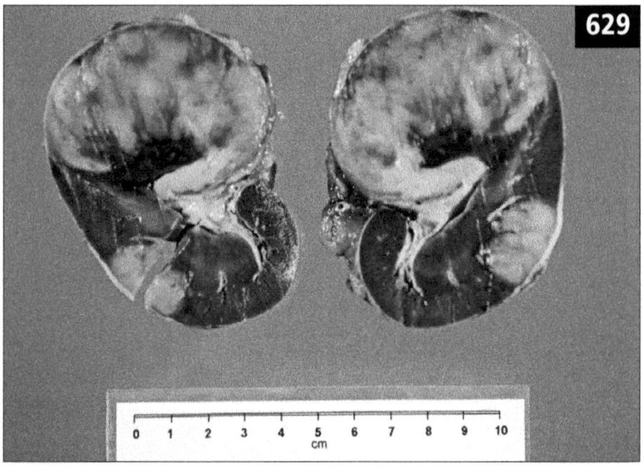

629 Solitary lymphoma. Kidney from an eight-year-old neutered female Labrador Retriever with extensive infiltration by neoplastic lymphoid cells. Other viscera were unaffected and the dog had secondary absolute polycythaemia related to inappropriately elevated production of erythropoietin.

- **Cutaneous:** involves either the dermis (dermal lymphoma) or epidermis (epitheliotropic lymphoma). In epitheliotropic lymphoma the neoplastic infiltrate is primarily epidermal and only in the latter stages of disease is the dermis involved.

In dogs, multicentric lymphoma is more common than alimentary lymphoma and thymic lymphoma is rare. In recent years there has been increased recognition of canine epitheliotropic lymphoma. As discussed above, the prevalence of feline alimentary lymphoma has increased with the increased prevalence of non-FeLV-associated tumours. Solitary lymphoma is less common and cutaneous lymphoma is rare in the cat. Dogs and cats with lymphoma generally do not have circulating neoplastic lymphocytes, and the blood lymphocyte count is often normal or reduced. However, in late stage disease there may be involvement of blood and bone marrow (leukaemic lymphoma).

The lesions of lymphoma generally appear as distinct, firm, cream-coloured, nodular masses within affected viscera. In some instances there may be diffuse infiltration of an organ (630). The distribution and extent of visceral involvement will determine the clinical presentation and laboratory findings. For example, the most common presenting feature of multicentric lymphoma is localized or generalized lymphadenomegaly. Thymic lymphoma is associated with dyspnoea, reduced exercise tolerance, dysphagia or regurgitation, whereas alimentary lymphoma may present as chronic vomiting, diarrhoea and weight loss. Schemes for clinical staging of canine multicentric lymphoma have been described (*Table 21*). Some lymphomas secrete parathyroid hormone-like substances, causing mobilization of calcium from bone and leading to hypercalcaemia. B cell lymphoma or lymphocytic leukaemia may be associated with monoclonal gammopathy or secondary autoimmune disease (particularly IMHA or IMTP).

Diagnosis of lymphoma in the dog and cat

The high prevalence of lymphoma, and the wide spectrum of possible visceral and paraneoplastic involvement, means that this disease frequently appears on lists of differential diagnoses for many conditions. The diagnostic approach to each case will depend, therefore, on the system(s) affected and the range of clinical signs that the animal displays (631–634). This may include:

630

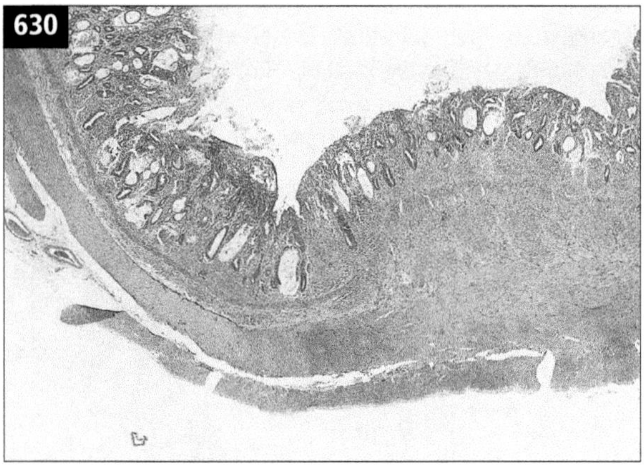

630 Alimentary lymphoma. Section of intestine from a ten-year-old Jack Russell Terrier with a four-week history of vomiting, diarrhoea and weight loss. At necropsy examination there was no evidence of gross thickening of the intestinal wall, but microscopic examination confirms the presence of alimentary lymphoma that diffusely infiltrates the mucosa and displaces normal structure.

Table 21: Clinical staging of canine multicentric lymphoma. (After Owen LN (1980) *The TNM Classification of Tumours in Domestic Animals* (1st edn). WHO, Geneva.)

Stage I	Disease confined to one lymph node or organ.
Stage II	Disease confined to multiple lymph nodes within one area of the body.
Stage III	Generalized peripheral and internal lymph node involvement.
Stage IV	Generalized peripheral and internal lymph node involvement with hepatic or splenic tumour.
Stage V	Involvement of multiple other organs, or bone marrow and blood.

- Haematological assessment to detect abnormality of leukocyte, erythrocyte or platelet number or morphology.
- Bone marrow aspiration or biopsy to determine marrow involvement.
- Serum biochemistry to define the extent of visceral damage, to identify paraneoplastic hypercalcaemia and to assess gammaglobulin concentration. Recent studies have shown the utility of measurement of serum concentration of thymidine kinase 1 (TK1) in the serum of dogs with lymphoma. Elevated concentrations of TK1 reflect cytoplasmic leakage from actively cycling cells, and concentrations normalize when dogs are in remission. Other serum biomarkers are also being evaluated.

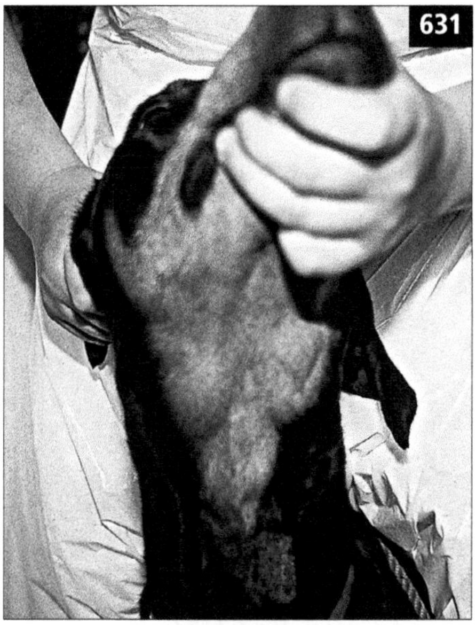
631

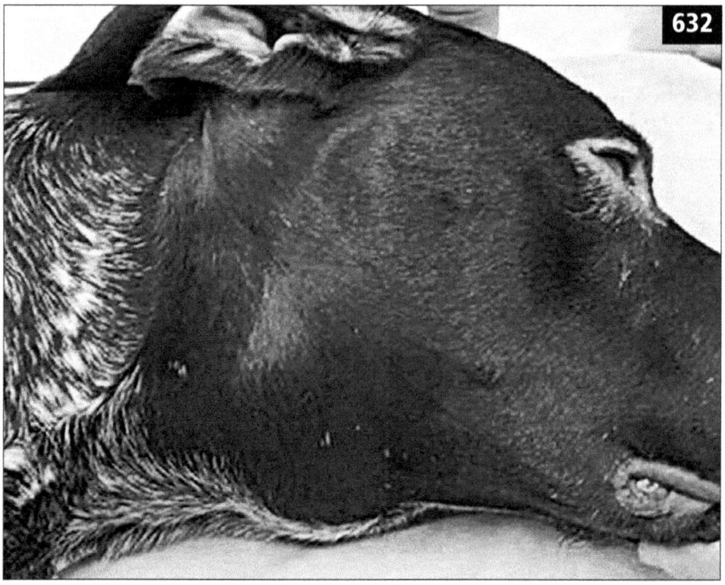
632

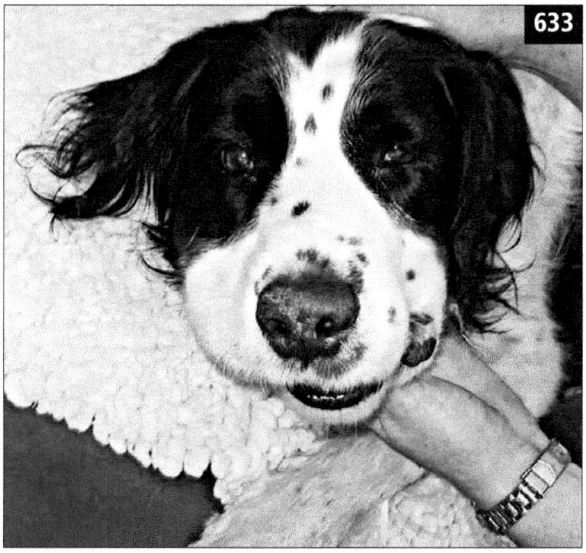
633

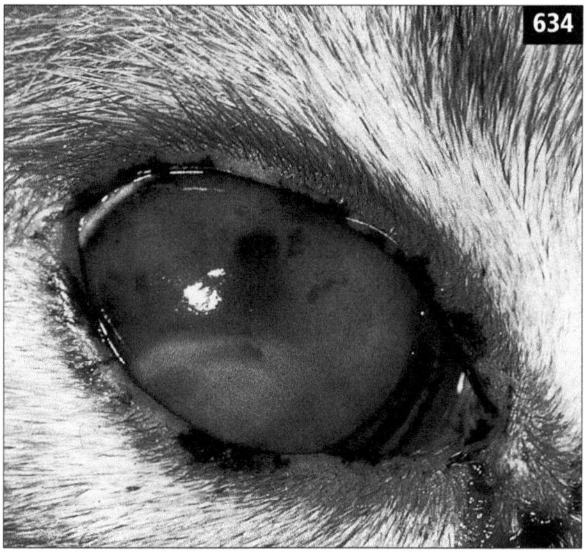
634

631–634 Clinical presentation of lymphoma. (**631**) Middle-aged female Dobermann with multicentric lymphoma. All superficial lymph nodes were grossly enlarged, as shown by the submandibular nodes in this photograph. (**632**) Similar generalized peripheral lymphadenomegaly is present in this middle-aged Pointer. (**633**) An eight-year-old Border Collie with facial swelling and oedema due to lymphomatous enlargement of submandibular and retropharyngeal lymph nodes, with subsequent obstruction to lymphatic drainage. (**634**) Cat with intraocular lymphoma. There is infiltration of the iris and a lymphomatous cellular precipitate in the anterior chamber. (Photograph courtesy D.E. Bostock.)

- Assessment of FeLV and FIV status in the cat.
- Imaging examinations (radiography or ultrasound) to identify visceral involvement (**635–638**). CT and MRI are not generally indicated for imaging visceral organs, but they may play a role in cases with suspected CNS involvement.
- Cytological examination of fine needle aspirated lesions or thoracic/abdominal fluids.
- Excisional biopsy of peripheral lymph nodes or accessible viscera.
- Immunophenotypic studies by immunocytochemistry or immunohistochemistry.
- Molecular studies to determine genetic rearrangements in neoplastic lymphocytes.

Cytology of lymphoma

Cytology is of major importance in the investigation of lymphoma, as diagnostic samples are often obtained by fine needle aspiration of lymph nodes or internal viscera or by sampling thoracic or abdominal fluid that may contain exfoliated tumour cells (**639–641**).

Histopathology of lymphoma

Lymphoma presents as a **diffuse** infiltration of neoplastic cells that obliterates normal structure of the affected lymph node or organ (**642, 643**); however, some tumours (particularly within

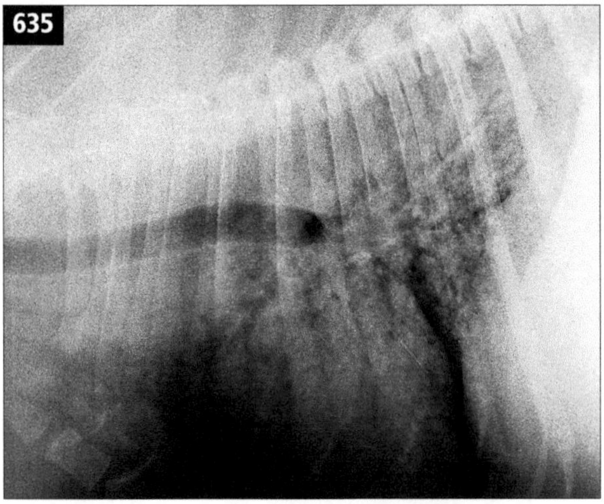

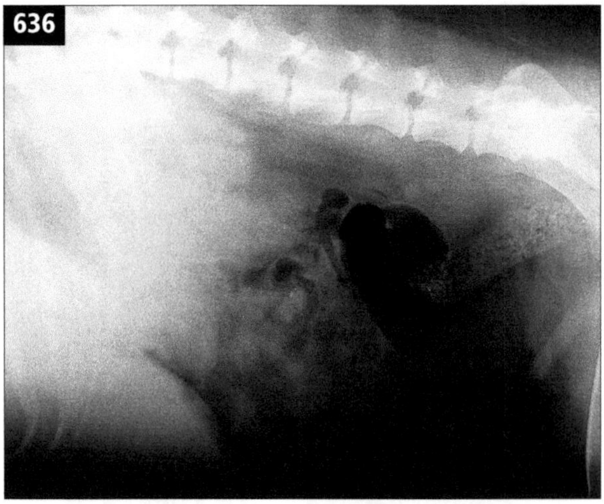

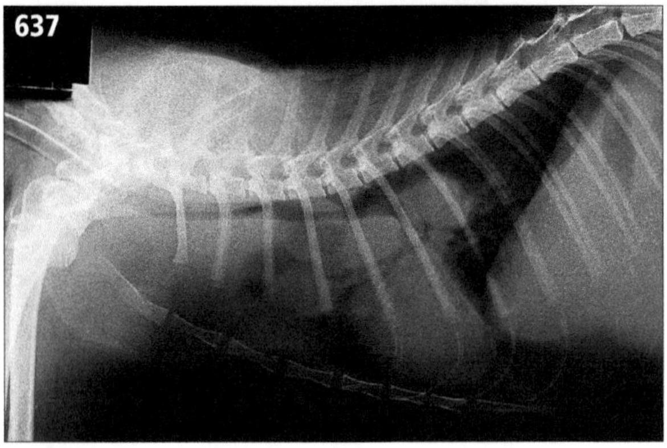

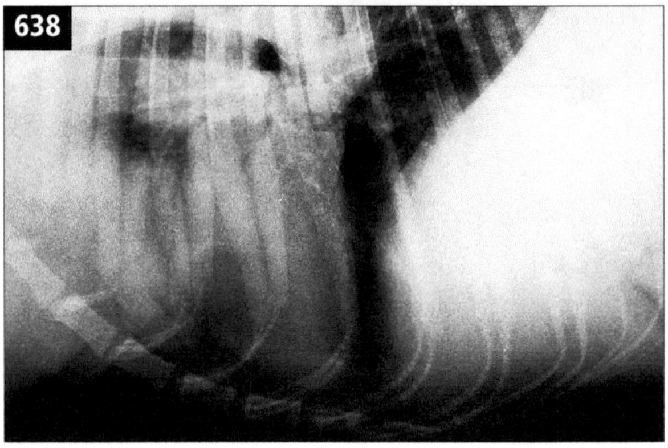

635–638 Imaging in the diagnosis of lymphoma. (**635**) Lateral thoracic radiograph from a dog with multicentric lymphoma. There is increased interstitial pattern within the lung fields, which is characteristic of pulmonary involvement in lymphoma occurring as a diffuse infiltrate rather than as discrete tumour nodules. (**636**) Lateral abdominal radiograph of a dog with stage IV multicentric lymphoma. Hepatosplenomegaly and sublumbar lymphadenopathy may be detected on plain abdominal radiographs. (**637**) Lateral thoracic radiograph of a cat with multicentric lymphoma showing several enlarged mediastinal lymph nodes. (**638**) Lateral thoracic radiograph of a dog with multicentric lymphoma. Presternal and tracheobronchial lymph node enlargement may be detected on plain thoracic films.

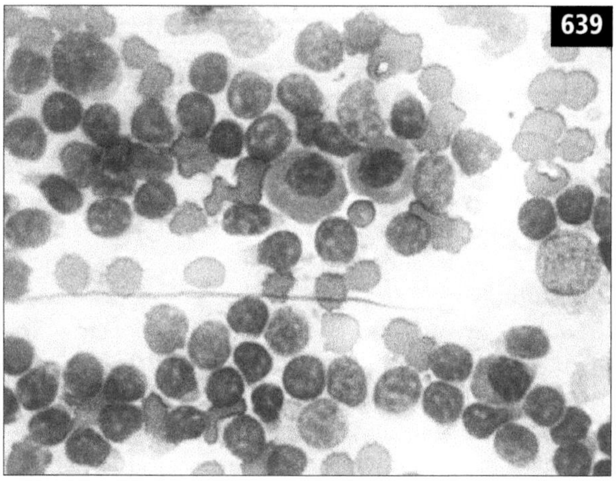

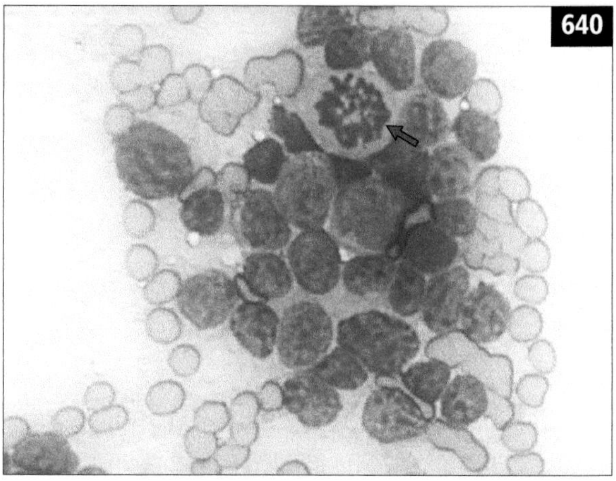

639–641 Cytological appearance of lymphoma. (**639**) Fine needle aspirate from a reactive canine submandibular lymph node. A range of cytologically normal cell types are present, including small lymphocytes (in greatest number), lymphoblasts and plasma cells. (**640**) Fine needle aspirate from a lymph node of a cat with generalized lymphadenopathy due to lymphoma. There is a background content of blood, with a predominant population of uniform, lymphoblastic cells with aggregated nuclear chromatin. A prominent irregular mitotic figure is present (arrowed). (**641**) Ultrasound-guided fine needle aspirate of a nodular mass in the liver of a cat. There is a population of pleomorphic lymphoblasts, with prominent single nucleoli and a mitotic figure within one of the cells (arrow).

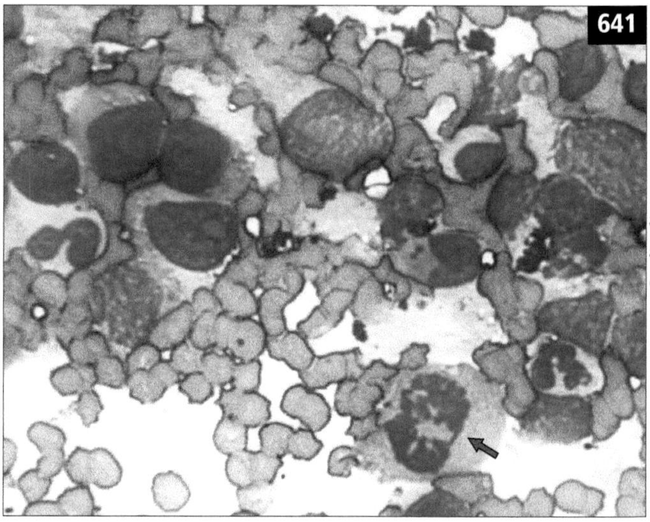

arroow added to 641

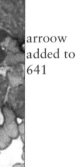

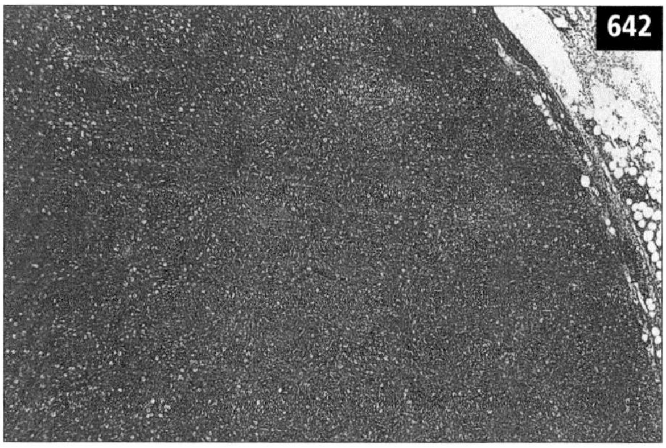

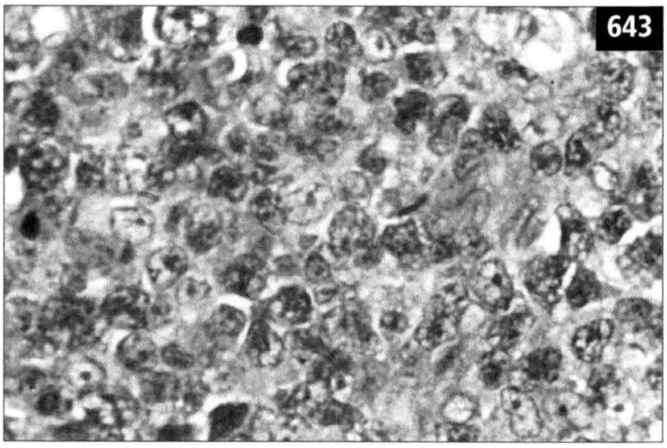

642, 643 Histological appearance of diffuse lymphoma. (**642**) Section of lymph node from a dog with lymphoma. There is complete obliteration of normal corticomedullary structure, which is replaced by a dense sheet of neoplastic lymphoid cells that are also present in the extranodal adipose tissue. The small spaces within the infiltrate give the impression of a 'starry sky' and are places where degenerate lymphocytes have been phagocytosed by macrophages. (**643**) High power magnification of a section of feline nasal lymphoma. There is a closely packed population of lymphoblastic cells, with an oval, occasionally convoluted, vesicular nucleus with central prominent nucleolus and relatively abundant eosinophilic cytoplasm. (From Day MJ, Henderson SM, Belshaw Z *et al.* [2004] An immunohistochemical investigation of 18 cases of feline nasal lymphoma. *Journal of Comparative Pathology* **130:**152–161, with permission.)

644

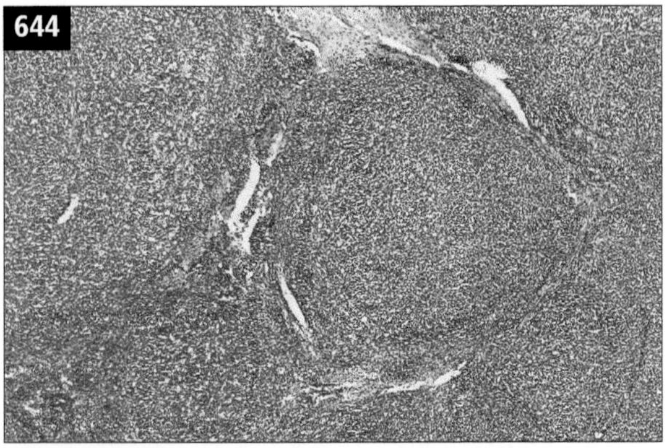

644 Histological appearance of follicular lymphoma. Section of lymph node from a dog with follicular lymphoma. The neoplastic lymphocytes are arranged in distinct follicular aggregates. This microscopic appearance is much less common than diffuse lymphoma in dogs and cats.

lymphoid tissue) may have an irregular **follicular** arrangement (**644**). Although once considered rare, a recent study of canine 'indolent nodular lymphoma' suggests that the range of follicle-associated patterns (follicular lymphoma, mantle cell lymphoma, marginal zone lymphoma and T-zone lymphoma) may have been underrecognized. This group of tumours is generally associated with indolent behaviour and good clinical survival. In addition to assessing the distribution and invasiveness of neoplastic lymphoid cells, the pathologist will also examine whether the neoplastic cells are well-differentiated or poorly differentiated; have the appearance of small lymphocytes, lymphoblasts or histiocytic cells; have irregularities of the nucleus, nucleoli or nuclear chromatin; and are of low or high mitotic rate.

Immunophenotyping of lymphoma

Diagnostic immunophenotyping of canine and feline lymphoma is a useful adjunct to cytological or histological procedures. The most commonly used approach involves the use of formalin-fixed tissue biopsies. Following standard histopathological examination, additional sections may be cut from the block of fixed tissue for immunohistochemical labelling for tumour markers. At present the range of antisera appropriate for use with fixed tissue is limited to detection of molecules such as CD3 (T cells), SmIg and CD79a (B cells), MHC class II (B cells and APCs) and MAC387 (myelohistiocytic cells) (**645–647**). A separate sample of fresh tissue (snap frozen in cryopreservative medium) would be required for more detailed analysis of expression of molecules such as CD4 or CD8. In research studies the expression of various molecules associated with cellular proliferation (e.g. Ki67) or apoptosis (e.g. p53) has been examined by immunohistochemistry. Immunophenotypic studies may also be performed on cytological preparations (immunocytochemistry), although this is less frequently available. The same antisera may be used to label neoplastic cells in blood or fluid samples by lymphocyte isolation, labelling and flow cytometry, (Chapter 12). Flow cytometric diagnosis has also been applied to cell suspensions prepared by disaggregating lymph node biopsies. Immunophenotyping studies are used to distinguish T cell from B cell lymphoma, but occasional tumours may express neither ('null cell lymphoma') or both antigens.

There is no clear relationship between the cytological or histological morphology of canine and feline lymphoma and cellular phenotype. Studies of the prognostic value of immunophenotyping are still in their infancy. It is established that canine T cell lymphoma generally carries a less favourable prognosis than B cell lymphoma, but recently subtypes have been identified within each category that defy this general rule. Small clear T cell lymphoma carries a favourable prognosis and Burkitt-type B cell lymphoma carries a very poor prognosis. In feline lymphoma overall, expression of CD3 or proliferation markers does not appear to be of prognostic value, but factors such as FeLV status, clinical substage and response to therapy are predictive of outcome. In contrast, low grade alimentary lymphoma of cats is a T cell tumour, while B lymphoblastic alimentary tumours are more aggressive.

Molecular characterization of lymphoma

Molecular studies of canine T cell lymphoma, leukaemia and epitheliotropic lymphoma have demonstrated rearrangements in the TCRβ, and TCRγ chain genes, and rearrangements in heavy chain genes have been recorded in B cell lymphoma. TCRβ and Ig heavy chain gene rearrangements also occur in feline spontaneously arising and experimentally induced lymphoma. The most recent advance in lymphoma diagnostics is the availability of 'clonality testing', which examines such molecular rearrangements amongst a population of lymphocytes in order to determine whether the population comprises cells of

645–647 Immunophenotyping of lymphoma. (**645**) Section of small intestine from a cat with alimentary lymphoma. The infiltrating lymphocytes uniformly express membrane CD3, characterizing this as T cell lymphoma. (**646**) Section from feline nasal lymphoma demonstrating cytoplasmic expression of CD79a by the neoplastic population and characterizing this as B cell lymphoma. (**647**) From a different case of feline nasal B cell lymphoma in which the neoplastic B cells also have membrane expression of MHC class II, as depicted here. (**646** and **647** from Day MJ, Henderson SM, Belshaw Z *et al.* [2004] An immunohistochemical investigation of 18 cases of feline nasal lymphoma. *Journal of Comparative Pathology* **130:**152–161, with permission.)

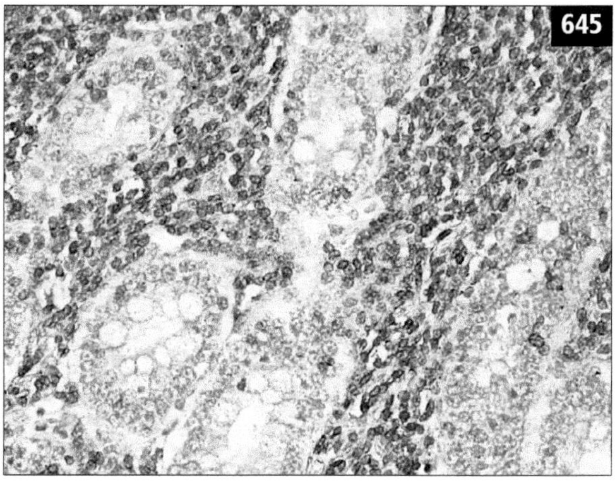

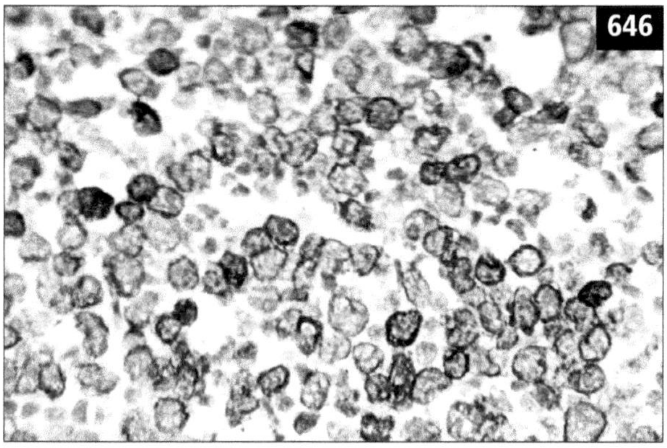

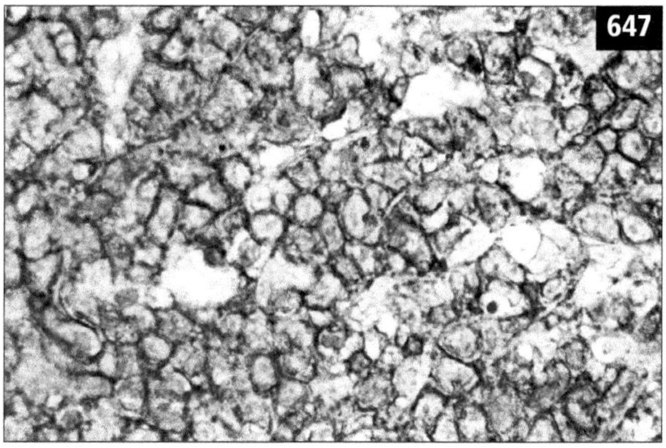

numerous specificities (i.e. a reactive population) or a clonal population that has arisen from a single lymphoid precursor (i.e. a neoplastic population). Although these tests may also distinguish the phenotype of neoplastic lymphocytes, their more useful application is in the distinction between a reactive or neoplastic lymphoid infiltration. There are situations where it is difficult to distinguish between these possibilities at the histopathological level, in particular in the case of alimentary lymphoma, which may be preceded by lymphoplasmacytic inflammation. In a recent immunohistochemical study of feline alimentary lymphoma, a series of biopsy samples previously diagnosed as being neoplastic, were re-evaluated by immunohistochemistry. A proportion of these had mixed lymphoid infiltration more consistent with inflammation than neoplasia. Clonality testing may also be used in this context to distinguish between these possibilities; optimally, both methodologies would be applied. Clonality testing may also be used for monitoring the progress of therapy for lymphoma, as it provides a very sensitive means of establishing whether there is a residual neoplastic population within blood or lymphoid tissue. This methodology would also enable questions concerning the pathogenesis of lymphoma to be addressed; for example, whether a neoplastic population has arisen from one or more clones of lymphoid cells or whether a neoplastic population evolves by serial transformation of an initial neoplastic clone. One drawback to clonality testing is the potential for false-positive results in diseases such as monocytic ehrlichiosis or leishmaniosis, where there may be monoclonal expansion of lymphocytes.

Classification schemes for lymphoma

For many years, veterinary pathologists have devised schemes to classify canine and feline lymphoma with a view to correlating such classification with the biological behaviour of the tumours. These schemes have generally been modifications of human histopathological grading systems that have been in vogue at different times. For example, the Rappaport Classification, Kiel Classification and National Cancer Institute

Table 22: Current World Health Organization classification of human lymphoid and haemopoietic neoplasia. This Table, adapted by the WHO from the Revised European and American Lymphoma (REAL) Classification, presents the most recent classification for human lymphoid and haemopoietic neoplasia. This scheme is based on the combined clinical, histopathological, cytological, cytogenetic, immunohistochemical and molecular characteristics of each entity. Classification schemes for canine and feline lymphoma are generally based on such human schemes and there are direct equivalents for many of the entities listed here in veterinary medicine. Many of these tumour types are described in this chapter as spontaneously-arising diseases of the dog and cat. (Data from Lu P (2005) Staging and classification of lymphoma. *Seminars in Nuclear Medicine* **35:**160–164.)

Hodgkin's lymphoma	**B cell neoplasms**	**T cell and NK cell neoplasms**
1. Nodular lymphocyte-predominant Hodgkin's lymphoma	**1. Precursor B cell neoplasms**	**1. Precursor T cell neoplasms**
2. Classic Hodgkin's lymphoma	Precursor B lymphoblastic leukaemia/lymphoma	Precursor T lymphoblastic leukaemia/lymphoma
Nodular sclerosis classical Hodgkin's lymphoma		Blastic NK cell lymphoma
Lymphocyte-rich classic Hodgkin's lymphoma	**2. Mature B cell neoplasms**	**2. Mature T cell and NK cell neoplasms**
Mixed cellularity classic Hodgkin's lymphoma	Chronic lymphocytic leukaemia/small lymphocytic lymphoma	T cell prolymphocytic leukaemia
Lymphocyte-depleted classic Hodgkin's lymphoma	B cell prolymphocytic leukaemia	T cell large granular lymphocytic leukaemia
	Lymphoplasmacytic lymphoma	Aggressive NK cell leukaemia
	Splenic marginal zone lymphoma	Adult T cell leukaemia/lymphoma
	Hairy cell leukaemia	Extranodal NK/T cell lymphoma, nasal type
	Plasma cell myeloma	Enteropathy-type T cell lymphoma
	Solitary plasmacytoma of bone	Hepatosplenic T cell lymphoma
	Extraosseous plasmacytoma	Subcutaneous paniculitis-like T cell lymphoma
	Extranodal marginal zone B cell lymphoma of mucosa-associated lymphoid tissue (MALT-lymphoma)	Mycosis fungoides
	Nodal marginal zone B cell lymphoma	Sézary syndrome
	Follicular lymphoma	Primary cutaneous anaplastic large cell lymphoma

Table 22: (*Continued*)

	Mature B cell neoplasms (*continued*)	**Mature T cell and NK cell neoplasms (*continued*)**
	Mantle cell lymphoma	Peripheral T cell lymphoma, unspecified
	Diffuse large B cell lymphoma	Angioimmunoblastic T cell lymphoma
	Mediastinal (thymic) large B cell lymphoma	Anaplastic large cell lymphoma
	Intravascular large B cell lymphoma	
	Primary effusion lymphoma	
	Burkitt lymphoma/leukaemia	
	3. B cell proliferations of uncertain malignant potential	**3. T cell proliferation of uncertain malignant potential**
	Lymphomatoid granulomatosis	Lymphomatoid papulosis
	Post-transplant lymphoproliferative disorder, polymorphic	

NK: natural killer (cell).

Working Formulation (NCIWF) have all been adapted for this purpose. These various schemes fundamentally aim to describe the cellular distribution and morphological features of the neoplastic cells.

Using the NCIWF, two thirds of canine lymphomas are reported to be high-grade tumours, approximately one third are intermediate and relatively few are low grade. The distribution is similar for the cat (54% high grade, 33% intermediate, 12% low grade), with a greater proportion of immunoblastic tumours. In one study, high-grade canine lymphoma (Kiel Classification) had a more favourable response to chemotherapy, but relapsed within a shorter time period, whereas high-grade lymphoma (NCIWF) was associated with shorter survival time.

The most recent evolution of human lymphoma classification schemes is the WHO modification of the Revised European and American Lymphoma (REAL) Classification, which defines lymphoid neoplasia based on the combination of clinical, histopathological and cytological appearance, together with immunophenotype, cytogenetics and molecular characteristics (*Table 22*). This scheme has formed the basis for the most recent WHO classification system for canine and feline lymphoma, and the applicability of this system has been reported by an international working party of veterinary pathologists. As with all such grading schemes, what is still required in veterinary medicine are good data relating these laboratory features to clinical outcome following chemotherapy.

Treatment and prognosis of canine and feline lymphoma

Solitary lesions may be treated by surgery or radiotherapy, but systemic chemotherapy is indicated for most forms of lymphoma. Combination chemotherapy is usually more effective than the use of single agents, and

Table 23: Semi-continuous protocol for the treatment of lymphoma.

Induction	
COP (low dose)	
Cyclophosphamide	50 mg/m^2 p/o every 48 hours or for the first 4 days of each week.
Vincristine	0.5 mg/m^2 i/v every 7 days.
Prednisolone	40 mg/m^2 p/o daily for 7 days then 20 mg/m^2 p/o every 48 hours (with cyclophosphamide).
Maintenance	
COP	After 8 weeks of induction with COP, continue as alternate week treatment for 4 months, then 1 week in 3 for 6 months, and reduce to 1 week in 4 after 1 year.
or	
MOP	As for COP, but to reduce the risk of haemorrhagic cystitis, substitute melphalan (5 mg/m^2 by mouth) for cyclophosphamide after 6 months.

Table 24: Chemotherapy protocols for the treatment of lymphoma (21-day cycles).

Induction	
COP (high dose)	
Cyclophosphamide	250–300* mg/m^2 p/o every 21 days.
Vincristine	0.75 mg/m^2 i/v every 7 days for 4 weeks, then every 21 days.
Prednisolone	1 mg/kg p/o daily for 4 weeks, then every 48 hours.
CHOP	
Cyclophosphamide	100–150 mg/m^2 i/v on day 1.
Doxorubicin	30 mg/m^2 i/v on day 1.
Vincristine	0.75 mg/m^2 i/v on days 8 and 15.
Prednisolone	40 mg/m^2 daily for 7 days, then 20 mg/m^2 every 48 hours, days 8–21.
(Potentiated sulphonamides)	Protocol very myelosuppressive, therefore antibiotic cover advised.
Maintenance	
COP	After 1 year of induction with COP (high dose), use the same cycle every 4 weeks for another 6 months.
CHOP	After 12 weeks of induction with CHOP, change to low dose COP or LMP for maintenance.
LMP	
Chlorambucil	20 mg/m^2 by mouth every 14 days.
Methotrexate	2.5 mg/m^2 by mouth 2 to 3 times per week.
Prednisolone	20 mg/m^2 by mouth every 48 hours.

*The maximum recommended dose of cyclophosphamide in the dog is 250 mg/m^2.

Table 25: Chemotherapy protocols for treatment of lymphoma. Cyclic combination/pulse treatment of lymphoma (Madison-Wisconsin Protocol).

Induction

Week 1 (day 1)	Vincristine, L-asparaginase, ± prednisolone	0.5–0.75 mg/m^2 i/v 400 IU/kg i/m 2.0 mg/kg p/o q24h
Week 2 (day 8)	Cyclophosphamide, ± prednisolone	200 mg/m^2 i/v or p/o 1.5 mg/kg p/o q24h
Week 3 (day 15)	Vincristine, ± prednisolone	0.5–0.75 mg/m^2 i/v 1.0 mg/kg p/o q24h
Week 4 (day 22)	Doxorubicin, ± prednisolone	30 mg/m^2 i/v 0.5 mg/kg p/o q24h
Week 5 (day 29)	No treatment	
Week 6 (day 36)	Vincristine	0.5–0.75 mg/m^2 i/v
Week 7 (day 43)	Cyclophosphamide	200 mg/m^2 i/v or p/o
Week 8 (day 50)	Vincristine	0.5–0.75 mg/m^2 i/v
Week 9 (day 57)	Doxorubicin	30 mg/m^2 i/v
Week 10 (day 64)	No treatment	

Maintenance

Repeat the cycle twice with an interval of 2 weeks between each drug administration. Some authorities recommend stopping at week 25 if patient is in remission; others continue with three-week intervals between treatments.

Recently a maintenance-free 12-week protocol has been claimed to be of equal efficacy to 25 weeks (Simon D, Nolte N, Eberle N *et al.* (2006) Treatment of dogs with lymphoma using a 12-week, maintenance-free combination chemotherapy protocol. *Journal of Veterinary Internal Medicine* **20**:948–954.)

Note: The addition of a single dose of L-asparaginase has been called into question by recent reports showing no survival advantage (MacDonald VS, Thamm DH, Kurzman ID *et al.* (2005) Does L-asparaginase influence efficacy or toxicity when added to a standard CHOP protocol for dogs with lymphoma? *Journal of Veterinary Internal Medicine* **19**:732–6; and Jeffreys AB, Knapp DW, Carlton WW *et al.* (2005) Influence of asparaginase on a combination chemotherapy protocol for canine multicentric lymphoma. *Journal of the American Animal Hospital Association* **41**:221–226.)

numerous protocols are described using combinations of vincristine, cyclophosphamide, cytarabine, L-asparaginase, doxorubicin and prednisolone (*Tables 23–25*). Regardless of the protocol used, approximately 70–80% of dogs with multicentric lymphoma achieve remission and remain in remission for a mean of 6–12 months. Survival times, however, range from one week to several years and prognosis varies with different anatomical forms of the disease. Survival times are far shorter in alimentary lymphoma. In most cases the disease eventually relapses and this is often associated with development of resistance to cytotoxic drugs. A variety of strategies may be followed for 'rescue' treatment in such cases (*Table 26*), but it should be recognized that the rate and duration of second and subsequent remissions is much lower than the first response. PCR testing can be used to monitor 'minimal residual disease' during therapy and remission. Cats with lymphoma may be treated with similar protocols. Tablet size presents a problem in dosing cats with alternate day cyclophosphamide, and it may be more practical to use weekly or three-weekly pulse regimes (*Tables 24* and *25*).

Cutaneous lymphoma

Cutaneous lymphoma is more commonly recognized in the dog than the cat, but dermal and epitheliotropic forms occur in both species. Cats

Table 26: Rescue chemotherapy for relapsed cases of lymphoma.
If response to initial treatment was good, return to original induction protocol until remission achieved and then use maintenance protocol. If response to initial treatment was slow, or for a second relapse, change to new drugs for rescue. Return to maintenance once remission complete.

Single agents	
Doxorubicin	30 mg/m^2 i/v every 21 days
L-asparaginase	10,000–20,000 IU/m^2 i/m every 14–21 days
Lomustine (CCNU)	50–70 mg/m^2 p/o every 3–4 weeks
Rescue combinations:	
D-MAC (14 day cycle)	
Dexamethasone	0.23 mg/kg p/o or s/c on days 1 and 8
Actinomycin D	0.75 mg/m^2 as i/v push day 1
Cytosine arabinoside	200–300 mg/m^2 as i/v drip over 4 hours or s/c on day 1
Melphalan	20 mg/m^2 p/o on day 8
ADIC	
Doxorubicin and	30 mg/m^2 i/v every 21 days
dacarbazine	1,000 mg/m^2 i/v infusion (over 6–8 hours) every 21 days
CHOP	See *Table 24* (p. 328)

648

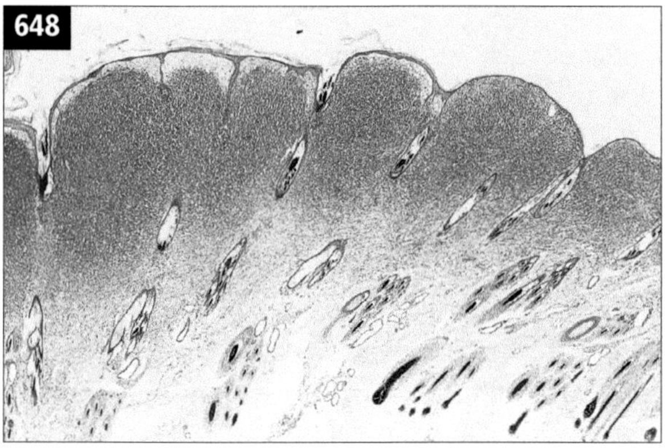

649

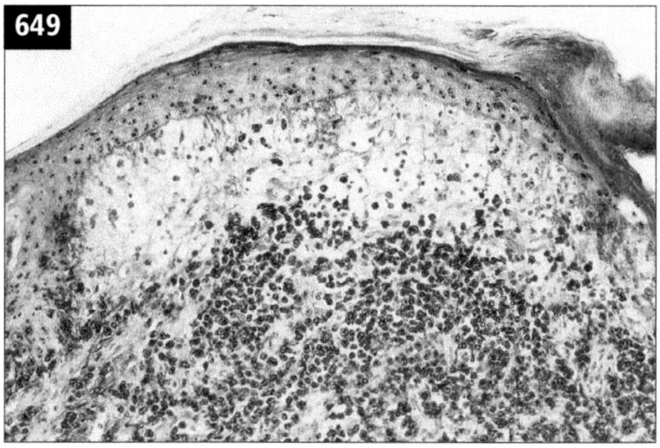

648–649 Dermal lymphoma. (**648**) Histopathological appearance of canine dermal lymphoma. There is a dense infiltration of neoplastic lymphocytes into the superficial dermis, with a distinct Grenz zone between the infiltrate and the epidermis. There is partial preservation of pilosebaceous units within the infiltrate. (**649**) Immunoperoxidase labelling demonstrates uniform expression of CD3 by the neoplastic population in the absence of labelling for canine γ, μ, κ or λ chains.

with cutaneous lymphoma are consistently FeLV negative, but FeLV proviral DNA can be identified within tumour tissue by PCR. In dermal lymphoma, neoplastic lymphocytes are restricted to the dermis, where they infiltrate widely and may obliterate adnexal structures. There is often a distinct 'Grenz zone' between the infiltrating cells and the epidermis (**648–651**). A range of cytological forms is recognized, but large cell and lymphoblastic types predominate. Although it was once suggested that dermal lymphomas were primarily B cell tumours, recent studies have shown that most are of T cell origin, expressing CD3 and either an $\alpha\beta$ or $\gamma\delta$ TCR (rarely, no TCR). The cells may be $CD4^+$ or $CD8^+$, but most often express neither marker. Dermal lymphoma may be a primary cutaneous disease or part of multicentric lymphoma, and it presents as one or more nodular ulcerated masses or plaques of the trunk, head or extremities (**652–654**). Solitary tumours in the dog may be surgically excised

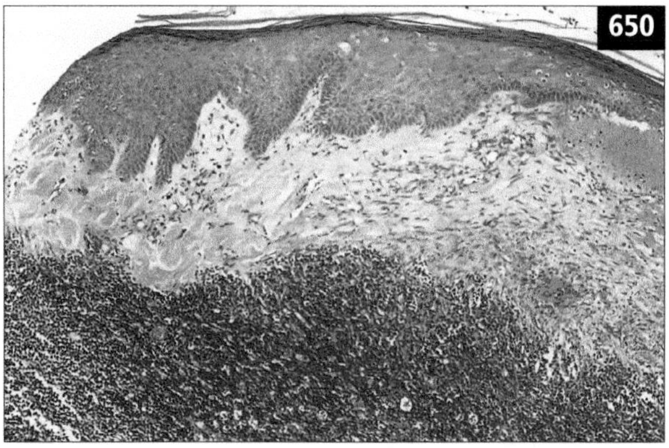

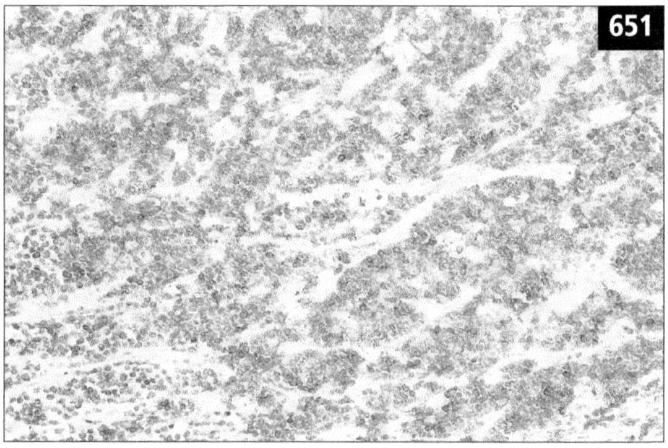

650–651 Dermal lymphoma. (**650**) Canine dermal lymphoma. In this case the neoplastic cells uniformly express the B cell marker CD79 (**651**) in addition to MHC class II and λ light chain. There was no expression of CD3.

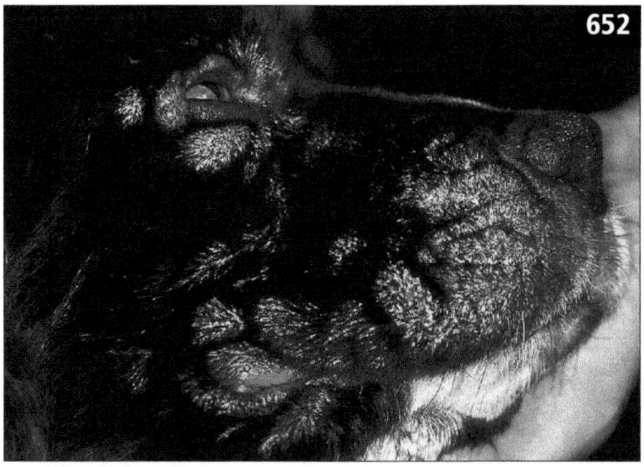

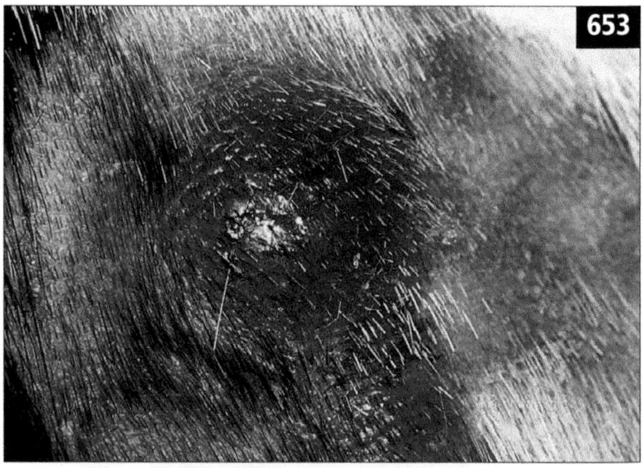

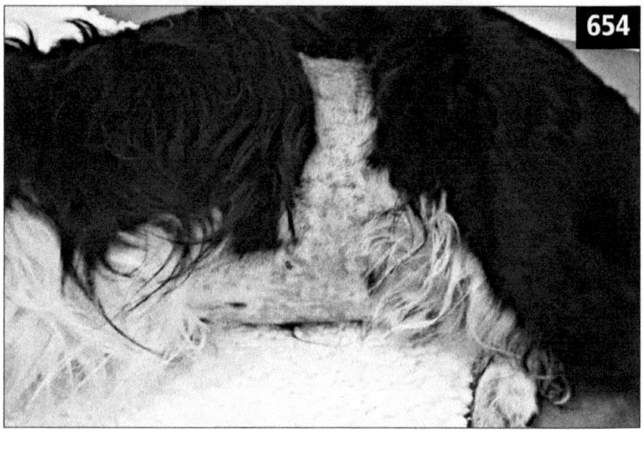

652–654 Clinical presentation of dermal lymphoma. (**652**) An 11-year-old Springer Spaniel presented with a three-month history of skin disease and recent lymphadenopathy. There were erythematous plaque-like lesions affecting the eyelids and lips, with surrounding oedema. Skin biopsies showed dermal lymphoma. (**653**) Erythematous dermal nodules in a case of dermal lymphoma. (**654**) Erythematous plaques resulting from diffuse infiltration of the skin of the ventral abdomen of the Border Collie shown in **633**.

without recurrence, but excised tumours commonly recur in the cat. Non-epitheliotropic dermal lymphoma with concurrent lymphoid leukaemia is described in the dog.

Epitheliotropic lymphoma (mycosis fungoides) is recognized with increasing frequency in the dog, but remains rare in the cat. The disease is characterized by progressive infiltration of epidermis and adnexal epithelium by neoplastic lymphocytes, with the formation of intraepidermal aggregates (Pautrier's microabscesses) (**655, 656**). Mucocutaneous (buccal) (**657**) and alimentary (**658**) forms of epitheliotropic T cell lymphoma have been described in the dog and, in some cases, cutaneous and alimentary epitheliotropic lymphoma has occurred concurrently. Similarly,

655

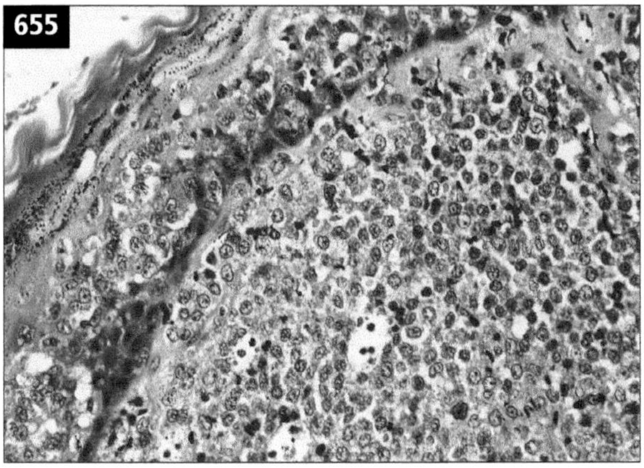

656

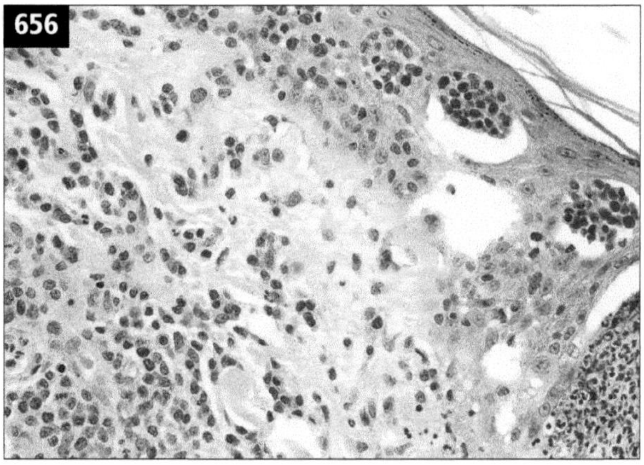

655, 656 Epitheliotropic lymphoma. (**655**) Skin biopsy of a recurrent nodule on the ear of a six-year-old English Cocker Spaniel with epitheliotropic lymphoma. Neoplastic lymphocytes closely abut, and infiltrate into, the epidermis. (**656**) Skin biopsy from a dog with epitheliotropic lymphoma demonstrating clusters of neoplastic lymphocytes within Pautrier's microabscesses in the epidermis.

657

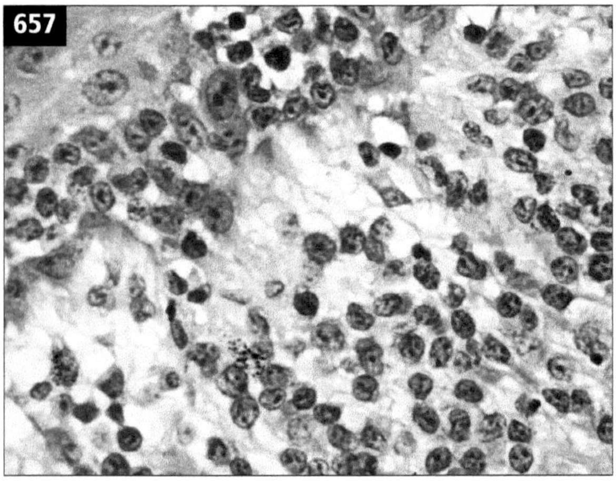

657 Buccal epitheliotropic lymphoma. Biopsy from the lip of a ten-year-old Cocker Spaniel with melaena and infiltrative lesions of the mucous membranes and footpads. The appearance is consistent with epitheliotropic lymphoma, showing infiltration of neoplastic cells into the overlying squamous epithelium.

658

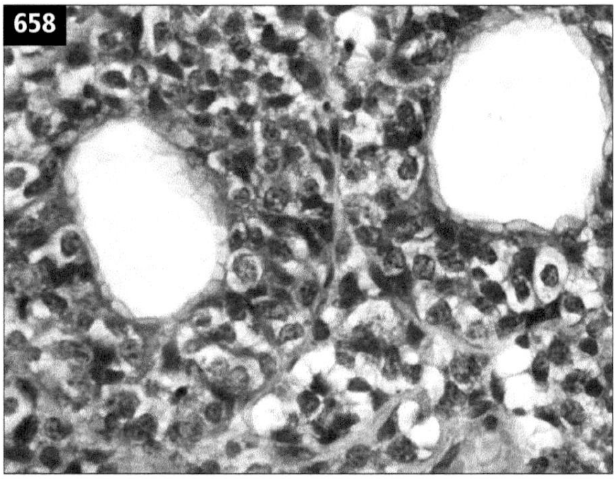

658 Alimentary epitheliotropic lymphoma. Biopsy of gastric mucosa from the dog described in **657**. The dog has alimentary, in addition to mucocutaneous, epitheliotropic lymphoma. There is almost complete obliteration of the gastric epithelium by infiltrating neoplastic cells, which have a relatively abundant, vesicular cytoplasm.

alimentary epitheliotropic lymphoma is described in the cat. This is exclusively a T cell tumour, and recent studies in the dog have shown that the cells uniformly express CD3 (with γδ TCR more frequent than αβ TCR) and CD45, together with CD8 (commonly), CD4 (occasionally) or neither of these molecules ($CD4^-CD8^-$) (**659, 660**). There is lack of expression of CD45RA and high expression of surface β_1 integrin, consistent with a memory phenotype. The cells often have a distinctive convoluted nucleus (**661**). The tropism for epithelium is likely due to expression of adhesion molecules by the neoplastic cells that bind ligands on keratinocytes.

Early lesions of epitheliotropic lymphoma include generalized, erythematous, exfoliative dermatitis or oral plaque formation in the buccal form. At a later stage, multiple coalescing plaques

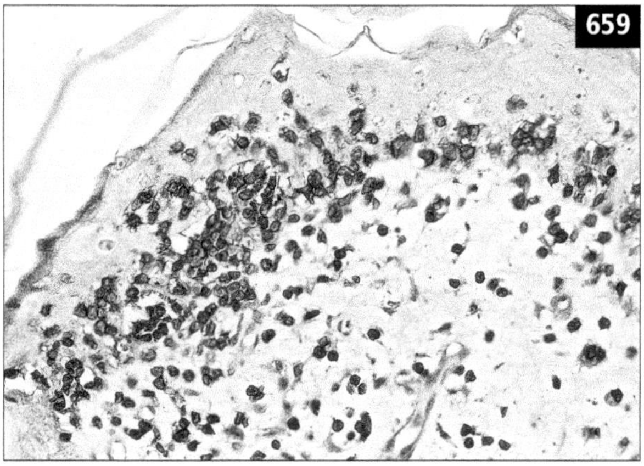

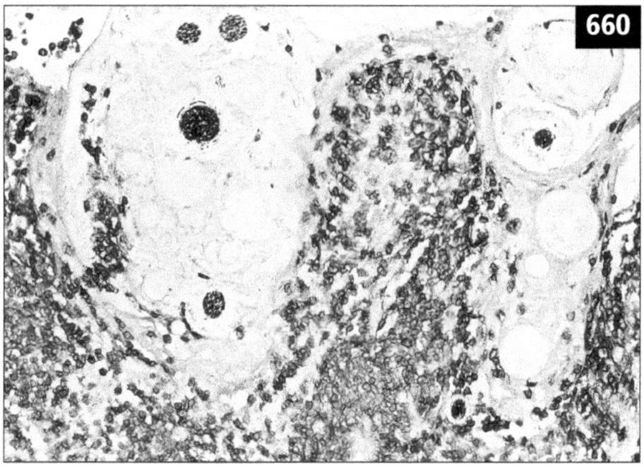

659, 660 Epitheliotropic lymphoma. (**659**) Skin biopsy from a six-year-old English Cocker Spaniel with multifocal areas of crusting over the dorsum of four months' duration. This slide demonstrates the very early changes of epitheliotropic lymphoma, with epidermal infiltration by lymphocytes expressing CD3. (**660**) Late stage epitheliotropic lymphoma in a ten-year-old English Cocker Spaniel with pinnal lesions, demonstrating infiltration of dermis by CD3-positive lymphocytes that have tropism for follicular epithelium.

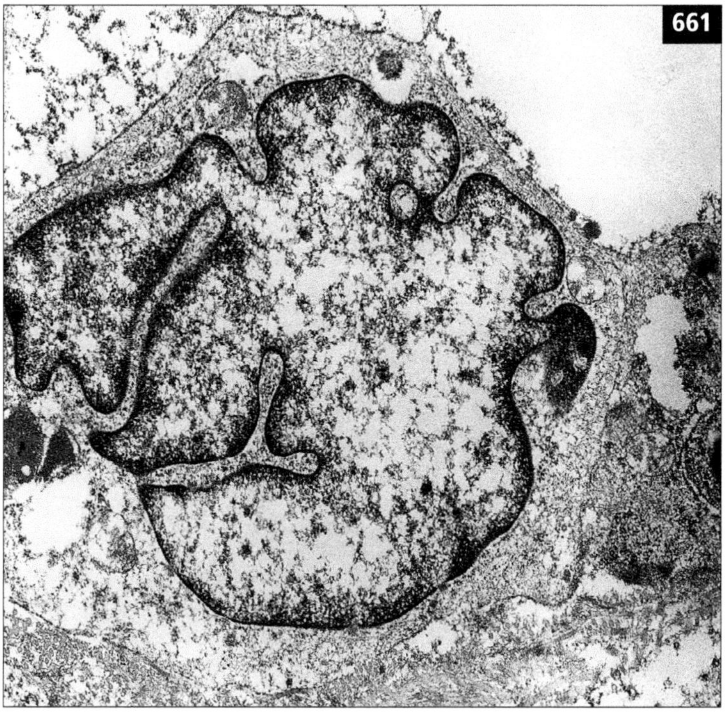

661 Lymphocyte ultrastructure in epitheliotropic lymphoma. Transmission electron micrograph of a neoplastic T lymphocyte in canine epitheliotropic lymphoma. The nucleus has a characteristic convoluted appearance.

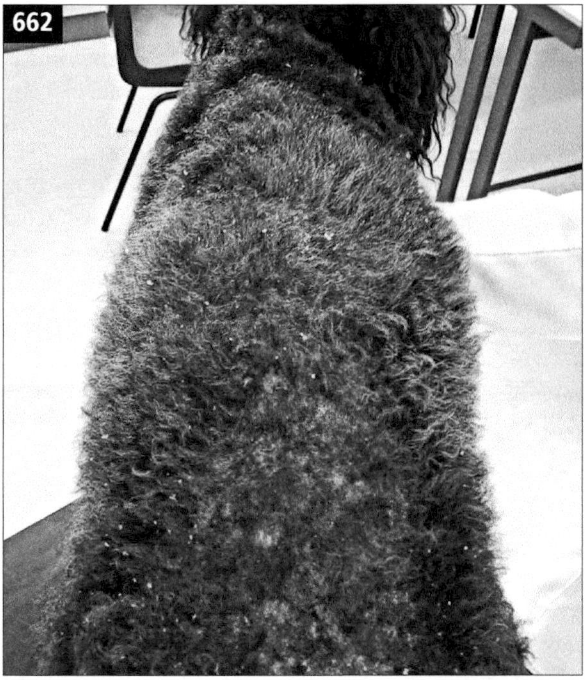

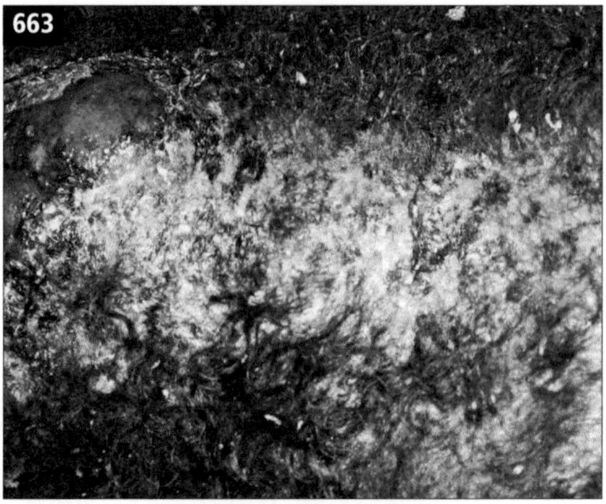

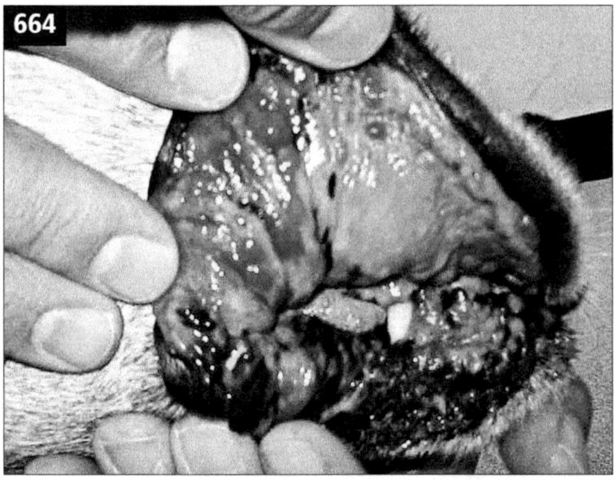

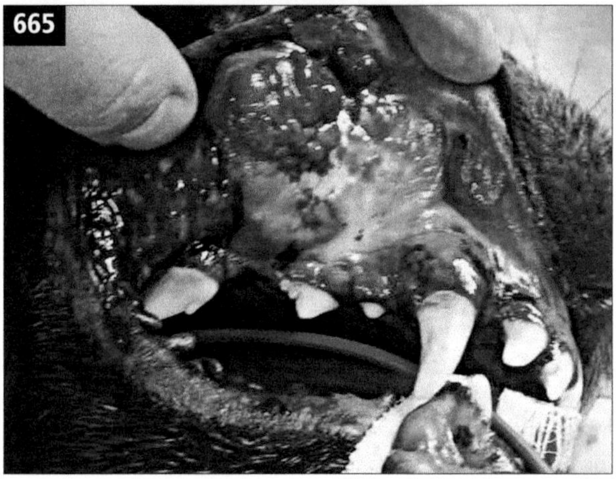

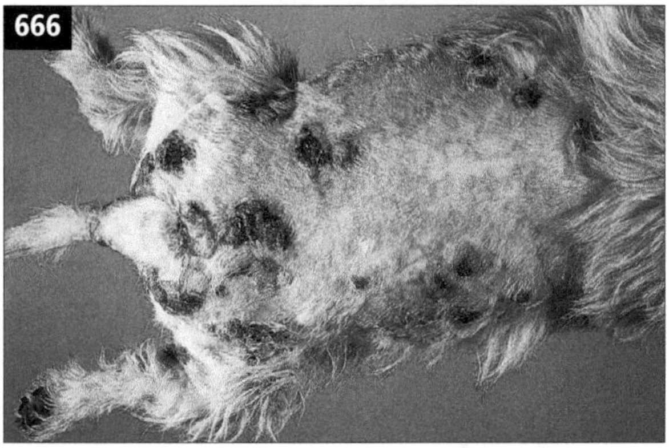

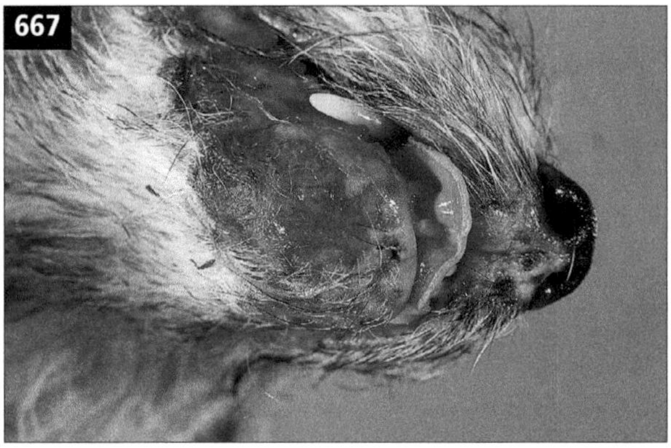

662–667 Clinical presentation of epitheliotropic lymphoma. (**662**) Middle-aged Miniature Poodle with epitheliotropic lymphoma. The early stage of disease (shown here) was characterized by erythematous, scaly, alopecic and pruritic skin lesions, particularly affecting the dorsum. (**663**) The disease progressed to form more distinct ulcerated plaques. (**664**) Buccal epitheliotropic lymphoma presenting as raised, erythematous nodules of the mucosal surface of the lips of a nine-year-old Boxer dog. (**665**) Similar lesions of buccal epitheliotropic lymphoma in a Labrador Retriever dog. (**666**) Late stage canine epitheliotropic lymphoma showing generalized plaques and ulcerated nodular skin lesions. (**667**) Involvement of the mucocutaneous junctions in the dog shown in **666**.

or nodules may develop in haired skin or at mucocutaneous junctions (662–667). Epitheliotropic lymphoma may progress to involve regional lymph nodes and occasional dogs have also had circulating malignant lymphocytes, a state resembling human Sézary syndrome.

Cutaneous forms of lymphoma are usually treated with chemotherapy, using the protocols previously outlined (*Tables 23–26*, pp. 328–330). Dermal lymphoma is a highly aggressive tumour and although the initial response to therapy may be favourable, this is usually short lived. Average survival times are in the order of 2–3 months. Systemic chemotherapy can also be used to treat the tumour phase of epitheliotropic lymphoma, but the response is variable and often disappointing. Recently there have been reports of durable responses to the alkylating agent lomustine (CCNU). Topical chemotherapy with mechlorethamine is not recommended in animals because of the hazardous nature of this agent. In cases where lesions are localized (e.g. oral lesions), radiotherapy may be indicated. Retinoids are reported to be useful in the management of human and generalized canine epitheliotropic lymphoma. In the absence of an effective treatment for widespread disease, the prognosis is guarded to poor.

Cutaneous lymphocytosis

Benign cutaneous lymphocytosis has been reported in both the dog and cat and must be distinguished from the neoplastic lesions described above. Although such lesions likely have an antigenic stimulus, initiating factors have not been described. Feline cutaneous lymphocytosis presents in older cats with solitary nodular lesions, often involving the extremities. The nodules are generally no larger than 1 cm in diameter and are not invasive or metastatic. Alternatively, solitary or multiple areas of erythema, plaques or papules may be seen. Histologically there are dermal follicle-like aggregates of lymphocytes that may display mild epitheliotropism. The lymphocytes are of mixed phenotype ($CD3^+$, $CD4^+$, $CD8^+$, $CD5^+$, $CD21^+$ and $CD79a^+$) and may be polyclonal or of restricted clonality. The lesions may remain stable, wax and wane, regress or recur. Cutaneous lymphocytosis is rare in the dog and presents as erythematous plaques comprised of $CD3^+$ T cells of mixed phenotype.

Hodgkin's-like lymphoma

This rare form of canine lymphoma is characterized by the presence of large 'Reed-Sternberg' cells with deeply lobulated nuclei, prominent nucleoli and abundant cytoplasm. These are scattered amongst a background population of neoplastic lymphocytes and there may be infiltration by plasma cells, eosinophils and neutrophils. The tumour generally involves the lymph nodes, liver, spleen and lungs.

T cell-rich B cell lymphoma

This form of lymphoma has recently been characterized in older cats that present with focal enlargement of submandibular or cervical lymph nodes (668). The lesions consist of a population of

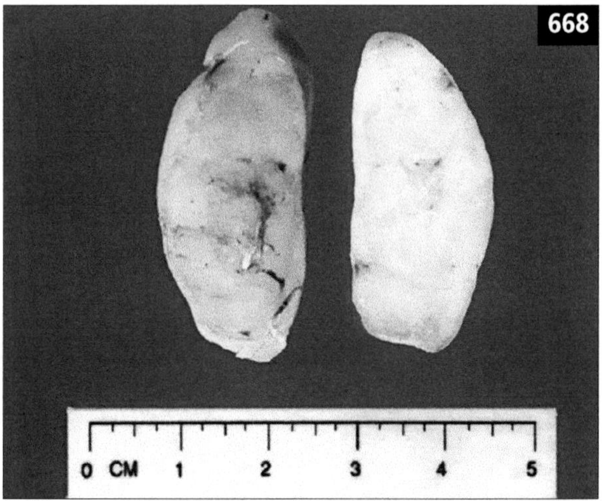

668 T cell-rich B cell lymphoma. Excisional biopsy of an enlarged cervical lymph node from a cat with T cell-rich B cell lymphoma. The cut surface is diffusely white in colour, with an absence of corticomedullary architecture.

cytologically bizarre giant B cells mixed with a background of small T and B lymphocytes (669, 670). The tumour is not associated with FeLV or FIV and carries a favourable prognosis following complete surgical excision of the lesions. There is debate in the literature as to whether this entity is actually a form of feline Hodgkin's-like lymphoma that lacks classic Reed-Sternberg cells, and the alternative nomenclature 'lymphocyte predominance Hodgkin's disease with lymphohistiocytic (L+H) Reed-Sternberg variants' has been proposed.

Feline large granular lymphocyte lymphoma

Large granular lymphocytes (LGLs) are a distinctive subpopulation of lymphocytes with cytoplasmic azurophilic granules. LGLs normally circulate in low numbers, but they are a prominent subset of IELs (see Chapter 7, p. 203), particularly in the cat. In the dog, neoplasia of LGLs most frequently presents as chronic leukaemia (see below), but in cats, immunophenotyping has recently defined a LGL lymphoma of the intestinal tract (which may also involve other abdominal viscera), with secondary leukaemia (and sometimes involvement of the bone marrow). This form of lymphoma presents in older cats (mean age 9.3 years) and has an aggressive course with a mean survival time of 18 days post diagnosis. The neoplastic cells are often epitheliotropic and generally $CD3^+$ with a $CD8\alpha\alpha^+$ phenotype in most cases. This neoplasm likely arises from the intestinal LGL IEL population.

Canine large granular lymphocyte lymphocytosis

LGL lymphocytosis has been documented in a series of older, large breed dogs with persistent elevation of blood LGLs. A proportion of these dogs also had splenomegaly. The circulating LGLs are genetically and phenotypically T cells that also express CD11a and the leukointegrin $\alpha_4\beta_2$, and they are thought to originate in the spleen. LGL lymphocytosis has a variable clinical outcome ranging from a benign reactive lymphocytosis, to persistent lymphocytosis with or without concurrent anaemia, to acute LGL leukaemia with widespread dissemination and a poor prognosis.

669

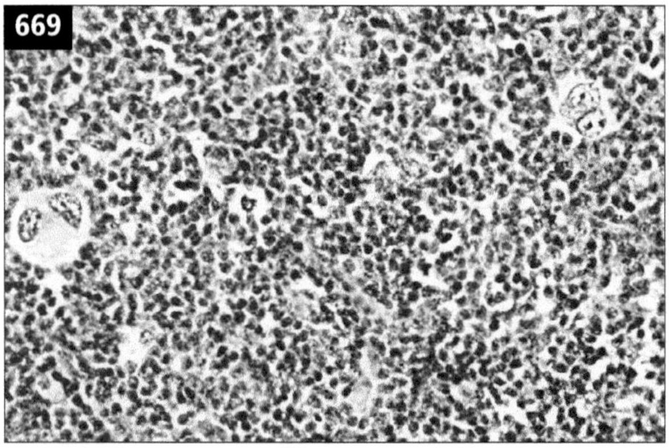

670

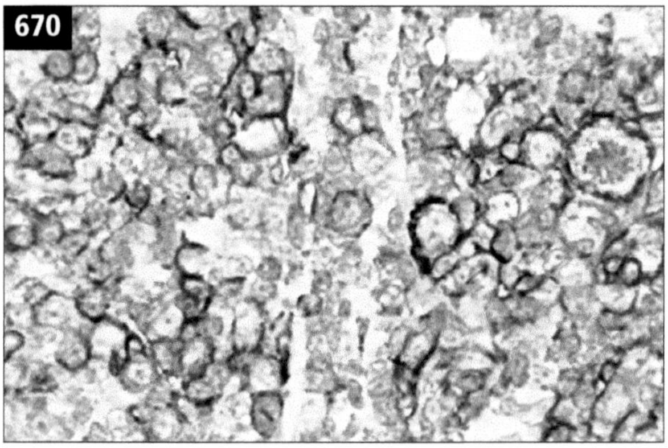

669, 670 T cell-rich B cell lymphoma. (**669**) This section displays the characteristic features of this tumour, with the presence of occasional large 'popcorn' cells amidst a background of smaller lymphocytes. The former cells have one or more, giant, vesicular nuclei and abundant cytoplasm. (**670**) Immunohistochemical characterization of this tumour reveals that the majority of cells, including the 'popcorn' cells, are of the B cell lineage and express the marker BLA-36.

LYMPHOMATOID GRANULOMATOSIS

Lymphomatoid granulomatosis is a rare lymphohistiocytic proliferative disease of the skin and viscera (particularly lungs, lymph nodes and spleen) of the dog. The lesions are characterized by mixed infiltrates of cells (small, large and atypical lymphocytes; plasma cells and macrophages) that target and destroy blood vessels, resulting in areas of ischaemic necrosis (**671–674**). The lymphoid cells express CD3, suggesting that the disease may be an atypical form of T cell lymphoma. A recent case is described in which neoplastic B cells were also identified, together with occasional Reed-Sternberg-like cells.

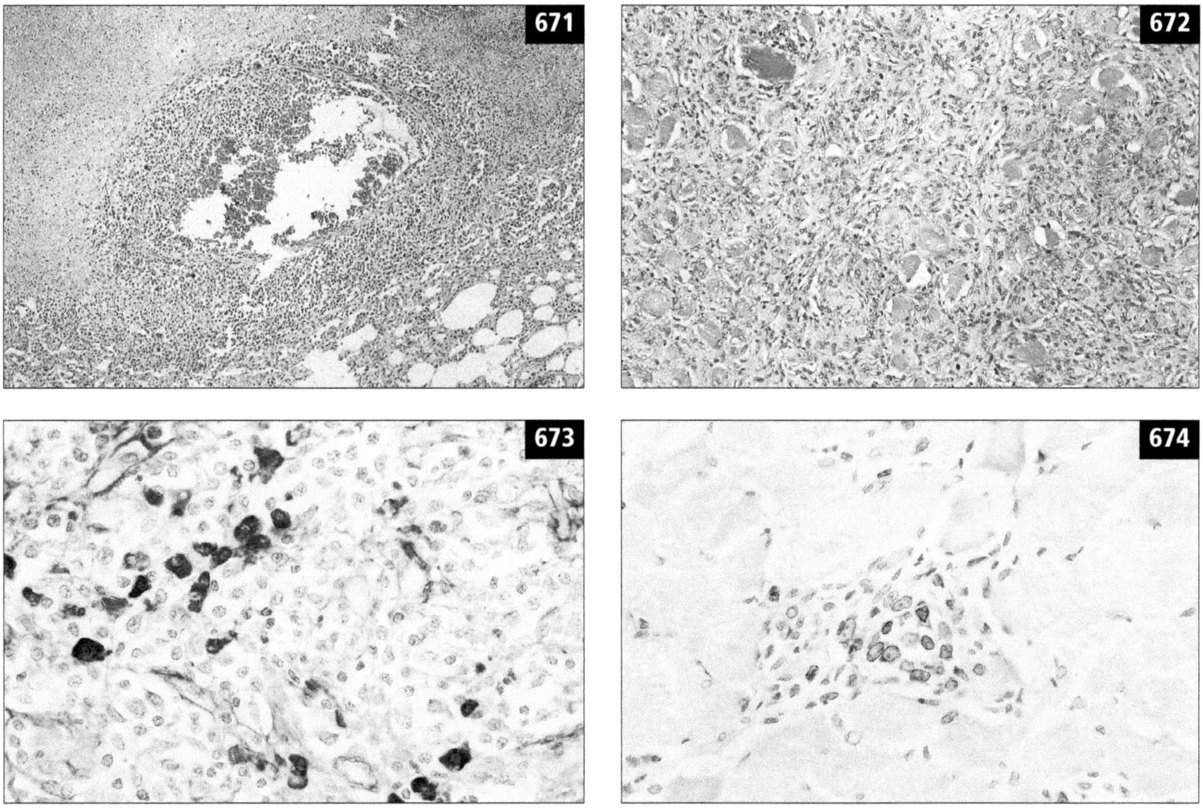

671–674 Lymphomatoid granulomatosis. Sections of lung (**671**) and muscle (**672**) from a dog with lymphomatoid granulomatosis. There is an angiocentric infiltration of mixed mononuclear populations including T lymphocytes, macrophages and plasma cells. The lesions contain cells that label positively by immunohistochemistry for IgG, IgM, IgA (**673**, section of lung) and CD3 (**674**, section of muscle).

LYMPHOID LEUKAEMIA

Lymphoid leukaemia is uncommon in the dog and cat and is defined by primary involvement of bone marrow and blood (abnormal circulating lymphocytes with or without lymphocytosis) (**675, 676**), with secondary seeding to the spleen, liver, lymph nodes and other viscera (**677, 678**). Lymphoid leukaemia may be divided into acute and chronic forms:

- **Acute lymphoblastic leukaemia** (ALL) is often a disease of young cats less than one year of age. It may occur in young dogs, although the mean age is generally 7–8 years. Most cases of canine ALL are B cell tumours. Feline ALL is caused by FeLV. A grading system for the cytological appearance of the leukaemic cells has been applied to ALL (L1 microlymphoblastic, L2 prolymphocytic, L3 lymphoblastic).
- **Chronic lymphocytic leukaemia** (CLL) occurs in older dogs and cats (8–10 years of age) and is a slowly progressive disease that may be associated with concurrent IMHA or monoclonal gammopathy. Although assumed to be a B cell tumour, recent studies have shown that 70% of canine CLL cases are of the T cell lineage (and many are large granular lymphocytes) and 30% are B lymphoid. The relatively high proportion of γδ TCR T cell CLL may suggest a primary splenic rather than bone marrow origin for some of these tumours, as the canine spleen is rich in γδ T cells. A recent study shows that dogs with T cell CLL have more favourable outcome.

Therapy for lymphoid leukaemia is aimed at destroying the leukaemic cells and allowing normal haemopoiesis to resume. In ALL, induction protocols are usually based on vincristine and prednisolone, with the addition of cyclophosphamide and/or cytarabine if the animal is not too neutropenic. These are used until the WBC count returns to the normal range and circulating blast cells are no longer seen. In theory, drug doses and frequencies can then be reduced to maintenance levels, but in practice this is rarely achieved. The use of chemotherapy is severely hampered by the myelosuppression and organ dysfunction that is often present and by the inability to preserve sufficient levels of normal blood cells during treatment. The prognosis for ALL is poor; survival times rarely exceed three months.

In contrast, treatment may not be required for asymptomatic cases of CLL, although frequent haematological monitoring is advised. Chemotherapy with chlorambucil and prednisolone is recommended for symptomatic cases. The aim is to restore the peripheral blood counts to the normal range, and response to treatment is monitored by haematology. Once remission is achieved, maintenance therapy is continued in order to keep the WBC counts within the normal range. The prognosis for CLL is much more favourable, with some patients surviving in excess of 1–2 years.

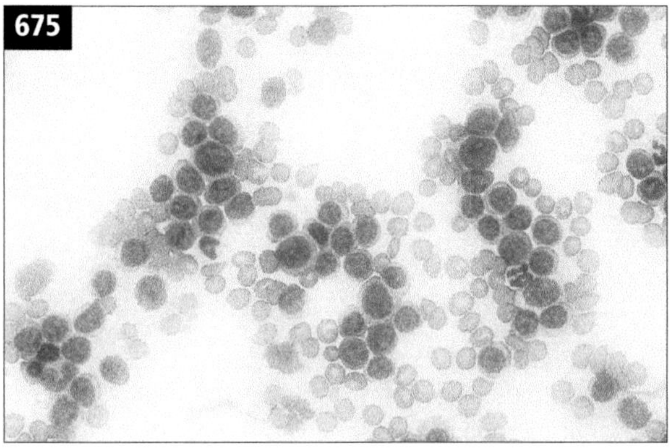

675 Lymphoid leukaemia. Blood smear from a dog with lymphoid leukaemia demonstrating large numbers of lymphocytes within the circulation.

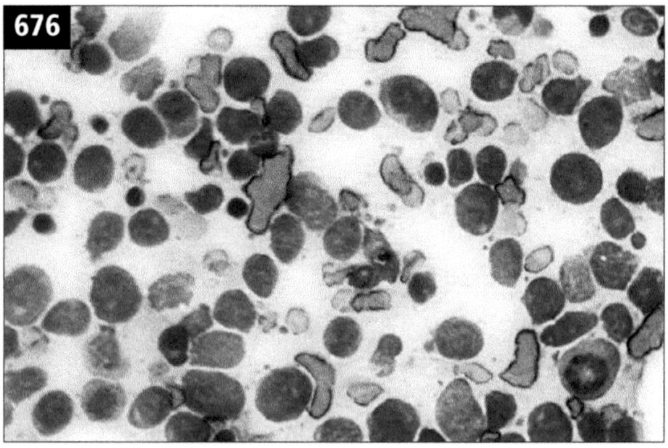

676 Lymphoid leukaemia. Bone marrow aspirate from a five-year-old GSD with lymphoid leukaemia. There are numerous lymphoblastic cells, with evidence of active mitosis, and similar cells were found in the circulating blood. Immunophenotyping of a core biopsy of bone marrow revealed the neoplastic population to be $CD3^+$ T lymphocytes.

MULTIPLE MYELOMA

Multiple myeloma is an uncommon plasma cell tumour of middle-aged to older dogs and cats. Most cats with myeloma are FeLV negative. The neoplastic cells most commonly occupy bone marrow (long bones, vertebrae or ribs), where they can release parathyroid hormone-like factors, which mobilize calcium from bone (often resulting in hypercalcaemia) and cause small, focal 'punched out' osteolytic lesions (**679**). Large osteolytic lesions may sometimes be observed with clinical presentation referable to the skeletal system. The tumour within bone marrow also has a myelophthisic effect; dogs often present with mild cytopenia and numerous irregular plasma cells may be identified on marrow biopsy (**680, 681**). In the dog there is rarely involvement of lymph nodes, liver, spleen, kidney and alimentary tract; however, recent reviews of feline myeloma have

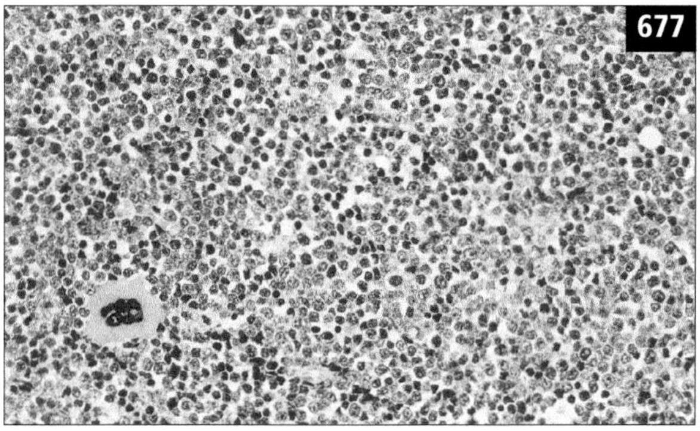

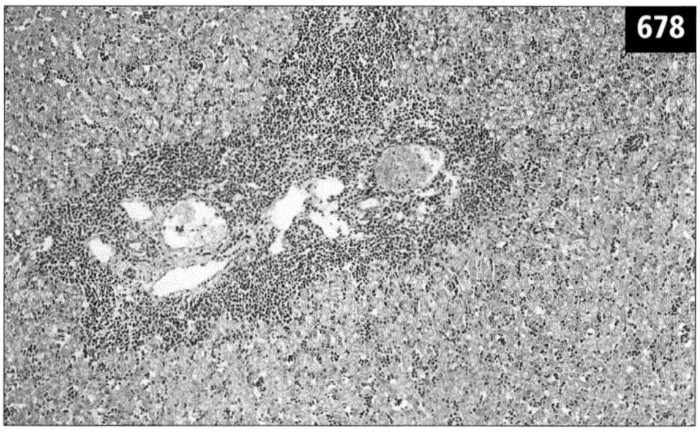

677, 678 Lymphoid leukaemia. Experimentally induced lymphoid leukaemia in a cat infected with FeLV. (**677**) Normal haemopoietic elements within the bone marrow are almost obliterated by neoplastic lymphoid cells that circulate and establish within the spleen and around the portal tracts of the liver (**678**).

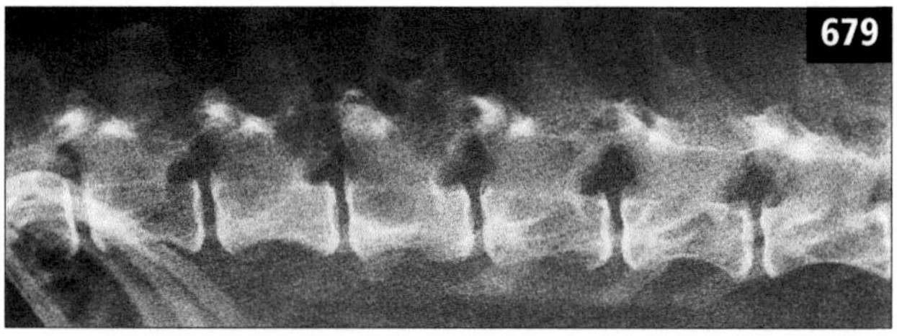

679 Radiographic appearance of multiple myeloma. Radiograph of the lumbar spine of a West Highland White Terrier, which presented with pyrexia, depression and back pain. The radiograph shows multiple 'punched out' osteolytic lesions in the dorsal spinous processes of the lumbar vertebrae. (Photograph courtesy S. Gould)

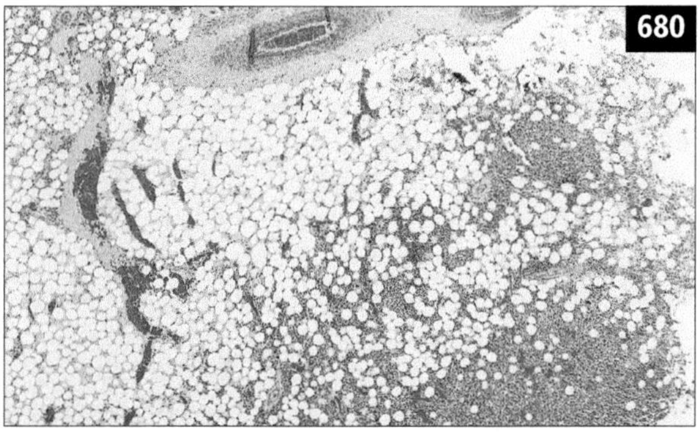

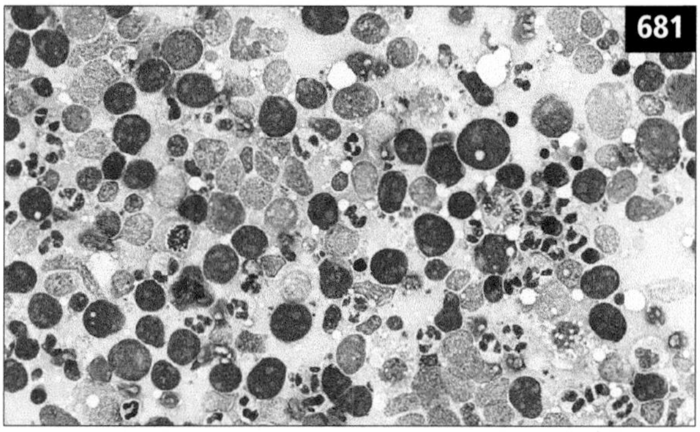

680, 681 Bone marrow in multiple myeloma. (**680**) Core biopsy of bone marrow from a 12-year-old Golden Retriever dog with serum globulin of 111 g/l (11.1 g/dl), subsequently characterized as an IgM paraprotein. (**681**) Aspirate of bone marrow from a four-year-old crossbred dog with multiple myeloma. There are numerous, large and irregular plasma cells, which are associated with a concurrent proliferation of eosinophils.

noted that in this species the disease may primarily affect the viscera (liver and spleen) in the absence of bone marrow involvement (**682–684**). Renal disease is common in multiple myeloma and has a complex pathogenesis that involves factors other than neoplastic infiltration.

Usually, the neoplastic plasma cells also produce large quantities of a structurally abnormal Ig termed 'paraprotein'. Occasionally, there is asynchronous synthesis of more light chain than heavy chain, with release of free light chain. Rarely, synthesis of heavy chain alone may occur. Some cases of 'non-secretory' myeloma are documented in the dog. The secreted paraprotein results in marked hyperproteinaemia and a monoclonal spike on serum protein electrophoresis (monoclonal gammopathy) (**685**). The class of Ig can be determined by agar gel diffusion, immunofixation, immunoelectrophoresis (IEP) or western blotting, and the latter three methods will also demonstrate the irregular nature of the molecule (**686–688**). Immunohistochemical studies of biopsy material can also define the clonal nature of plasmacytic infiltrates, which will show cytoplasmic expression of the same class of immunoglobulin heavy chain as the secreted paraprotein. Clonality testing (see above) has also been recently applied to the lesions of multiple myeloma, and in one canine case has been used to demonstrate the evolution of B cell lymphoma to myeloma.

The most common paraproteins are IgG and IgA, and occasional biclonal gammopathies are identified. IgM paraprotein (macroglobulinaemia) is uncommon and may act as a cryoglobulin that reversibly precipitates or gels at temperatures below 37°C (cryoglobulinaemia). Less commonly, aggregated IgA or IgG acts as a cryoglobulin. Macroglobulinaemia or cryoglobulinaemia may be associated with a serum hyperviscosity syndrome involving cardiac and renal dysfunction, haemorrhages, ischaemic necrosis of peripheral cutaneous sites, retinopathy and neurological disturbance. The quantity of the paraprotein may be determined by SRID (see Chapter 12, p. 293) and there is often reduced concentration of other Ig classes. Whilst monoclonal gammopathy is usually indicative of immune system neoplasia, it may occur in non-neoplastic disease with chronic immune stimulation (e.g. *Ehrlichia* or *Leishmania* infection in the dog, FIP virus infection in the cat). Circulating Ig light chains (Bence-Jones protein) may pass the glomerular filter and be identified in the proteinuric animal by heat precipitation of the urine or by IEP of a concentrated urine sample. Amyloid deposition (generally AL amyloid) is not often associated with multiple myeloma in dogs and cats.

682

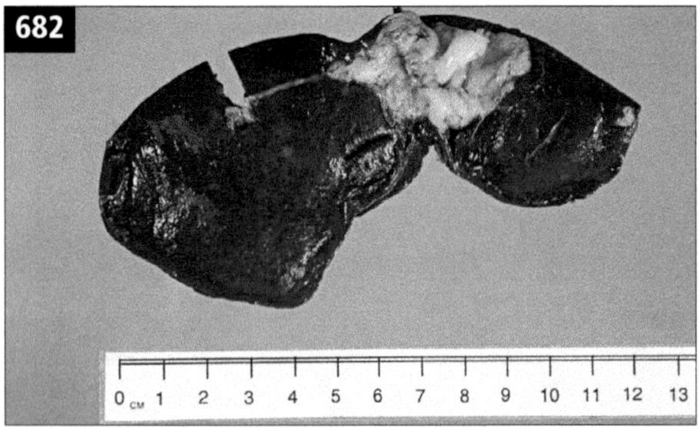

683

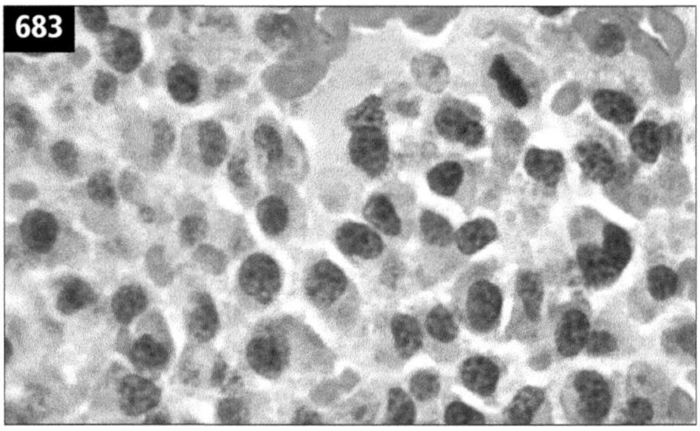

684

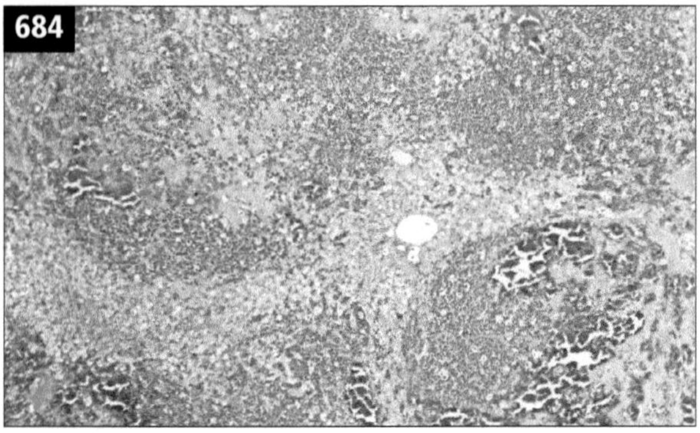

682–684 Visceral lesions in multiple myeloma. (**682**) Spleen removed from a 12-year-old DSH cat with an IgG paraproteinaemia. (**683**) A section taken from the spleen reveals the presence of a sheet of pleomorphic plasmacytic cells. Occasional cells are binucleate and mitotic activity is present. (**684**) Section of liver from a four-year-old DSH cat with multiple myeloma. Most of the hepatic architecture has been replaced by infiltrating sheets of neoplastic plasma cells, with associated zones of haemorrhage.

Diagnosis requires satisfaction of at least two of the following criteria:

- Abnormal plasma cells in bone marrow.
- Monoclonal gammopathy (non-IgM).
- Bence-Jones proteinuria.
- Osteolytic bone lesions.

In canine myeloma, hypercalcaemia, Bence-Jones proteinuria and extensive bony lesions have been correlated with shorter survival times after diagnosis.

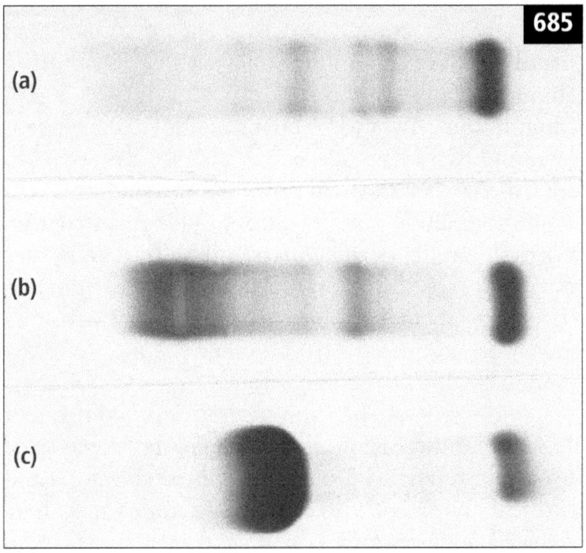

685 Monoclonal gammopathy in multiple myeloma. Protein electrophoresis of serum from **(a)** a normal dog, **(b)** a dog with polyclonal hypergammaglobulinaemia, and **(c)** a dog with IgA myeloma demonstrating a prominent monoclonal gammopathy in the β globulin region.

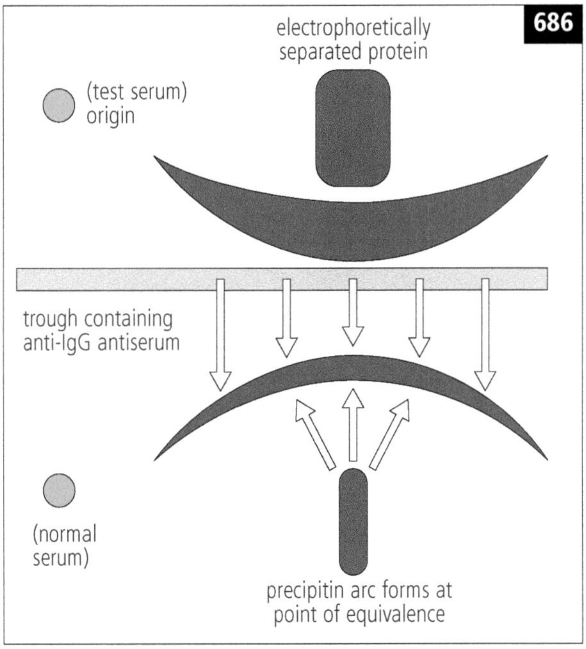

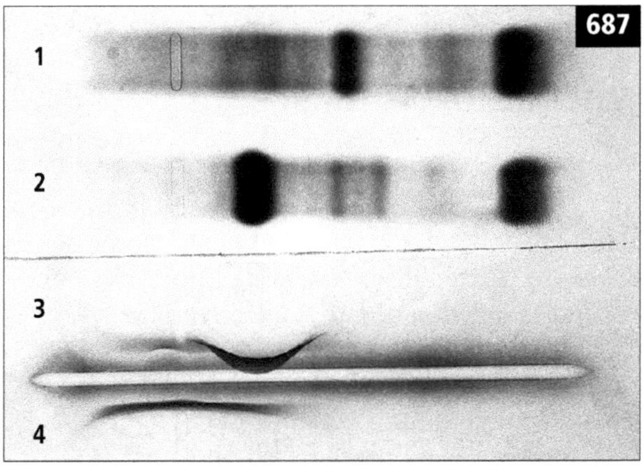

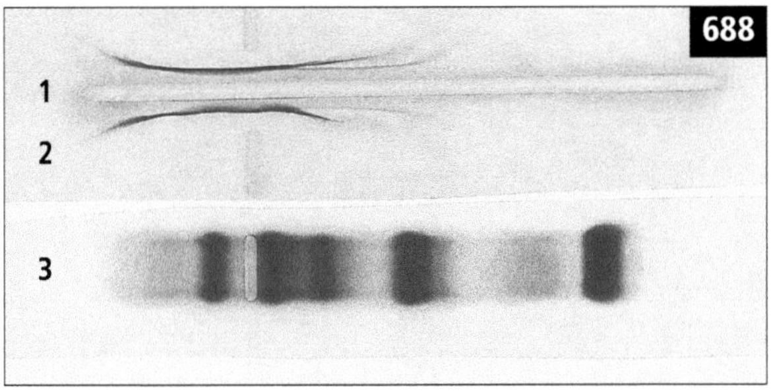

686–688 Immunoelectrophoresis. (**686**) Following electrophoretic separation of serum proteins, troughs are cut into the agarose gel parallel to the separated serum proteins. Antisera specific for each of the major Ig classes or light chain types are loaded into the troughs and the gel incubated for 24 hours. The antiserum diffuses from the trough and forms an arc of precipitation where it encounters specific antigen. The technique is used to determine the class of paraprotein and to demonstrate the abnormal nature of this Ig through altered electrophoretic mobility (altered charge) or distortion of the precipitin arc relative to that obtained with control normal serum. (Reproduced from Davidson M, Else R, Lumsden J [1998] *Manual of Small Animal Clinical Pathology*. BSAVA Gloucester, with permission.) (**687**) SPE and immunoelectrophoresis of serum from a dog with IgG myeloma (lanes 2 and 3) and a normal dog (lanes 1 and 4) against antiserum specific for IgG. The precipitin arc has an irregular appearance relative to that obtained with normal serum immunoglobulin, and it has altered electrophoretic mobility. (**688**) SPE and immunoelectrophoresis of serum from a dog with IgG myeloma. The biclonal gammopathy evident in the serum electrophoretic trace (lane 3) is mirrored in the irregular IgG precipitin arc obtained with this serum (lane 2) relative to normal dog serum (lane 1).

Chemotherapy is the treatment of choice and usually involves induction with combination chemotherapy based on an alkylating agent (melphalan or cyclophosphamide) and prednisolone, with or without vincristine. Response to treatment is assessed by monitoring plasma immunoglobulin concentration. Once this is within normal limits, drug doses and frequency are reduced to maintenance levels. Supportive treatment including fluid therapy and antibiotics may be required to manage some of the complications of the condition. Over 75% of cases respond to treatment, with median survival times of 12–18 months. Radiotherapy may be considered for palliation of painful solitary skeletal lesions and medical treatment with bisphosphonates may help reduce bone lysis and pain in cases with widespread skeletal lesions.

WALDENSTRÖM'S MACROGLOBULINEMIA

Waldenström's macroglobulinemia is a rare form of B cell lymphoma that is described in the dog. Although this entity falls within the spectrum of myeloma-related disorders, it is characterized by:

- Transformation of late stage B lymphocytes ('plasmacytoid lymphocytes').
- Serum monoclonal IgM with hyperviscosity.
- Infiltration of bone marrow and lymphoid tissues but without osteolysis and hypercalcaemia.

PLASMACYTOMA

Plasmacytoma is a benign plasma cell tumour of the skin (occasionally oral or rectal mucosa) of the dog and, less commonly, the cat. The lesions are usually solitary, domed, alopecic nodules up to 2 cm in diameter, and they occur most frequently on the ears, face (lip) and feet. The histological appearance is of a circumscribed, nodular aggregate of well-differentiated plasma cells, with occasional large multinucleate cells and an eosinophil infiltrate (689, 690). The lesions rarely recur after excision. Intralesional AL amyloid deposition is occasionally recorded and may be associated with a greater risk of recurrence. There is no paraproteinaemia and no clear relationship to multiple myeloma, although isolated cases with concurrent or subsequent myeloma are documented. Plasmacytoma is also reported to arise in the bone of some dogs (solitary plasmacytoma of bone) and although these tumours may initially respond to surgical excision (where possible), chemotherapy and radiotherapy, in most cases the patients have gone on to develop multiple myeloma. Solitary plasmacytoma of bone has been documented in two cats that had good clinical response to radiotherapy or chemotherapy (one case each). Plasmacytoma affecting the gastrointestinal tract is rare, but can follow a more malignant course.

MYELOPROLIFERATIVE DISEASE

Myeloproliferative disease is a primary tumour of haemopoietic precursor cells (non-lymphoid) and may affect any one, or more, bone marrow lineages at any stage of differentiation (*Table 27*). It is an uncommon disease of the dog and cat; feline myeloproliferative disease is generally a manifestation of FeLV infection. In all cases there is involvement of bone marrow and peripheral blood (691–693), with seeding of tumour to areas such as

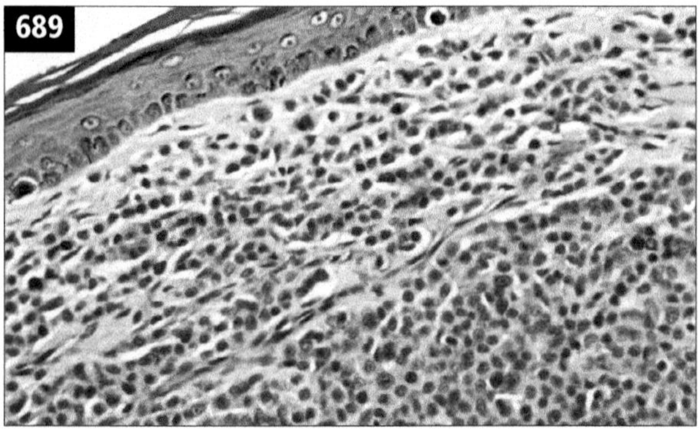

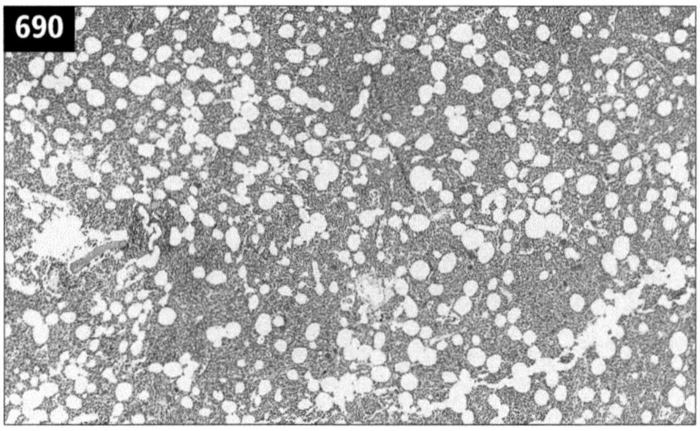

689, 690 Plasmacytoma. High (**689**) and low (**690**) power histological appearance of plasmacytoma removed from the ear of an eight-year-old Dachshund. A sheet of plasmacytoid cells obliterates the dermal microarchitecture and occasional cells with giant or multiple nuclei are present.

Table 27: Subgroups of myeloproliferative disease. The term 'myeloproliferative disease' encompasses a spectrum of tumours of bone marrow haemopoietic precursor cells that seed to the blood and viscera. Myeloproliferative diseases may run an acute or chronic course, and particular types of tumour more frequently fall into either of these two categories. Myeloproliferative disease may involve a single precursor type or more than one lineage.

Lineage	Acute myeloproliferative disease	Chronic myelproliferative disease
Granulocyte, monocyte	• Acute myeloid leukaemia • Acute myelomonocytic leukaemia • Acute monocytic and monoblastic leukaemia	• Chronic granulocytic/myeloid leukaemia • Chronic myelomonocytic leukaemia
Erythroid	• *Erythremic myelosis* and *erythroleukaemia*	• Primary polycythaemia
Megakaryocytic	• *Acute megakaryoblastic leukaemia*	• Essential thrombocytosis

Conditions in italics are very rare in animals.

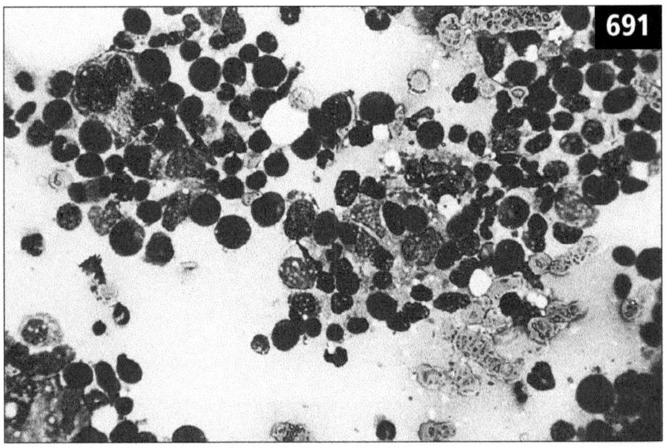

691 Myeloproliferative disease. Photomicrograph of bone marrow from a Bernese Mountain Dog with presumed AML, showing a predominance of early myeloid cells.

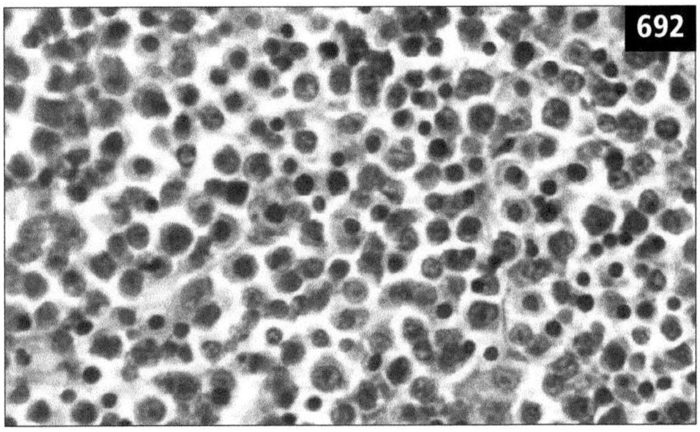

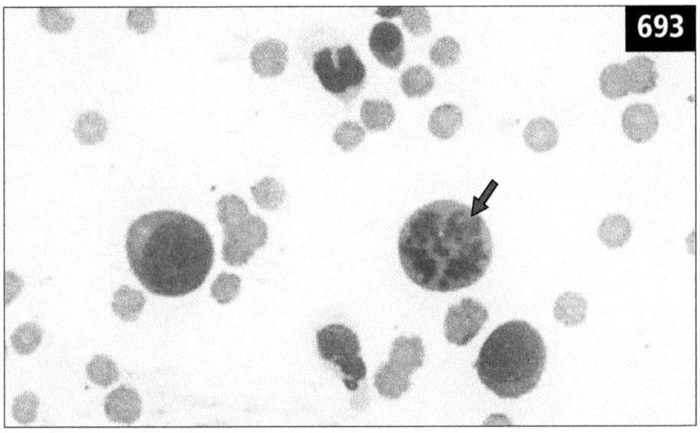

692–693 Myeloproliferative disease. (**692**) Bone marrow and (**693**) blood smear from a seven-year-old DSH cat with erythremic myelosis. There are numerous erythroblastic cells within the bone marrow and peripheral blood (note the mitosis in one circulating cell [arrowed]), and in this cat the tumour had seeded to the liver, spleen and kidney.

the spleen, liver and lung (**694–697**). Secondary immune-mediated disease (e.g. IMHA) may occur in both dogs and cats. Myeloproliferative disease may be acute (AMD), involving early stage, immature cells (with survival time of 2–3 months after diagnosis), or chronic (CMD), involving late stage, relatively mature cells (survival time of 1–3 years after diagnosis).

Treatment of AMD is difficult and often impractical. Attempts have been made to treat AMD using antimetabolites (cytarabine, thioguanine or mercaptopurine), prednisolone or the anti-tumour antibiotic doxorubicin. The outcome in most cases is disappointing, with the animal succumbing to overwhelming sepsis, organ failure or DIC. Survival times for AMD are generally less than those for ALL.

The prognosis for CMD is more favourable. Chemotherapy is recommended in most cases, with the aim of restoring the peripheral blood counts to the normal range. Choice of agent depends on the cell lineage affected; for example, busulphan is the drug of choice for chronic granulocytic leukaemia (CGL) as it has specific action on the neutrophil series. Hydroxyurea is usually recommended for treatment of polycythemia vera. The prognosis for long-term control of CMD is usually fair, but some cases of CGL may revert to an acute form in what is termed 'blast cell crisis'.

HISTIOCYTOMA

Histiocytoma is the most common canine skin tumour and occurs as a solitary (occasionally multiple), domed, alopecic and erythematous mass (0.5–1.5 cm diameter) anywhere on the body (**698**). The tumour arises most frequently in dogs under two years of age, is well circumscribed, grows

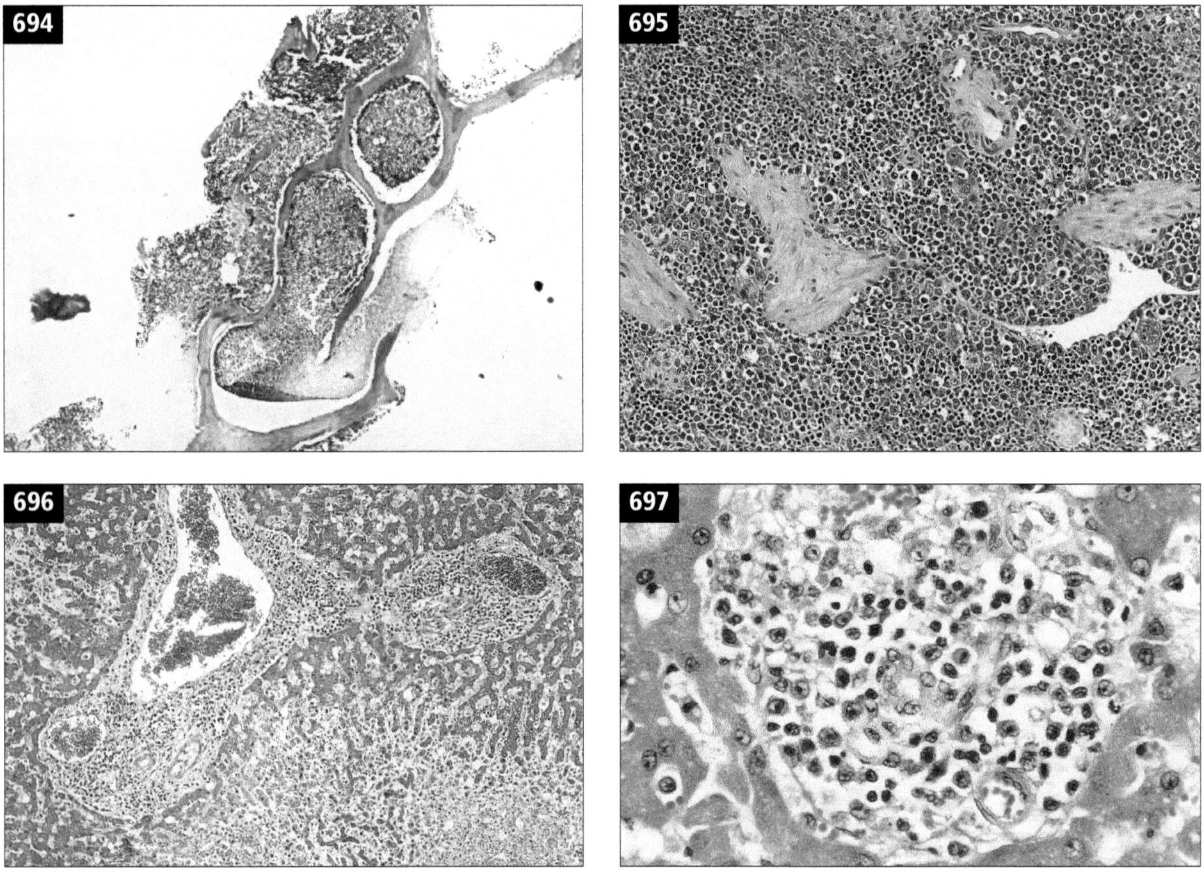

694–697 Myeloproliferative disease. Myeloproliferative disease in a ten-year-old DSH cat with pyrexia, weight loss and renal and hepatic failure. Necropsy examination confirms involvement of the bone marrow (**694**) and spleen (**695**). (**696, 697**) Myeloproliferative disease in a three-year-old DSH cat that has seeded to the periportal areas of the liver. The infiltrates comprise mitotic myeloid precursors.

rapidly but may spontaneously regress (in weeks to months), and generally does not recur after excision. Less commonly, histiocytomas may occur in older dogs or they appear as multiple lesions with delayed regression, a presentation that is more often reported in Shar Pei dogs. Migration of histiocytomas to regional draining lymph nodes has also been reported. Rarely, there may be confluent cutaneous lesions in multiple cutaneous sites, with rapid systemic spread. These less common variants of histiocytoma are now described as examples of Langerhans cell histiocytosis.

Histologically, histiocytoma is characterized by a dense infiltrate of highly mitotic, epidermotropic histiocytic cells that may efface dermal structures (699–701). The tumour has been determined to be

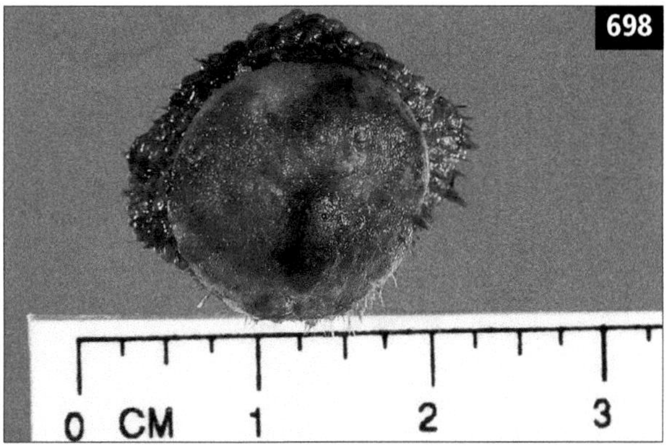

698 Canine histiocytoma. Surgically excised histiocytoma from the skin of a 16-month-old Shar Pei. There is a well-circumscribed raised nodular mass of 1 cm diameter, with a red-tan surface.

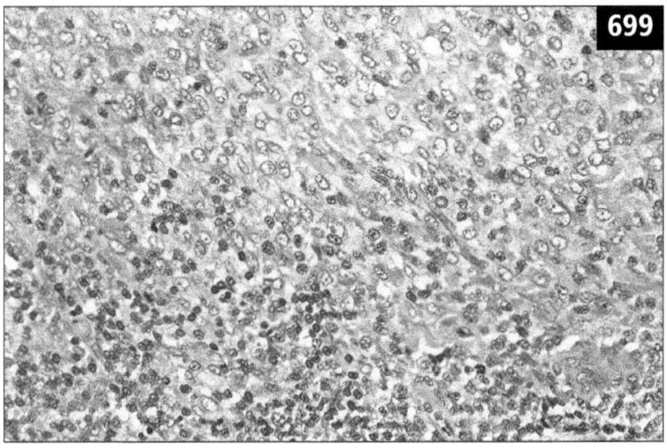

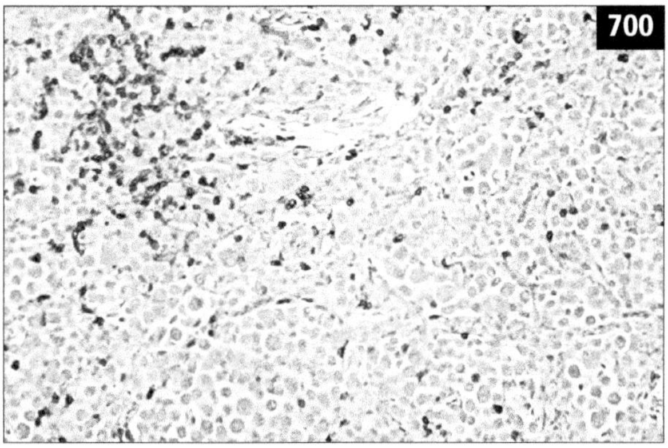

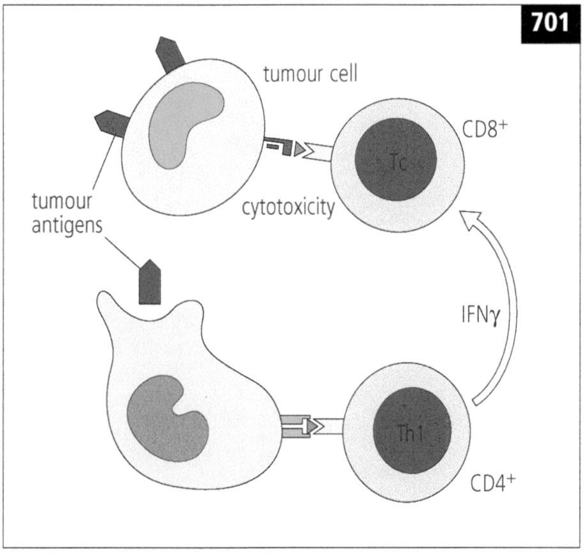

699–701 Canine histiocytoma. Microscopic appearance of a histiocytoma removed from the pinna of a two-year-old Boxer. (**699**) There is a diffuse infiltrate of large histiocytic cells, with abundant eosinophilic cytoplasm and a high mitotic rate. The infiltrate effaces follicles and other adnexae and there is surface ulceration (not shown). At the deep margin of the tumour are aggregates of small lymphocytes. (**700**) Section of histiocytoma labelled to show infiltrating T lymphocytes. These are known to be predominantly of the CD8 phenotype and may be involved in mediating the spontaneous regression that is characteristic of these tumours via the mechanism depicted in **701**.

of Langerhans cell origin (bearing CD1a, b and c, CD11a and c, CD18, CD45, MHC class II, ICAM-1, E-cadherin and CD14). The spontaneous regression is likely to be mediated by an initial infiltration of Th1 $CD4^+$ T cells that express IL-2 and IFNγ and further recruit $CD8^+$ T cells and normal myelohistiocytic cells. Histiocytoma has not been clearly documented in the cat.

CUTANEOUS AND SYSTEMIC HISTIOCYTOSIS

Canine cutaneous and systemic histiocytosis form a spectrum of reactive, rather than neoplastic, histiocytic proliferative disease and are collectively termed canine reactive histiocytosis. Cutaneous histiocytosis involves the formation of multiple, non-painful, non-pruritic nodules over the head, neck and extremities, which may spontaneously regress or slowly progress. In contrast, systemic histiocytosis affects skin (and ocular and nasal mucosae) in addition to lymph nodes and a range of other organ systems (e.g. liver, spleen, lungs and bone marrow). Related Bernese Mountain Dogs (particularly males) develop systemic histiocytosis, although a number of other breeds (e.g. Golden Retriever, Labrador Retriever, Boxer and Rottweiler) may be affected. The diseases have identical histopathology, characterized by angiocentric aggregates of mixed histiocytes, lymphocytes, neutrophils and eosinophils (702). Phenotypic studies have shown the histiocytes to be of activated interstitial dendritic cell origin ($CD1^+$, $CD11b^+$, $CD11c^+$, MHC class II^+, $CD4^+$, ICAM-1^+, CD90(Thy-1$)^+$), with the T cell component expressing predominantly CD3, CD8 and αβ TCR. It has been suspected that these diseases involve a persistent antigenic stimulation, but as no antigen has been readily identified, recent hypotheses suggest a T cell-driven immune dysregulation with failure of inhibition through the CD80/86:CTLA4 interaction. The diseases respond variably to immunosuppressive therapy. Some respond to glucocorticoids and successful management of persistent lesions with ciclosporin or leflunomide has been reported.

HISTIOCYTIC SARCOMA

Localized and disseminated histiocytic sarcomas (the latter previously called malignant histiocytosis) form a spectrum of malignant histiocytic tumours of the dog. Cats are rarely reported to develop histiocytic sarcoma (localized or generalized).

Localized histiocytic sarcoma

Localized histiocytic sarcoma is a solitary, locally invasive tumour that arises from skin and subcutaneous tissue, particularly on extremities and often near joints. A proportion of neoplasms previously diagnosed as 'synovial sarcoma' have now been shown immunophenotypically to be

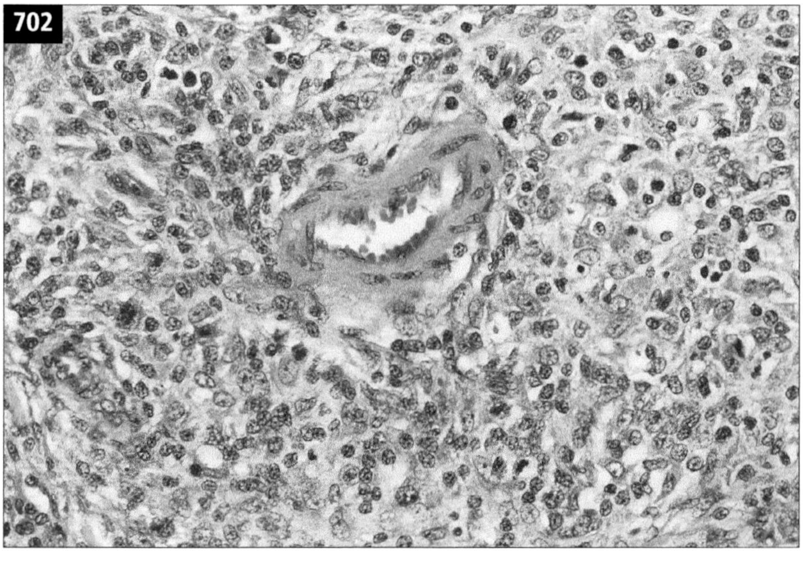

702 Systemic histiocytosis. Skin biopsy from a two-year-old Border Collie with nodular skin lesions and generalized lymphadenopathy, both of which have a waxing and waning course. There is a background of actively mitotic histiocytic cells, together with an infiltrate of lymphocytes, plasma cells and neutrophils. The cells closely abut blood vessels, but do not clearly infiltrate them. A similar appearance was present in lymph node.

histiocytic sarcoma. The tumours can metastasize to regional lymph nodes and can also develop in spleen, liver, CNS, stomach and tongue. The disease is recognized in Bernese Mountain Dogs, Flat Coated Retrievers, Golden Retrievers, Labrador Retrievers and Rottweilers. There is some breed variation in the behaviour of these tumours; for example, in the Flat Coated Retriever up to 75% of localized histiocytic sarcomas may metastasize. The histological appearance is of pleomorphic round cells or densely packed spindle cells with multinucleate histiocytic cells and bizarre mitoses. The prognosis is guarded if metastasis has occurred, but surgical excision and/or radiotherapy may be curative for localized tumours.

Disseminated histiocytic sarcoma

Disseminated histiocytic sarcoma is documented in related Bernese Mountain Dogs in addition to Rottweilers, Golden Retrievers, Labrador Retrievers and Flat Coated Retrievers. A polygenic mode of inheritance has been suggested for the Bernese Mountain Dog. There are multicentric nodular masses that may involve lung, lymph nodes, liver, kidneys, CNS, muscle, alimentary tract, heart, bone marrow and spleen (703, 704). The skin is rarely involved. The histological appearance is of pleomorphic and phagocytic histiocytes, together with scattered multinucleate giant cells with bizarre mitoses (705). The histiocytic cells in both tumours express phenotypic

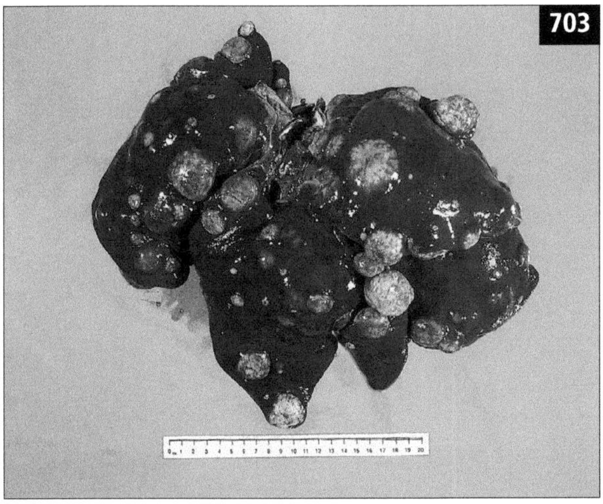

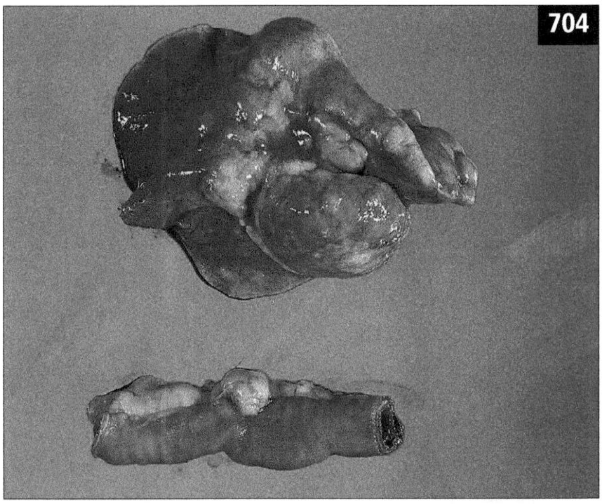

703, 704 Disseminated histiocytic sarcoma. Liver, lungs and small intestine from a seven-year-old male Bernese Mountain Dog with a two-week history of anorexia and weight loss. There are multiple, firm, cream nodules scattered throughout all the liver lobes and the lung, with enlargement of mesenteric lymph nodes.

705 Disseminated histiocytic sarcoma. The microscopic appearance of the lesions in the Bernese Mountain Dog described in **703** is of a diffuse infiltrate of pleomorphic histiocytes, with scattered multinucleate giant cells with numerous mitotic figures (arrowed).

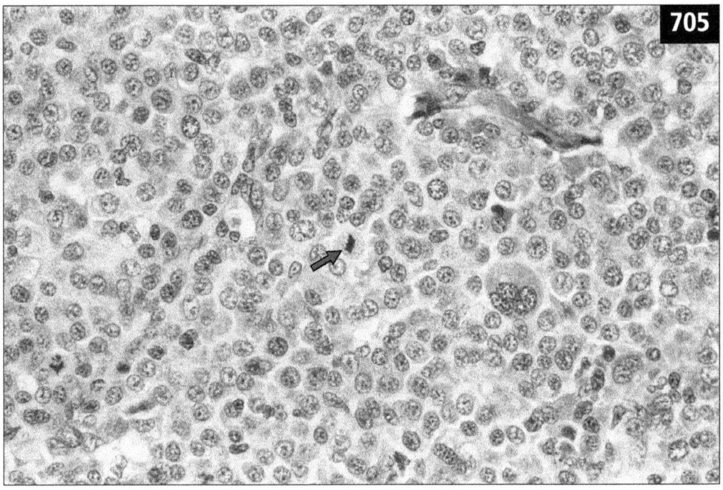

markers consistent with a dendritic cell origin (CD1, CD11c, MHC class II, ICAM-1 and less commonly CD4 and CD90). The lack of CD4 expression is consistent with the hypothesis that these dendritic cells are not activated and, therefore, may induce T cell anergy rather than stimulation, accounting for the aggressive biological behaviour of the tumour. Disseminated histiocytic sarcoma is rapidly progressive and carries a poor prognosis.

Haemophagocytic histiocytic sarcoma

A newly characterized subset of histiocytic sarcoma is haemophagocytic histiocytic sarcoma, which is also a rapidly progressive neoplastic disorder. These cells are phenotypically of macrophage rather than dendritic cell origin ($CD11d^{+}$) and may be actively erythrophagocytic. The neoplastic proliferation is typically associated with striking extramedullary haematopoiesis. The tumour generally arises in the spleen and spreads to the liver, where it diffusely infiltrates portal areas and sinusoids. Affected dogs are characteristically anaemic and thrombocytopenic, but lack erythrocyte- or platelet-bound antibodies. Cats are rarely reported to develop haemophagocytic histiocytic sarcoma.

Feline histiocytic proliferative disease

Histiocytic proliferative disease is rarely documented in the cat, although a recent report details information on 30 cases. The entity termed 'feline progressive histiocytosis' forms a clinical spectrum involving proliferation of cells of interstitial dendritic phenotype (expressing CD1a, CD1c, CD18 and MHC class II). In early stages there are cutaneous nodules, papules or plaques, which often affect the feet, limbs and face (706, 707). Although the disease may remain restricted to the skin for prolonged periods, in some cats there is terminal involvement of the viscera. The disease fails to respond to immunotherapy of various types, suggesting that the pathogenesis involves progressive histiocytic neoplasia rather than aberrant antigenic stimulation (708).

MAST CELL TUMOUR

Mast cell tumours occur in both the cat and dog and primarily involve the skin (common) or alimentary tract (rare) (709, 710).

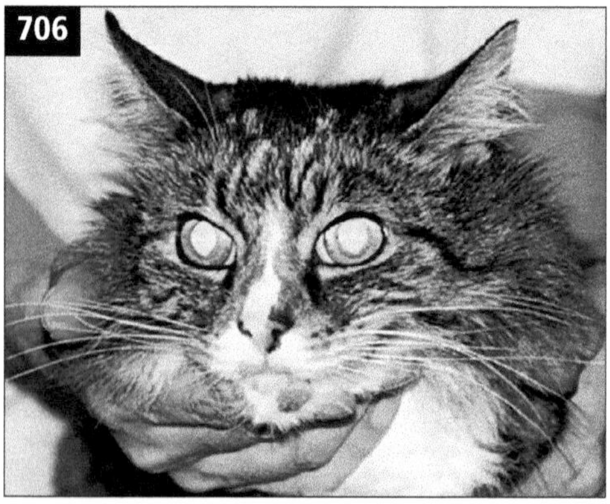
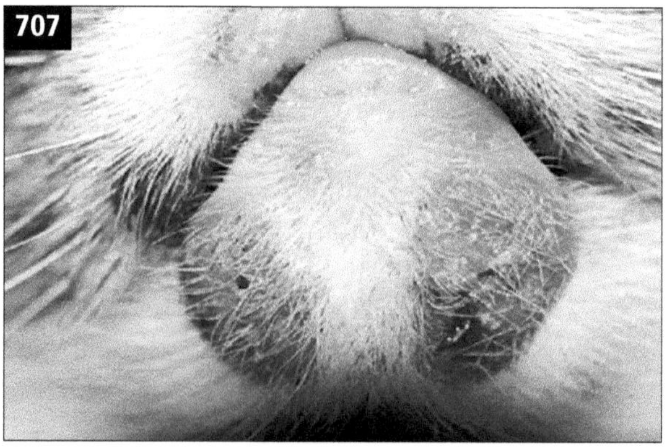

706, 707 Feline progressive histiocytosis. A 15-year-old DLH cat with slowly progressive multiple cutaneous nodular masses. Microscopically these comprise an infiltrate of MHC class II expressing histiocytic cells, with perivascular T cell aggregation. Although initially described as 'multiple histiocytomas', this case is compatible with the recently described entity of 'feline progressive histiocytosis'.

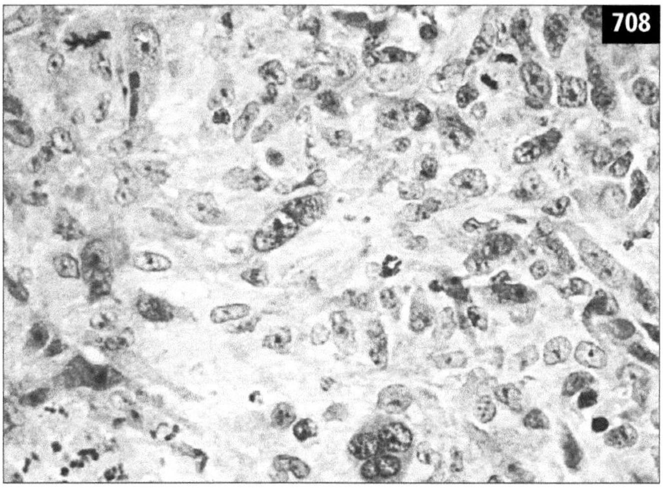

708 Feline progressive histiocytosis. Biopsy from a cat with multiple cutaneous nodular masses comprised of pleomorphic histiocytic cells. The population includes cells with giant or multiple nuclei; numerous bizarre mitoses are also present.

709, 710 Alimentary mast cell tumour. (**709**) Portion of colon and associated mesenteric lymph nodes from an eight-year-old Labrador Retriever with a history of diarrhoea and melaena. There is a large oval shaped mass that arises from the colonic mucosa and virtually occludes the gut lumen. (**710**) Microscopic examination confirms the presence of a sheet of poorly differentiated mast cells that stain variably by toluidine blue, together with numerous eosinophils. There is metastasis to the regional lymph nodes.

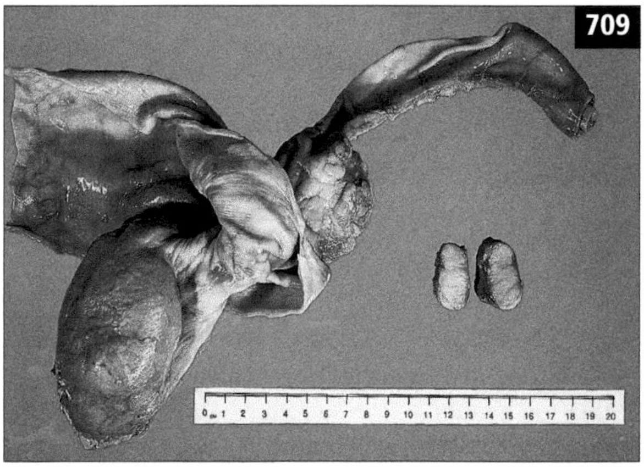

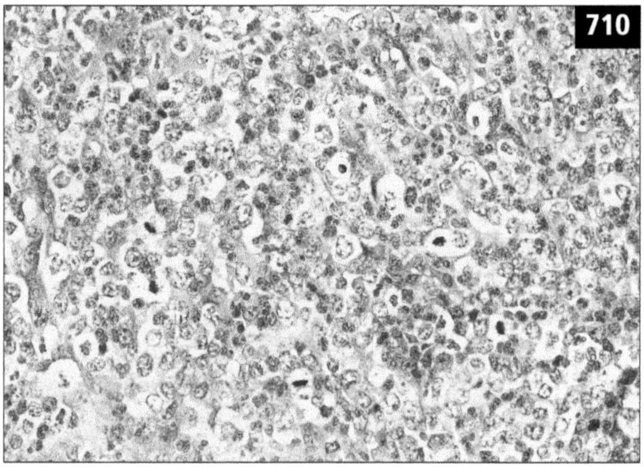

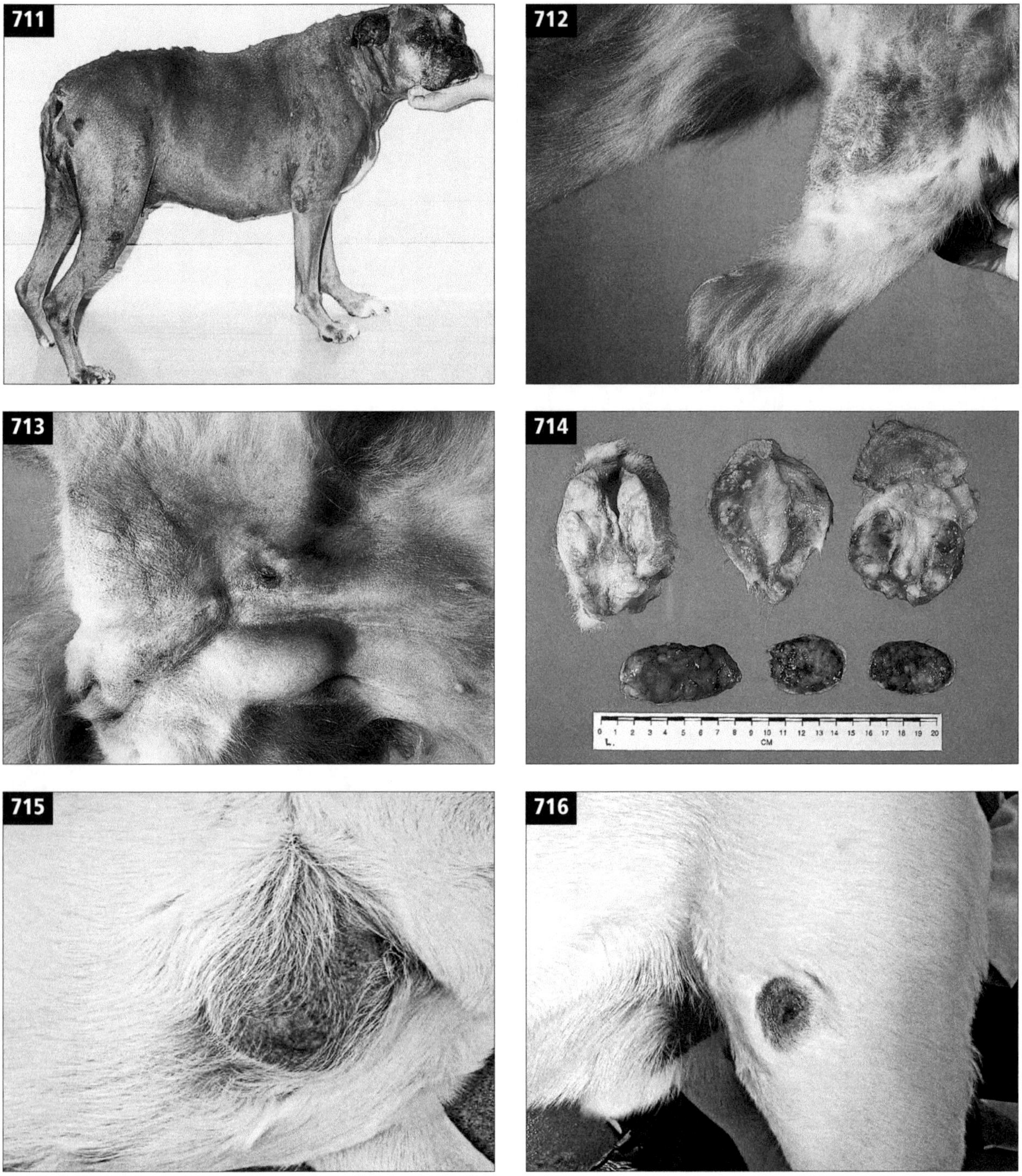

711–716 Canine cutaneous mast cell tumour. (**711**) A Boxer with multiple cutaneous nodules of mast cell tumour over the face, limbs and body. (Photograph courtesy S.E. Shaw.) (**712, 713**) Hindlimb and groin of a ten-year-old Golden Retriever with large subcutaneous masses in the limbs and marked enlargement of the inguinal lymph nodes. (**714**) On necropsy examination this was revealed to be a locally infiltrative mast cell tumour (upper specimens) that had metastasized to regional lymph nodes (lower specimens). There was no visceral involvement. (**715**) A large subcutaneous mast cell tumour in the axilla of a ten-year-old Labrador Retriever. (**716**) An intermediate grade dermal mast cell tumour in the skin of the lateral thigh of a six-year-old Labrador Retriever.

Mast cell tumours in the dog

Cutaneous mast cell tumour in the dog presents as single or multiple, alopecic, erythematous and oedematous nodules up to several centimetres in diameter (711–716). They may arise at any site, but are frequently documented on the limbs or trunk. Perineal, scrotal, preputial or digital mast cell tumours may be more malignant. Particular breeds of dog appear predisposed to mast cell tumour (e.g. Boxer, Boston Terrier, Bull Terrier, Golden Retriever) and middle-aged dogs are affected most often.

The tumours may be diagnosed by fine needle aspiration (717) or by biopsy (718–721). Confirmation of mast cell lineage can be made by staining with toluidine blue or by immunohistochemical labelling for expression of chymase or

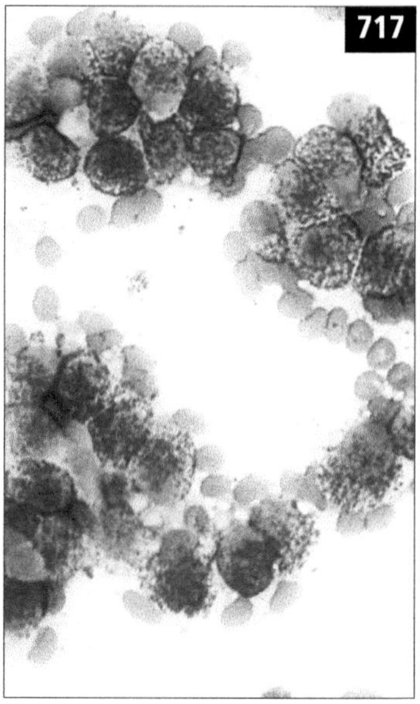

717 Cytological appearance of mast cell tumour. Fine needle aspirate from a canine cutaneous mast cell tumour. There are large numbers of well-differentiated mast cells with granular cytoplasm.

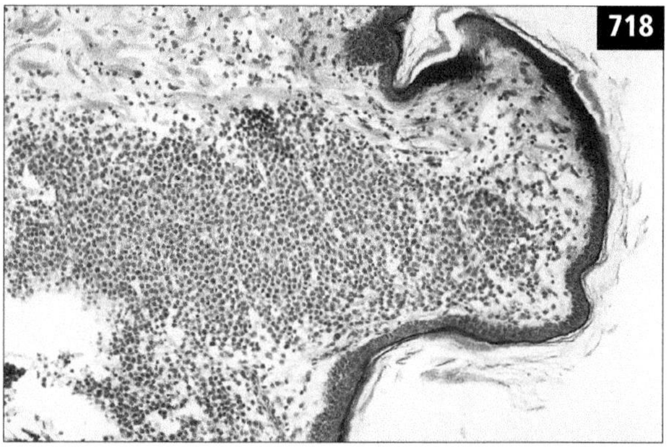

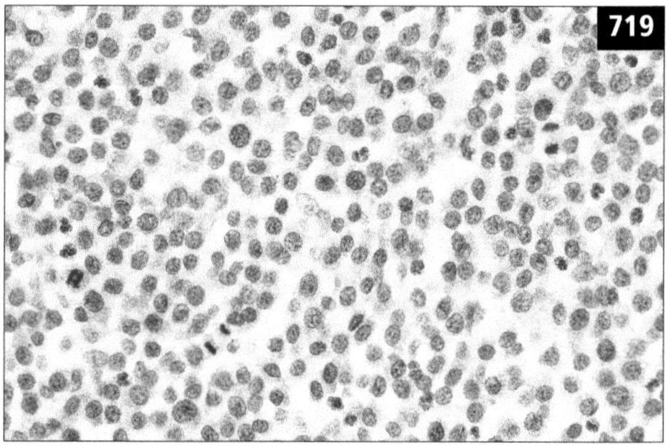

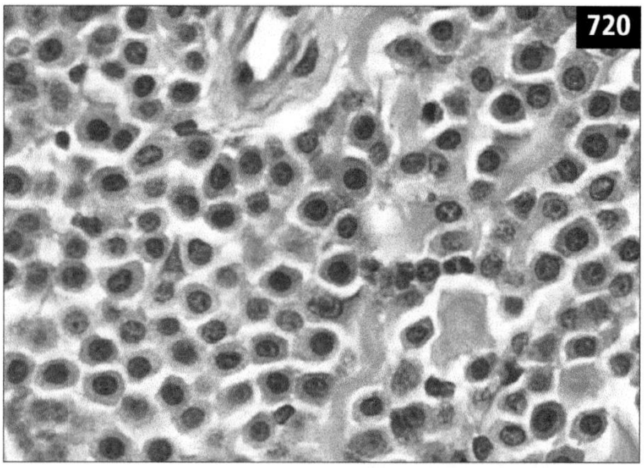

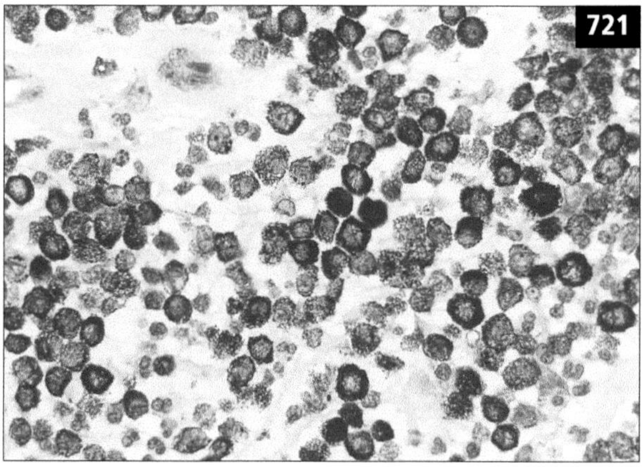

718–721 Histological appearance of canine mast cell tumour. (**718**) Section of skin from a nine-month-old Labrador Retriever with multiple small skin nodules. There are well-circumscribed, small dermal foci of well-differentiated mast cells with numerous mitoses (**719**). (**720**) Section of skin from a canine mast cell tumour. The cells are uniform and well-differentiated, with scattered eosinophils throughout. (**721**) The neoplastic mast cells stain positively by toluidine blue.

tryptase. A histopathological grading scheme for mast cell tumour is often used:

- Grade 1 (well-differentiated) tumours are most common and comprise a circumscribed dermal infiltrate of well-differentiated mast cells, together with an accompanying infiltrate of eosinophils.
- Grade 2 (intermediate) tumours are less well-circumscribed ulcerated lesions that infiltrate the deep dermis to subcutis. There is a degree of cellular pleomorphism and less eosinophil infiltration.
- Grade 3 (poorly differentiated) tumours are ulcerated, extensively infiltrative lesions comprised of highly pleomorphic and mitotic mast cells that may stain poorly with toluidine blue. Eosinophil infiltration may be variable.

Mast cell tumours are clinically significant due to their potential for local recurrence after excision and metastasis to regional lymph nodes (and occasional systemic metastasis), and for the production of clinical signs secondary to release of vasoactive factors. There is correlation between histopathological grade and the potential for local infiltration and metastasis.

The majority of mast cell tumours are best treated by surgical resection. Well-differentiated tumours are generally benign and carry a favourable prognosis; 90% of cases are cured by surgical excision. Moderately differentiated tumours are intermediate in histological appearance and behaviour; however, about 70–75% follow a relatively benign course. Poorly differentiated tumours are invasive, with a high rate of metastasis and therefore a poor prognosis; less than 25% of cases survive more than 12 months and most animals succumb to the disease within the first six months following diagnosis, irrespective of treatment. Low-grade and intermediate-grade tumours that by virtue of their site cannot be excised with adequate margins may be managed successfully with postoperative radiotherapy. The use of cytotoxic drugs in the treatment of mast cell tumours is controversial. Empirical clinical evidence shows that some mast cell tumours undergo temporary regression in response to high-dose corticosteroid treatment (prednisolone). Currently, a combination of prednisolone and vinblastine appears to be the treatment of choice for unresectable or disseminated high-grade mast cell tumours, but responses are variable and often short lived.

Mast cell tumours in the cat

Feline cutaneous mast cell tumours occur predominantly in middle-aged cats and generally present as multiple, discrete, firm, tan coloured nodules (up to 2 cm diameter) anywhere on the skin (722). Local recurrence or distant metastasis of

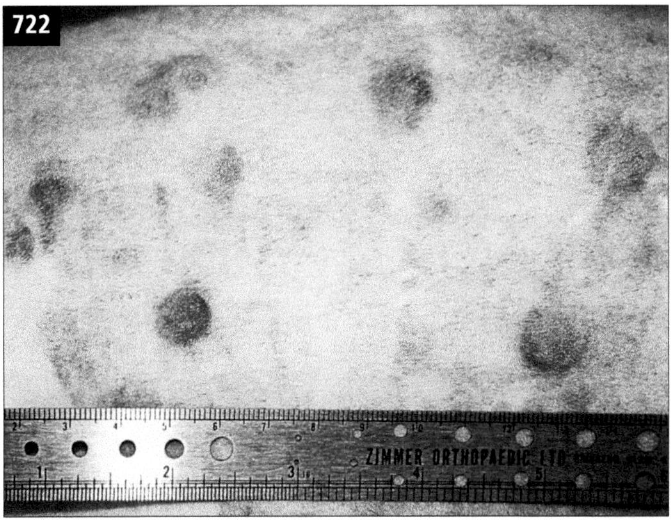

722 Feline cutaneous mast cell tumour. Cutaneous mast cell tumour in a six-year-old DSH cat, presenting as multiple, discrete, firm tan nodules over the flank.

these tumours is uncommon. Histologically most consist of dermal infiltrates of well-differentiated mast cells, with few eosinophils and occasional lymphoid aggregates (723, 724). An anaplastic form of feline cutaneous mast cell tumour is recognized that demonstrates deep dermal infiltration. Young Siamese cats appear predisposed to a unique form of mast cell tumour that appears as coalescing, papular to nodular lesions on the head. The mast cells have a poorly differentiated histiocytic appearance, but lesions generally regress spontaneously.

Surgery is the treatment of choice for feline cutaneous mast cell tumours. Most are behaviourally benign and have a fair prognosis, and surgical margins may not be as critical as in the dog. The value of chemotherapy and radiotherapy as alternative or adjunctive treatment in the cat is not known.

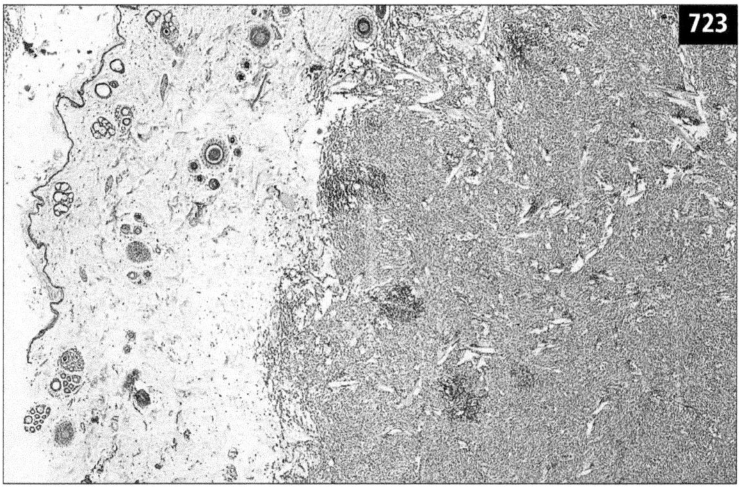

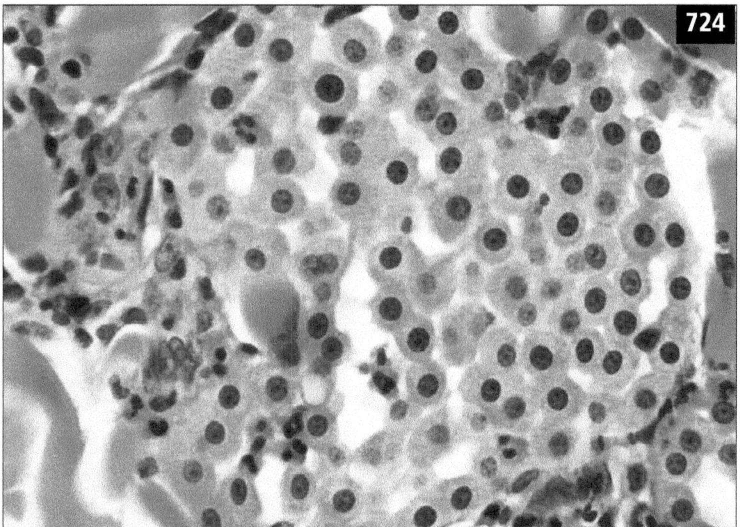

723, 724 Feline cutaneous mast cell tumour. (**723**) Section of mast cell tumour from the cat described in **722**. There is a circumscribed infiltrate of well-differentiated mast cells and eosinophils, with aggregates of small lymphocytes scattered throughout. (**724**) High power detail of the cellular morphology of a feline mast cell tumour is shown.

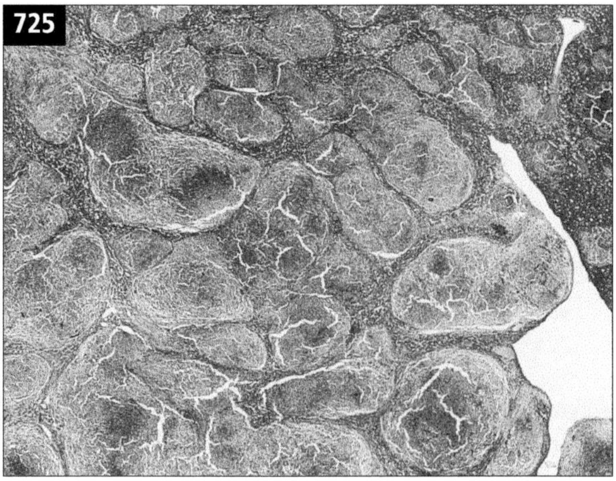

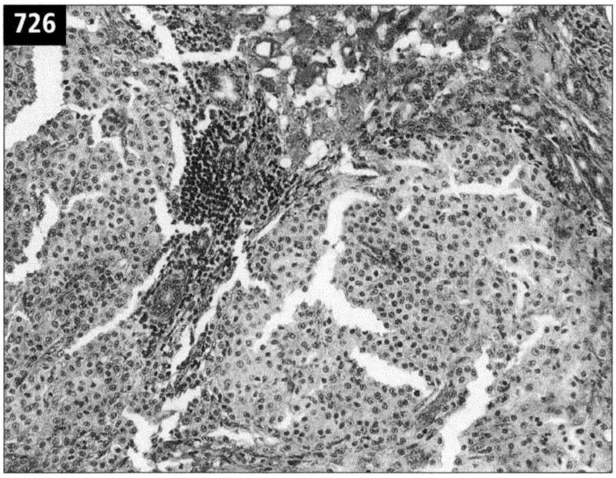

725, 726 Systemic mastocytosis. Section of liver from a cat with systemic mastocytosis. Normal hepatic tissue is almost obliterated by multiple nodular aggregates of well-differentiated mast cells that stain positively by toluidine blue.

SYSTEMIC MASTOCYTOSIS

Recognized in the cat, but extremely rare in the dog, systemic mastocytosis occurs independently of cutaneous or alimentary mast cell tumour. There may be intermittent mastocytaemia associated with mast cell infiltration of spleen, liver, kidney, bone marrow and other viscera (725, 726). The clinical presentation is often of vomiting, with gastric and duodenal ulceration (secondary to histamine production and release of HCl from gastric parietal cells) and splenomegaly. Systemic mastocytosis in the cat appears not to be caused by FeLV.

FURTHER READING

Affolter VK, Moore PF (2002) Localized and disseminated histiocytic sarcoma of dendritic cell origin in dogs. *Veterinary Pathology* **39**:74–83.

Affolter VK, Moore PF (2006) Feline progressive histiocytosis. *Veterinary Pathology* **43**:646–655.

Bertone ER, Snyder LA, Moore AS (2002) Environmental tobacco smoke and risk of malignant lymphoma in pet cats. *American Journal of Epidemiology* **156**:268–273.

Bridgeford EC, Marini RP, Feng Y *et al.* (2008) Gastric *Helicobacter* species as a cause of feline gastric lymphoma: a viable hypothesis. *Veterinary Immunology and Immunopathology* **123**:106–113.

Comazzi S, Gelain ME, Martini V *et al.* (2011) Immunophenotype predicts survival time in dogs with chronic lymphocytic leukemia. *Journal of Veterinary Internal Medicine* **25**:100–106.

Dobson J, Hoather T, McKinley TJ *et al.* (2009) Mortality in a cohort of float-coated retrievers in the UK. *Veterinary and Comparative Oncology* **7**:115–121.

Fontaine J, Heimann M, Day MJ (2010) Canine cutaneous epitheliotropic T-cell lymphoma: a review of 30 cases. *Veterinary Dermatology* **21**:267–275.

Fontaine J, Heimann M, Day MJ (2011) Cutaneous epitheliotropic T-cell lymphoma in the cat: a review of the literature and five new cases. *Veterinary Dermatology* (in press).

Gavazza A, Presiuttini S, Barale R *et al.* (2000) Association between canine malignant lymphoma, living in industrial areas, and use of chemicals by dog owners. *Journal of Veterinary Internal Medicine* **15**:190–195.

Giraudel JM, Pages J-P, Guelfi J-F (2002) Monoclonal gammopathies in the dog: a retrospective study of 18 cases (1986–1999) and literature review. *Journal of the American Animal Hospital Association* **38**:135–147.

Kaim U, Moritz A, Failing K *et al.* (2006) The regression of canine Langerhans cell tumour is associated with increased expression of IL-2, TNF-α, IFN-γ and iNOS mRNA. *Immunology* **118**:472–482.

Kiupel M, Smedley RC, Pfent C *et al.* (2011) Diagnostic algorithm to differentiate lymphoma from inflammation in feline small intestinal biopsy samples. *Veterinary Pathology* **48**:212–222.

Krick EL, Little L, Patel R *et al.* (2008) Description of clinical and pathological findings, treatment and outcome of feline large granular lymphocyte lymphoma (1996–2004). *Veterinary and Comparative Oncology* **6**:102–110.

Lingard AE, Briscoe K, Beatty JA *et al.* (2009) Low-grade alimentary lymphoma: clinicopathological findings and response to treatment in 17 cases. *Journal of Feline Medicine and Surgery* **11**:692–700.

Louwerens M, London CA, Pedersen NC *et al.* (2005) Feline lymphoma in the post-feline leukemia virus era. *Journal of Veterinary Internal Medicine* **19**:329–335.

Marconato L, Leo C, Girelli R *et al.* (2009) Association between waste management and cancer in companion animals. *Journal of Veterinary Internal Medicine* **23**:564–569.

Marconato L, Stefanello D, Valenti P *et al.* (2011) Predictors of long-term survival in dogs with high-grade multicentric lymphoma. *Journal of the American Veterinary Medical Association* **238**:480–485.

Mellor PJ, Haugland S, Murphy S *et al.* (2006) Myeloma-related disorders in cats commonly present as extramedullary neoplasms in contrast to myeloma in human patients: 24 cases with clinical follow up. *Journal of Veterinary Internal Medicine* **20**:1376–1383.

Mellor PJ, Haugland S, Smith KC *et al.* (2008) Histopathological, histochemical, immunohistochemical and cytological analysis of feline myeloma-related disorders: further evidence for primary extramedullary development in the cat. *Veterinary Pathology* **45**:159–173.

Modiano JF, Breen M, Burnett RC *et al.* (2006) Distinct B-cell and T-cell lymphoproliferative disease prevalence among dog breeds indicates heritable risk. *Cancer Research* **65**:5654–5661.

Moore PF, Woo JC, Vernau W *et al.* (2005) Characterization of feline T cell receptor gamma (TCRG) variable region genes for the molecular diagnosis of feline intestinal T cell lymphoma. *Veterinary Immunology and Immunopathology* **106**:67–178.

Pastor M, Chalvet-Monfray K, Marchal T *et al.* (2009) Genetic and environmental risk indicators in canine non-Hodgkin's lymphomas: breed associations and geographic distribution of 608 cases diagnosed throughout France over 1 year. *Journal of Veterinary Internal Medicine* **23**:301–310.

Pohlman LM, Higginbotham ML, Welles EG *et al.* (2009) Immunophenotypic and histologic classification of 50 cases of feline gastrointestinal lymphoma. *Veterinary Pathology* **46**:259–268.

Ponce F, Marchal T, Magnol JP *et al.* (2010) A morphological study of 608 cases of canine malignant lymphoma in France with a focus on comparative similarities between canine and human lymphoma morphology. *Veterinary Pathology* **47**:414–433.

Roccabianca P, Vernau W, Caniatti M *et al.* (2006) Feline large granular lymphocyte (LGL) lymphoma with secondary leukemia: primary intestinal origin with predominance of a CD3/CD8αα phenotype. *Veterinary Pathology* **43**:15–28.

Stein TJ, Pellin M, Steinberg H *et al.* (2010) Treatment of feline gastrointestinal small-cell lymphoma with chlorambucil and glucocorticoids. *Journal of the American Animal Hospital Association* **46**:413–417.

Tasca S, Carli E, Caldin M *et al.* (2009) Hematologic abnormalities and flow cytometric immunophenotyping results in dogs with hematopoietic neoplasia: 210 cases (2002–2006). *Veterinary Clinical Pathology* **38**:2–12.

Valli VE, Vernau W, De Lorimier L-P *et al.* (2006) Canine indolent nodular lymphoma. *Veterinary Pathology* **43**:241–256.

Valli VE, San Myint M, Barthel A *et al.* (2011) Classification of canine malignant lymphomas according to the World Health Organization criteria. *Veterinary Pathology* **48**:198–211.

Vezzali E, Parodi AL, Marcato PS *et al.* (2010) Histopathologic classification of 171 cases of canine and feline non-Hodgkin lymphoma according to the WHO. *Veterinary and Comparative Oncology* **8**:38–49.

Von Euler HP, Rivera P, Aronsson A-C *et al.* (2008) Monitoring therapy in canine malignant lymphoma and leukemia with serum thymidine kinase 1 activity – evaluation of a new, fully automated non-radiometric assay. *International Journal of Oncology* **34**:505–510.

Weiss ATA, Klopfleisch R, Gruber AD (2010) Prevalence of feline leukaemia provirus DNA in feline lymphomas. *Journal of Feline Medicine and Surgery* **12**:929–935.

Yamazaki J, Takahashi M, Setoguchi A *et al.* (2010) Monitoring of minimal residual disease (MRD) after multidrug chemotherapy and its correlation to outcome in dogs with lymphoma: a proof-of-concept pilot study. *Journal of Veterinary Internal Medicine* **24**:897–903.

14 MULTISYSTEM AND INTERCURRENT IMMUNE-MEDIATED DISEASE

Michael J. Day

INTRODUCTION

The major types of immune-mediated disease (hypersensitivity, autoimmunity, immunodeficiency, immune system neoplasia) are intrinsically linked, and immune-mediated disease of one type may be accompanied by one or more other immunological irregularities, expressed concurrently or sequentially (see Chapter 3, p. 75). For example, dogs with AIHA may subsequently (months to years later) develop other manifestations of autoimmunity (including AITP, autoimmune skin disease or lymphocytic thyroiditis), and atopic dermatitis may be complicated by other allergic disease. This chapter gives examples of multisystem or intercurrent immune-mediated diseases in dogs and cats.

SYSTEMIC LUPUS ERYTHEMATOSUS

Pathogenesis

SLE is the prototype multisystem autoimmune disease; it is at best uncommon in dogs and rare in cats. Numerous criteria for the diagnosis of canine SLE have been proposed (*Table 28*), but the most commonly accepted are that there should be at least two clinical manifestations of autoimmunity supported by laboratory evidence that the processes are immune-mediated, together with high titred serum ANA. Occasionally, animals may only partially satisfy these criteria; for example, by having two autoimmune processes but no serum ANA (approximately 10% of dogs with SLE are reported to be seronegative). Similarly, a syndrome of ANA-positive, immune-mediated polyarthritis and non-specific systemic illness is recognized in the GSD. Such cases may not necessarily be diagnosed as SLE, but they still fall within the same spectrum of disease and are thus considered 'SLE-overlap syndromes'. In similar vein, two studies of canine 'pyrexia of unknown origin' have now concluded that a high proportion of animals with this clinical diagnosis are likely to have an immune-mediated disease and be ANA-positive.

The aetiopathogenesis of SLE is poorly understood, but predisposing factors and immunological mechanisms will be similar to those discussed in Chapter 3. A role for viruses in the induction of canine SLE has been proposed. Antigens that cross-react with c-type retrovirus have been identified on the surface membrane of blood lymphocytes from affected dogs, and the serological abnormalities (but not clinical signs) of SLE can be transferred to normal dogs and mice by administration of cell-free extracts. However, these findings have not been widely corroborated and virus has not been isolated from the tissue of canine SLE patients. The arthropod-borne infectious diseases (particularly leishmaniosis and monocytic ehrlichiosis) are excellent clinical and serological mimics for canine SLE. A recent report described three cats with pyrexia, lethargy, inappetence, polyarthritis, anaemia, thrombocytopenia, neutropenia and serum ANA. In each case the disease was associated with molecular evidence of infection by an *Ehrlichia canis*-like organism and there was clinical response to antimicrobial therapy. ANA has been experimentally induced in dogs with the drug hydralazine. The antithyroid drug propylthiouracil can induce a disease in cats characterized by lethargy, weight loss, lymphadenopathy, Coombs-positive haemolytic anaemia and serum ANA. A similar spectrum of adverse effects is recorded in hyperthyroid cats treated with methimazole or carbimazole. Whilst human SLE is more prevalent in females, there is no clear evidence of gender influence in the dog or cat. SLE generally occurs in middle-aged dogs (age range two months to 13 years) and cats (age range one to 11 years).

Canine SLE is clearly inherited (but not by a simple mechanism) and associations with the MHC (DLA) are documented. Predisposition for GSDs, Shetland Sheepdogs, Collies, Beagles and Poodles is proposed. The earliest colony of dogs with SLE was established by Lewis and Schwartz in 1965. Three inbred lines of dogs were derived from parents with clinical and serological evidence of SLE (*Table 29*). Many offspring developed serum ANA but did not have clinical signs of autoimmune disease, likely due to the relatively young age of the dogs (less than three years) when reported. Thirteen of 33 dogs kept for long-term study developed autoimmune diseases including SLE, RA and lymphocytic thyroiditis. More recently, a colony of GSDs with SLE was established in France (see Chapter 3, p. 80)

Table 28: Diagnostic criteria for systemic lupus erythematosus in the dog. The diagnostic criteria for canine and feline SLE have been modified from those given for humans by the American Rheumatism Association. Three such schemes are presented here as proposed by Drazner (Drazner FH (1980) Systemic lupus erythematosus in the dog. *Compendium on Continuing Education for the Practicing Veterinarian* **2:**243–254); Grindem and Johnson (Grindem CB, Johnson KH (1983) SLE: literature review and report of 42 new canine cases. *Journal of the American Animal Hospital Association* **19:**489–503); and Bennett (Bennett D (1987) Immune-based non-erosive inflammatory joint disease of the dog. 1. Canine systemic lupus erythematosus. *Journal of Small Animal Practice* **28:**871–889).

Drazner	Grindem and Johnson	Bennett
1. Skin disease	*Class I:*	*Class I:*
2. Polyarthritis	1. Serum ANA	1. Serum ANA
3. AIHA		
4. AITP	*Class II:*	*Class II:*
5. Glomerulonephritis	1. Polyarthritis	1. Polyarthritis
6. Myositis	2. Gomerulonephritis	2. AIHA
7. Myocarditis	3. AIHA	3. AITP
8. Interstitial pneumonitis	4. Skin disease	4. Immune leukopenia
	5. Pleuritis/pericarditis/ pneumonitis/myocarditis	5. Glomerulonephritis
		6. Polymyositis
	6. Petichiae (AITP)	7. Skin disease
		8. CNS disease
	Class III:	9. Pleuritis
	1. Generalized lymphadenopathy	10. Gastrointestinal disease
	2. Oral ulcers	
	3. Pyrexia	*Class III:*
	4. Polymyositis	Immunopathological features consistent with clinical signs (e.g. Coombs positive, lupus band)
	5. Convulsions	
	6. Non-haemolytic anaemia	
	7. Hypergammaglobulinaemia	
	8. Hypocomplementaemia	
	9. Cryoglobulinaemia	
Diagnosis requires ANA and one or more of above.	Diagnosis requires Class I with two or more Class II criteria. (NB: other minor Class III criteria were included.)	Definite SLE requires Class I with two or more Class II and Class III; probable SLE requires Class I with two or more Class II.

Table 29: Breeding studies of canine systemic lupus erythematosus. A breeding colony of dogs with SLE was established in 1965 by Lewis and Schwartz (Lewis RM, Schwartz RS (1971) Canine systemic lupus erythematosus: genetic analysis of an established breeding colony. *Journal of Experimental Medicine* **134:**417–437) in which 480 dogs were bred by brother-sister matings within three lines. There was a high incidence of serological abnormality (LE cell positivity and serum ANA) amongst the F1, F2 and F3 progeny and a range of autoimmune diseases developed in selected dogs kept for long-term study.

Line	Sire/dam	Progeny
Line A	Sire: clinically normal GSD Dam: GSD with ragweed hypersensitivity from two years of age; developed Coombs-positive AIHA, proteinuria and serum ANA at four years of age	F1 progeny 57% ANA positive F2 progeny 16% ANA positive

Continues on page 358

Table 29: Breeding studies of canine systemic lupus erythematosus. (*Continued*)

Line	Sire/dam	Progeny
Line B	Sire: developed AITP and serum ANA at three years of age Dam: GSD; developed AIHA; thrombocytopenia, leukopenia and serum ANA at six months of age	F1 progeny 31% ANA positive F2 progeny 45% ANA positive
Line C	Sire: clinically normal Poodle Dam: Poodle; progressive symmetrical polyarthritis, skin disease, leukopenia, hyperglobulinaemia and positive LE cell test from three years of age	F1 progeny 66% ANA positive F2 progeny 10% ANA positive F3 progeny 25% ANA positive

and the same authors reported spontaneously arising SLE in a second colony of GSDs. In this study, association between SLE and expression of the DLA allele DLA A7 was described, in addition to a negative ('protective') association with DLA A1 and DLA B5. An association with the MHC-encoded complement C4 allotype C4,4 has been proposed for an SLE-like disease in the dog characterized by non-erosive polyarthritis, pyrexia and ANA positivity. A genome-wide association study of an SLE-like canine disease is described in Chapter 3. There may be geographical influences (regional gene pools or environmental factors) in the expression of canine SLE.

A novel experimental model of canine SLE has recently been described in which Beagle dogs were repeatedly immunized over a six-week period with heparan sulphate in Freund's adjuvant. Heparan sulphate is a glycosaminoglycan component of the glomerular basement membrane and a target autoantigen for the renal component of SLE. These dogs developed a SLE-like disease characterized by cutaneous changes (alopecia, erythema, crusting, scaling and seborrhea), with lymphoplasmacytic dermal inflammation and BMZ deposition of IgM and complement C3, glomerular damage as assessed by elevated urine protein:creatinine ratio, and elevated serum ANA. The model was used to study the therapeutic potential of a novel peptide-vectored gene therapy, in which a construct encoding the canine CTLA-4 extracellular domain was coupled to canine immunoglobulin heavy chain C_H2-C_H3 domain sequence, and the peptide–gene construct was injected intravenously. CTLA-4 binds with high affinity to the APC co-stimulatory surface molecules CD80/86, thus preventing their ligation by T cell CD28 and activation of the T cell (see Chapter 1, p. 57). In treated dogs there was resolution of the clinical and serological abnormalities described above and the dogs failed to make an immune response to the therapeutic construct.

One study examined the phenotype of blood lymphocytes in 20 dogs with SLE. During active disease there was:

- Marked lymphopenia ($1.05 \pm 0.5 \times 10^9$/l [1,050 ± 500 cells/μl] versus $2.13 \pm 1.0 \times 10^9$/l [2,130 ± 1,000 cells/μl] in controls).
- An imbalance in the CD4:CD8 ratio (5.2 versus 2.25 in controls).
- Increased expression of a T cell activation marker (64% versus 46.5% in controls).

The CD4:CD8 ratio was corrected when treatment induced clinical remission, but remained abnormal in dogs that responded poorly to therapy.

There have been too few reported cases of feline SLE to suggest aetiopathological factors in this species. FeLV and FIV can induce a disease syndrome similar to SLE, and FeLV-infected cats may have serum ANA during early stages of disease. However, cats with true SLE should test negative for both viruses. The majority of cats with SLE have been purebred (Siamese, Persian and Persian-related).

Clinical signs

The spectrum of clinical presentation in SLE is broad, involving lesions of the joints, skin, haemopoietic system, kidneys, muscles, pleura and myocardium. The most commonly recorded manifestations of SLE in the dog and cat are polyarthritis (**727**), mucocutaneous lesions (of the face, ears, oral mucosa and limbs) (**728–731**),

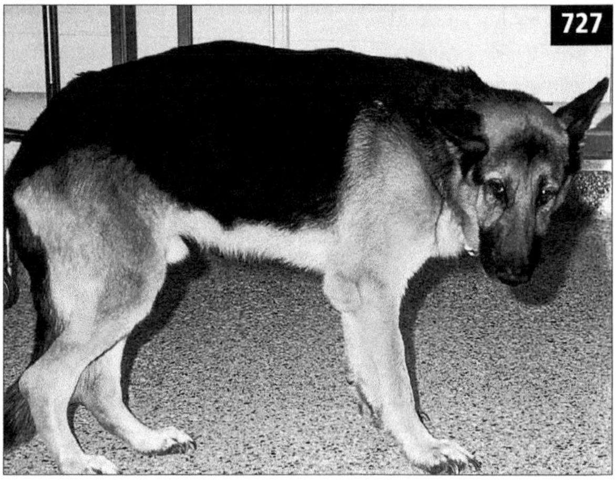

727 Canine systemic lupus erythematosus. A three-year-old male GSD with non-erosive polyarthritis, skin disease, leukopenia, hypergammaglobulinaemia and pyrexia. The dog was ANA positive but negative for serum RF. There was elevation of serum IgG concentration (24 mg/ml), reduced serum complement C4 concentration and normal levels of serum C3. The dog responded to treatment with immunosuppressive doses of glucocorticoids (tapered over 12 weeks) and subsequently went into remission until the disease recurred 284 weeks after initial diagnosis. The dog was maintained on glucocorticoids until it died from congestive heart failure at week 336. (Photograph courtesy W.T. Clark.)

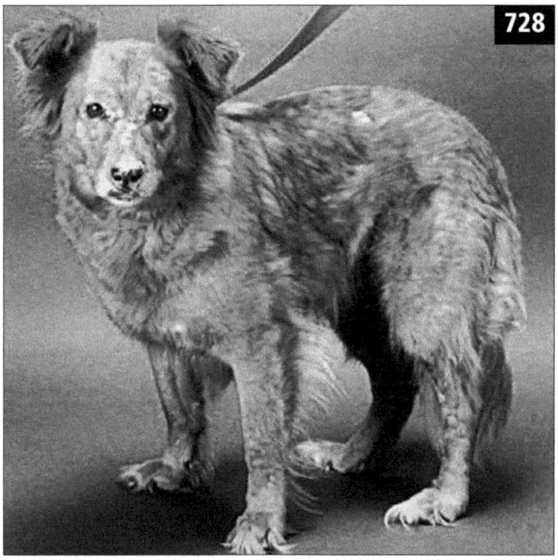

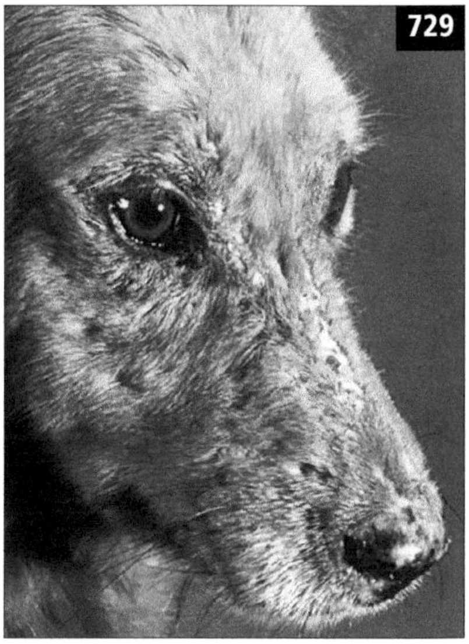

728, 729 Canine systemic lupus erythematosus. This dog has polyarthritis, skin lesions characterized histologically as 'interface dermatitis', glomerulopathy and serum antinuclear antibody. (Photographs courtesy S.E. Shaw.)

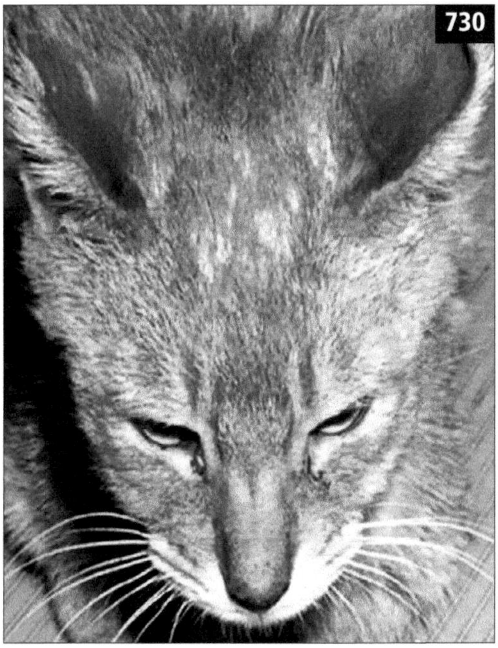

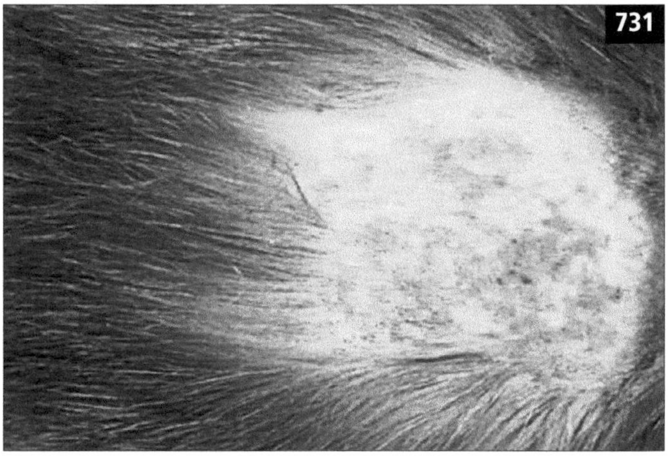

730, 731 Feline systemic lupus erythematosus. This cat has skin lesions characterized histologically as vasculitis, together with thrombocytopenia (presumptively in part immune-mediated), glomerulonephritis and serum antinuclear antibody. (Photographs courtesy S.E. Shaw.)

Table 30: Frequency of clinical findings in systemic lupus erythematosus. Published cases of SLE in 260 dogs and 21 cats were reviewed and the frequency of occurrence of the various clinical manifestations of SLE compiled. In both species, lesions of the joints, skin, kidney and haemopoietic system occur with greatest frequency.

Clinical finding	Dogs (n = 260) Percentage frequency	Cats (n = 21) Percentage frequency
Polyarthritis	75	43
Mucocutaneous lesions	49	48
Glomerular disease (proteinuria)	48	44
AIHA/AITP/leukopenia	43	57
Pleuritis/pericarditis	5.7	0
Neurological signs	4.9	29

proteinuria (glomerular disease) and anaemia or thrombocytopenia (*Table 30*). There are often periods of remission and relapse. Details of each of these individual entities are given elsewhere in this book.

Diagnosis

The complex presentation of SLE necessitates use of wide-ranging diagnostic procedures:

- Haematological profile to identify anaemia or thrombocytopenia, with a Coombs test or tests for platelet autoantibody if indicated. Not all cases of SLE have a Coombs-positive, regenerative, haemolytic anaemia. A proportion present with non-regenerative, Coombs-negative anaemia of chronic disease. Leukopenia may sometimes be present and is presumed to be secondary to the presence of leukocyte autoantibodies. Abnormalities in coagulation pathways may be identified (activated clotting time, activated partial thromboplastin time) due to the presence of 'lupus anticoagulant' anti-phospholipid antibody (see Chapter 4, p. 105).
- Serum biochemistry and urinalysis to identify glomerular immune complex deposition or polymyositis.
- Skin biopsy to demonstrate an interface dermatitis (rarely leukocytoclastic vasculitis or panniculitis) and immunohistochemistry to demonstrate deposition of immunoreactants (IgG, IgM, IgA, complement C3) at the BMZ (the 'lupus band' test). In some cases, interepithelial desmosomal labelling is reported and immunoreactants may also be associated with superficial dermal blood vessels. Positive immunolabelling is only documented within lesional skin of canine SLE, but in human patients, non-lesional skin may be affected. This suggests that immune complex deposition is not the primary causative event in the cutaneous lesions of SLE, which are more likely a manifestation of cytotoxic destruction of epidermal cells by infiltrating T lymphocytes (see Chapter 5, p. 158).
- Radiography to identify the characteristic articular changes of non-erosive polyarthritis with soft tissue swelling (erosive polyarthropathy has been documented in canine SLE).
- Synovial fluid cytology, mucin clot and culture, and synovial biopsy. Synovial fluid abnormalities may be present in animals (particularly cats) without clinical signs of joint disease.

The serological test of greatest importance is the ANA test (see Chapter 6, p. 179). Interpretation of serum ANA should be made with caution. Normal or chronically ill animals may have low titred ANA, but high titre is supportive of autoimmune disease. Animals suspected of having SLE, with clinical evidence of polyarthritis, should also be tested for serum RF (see Chapter 6, p. 178). Measurement of serum complement levels (see Chapter 12, p. 295) and CICs (see Chapter 5, p. 146) may be useful adjunct tests. Serum CH_{50}, as well as levels of C3 and C4 may be decreased due to utilization in

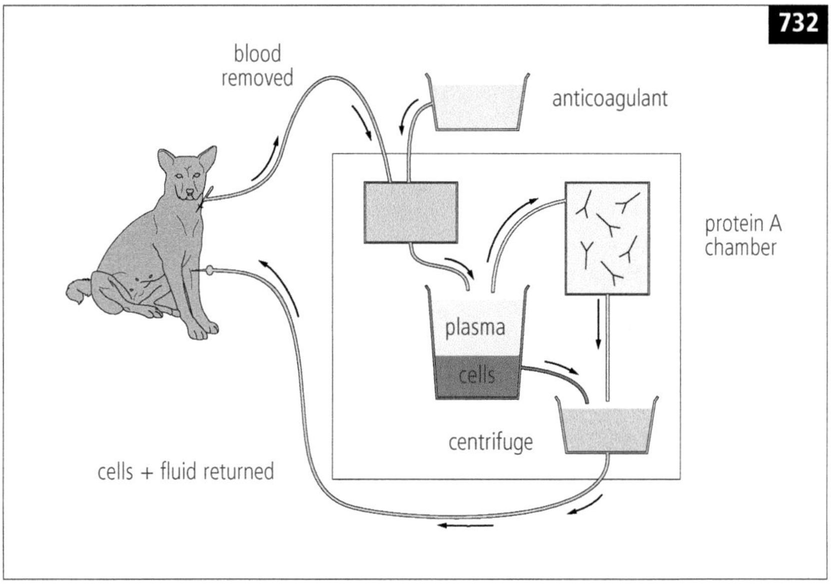

732 Plasmapheresis. Blood is withdrawn from the patient and mixed with anticoagulant before centrifugation to separate plasma from cells. The plasma is passed through staphylococcal protein A immunoadsorption chambers, which removes Ig (autoantibody) and immune complexes. The adsorbed plasma is returned to the patient together with the blood cells. In one case report the procedure was repeated eight times over a 45-day period, treating 1 litre of plasma on each occasion. Following plasmapheresis, serum levels of immune complexes decreased and there was elevation of complement CH_{50} and C3 to normal levels. Serum IgG concentration also decreased initially, with periods of moderate elevation attributed to a 'rebound phenomenon'. (Redrawn after Matus RE, Scott RC, Saal S *et al.* [1983] Plasmapheresis-immunoadsorption for treatment of systemic lupus erythematosus in a dog. *Journal of the American Veterinary Medical Association* **182:**499.)

immune complex clearance. (Hereditary complement component deficiency as documented in humans with SLE has not been reported in the dog.)

Treatment and prognosis

Reported therapy for canine SLE involves supportive care (e.g. dietary management, whole blood or platelet rich plasma transfusion) together with tapered immunosuppressive doses of glucocorticoids with or without cytotoxic drugs. The immunomodulatory drug levamisole was reported in one study to produce long-term remission in over 50% of dogs with SLE when administered at 3–7 mg/kg every 48 hours (to a maximum of 140 mg/dog) in combination with prednisolone (1–2 mg/kg q24h). Prednisolone is tapered over 1–2 months then discontinued, and levamisole is given continuously for four months then stopped. If disease recurs, levamisole alone is given for a further four-month period. However, there is little good scientific basis for the use of levamisole in this context and administration of this drug is often associated with cutaneous drug eruptions that may be immune-mediated in nature. Dogs with SLE have been treated by plasmapheresis (**732**) in combination with low dose prednisone, and ciclosporin has been successfully employed in the treatment of refractory cases.

Cats with SLE have been treated successfully with glucocorticoids (prednisolone) alone or in combination with cyclophosphamide or chlorambucil. More aggressive therapy is warranted when the presentation includes renal disease.

A range of parameters should be monitored in animals with SLE:

- CBC.
- Urinalysis.
- Synovial fluid analysis.
- Serum ANA. Autoantibody levels may fall with clinical improvement, but some animals may have persistent low titred serum ANA.

Table 31: Serial monitoring of canine systemic lupus erythematosus. Serial laboratory data from the case described in **727**. Serum complement C4 concentration was reduced at the time of initial diagnosis, returned to normal level with immunosuppressive therapy, and subsequently decreased when maintenance glucocorticoids were withdrawn. The dog remained ANA positive throughout the period of spontaneous remission from clinical signs.

Weeks after initial diagnosis	Serum C3 (normal ≥ 66 units)	Serum C4 (normal ≥ 65 units)	ANA	Treatment
0	>100	41	+	Immunosuppressive glucocorticoids initiated
11	>100	65	+	Maintenance glucocorticoids
70	>100	48	+	No treatment
147	>100	75	+	No treatment
336	>100	>100	Negative	Glucocorticoids reinstituted at week 284. Pre-euthanasia sample

733
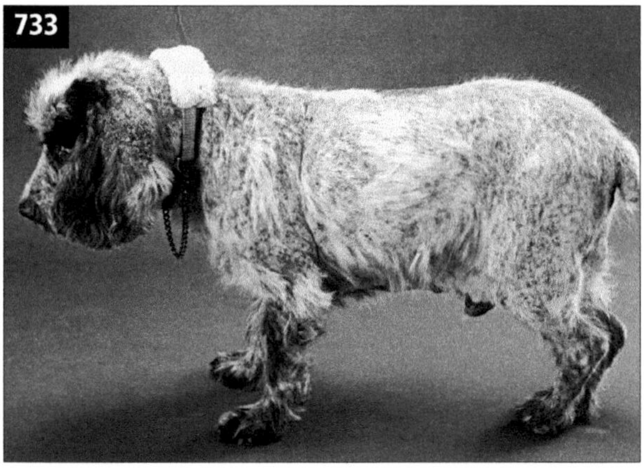

734
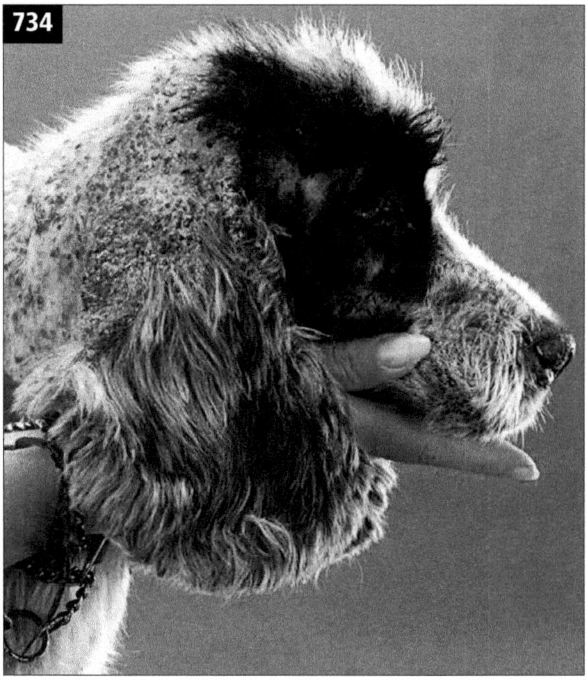

735
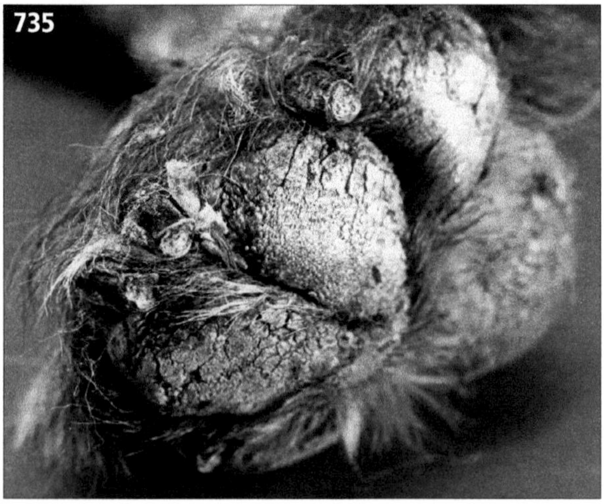

733–735 Autoimmunity and lymphoma. A seven-year-old male English Cocker Spaniel with keratoconjunctivitis sicca, pemphigus foliaceus (as shown in this series of photographs, and positive on immunohistochemistry for intraepidermal IgG deposition), lymphadenitis, Coombs-positive IMHA and presumptive IMTP. The dog had elevated concentration of serum IgG (26 mg/ml), was negative for serum rheumatoid factor, but had high titred (10,240) serum antinuclear antibody. The dog was successfully treated with immunosuppressive glucocorticoids, but seven months later developed B cell lymphoma. In this case the lymphoma may always have been present (but subclinical) or may have arisen subsequent to the multisystemic autoimmune disease (SLE). (From Foster AP, Sturgess CP, Gould DJ *et al.* [2000] Pemphigus foliaceus in association with systemic lupus erythematosus with subsequent lymphoma in a Cocker Spaniel dog. *Journal of Small Animal Practice* **41**:266–270, with permission.)

- CICs.
- Serum complement levels (*Table 31*). Normalization of serum CH_{50} with treatment is also recorded for feline SLE.

Immunosuppressive therapy may result in clinical remission, but affected animals should be monitored for recurrence. The long-term survival of dogs with SLE has not been well documented, but many cases have died from renal failure or secondary infection within 12 months of diagnosis.

AUTOIMMUNITY AND LYMPHOMA

Canine lymphoma may be associated with concurrent autoimmune disease (733–735). The US Veterinary Medical Data Program has been used to determine the concordance of lymphoma with lupus disorders, pemphigus disorders, autoimmune polyarthritis and IMHA or IMTP. In this study only dogs with IMTP had an increased odds ratio for the occurrence of lymphoma, but lymphoma is a well-recognized 'trigger-factor' for canine IMHA. Moreover, immune-mediated blood dyscrasias have also been documented in association with multiple myeloma, haemangiosarcoma and myeloproliferative disease in the dog (736–738). The mechanisms underlying such associations are not defined, but they may relate to loss of immunoregulatory cells following effacement of lymphoid structure by the tumour or production of cytokine or polyclonal immunoglobulin synthesis by the neoplastic lymphoid cells. In human medicine a subset of B cell

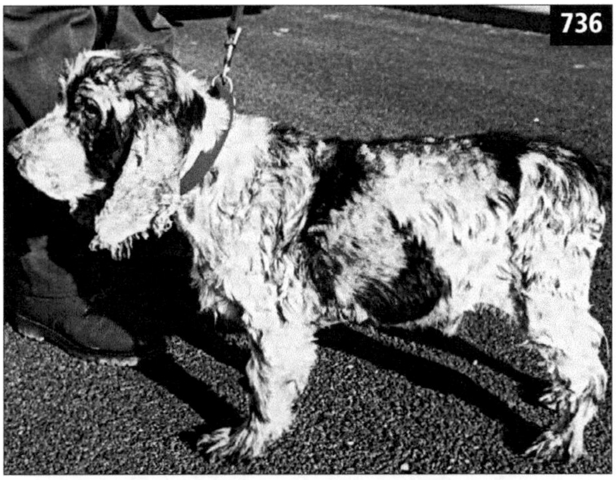

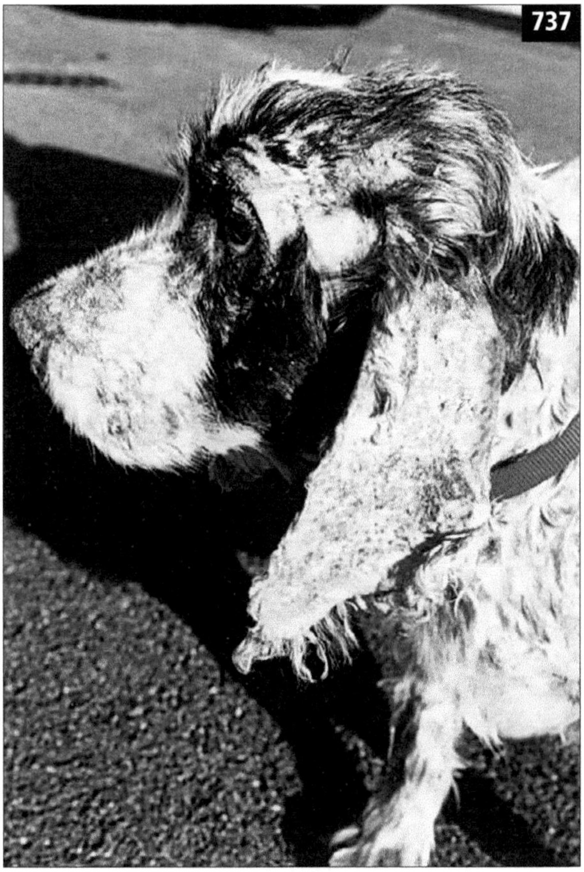

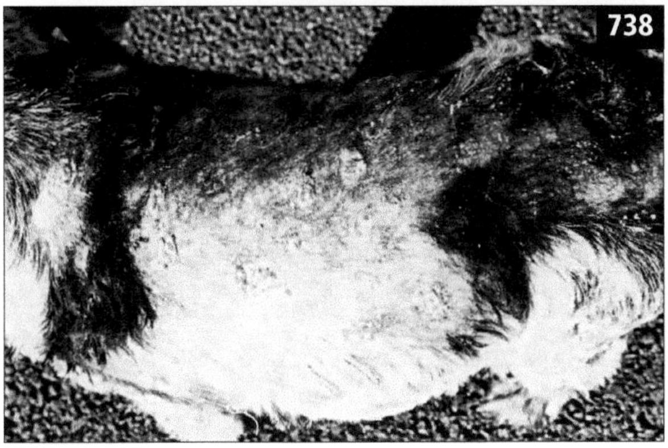

736–738 Autoimmunity and myeloproliferative disease. An eight-year-old male English Cocker Spaniel with pemphigus foliaceus (as shown in the photographs), Coombs-positive IMHA and presumptive IMTP. The dog was negative for serum antinuclear antibody. There was leukocytosis with circulating atypical cells and bone marrow aspiration suggested granulocytic leukaemia. The underlying neoplasia may have acted as a trigger for immune-mediated disease in this case.

lymphoma that is characterized by expression of CD5 is associated with IMHA, and the neoplastic cells are proposed to be the source of the autoantibody. In splenic haemangiosarcoma it is possible that traumatic fragmentation of erythrocytes leads to exposure of previously 'cryptic' erythrocyte membrane antigens, with subsequent triggering of autoimmunity.

MYASTHENIA GRAVIS AND THYMOMA

In humans and dogs there is a well-recognized association between myasthenia gravis (see Chapter 6, p. 193) and thymoma (see Chapter 15, p. 370), with or without concurrent polymyositis or non-thymic neoplasia (lymphoma, pulmonary adenocarcinoma, haemangiosarcoma). The association between thymoma and myasthenia may relate to expression of AChR by thymic myoid cells and titin epitopes by thymic epithelial cells, with the thymus acting as a site for sensitization of autoreactive T lymphocytes. Intrathymic expression of these self-epitopes may be triggered by prior viral infection. The occurrence of non-thymic neoplasia may relate to failure of immune surveillance. Five dogs have been reported with generalized myasthenia (including megaoesophagus and AChR antibody) and concurrent hypothyroidism (diagnosed by the TSH response test), with evidence of either polyneuropathy or polymyopathy in three cases. Thyroid disease (hyper- or hypothyroidism) is also recognized in human myasthenics, and the close embryological origin of the thyroid and thymus may permit expression of AChRs within the thyroid and initiation of an autoimmune response.

Thymoma-associated myasthenia is most commonly reported in GSDs and the clinical presentation relates both to the space-occupying nature of the mediastinal tumour (dyspnoea, regurgitation, dysphagia, cardiopulmonary dysfunction) and to the effects of localized (megaoesophagus) or generalized myasthenia (739, 740). Specific diagnostic tests for myasthenia gravis have been described (see Chapter 6, p. 194) and the diagnosis of thymoma may require thoracic imaging and thymic biopsy.

Concurrent thymoma and myasthenia gravis carries a poor clinical prognosis. The mean survival time of dogs with thymoma and myasthenia after surgical removal of the tumour is reported as

739

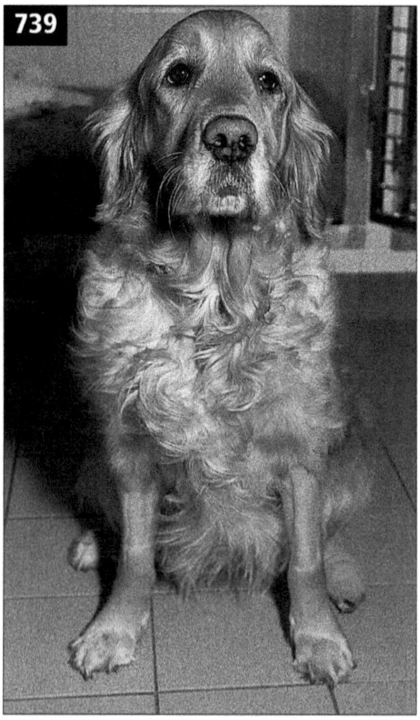

740

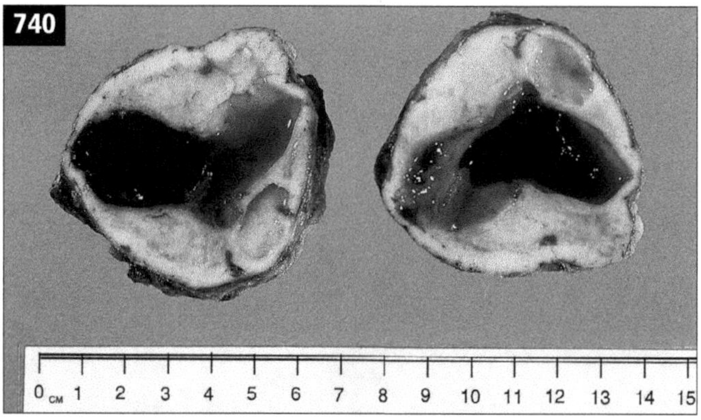

739, 740 Thymoma and myasthenia gravis in a dog. (**739**) A four-year-old Golden Retriever with clinical signs referable to megaoesophagus. An anterior mediastinal mass was identified on imaging examination and a Tru-cut biopsy confirmed that this was thymoma. The dog had an AChR autoantibody titre of 4.06 nmol/l (normal <0.6 nmol/l). The mass was surgically resected (**740**) and a cross-section (shown here) reveals a necrotic and haemorrhagic centre, surrounded by cream-coloured tumour tissue.

16 days (but individual dogs survive for up to 22 months), whereas the mean survival time for dogs with uncomplicated thymoma is 19 months. Most dogs die from postsurgical, megaoesophagus-related aspiration pneumonia, and AChR antibodies may persist, and often increase, after thymectomy. In one dog, removal of the thymoma resulted in resolution of the megaoesophagus, but there was persistence of high titred AChR autoantibodies and the dog died of a generalized, inflammatory myopathy 71 days after surgery. In one further case a dog developed myasthenia only after surgical removal of a thymoma, and in another case thymectomy resulted in localized myasthenia becoming generalized.

In cats, myasthenia gravis has been associated with thymoma and with cystic change within the thymus. Feline thymoma is also associated with a syndrome of polymyositis and myocarditis, or with polymyositis alone, or with progressive interface dermatitis (741, 742). A cat with cystic thymus was reported to have pemphigus foliaceus (see Chapter 5, p. 150) and a cat with thymic amyloidosis had superficial necrotizing dermatitis.

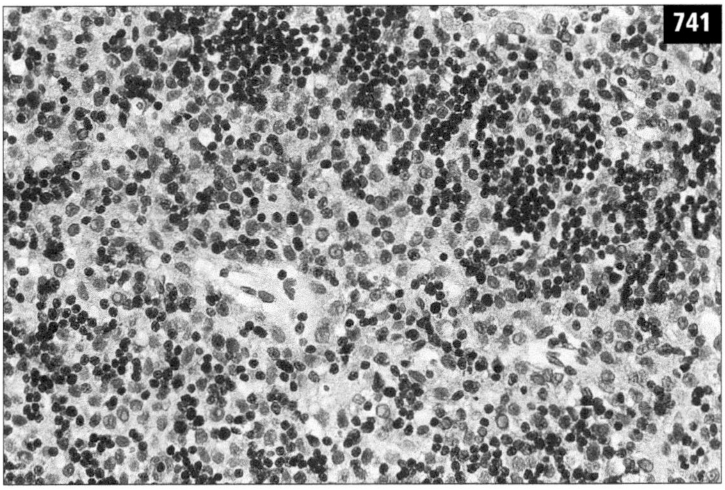
741

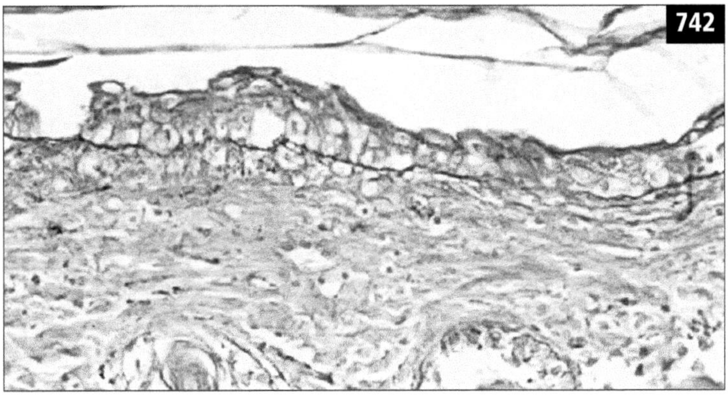
742

741, 742 Thymoma and interface dermatitis in a cat. (**741**) Core biopsy of thymus from a seven-year-old Siamese cat with thymoma and generalized crusting dermatitis. There is a population of neoplastic epithelioid cells, with focal aggregates of small lymphocytes. (From Day MJ [1997] A review of thymic pathology in 30 cats and 36 dogs. *Journal of Small Animal Practice* **38**:393–403, with permission.) (**742**) Affected skin had a mixed, mononuclear interface dermatitis with hydropic vacuolation of basal epithelial cells, extending to follicular epithelium. Immunohistochemical studies revealed the presence of IgG deposits at the BMZ.

743

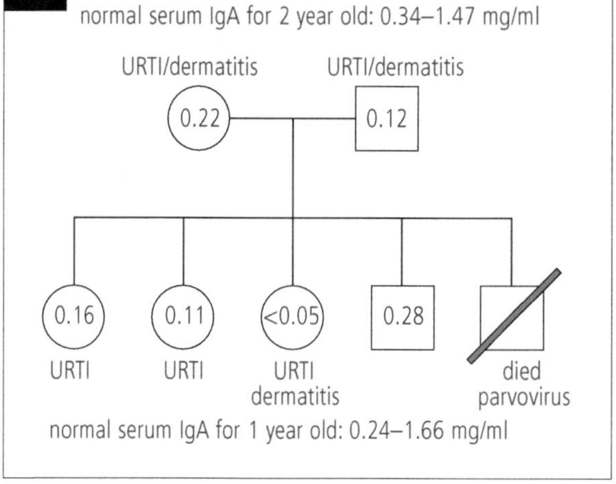

743 IgA deficiency in the dog. Family from a large colony of Beagles in which 1% of animals had undetectable serum IgA and 8% had reduced concentration of serum IgA. Affected animals had evidence of upper respiratory tract infection, dermatitis and serum rheumatoid factor. In this family, both sire and dam had upper respiratory tract infection and dermatitis, with reduced concentration of serum IgA. Three of the four offspring that survived to one year of age also had reduced serum IgA and clinical evidence of infection. (Data from Felsburg PJ, Glickman LT, Jezyk PF [1985] Selective IgA deficiency in the dog. *Clinical Immunology and Immunopathology* **36:**297–305.)

744

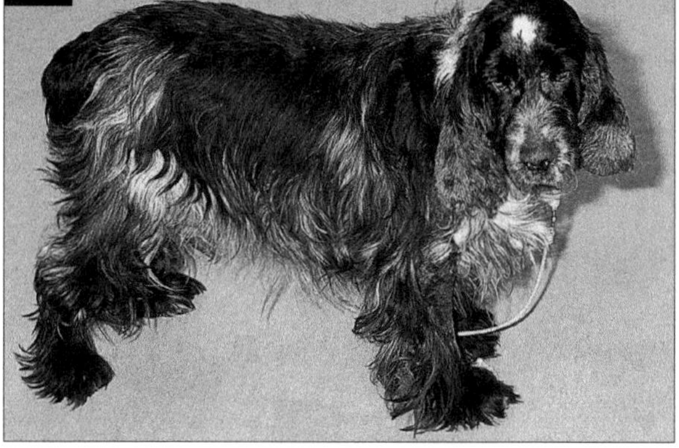

745

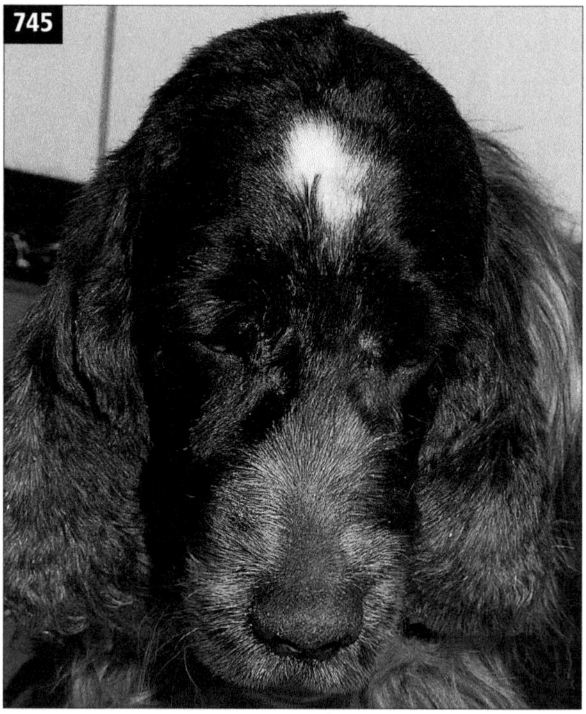

744, 745 Inherited IgA deficiency and autoimmunity. An English Cocker Spaniel from the kennel described in **746** and **747**. This seven-year-old bitch presented with acute onset, Coombs-positive haemolytic anaemia that responded to an immunosuppressive dose of glucocorticoids. There was elevated serum IgG (22 mg/ml), but no abnormality in serum IgM, IgA, C3 or C4 concentration, and the dog was negative for serum ANA. (**744**) Two years later the dog was represented with clinical signs of lethargy, obesity, alopecia and facial myxoedema (**745**). Hypothyroidism was diagnosed and confirmed as lymphocytic thyroiditis at necropsy examination. There was no abnormality in serum C3 or C4 concentration, but there was a significant serum titre of ANA.

IgA DEFICIENCY, HYPERSENSITIVITY AND AUTOIMMUNITY

IgA deficiency (see Chapter 12, p. 302) may lead to inadequate mucosal or cutaneous defence, with ensuing infectious disease. Additionally, reduced mucosal IgA concentration may enhance exposure to allergens, resulting in hypersensitivity disease, or to microbes that may trigger autoimmunity by bearing cross-reactive epitopes, expressing HSPs or acting as superantigens (see Chapter 3, p. 81).

There are several examples of such associations in the dog. Beagles with IgA deficiency (**743**) often have chronic upper respiratory tract infection and dermatitis. Some affected dogs have serum RF, although clinical autoimmunity is not present. Autoimmune disease (lymphocytic thyroiditis, lymphocytic orchitis, polyarteritis nodosa) is not uncommon in such Beagle colonies, and association with IgA deficiency may warrant further investigation.

A colony of English Cocker Spaniels has been described in which there was evidence of inherited idiopathic cardiomyopathy associated with anti-mitochondrial antibodies and other sporadic immune-mediated disease (lymphocytic thyroiditis, hypoadrenocorticism with lymphocytic infiltration of atrophic cortex, SLE, lymphoma) in different lines of inbred dogs (**744, 745**). In both lines there was also inheritance of serum ANA and reduced serum IgA concentration (**746, 747**).

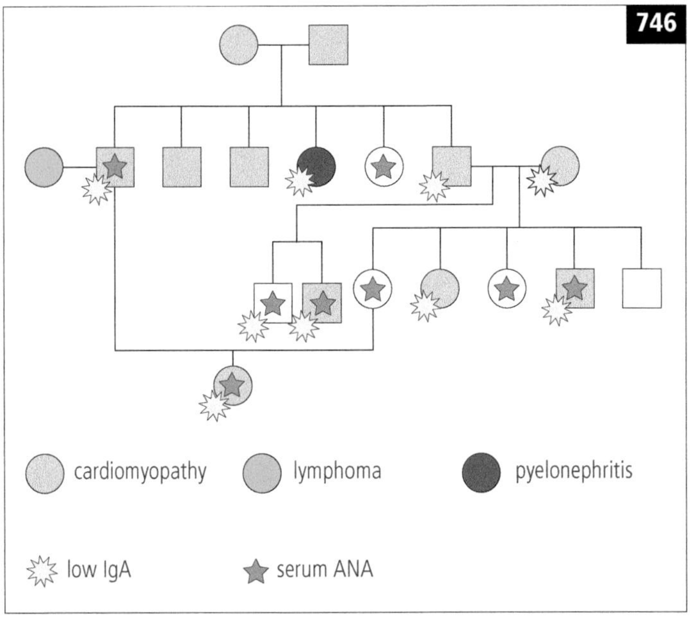

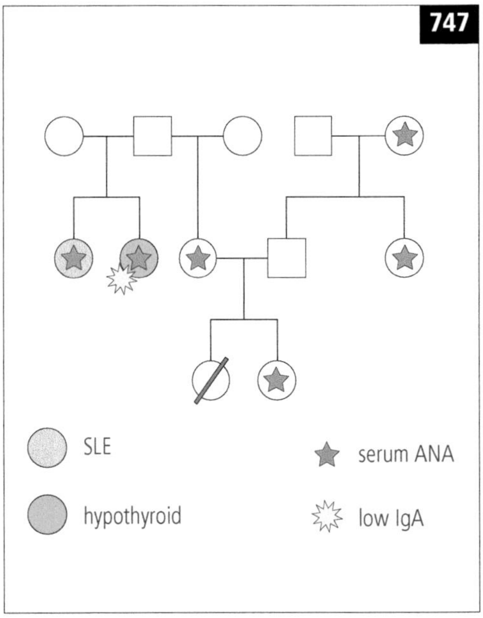

746, 747 Inherited IgA deficiency and autoimmunity. (**746**) Pedigree of English Cocker Spaniels with an idiopathic cardiomyopathy inherited through three generations. The cardiomyopathy may have an immune-mediated basis, as anti-mitochondrial antibodies are demonstrated in the serum of affected dogs. Dogs with cardiomyopathy and clinically normal dogs have either or both reduced serum IgA and serum ANA, and these abnormalities are present amongst four different litters. (**747**) Pedigree of a second breeding line from the same kennel. In these dogs there is no evidence of cardiomyopathy, but two siblings from one litter have autoimmune disease (SLE and hypothyroidism) associated with serum ANA (in both) and reduced serum IgA (in one). Related dogs that are clinically normal also have serum ANA. (Data from Day MJ [1996] Inheritance of serum autoantibody, reduced serum immunoglobulin A and autoimmune disease in a canine breeding colony. *Veterinary Immunology and Immunopathology* **53**:207–219.)

FURTHER READING

Choi E-W, Shin H-S, Youn H-Y *et al.* (2005) Gene therapy using non-viral peptide vector in a canine systemic lupus erythematosus model. *Veterinary Immunology and Immunopathology* **103**:223–233.

Foster AP, Sturgess CP, Gould DJ *et al.* (2000) Pemphigus foliaceus in association with systemic lupus erythematosus with subsequent lymphoma in a Cocker Spaniel dog. *Journal of Small Animal Practice* **41**:266–270.

Mellor PJ, Roulois AJA, Day MJ *et al.* (2005) Neutrophilic dermatitis and immune-mediated haematological disorders in a dog: suspected adverse reaction to carprofen. *Journal of Small Animal Practice* **46**:237–242.

Smee NM, Harkin KR, Wilkerson MJ (2007) Measurement of serum antinuclear antibody titer in dogs with and without systemic lupus erythematosus: 120 cases (1997–2005). *Journal of the American Veterinary Medical Association* **230**:180–1183.

15 DISEASES OF LYMPHOID TISSUE

Michael J. Day

INTRODUCTION

The major encapsulated lymphoid tissues (lymph nodes, spleen and thymus) may be involved in many primary immune-mediated diseases. In addition, these tissues are often the site of inflammatory, traumatic, developmental or neoplastic diseases that do not necessarily have an immunological pathogenesis. These diseases are summarized in this chapter.

DISEASES OF THE THYMUS

The overall prevalence of thymic disease in the dog and cat is summarized in *Table 32*. The thymus reaches maximum size during the neonatal period and involutes with age, so thymic tissue may be inapparent on necropsy of adult animals. In the Beagle, progressive thymic involution occurs between six and 23 months of age. Nodular hyperplasia of one or more thymic lobules has been reported in adult animals. The presence of secondary B cell follicles (follicular hyperplasia) (748) has been documented in dogs with AIHA and SLE; however, one study of experimental Beagles has suggested that such follicles are a normal feature of the canine thymus.

Table 32: Thymic pathology in the cat and dog. Breakdown of different forms of thymic disease recorded in dogs and cats over a 13-year period by a diagnostic histopathology laboratory. Thymic disease represented only 0.29% of diagnoses made in this time (n = 22,362). Thymic lymphoma was more commonly recognized in the cat, whereas thymoma was more frequently diagnosed in the dog. (Data from Day MJ (1997) Review of thymic pathology in 30 cats and 36 dogs. *Journal of Small Animal Practice* **38:**393–403.)

Diagnosis	**Cat**	**Dog**
Thymic lymphoma	19	12
Thymoma	5	18
Thymic cysts	1	4
Thymic hyperplasia	2	
Thymic hypoplasia	1	1
Thymic amyloidosis	1	
Thymic haemorrhage	1	1
Total	**30**	**36**

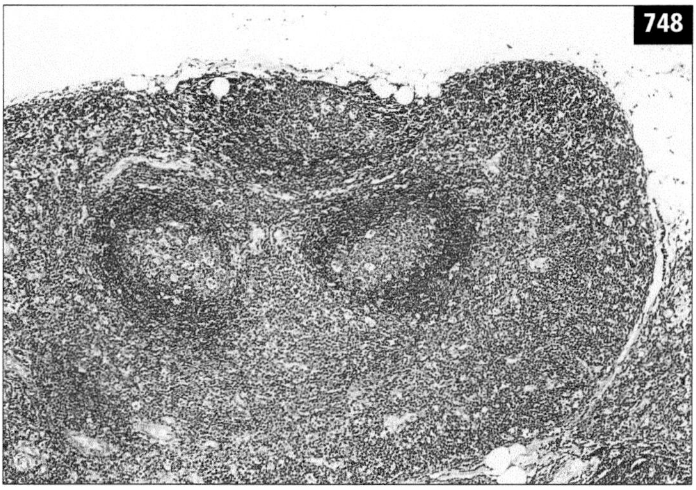

748 Thymic follicular hyperplasia. Section of thymus from a ten-year-old DSH cat with thymic enlargement. There is retention of normal thymic microarchitecture, but there are numerous lymphoid follicles with a distinct mantle zone and germinal centre at the corticomedullary junction.

Developmental abnormalities of the thymus lead to post-weaning immunodeficiency disease. Spontaneous thymic hypoplasia may occur in neonatal kittens (749–751), and thymic abnormalities may develop in dogs with X-SCID, Weimaraner pups or Mexican Hairless dogs (see Chapter 12). Thymic enlargement due to branchial cyst formation is recorded in the dog and cat (752).

Viral disease (e.g. FIE, FeLV, CDV, CPV) may cause thymic hypoplasia or atrophy as part of generalized lymphoid depletion. In such cases there is marked reduction in thymocyte numbers, with a residual rim of cortical thymocytes and prominent Hassall's corpuscles and stromal tissue (753). Thymic repopulation may occur in the chronic stages of distemper.

THYMOMA

Thymoma is a neoplasm of thymic epithelial cells that is generally associated with concurrent benign proliferation of lymphoid cells. Either of these two components may predominate within the tumour to form 'epithelial' or 'lymphoid' thymoma (754, 755). The epithelial cells may range in cytological appearance from epithelioid to spindle, to 'clear cells' with non-staining cytoplasm. The mitotic rate of thymoma is generally low, but rare

749

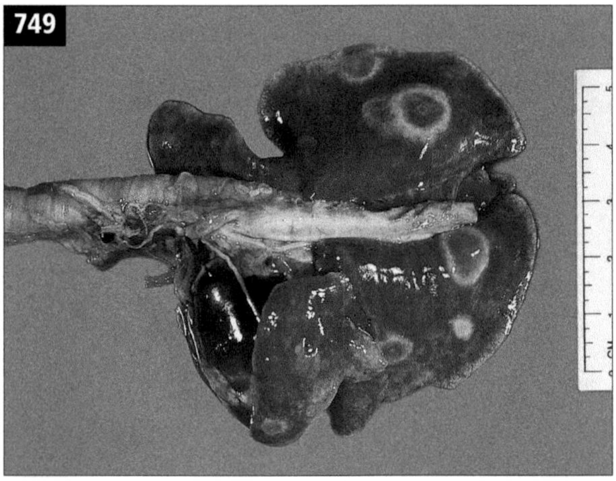

750

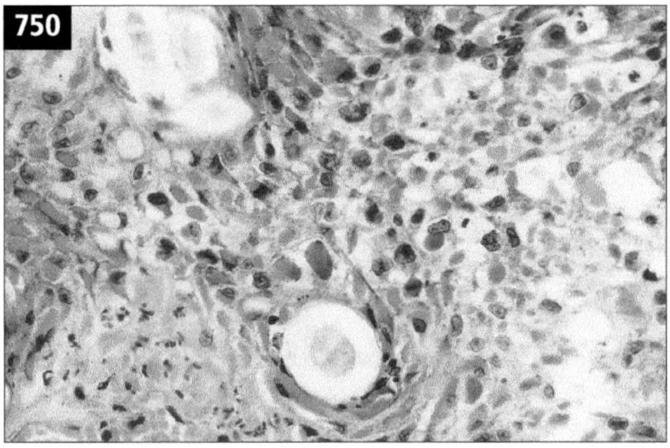

751

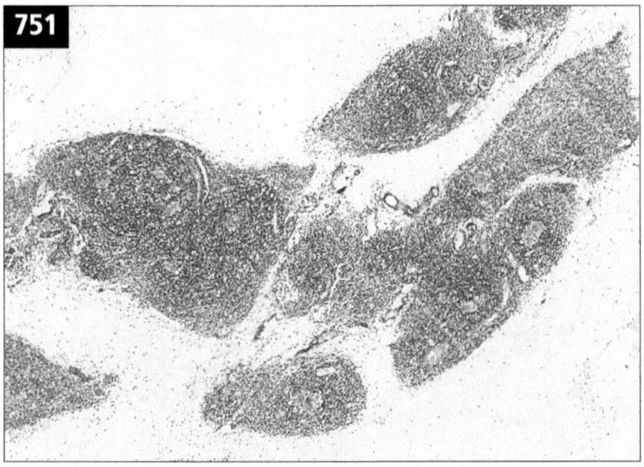

749–751 Thymic hypoplasia in the kitten. (**749**) Thoracic contents from a three-month-old DSH kitten with respiratory disease and generalized, nodular to ulcerative skin lesions. Multiple, cream coloured 'target' lesions are scattered throughout all lung lobes. Histopathological examination reveals widespread bronchopneumonia, with pox virus inclusions in macrophages and bronchial epithelia. The hyperplastic to ulcerative skin lesions also contain numerous pox virus inclusions (**750**). The findings were consistent with systemic pox virus infection. (**751**) Section of thymus from this kitten. The thymus was not grossly visible and this represents a section through anterior mediastinal adipose tissue. The entire thymus is present on this slide and consists only of a collection of small lobules with prominent Hassall's corpuscles. This change was not attributed to generalized lymphoid depletion, as there was marked follicular hyperplasia within the spleen and lymph nodes. It may be an example of primary, congenital thymic hypoplasia, with secondary, systemic viral infection.

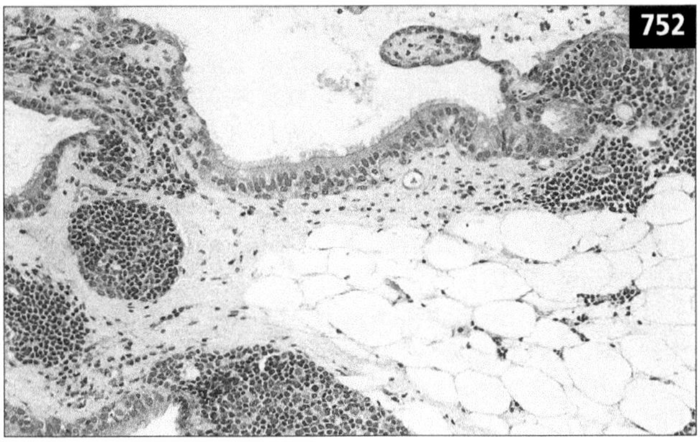

752 Thymic branchial cysts. Section of thymus from an 11-year-old Golden Retriever with a history of pericardial effusion. There is branchial cyst formation within the thymus, the cysts being lined by a columnar or pseudostratified, ciliated epithelium and separated by a connective tissue matrix containing small aggregates of mixed lymphoid cells.

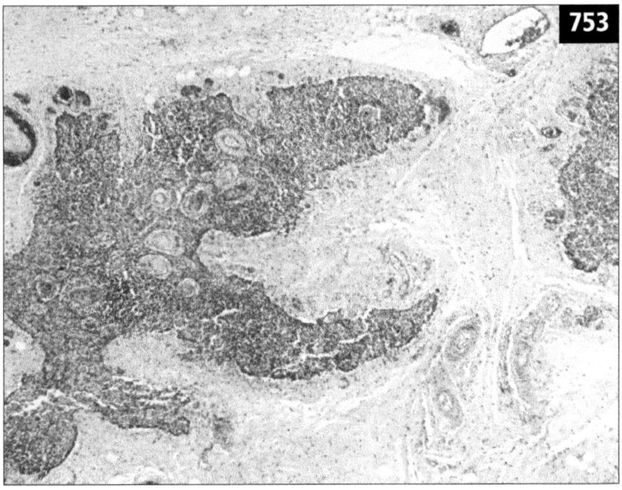

753 Thymic lymphoid depletion. Section of thymus from a puppy with canine parvovirus infection. There is marked reduction in the amount of thymic tissue, with lymphoid depletion of lobules leaving prominent residual Hassall's corpuscles.

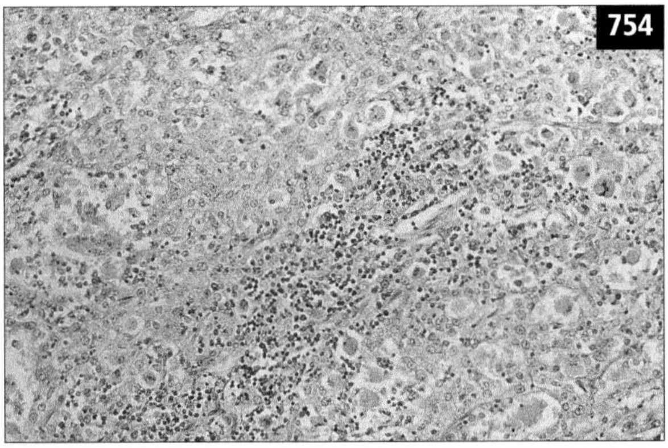

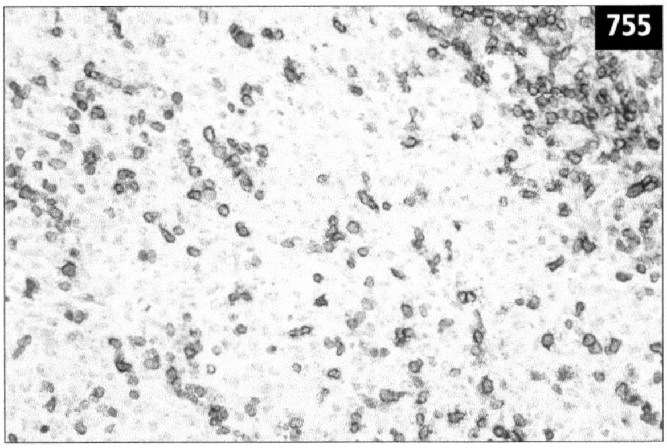

754, 755 Histology of thymoma. (**754**) Section from an anterior mediastinal mass in an 11-year-old Corgi-cross with recurrent thoracic effusion. There is a diffuse sheet of neoplastic epithelial cells, with occasional small clusters of lymphocytes (epithelial thymoma). (**755**) Immunohistochemical labelling for CD3 defines the positively labelled T lymphocytes amidst the unlabelled neoplastic thymic epithelial cells in the background.

cases of malignant thymoma may be locally invasive and disseminate widely throughout the body (756–758). Scattered melanocytes, mast cells or eosinophils may be recognized in thymoma (759), and mast cells appear within the normal feline thymus. Occasional thymomas have cystic spaces lined by attenuated, sometimes ciliated, epithelium (760).

Thymoma is uncommon in the dog and rare in the cat. Older dogs and cats, and GSDs and Labrador Retrievers are more frequently affected. Cats with thymoma are usually FeLV negative. The tumours are generally slow growing, encapsulated and multinodular (761, 762), and they may cause:

- Caudal displacement or compression of heart and lungs, with dyspnoea or tachypnoea.
- Protrusion through the thoracic inlet into the ventral neck.
- Subcutaneous oedema of ventral neck, pleural effusion.
- Oesophageal displacement with regurgitation or dysphagia.

A staging system has been described:

- Stage I: growth within the thymic capsule.
- Stage II: pericapsular spread to mediastinal fat, pleura or pericardium.
- Stage III: infiltration of surrounding organs or intrathoracic metastasis.
- Stage IV: extrathoracic metastasis.

Thymoma may also be associated with paraneoplastic effects including:

- Hypercalcaemia.
- Myasthenia gravis, polymyositis, myocarditis or immune-mediated skin disease (see Chapter 6, p. 193 and Chapter 14, p. 364).

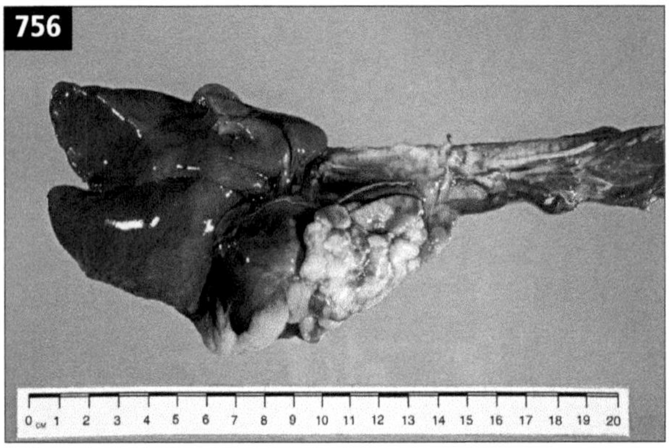

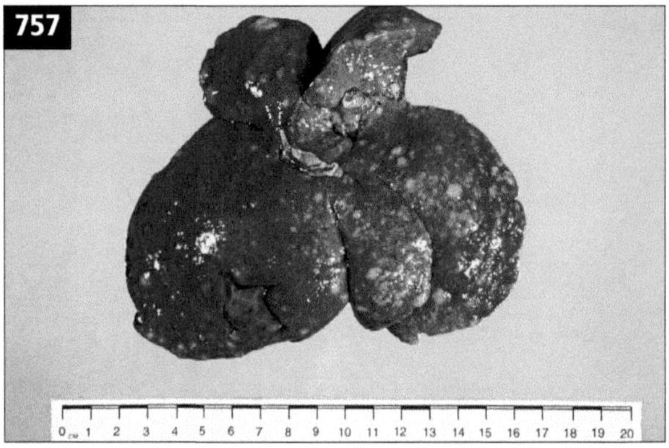

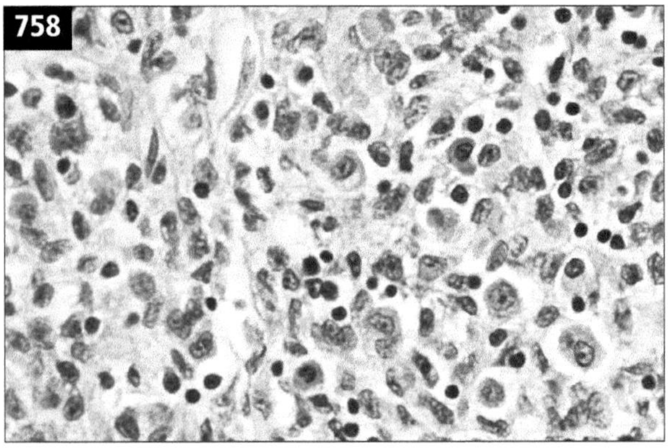

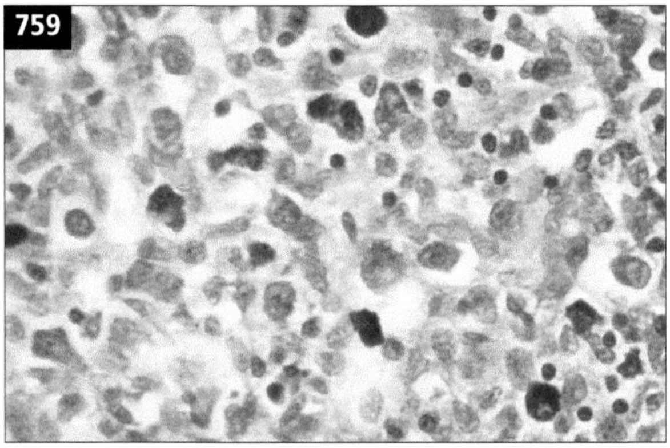

756–759 Malignant thymoma. A 16-year-old neutered female DSH cat was euthanased following a brief history of non-specific anorexia and lethargy. On necropsy examination there was a large, cream-coloured, multinodular anterior mediastinal mass (**756**) with diffusely scattered cream nodular masses within the liver (**757**). Microscopic examination of both sites revealed the presence of a pleomorphic population of spindle cells consistent with malignant thymoma (thymic carcinoma) (**758**). Toluidine blue-stained mast cells are scattered throughout the neoplastic population in both the thymus and liver (**759**).

Diagnosis of thymic disease

Differential diagnosis of thymic enlargement may involve:

- Thoracic imaging.
- Cytological examination of thoracic fluid or fine needle aspirate from the lesion (763).
- Thymic needle core biopsy taken under ultrasound guidance. Immunohistochemical studies have demonstrated that the neoplastic epithelia in feline thymoma express cytokeratins; in canine thymoma the neoplastic epithelia express cytokeratins and MHC class II.
- FeLV/FIV testing in the cat.
- Identification of paraneoplastic effects.

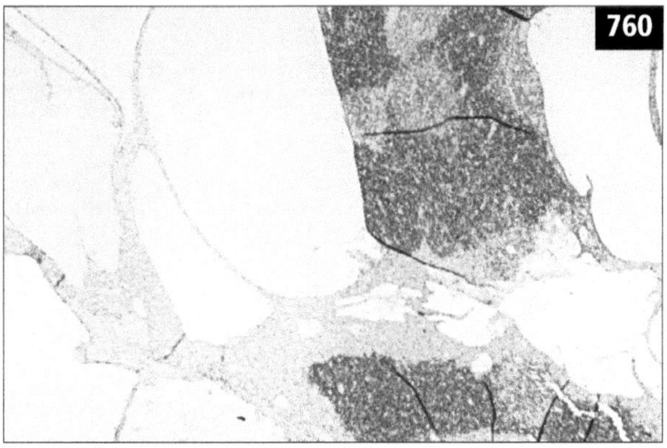

760 Cystic thymoma. Section of thymoma from a cat in which there were numerous cystic spaces lined by columnar ciliated epithelium consistent with branchial origin.

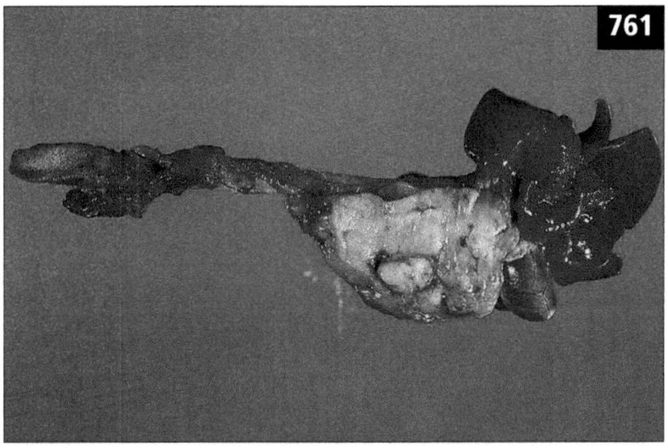

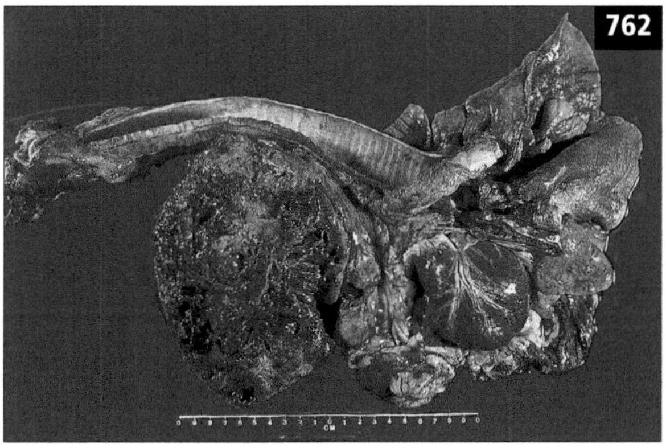

761, 762 Thymoma. (**761**) Thymoma in a 14-year-old Siamese cat with progressive dyspnoea and coughing. (From Day MJ [1997] A review of thymic pathology in 30 cats and 36 dogs. *Journal of Small Animal Practice* **38:**393–403, with permission.) (**762**) Thymoma in a 12-year-old GSD with dyspnoea and pleural effusion. In each case the anterior mediastinal mass causes caudal displacement of the heart and lungs; dorsal displacement of trachea and oesophagus is evident in the canine sample.

763 Cytological appearance of thymoma. Fine needle aspirate taken from the anterior mediastinal mass of the cat described in **761**. Within a background of blood and adipocytes, there is a scattering of large epithelial cells with occasional small lymphocytes. Needle core biopsy subsequently confirmed that this was a thymoma.

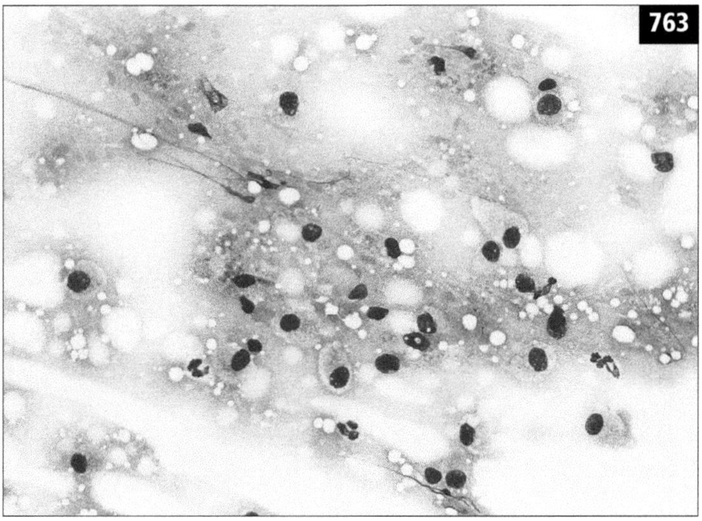

Treatment and prognosis

Management of thymoma may involve surgical excision of the tumour in combination with chemotherapy when complete removal is not possible. Management of paraneoplastic disease (e.g. myasthenia gravis) may be required. The prognosis for stage I thymoma without paraneoplastic disease is favourable.

LYMPH NODE DISEASES

Generalized lymphadenopathy (lymphadenomegaly), with or without other non-specific signs, is not an uncommon clinical presentation in dogs and cats. The most important differential is between lymphoma (see Chapter 13, p. 318) and other causes of lymph node enlargement, although feline lymphoma infrequently presents as generalized lymphadenopathy. A survey of canine primary lymphadenopathy demonstrated that lymphoma was the major cause of such presentation, but almost 40% of cases had other lymph node diseases (*Table 33*). Although the major abnormality of lymph nodes is enlargement, reduced size may occur in senile atrophy, with generalized lymphoid depletion in viral disease, stages of FIV infection or hyperadrenocorticism.

REACTIVE HYPERPLASIA

The most important cause of benign lymphadenopathy is the reactive hyperplasia that occurs as part of an immune response in infection, neoplasia or immune-mediated disease, or following vaccination (**764**). A range of histological and cytological changes characterize reactive hyperplasia (**765–769**). Two distinct feline idiopathic lymphadenopathy syndromes are documented:

- Young cats (five months to two years of age) with distorted lymph node microarchitecture (proliferation of macrophages, lymphocytes and plasma cells in the paracortex). These cats had either resolution, persistence or recurrence of lymphadenopathy. Most were positive for FeLV and one subsequently developed lymphoma.

Table 33: Causes of lymphadenopathy. The causes of primary, regional or generalized lymphadenopathy in 448 dogs from the UK are presented. The single most common cause of canine lymphadenopathy was lymphoma, but almost 40% of cases had other disease underlying this clinical presentation. Benign, reactive hyperplasia or lymphadenitis (with or without associated mineral deposition) were the second most frequent diagnoses. In some dogs there was gross evidence of lymph node enlargement, but no histological abnormality was found on biopsy. (Data from Day MJ, Whitbread TJ (1995) Pathological diagnoses in dogs with lymph node enlargement *Veterinary Record* **136**:72–73.)

Disease	Percentage of dogs (n = 448)
Lymphoma	62.5
Reactive hyperplasia	13
Metastatic neoplasia	9
Other pathology (mostly lymphadenitis)	7
Mineral-associated lymphadenopathy	6
Normal lymph node histology	2.5

764

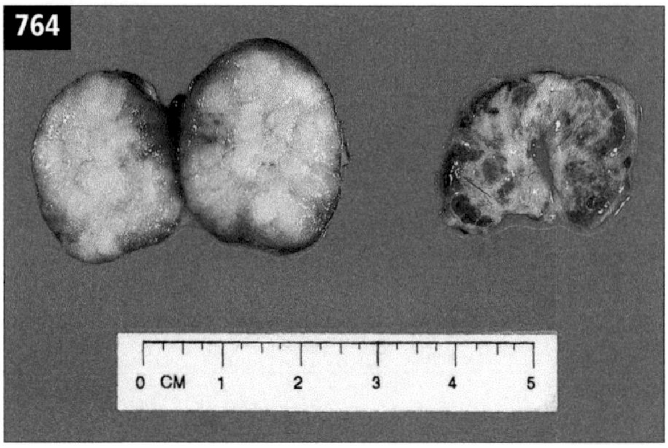

764 Metastatic neoplasia versus reactive hyperplasia of lymph nodes. Two palpably enlarged, hemisectioned peripheral lymph nodes from dogs. The one on the left has normal lymph node structure effaced by metastatic tumour (anaplastic sarcoma), with widespread distribution throughout the body. The lymph node on the right has microscopic evidence of reactive hyperplasia and gross corticomedullary distinction is preserved.

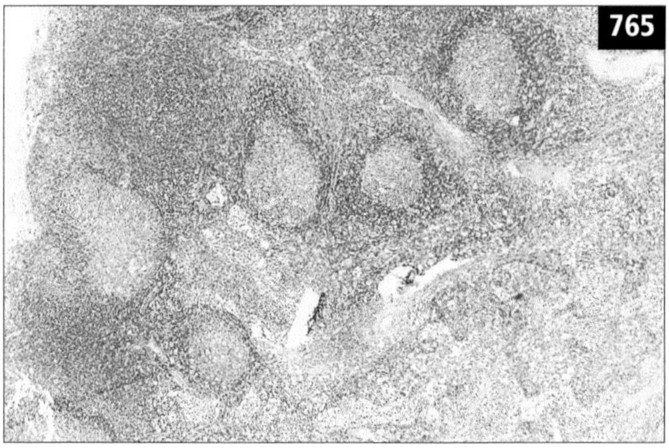

765 Reactive hyperplasia of lymph node. Reactive hyperplasia of a canine lymph node. There are numerous secondary follicles that orientate towards the medullary region, together with expansion of the paracortex and dilation and increased cellularity of the medullary sinuses.

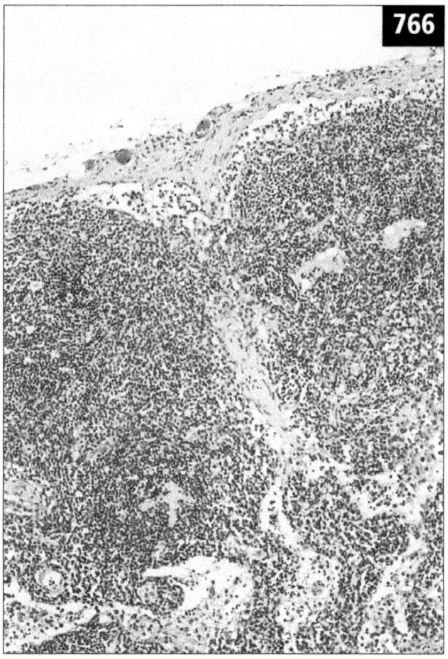

766 Sinus dilation in reactive hyperplasia. Section of lymph node from a cat with microscopic features of reactive hyperplasia. There is prominent dilation of the subcapsular and medullary sinuses and numerous macrophages are found within these channels (sinus histiocytosis). This is indicative of active transport of tissue-derived antigen to the draining lymph node in afferent lymph.

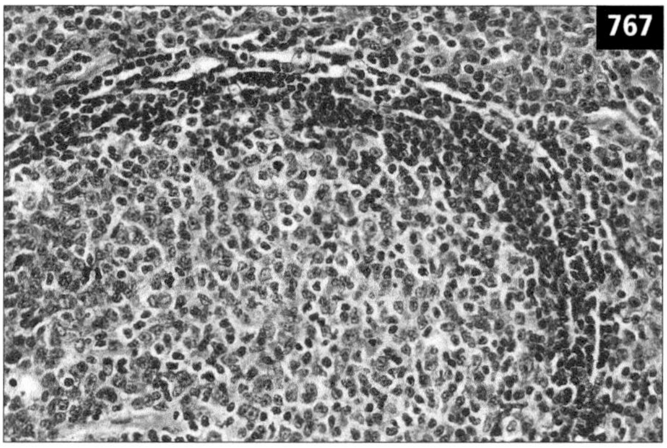

767 Follicular hyperplasia. The lymph node described in **766** also contained numerous secondary follicles, with an active germinal centre and surrounding mantle zone. These were often orientated towards and extending into the medullary region of the lymph node.

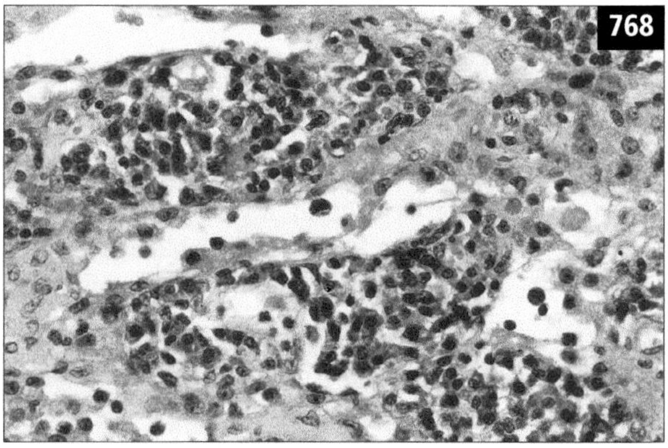

768 Expansion of medullary cords. The medullary cords in the lymph node described in **766** were expanded by mature plasma cells. Active lymph nodes may be a source of production of serum antibody. This accompanies a tissue immune response mediated by activated lymphoid cells that 'home' back to the inflamed tissue from the site of activation in the lymph node.

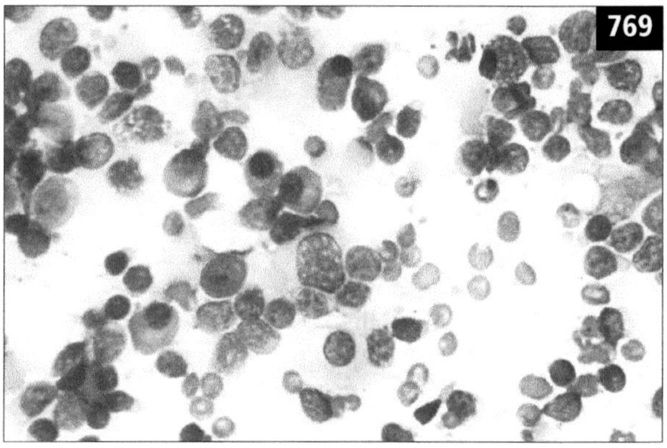

769 Cytology of nodal reactive hyperplasia. Fine needle aspirate from a dog with submandibular lymph node enlargement due to reactive hyperplasia. Small lymphocytes and lymphoblasts are present, but in this sample there is a dominant population of plasma cells.

- Young cats (1–4 years of age) with generalized lymphadenopathy and some histological features of lymphoma (expansion of paracortex and cortex by uniform, mitotic lymphocytes, and abnormal follicular aggregates), with other non-specific changes (reactive follicles, mixed cellularity of sinuses) within the same lymph node. These cats were FeLV negative and the lymphadenopathy resolved in 12–84 months.

LYMPHADENITIS

Lymph node enlargement may occur due to inflammation within the node (lymphadenitis). Lymphadenitis is generally secondary to infectious (e.g. *Mycobacterium*, *Leishmania*, *Bartonella*) or inflammatory disease in the site drained by the lymph node (770–776). Occasionally, aetiological agents cannot be identified by histochemical staining, culture or PCR of tissue and the process is

770
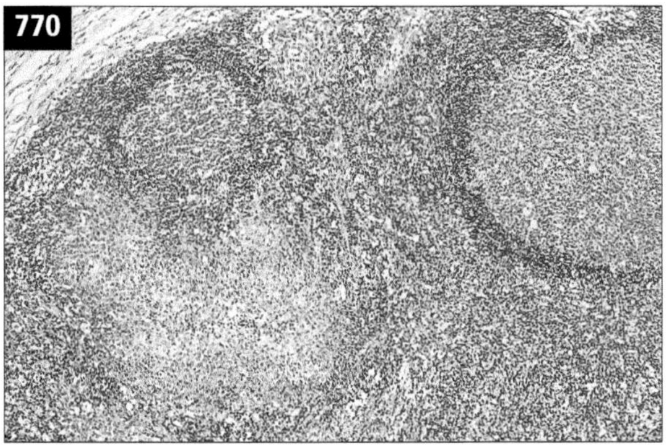

770 Lymphadenitis. Section of lymph node from a three-year-old Whippet with oral ulceration and submandibular lymphadenopathy. There is reactive change in this lymph node as evidenced by the formation of secondary lymphoid follicles; however, the area on the left is one of several zones of necrosis and mixed pyogranulomatous inflammation. Special stains did not reveal a specific aetiological agent in this case, and there was no evidence of crystalline material.

771
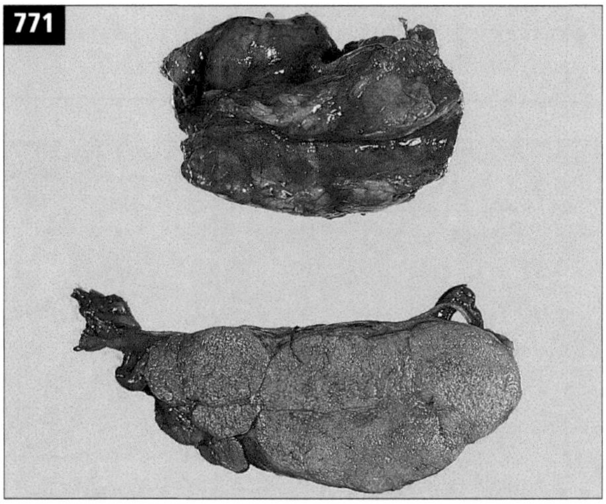

771 Fungal lymphadenitis. Enlarged lymph nodes from a GSD with disseminated aspergillosis (see Chapter 12, p. 304). Normal corticomedullary structure is replaced by coalescing granulomata centred upon hyphal elements of *Aspergillus terreus*. (Photograph courtesy Pathology Unit, Murdoch University.)

772
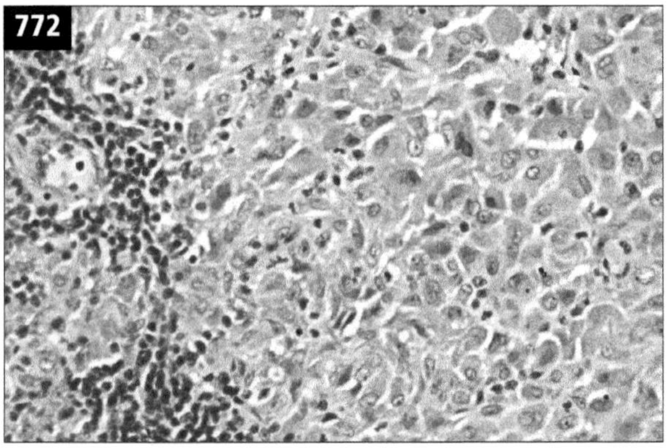

773
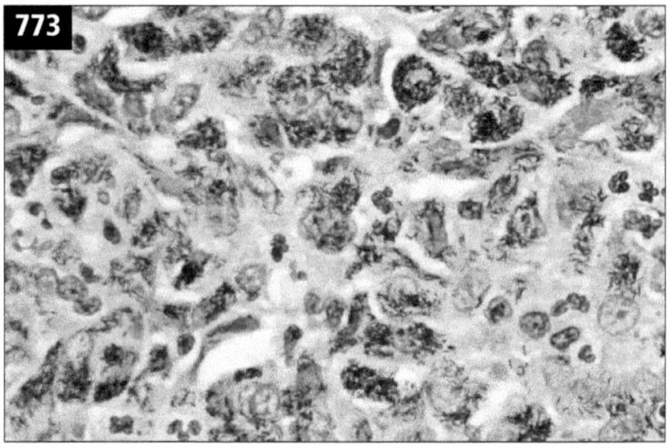

772, 773 Mycobacterial lymphadenitis. Section of lymph node from a four-year-old DSH with generalized lymphadenomegaly. There is a dense granulomatous inflammatory reaction throughout the node, with only marginal lymphoid cells remaining. ZN staining reveals these macrophages to contain large numbers of acid-fast bacteria.

described as a 'sterile lymphadenitis'. Recently, in the UK, a syndrome of 'sterile granulomatous lymphadenitis' has been recognized in English Springer Spaniels and this breed may also develop a sterile granulomatous disease of the skin, sclera and liver (777). Lymphadenitis may be acute, with microscopic evidence of oedema, hyperaemia, neutrophil extravasation and necrosis; in the chronic form there may be diffuse granulomatous inflammation, microgranulomas or fibrosis (granulation tissue).

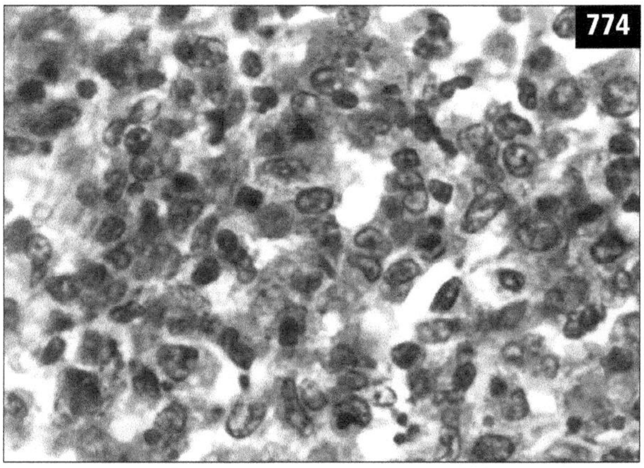

774 Leishmaniosis. Section of lymph node from an eight-year-old Greyhound dog imported from Italy into the UK. The dog had cutaneous and renal disease, with marked hypergammaglobulinaemia. On necropsy examination *Leishmania* organisms were identified in skin, lymph nodes and spleen. In this section of lymph node there is a granulomatous inflammatory focus, and amastigotes are present in the cytoplasm of some macrophages.

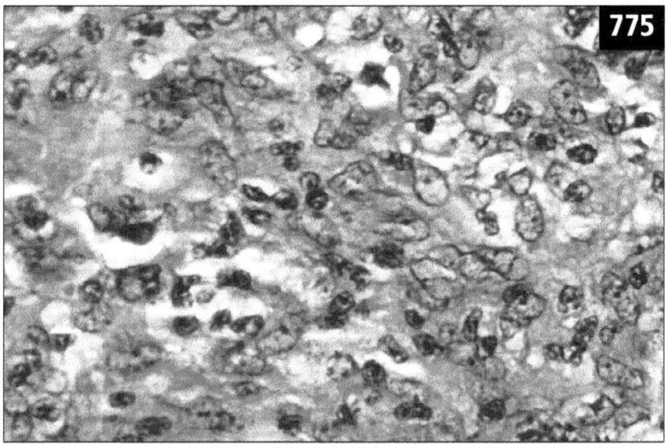

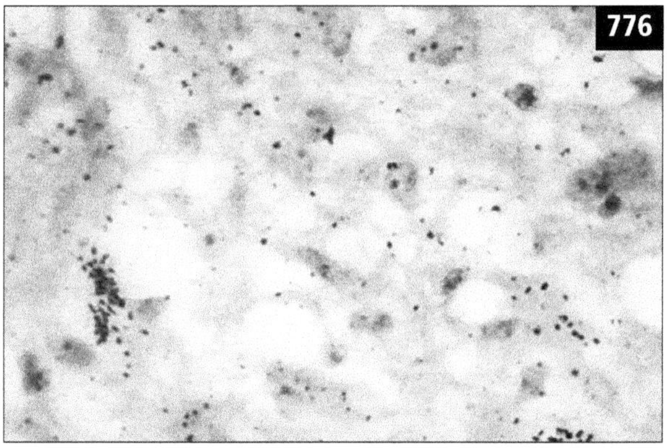

775, 776 Bartonellosis. Section of lymph node from a dog with granulomatous lymphadenopathy attributed to *Bartonella* infection (**775**). A serial section stained by Warthin–Starry silver stain reveals the presence of small colonies of organisms consistent with *Bartonella* (**776**).

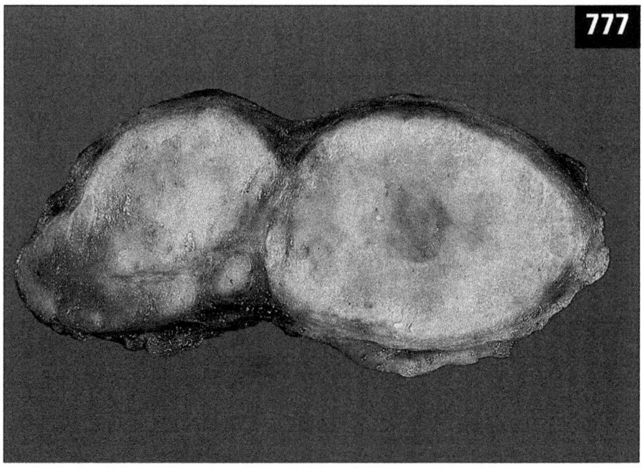

777 Sterile lymphadenitis. Sectioned submandibular lymph node from a five-month-old English Springer Spaniel. The cut surface demonstrates effacement of normal corticomedullary structure. Microscopically there is a diffuse sheet of admixed macrophages and neutrophils, but no specific aetiological agent was identified.

MINERAL-ASSOCIATED LYMPHADENOPATHY

Mineral-associated lymphadenopathy is a significant cause of primary lymph node disease of dogs in the UK. In this condition, large quantities of birefringent crystalline material accumulate within peripheral lymph nodes (most frequently the prescapular, axillary or popliteal) and induce a granulomatous response that may, in severe cases, obliterate normal lymph node structure (778, 779). Affected lymph nodes are often orange-brown in colour due to haemorrhage and accumulation of haemosiderin within sinus histiocytes (780).

The crystals range from small, dark, needle-like fragments (5–10 μm) within the cytoplasm of sinus macrophages, to large, angular, translucent and birefringent extracellular crystals (50 μm) in the midst of the granulomatous reaction (**781–784**). Electron-microprobe analysis has demonstrated the complex chemical nature of these crystals, which commonly contain Si, S, Cu, Ca, Al and P, and occasionally include Na, K, Fe, Mg, Ti, Ni or Cr (785). Similar crystals may be found within the lungs of dogs with or without mineral-associated lymphadenopathy. These are located in

778

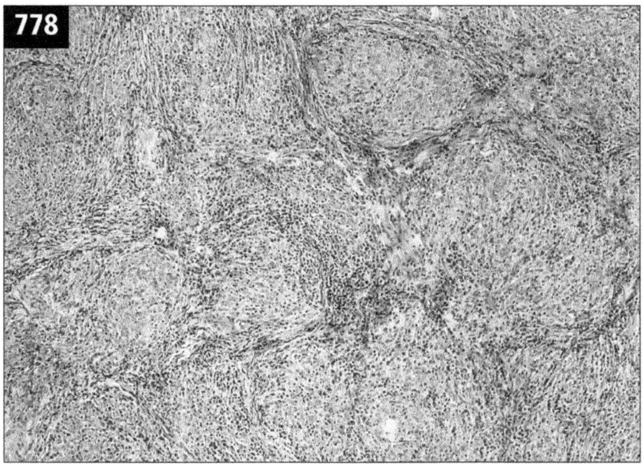

779

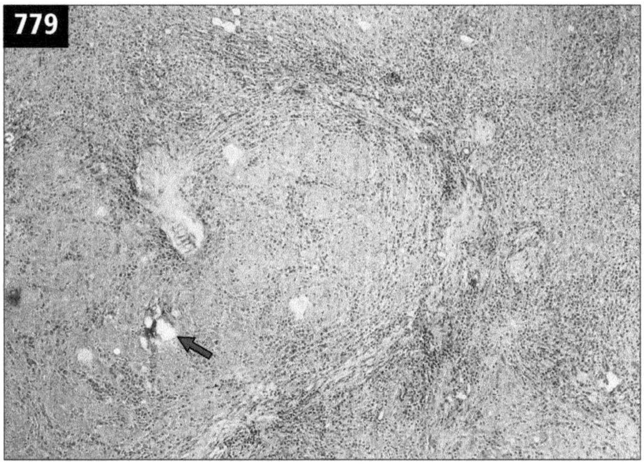

778, 779 Mineral-associated lymphadenopathy. (**778**) Section of lymph node from a ten-year-old Spaniel with generalized lymphadenopathy and pyrexia. Normal lymph node structure is effaced by a series of coalescing microgranulomas with peripheral fibrous connective tissue. (**779**) Under polarized light, large extracellular, birefringent crystalline fragments are seen (arrowed).

780

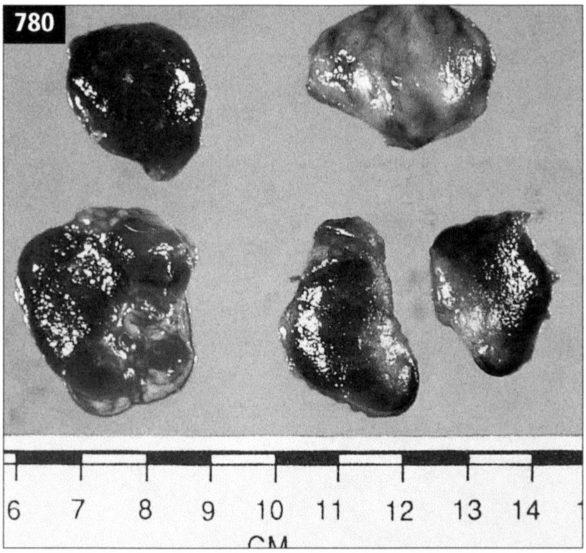

780 Mineral-associated lymphadenopathy. Prescapular, presternal and hilar lymph nodes from a 12-year-old German Shorthaired Pointer with chemodectoma and mineral material within lymph nodes and peribronchial mineral aggregates in the lung. The lymph nodes are enlarged and they are orange-red in colour due to the presence of haemorrhage and haemosiderin deposition.

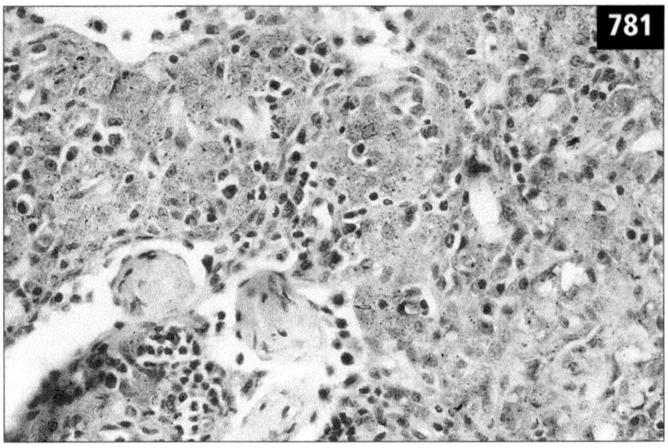

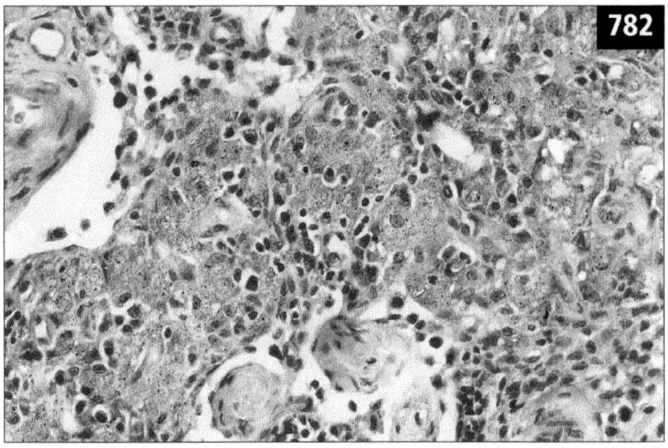

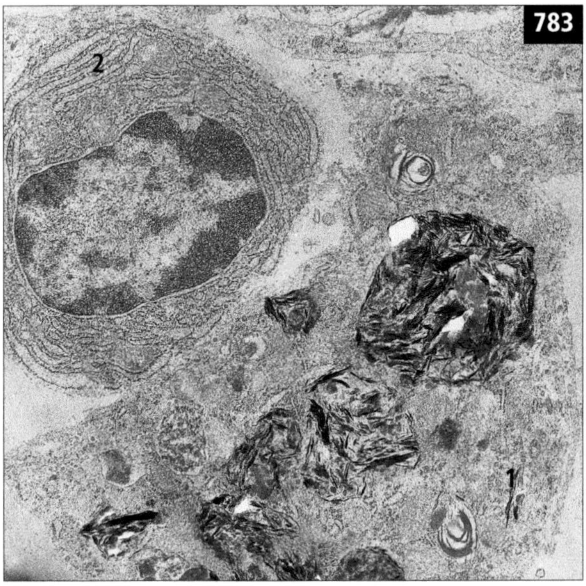

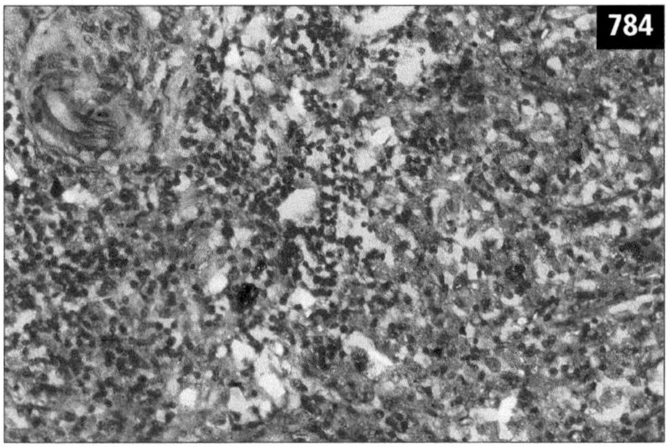

781–784 Mineral-associated lymphadenopathy. (**781**) Section of medullary region of a lymph node from a dog with Coombs-positive AIHA and generalized lymphadenopathy. There are numerous macrophages with markedly enlarged cytoplasm, each containing numerous small, needle-like crystalline fragments with some larger, extracellular crystals. (**782**) Under polarized light, many of these crystals are birefringent. (**783**) Transmission electron micrograph of a macrophage (1) from such a lymph node, with distinct cytoplasmic compartments that are filled by needle-like crystalline fragments. A plasma cell (2) is adjacent. (**784**) Section of lymph node from a seven-year-old English Springer Spaniel with scirrhous adenocarcinoma metastatic to prescapular lymph node; the section also contains large quantities of birefringent crystalline material (polarized light microscopy).

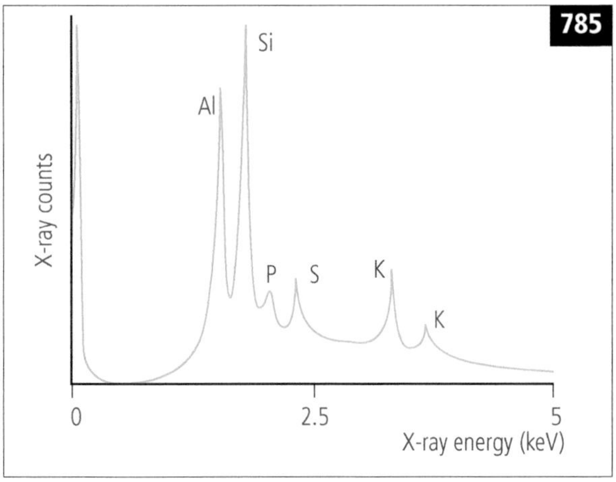

785 Mineral-associated lymphadenopathy. Electron microprobe analysis of a single crystal within the lymph node of a dog with mineral-associated lymphadenopathy. Numerous elements are identified within the crystal, and individual crystals within the same lymph nodes produce a different spectrum of elemental composition. (From Day MJ, Pearson GR, Lucke VM *et al.* (1996) Lesions associated with mineral deposition in the lymph node and lung of the dog. *Veterinary Pathology* **33**:29–42, with permission.)

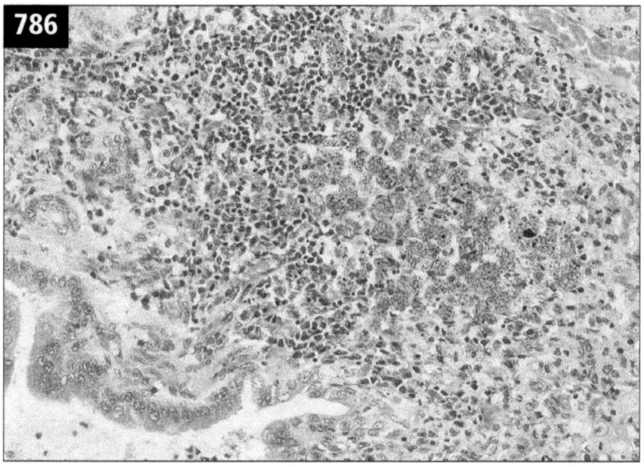

786 Peribronchiolar mineral deposition. Section of lung from a dog with aspiration pneumonia and prominent peribronchiolar lymphoplasmacytic aggregation. As an incidental finding there is a cluster of peribronchiolar macrophages with expanded cytoplasm that contain quantities of birefringent crystal fragments. These are likely to have been inhaled and may translocate to regional lymph nodes.

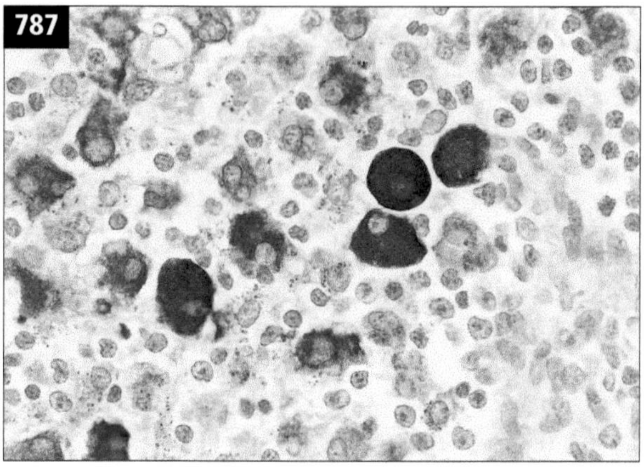

787 Cytokine expression in mineral associated lymphadenopathy. Section of popliteal lymph node from a five-year-old Rottweiler with mineral-associated lymphadenopathy. Macrophages within a medullary area of mineral deposition express cytoplasmic TNFα, as demonstrated by immunohistochemistry with specific antiserum to this cytokine. Phagocytosis of mineral may induce the production of an array of inflammatory cytokines (TNFα, IL-1, IL-6) by activated macrophages, and these in turn may underlie the onset of non-specific clinical signs such as pyrexia in affected dogs.

peribronchiolar regions and are often associated with anthracotic deposits (786). The analyses suggest that many of the minerals are inhaled environmental materials, either natural (e.g. clay minerals) or synthetic (e.g. cement dust), that translocate from the lungs (or skin in some cases) to the lymph node. Additionally, there are some unique mineral types that may represent chemical modification of absorbed mineral within the body to create *de novo* 'biominerals'.

There is no apparent geographical localization of cases and few data to demonstrate the origin of mineral or the pathogenesis of disease. Affected lymph nodes are a source of inflammatory cytokine production (IL-1, TNFα). This might underlie the non-specific clinical signs (pyrexia, anorexia, polyuria/polydypsia, weight loss) that accompany the lymph node pathology (787). Affected dogs may have concurrent autoimmune disease, lymphoma or other tumours. In rodent models of silica absorption and in humans with industrial diseases, such minerals may induce immunological dysfunction or chromosomal abnormalities, resulting in neoplasia.

Dogs with mineral-associated lymphadenopathy respond to palliative anti-inflammatory therapy and with time (months) the mineral may degrade and the lymphadenopathy resolve.

OTHER LYMPH NODE DISEASES

Other lymph node diseases recognized in the dog and cat includes:

- The spectrum of changes induced by FIV (see Chapter 12, p. 288).
- Lymph node haemorrhage or haemorrhage within the tissue drained by the lymph node (788).
- Lymph node oedema following obstruction to efferent outflow.
- Lymph node infarction following compromise of blood supply.
- Lymphadenopathy secondary to tumour metastasis (789).

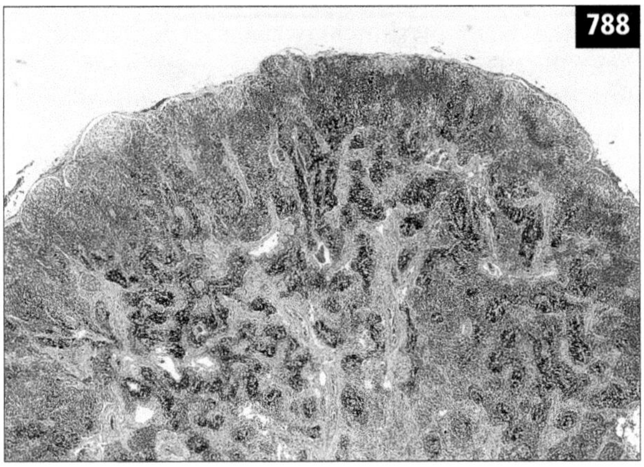

788 Haemosiderin deposition in lymph node. Section of lymph node from a six-year-old crossbred dog with a fibrosarcoma arising from the thoracic intercostal area and enlarged mediastinal lymph nodes. There is marked accumulation of granular, brown pigment (haemosiderin) within medullary sinus macrophages of one of the mediastinal nodes, consistent with previous haemorrhage within the lymph node or the tissues drained by it.

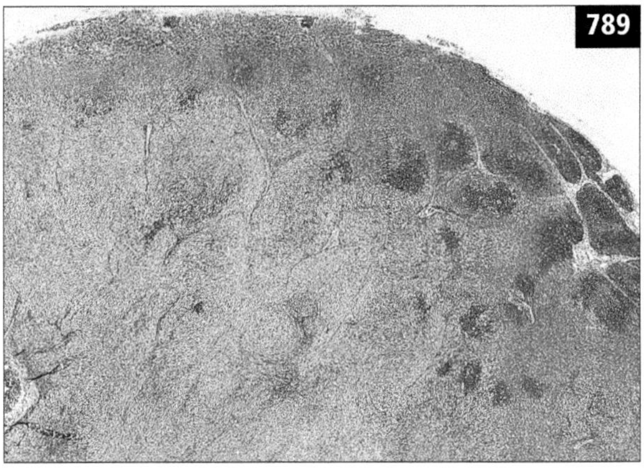

789 Metastasis to lymph node. Section taken from the lymph node shown in **764**. Normal microarchitecture has been effaced by the neoplastic infiltrate and there remain only small lymphoid aggregates in the outermost cortical region.

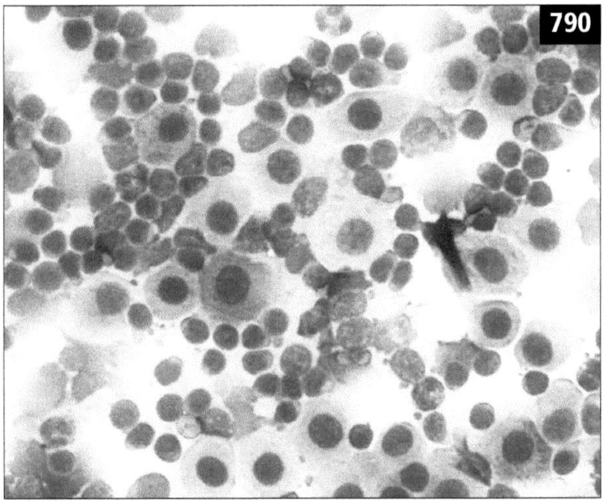

790 Lymph node cytology. Fine needle aspirate from an axillary lymph node enlarged due to metastatic spread of mast cell tumour from the digit of that limb. The field includes neoplastic mast cells and accompanying eosinophils admixed with the lymphoid population.

DIFFERENTIAL DIAGNOSIS OF LYMPHADENOPATHY

The diagnostic approach to lymphadenopathy may involve:

- General assessment (e.g. haematology, serum biochemistry, urinalysis, serology or PCR for detection of infectious disease agents, imaging examination) to identify underlying disease.
- Fine needle aspiration of the lymph node and examination of a stained smear (790), or evaluation of the aspirate by antibody labelling and flow cytometry or immunocytochemistry (see Chapter 13, p. 324).
- Needle core biopsy.
- Partial or complete excisional biopsy.

DISEASES OF LYMPHATIC VESSELS

Primary disease of lymphatic vessels is uncommon in the dog and cat. Lymphoedema due to obstructed lymphatic outflow may involve both lymphatics and lymph nodes (**791**). A specific example of this is lymphangiectasia, where there is lacteal dilatation and loss of protein-rich fluid and cells into the intestinal lumen (**792, 793**). Congenital defects of lymphatic vessels producing primary lymphoedema are documented in dogs and cats and autosomal dominant inheritance is proposed. The most common presentation is of pitting oedema of one or more extremities, often the hindlimbs. Regional lymph nodes may be absent or hypoplastic. A useful diagnostic procedure is the dye absorption test. In an anaethesized animal, a sterile 5–10% solution of patent blue violet dye is injected subcutaneously into the webs of skin between the digits. Diffuse spreading of the dye indicates absence of adequate lymphatic drainage. Both conservative (bandaging, antibiotics) and surgical approaches to therapy have been attempted, but the long-term outcome is generally unfavourable and chronic infection and fibrosis may develop.

Other diseases of lymphatic vessels include:

- Traumatic rupture or increased permeability (due to a range of underlying causes) of the thoracic duct with chylothorax (**794**).
- Lymphangioma and lymphangiosarcoma, rare tumours most frequently documented in the skin. These tumours are similar in structure and behaviour to those of vascular endothelium, but they have ultrastructural differences and do not express the vascular endothelial marker, factor VIII-related antigen (**795, 796**).

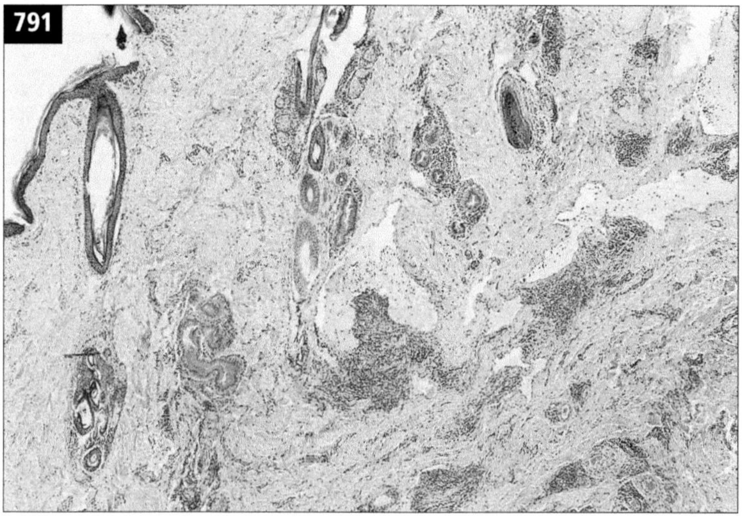

791 Lymphoedema. Skin biopsy from a six-year-old Weimaraner with chronic lymphoedema of both hindlimbs. There is prominent dilatation of dermal lymphatic vessels and an associated, mixed mononuclear inflammatory infiltrate adjacent to these. The cause of this lymphoedema was mineral-associated lymphadenopathy of the popliteal lymph nodes, which had interfered with lymphatic drainage.

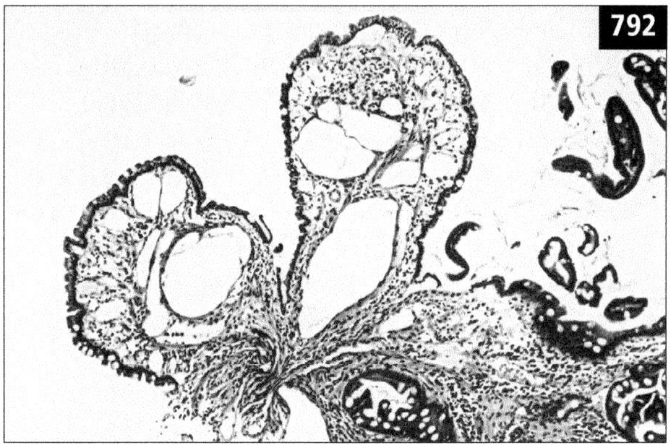

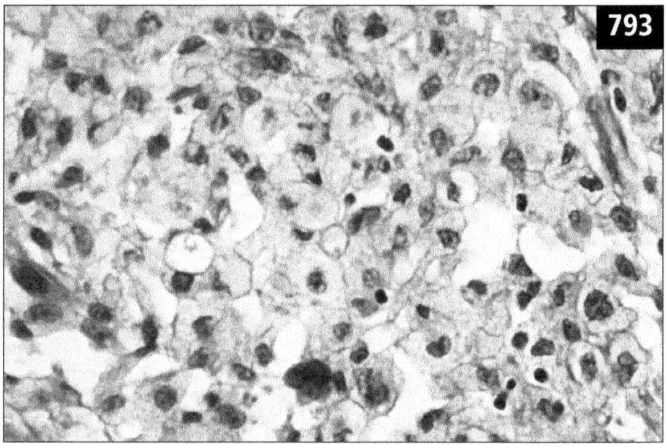

792, 793 Intestinal lymphangiectasia. (**792**) Endoscopic biopsy of duodenum from a dog with protein losing enteropathy, ascites and pleural effusion. There is marked dilatation of the lacteals, with oedema of the surrounding villus lamina. A cause for this was not ascertained. (**793**) In this full-thickness intestinal biopsy from another dog with lymphangiectasia there is a series of granulomatous foci within the submucosa. These comprise highly vacuolated macrophages and such lipogranulomas have been proposed to be an underlying cause of lymphangiectasia.

794 Chylothorax. Cytological appearance of thoracic fluid from a three-year-old DSH cat with increasing dyspnoea over the past seven days. Approximately 120 ml of milky white, chylous fluid was drained from the chest. There is some blood contamination of the sample, which otherwise contains an almost pure population of small lymphocytes derived from the thoracic duct.

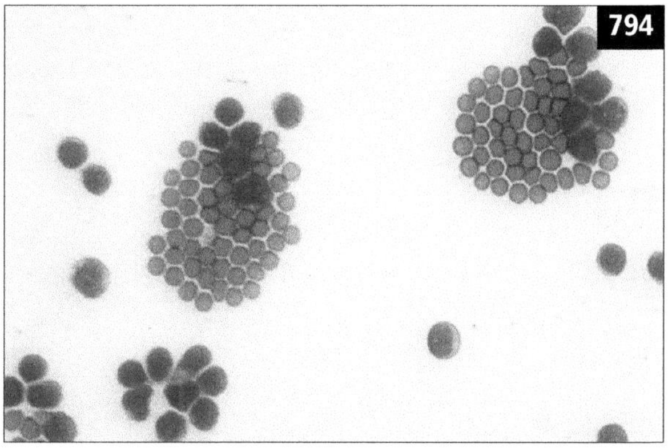

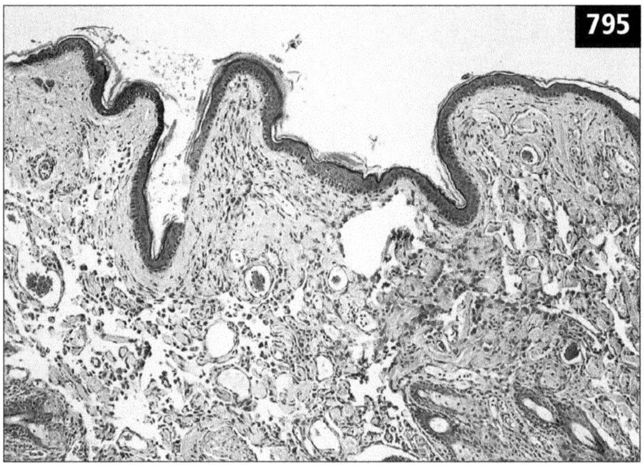

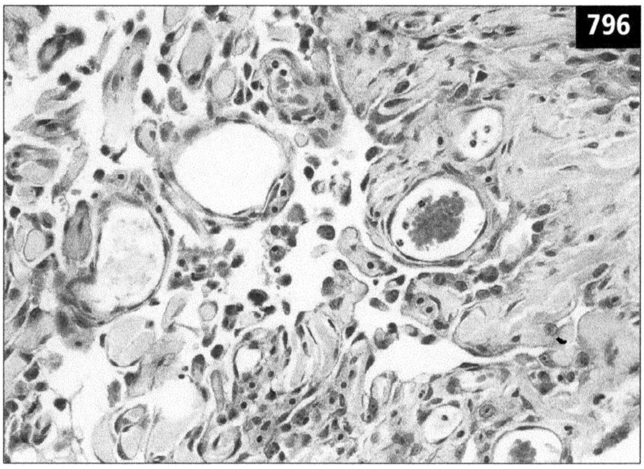

795–796 Cutaneous lymphangiosarcoma. (**795**) Skin biopsy from a ten-year-old DSH cat with a fluid filled mass on the ventral abdomen and recent development of pleural effusion. Within the dermis there is a network of lymphatic vessels, which on high power examination (**796**) are seen to be lined by large, plump endothelial cells, with occasional mitosis.

DISEASES OF THE TONSIL

Tonsillar enlargement may reflect reactive hyperplasia in response to oral inflammation (797), infectious tonsillitis (798) or primary or metastatic neoplasia. The tonsil may be involved in oral squamous cell carcinoma or be a primary site of development of this tumour (799, 800). Tonsillar carcinoma is more frequently documented in urban areas and may be associated with environmental pollution. Tonsillar melanoma (dog) and tonsillar lymphoma (dog and cat) are recognized. Tonsillar lymphoid depletion may occur with canine or feline parvovirus or canine distemper virus infections, but there may be lymphoid regeneration during the postviraemic phases of distemper.

DISEASES OF THE SPLEEN

Splenic disease is not uncommon in the dog and neoplasia accounts for the majority of cases (*Table 34*).

797

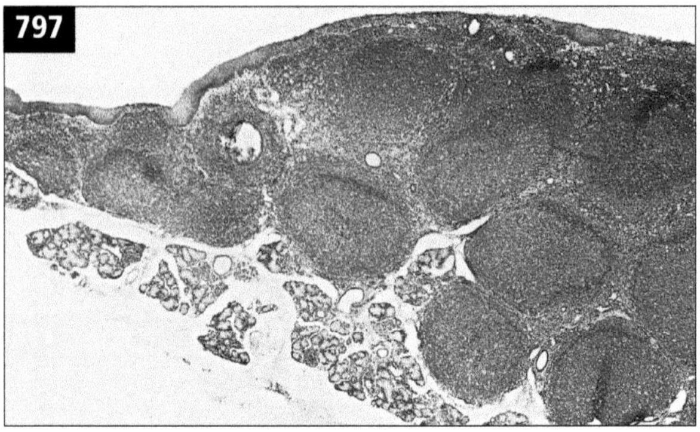

797 Tonsillar hyperplasia. Section of tonsil from a two-year-old Beagle with enlarged tonsils. There is marked follicular hyperplasia indicative of reactive change.

798

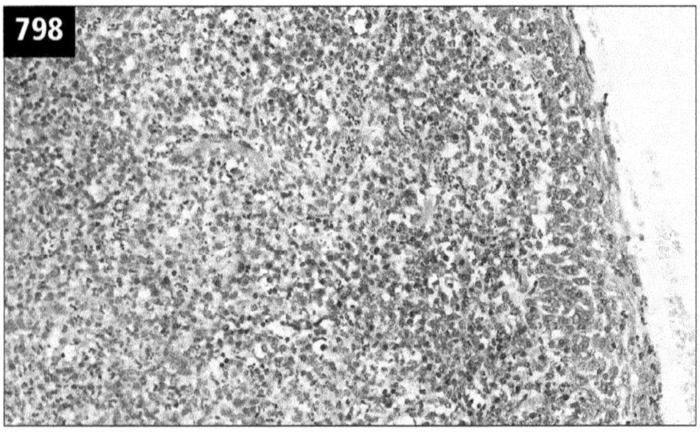

798 Tonsillitis. Section of enlarged tonsil from a ten-year-old crossbred dog with retching and gagging. There is diffuse pyogranulomatous inflammation of undetermined cause.

Splenic enlargement (splenomegaly) may be broadly considered as diffuse or nodular in nature. The major causes of diffuse splenomegaly include:

- Passive venous congestion following barbiturate anaesthesia or euthanasia, or blocking venous outflow of the splenic vein (e.g. splenic or gastrosplenic torsion, splenic vein thrombosis, rarely portal hypertension).
- Acute or chronic infectious or inflammatory disease (801).
- Expansion of white pulp during an immune response (802).
- Extramedullary haemopoiesis, erythrophagocytosis and haemosiderin deposition (see Chapter 4, p. 96).
- Amyloidosis (803).

Table 34: Splenic disease in the dog. Causes of splenic disease in 87 dogs were compiled from the records of a diagnostic histopathology laboratory. Splenic neoplasia was the most common diagnosis and the most frequently recognized tumour was haemangiosarcoma. No cases of splenic lymphoma were recorded, most likely because the study considered only biopsy (primarily splenectomy) specimens from cases of apparent primary splenic disease. (Data from Day MJ, Lucke VM, Pearson H (1995) A review of pathological diagnoses made from 87 canine splenic biopsies. *Journal of Small Animal Practice* **36:**426–433.)

Diagnosis	Number of cases
Haemangiosarcoma	17
Haematoma	16
Non-specific changes including congestion, haemorrhage, extramedullary haemopoiesis and haemosiderin deposition	14
Thrombosis and infarction	7
Nodular hyperplasia	6
Anaplastic sarcoma	6
Haemangioma	4
Torsion, thrombosis and infarction	3
Fibrosarcoma	3
Abscessation	2
Lipoma	2
Sarcoma with giant cells	2
Liposarcoma	1
Leiomyosarcoma	1
Myeloproliferative disease	1
Capsular seeding of adenocarcinoma	1
Mast cell proliferation	1
Total	**87**

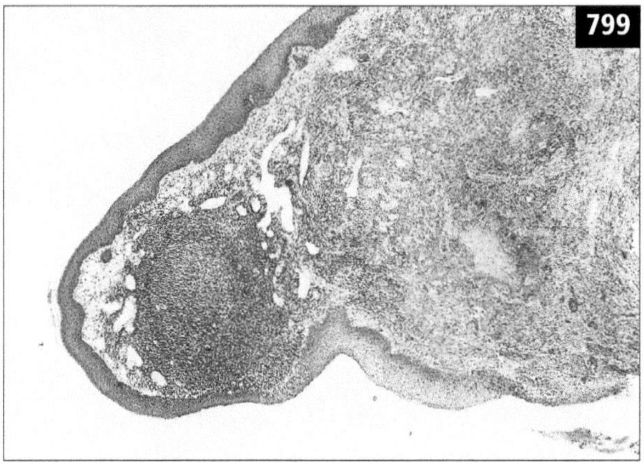

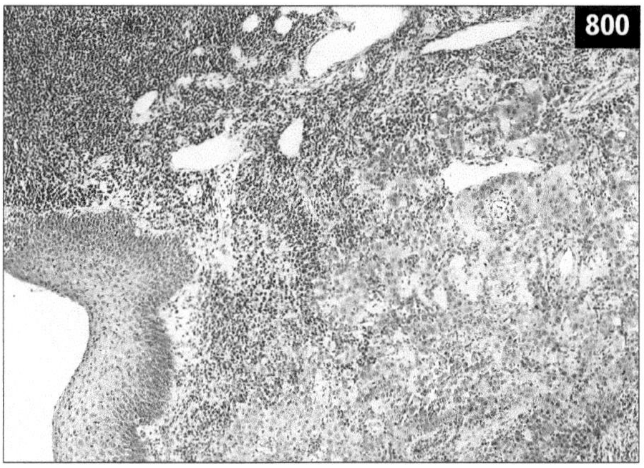

799, 800 Tonsillar carcinoma. Section of tonsil from an 11-year-old dog with tonsillar enlargement and intermittent coughing. In addition to a region of active tonsillar lymphoid tissue, there is infiltration by neoplastic squamous epithelial cells.

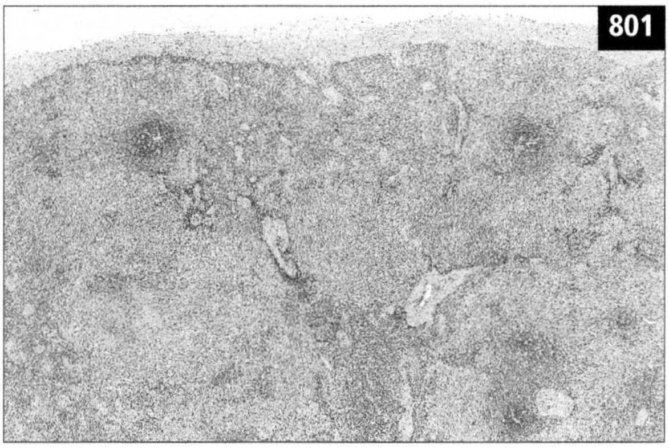

801 Granulomatous splenitis. Section of grossly enlarged spleen from a 15-year-old DLH cat with effusive FIP virus infection. There was a quantity of viscous, yellow fluid in the abdomen and the abdominal serosae were covered by pinpoint white foci. Additionally, most of the splenic red pulp was replaced by extensive pyogranulomatous inflammatory infiltration, with regions of necrosis.

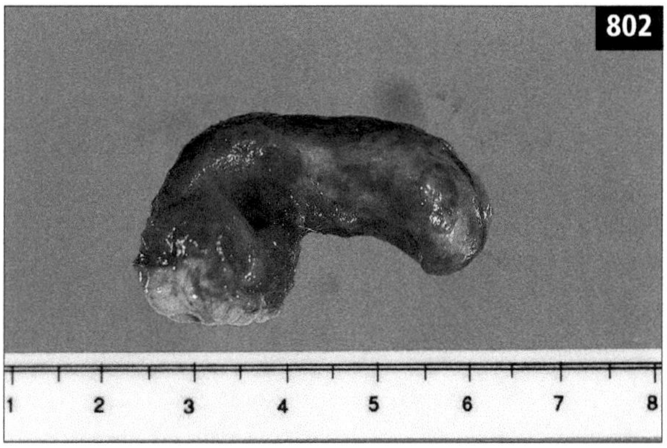

802 Splenic lymphoid hyperplasia. Grossly enlarged spleen from a nine-year-old DSH cat with a hepatic vascular anomaly and clinical signs of hepatic encephalopathy. Microscopic examination revealed the presence of marked hyperplasia of white pulp, with expansion of PALS and numerous, prominent secondary lymphoid follicles.

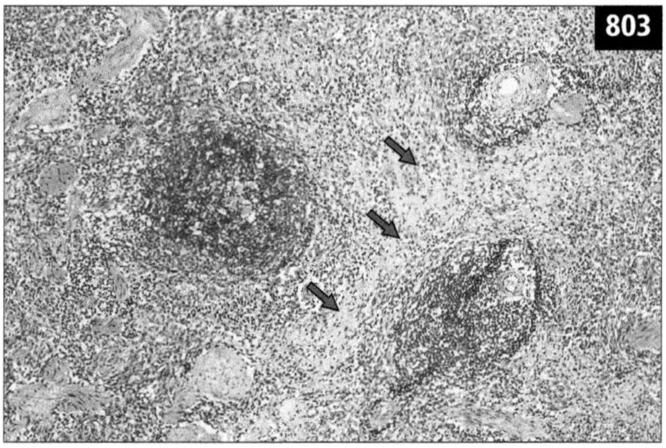

803 Splenic amyloidosis. Section of spleen from a five-year-old Siamese cat with systemic amyloidosis involving the spleen, liver, thyroid, kidney and adrenal cortex. The pale, eosinophilic material within the red pulp (arrowed) stains by Congo red.

804
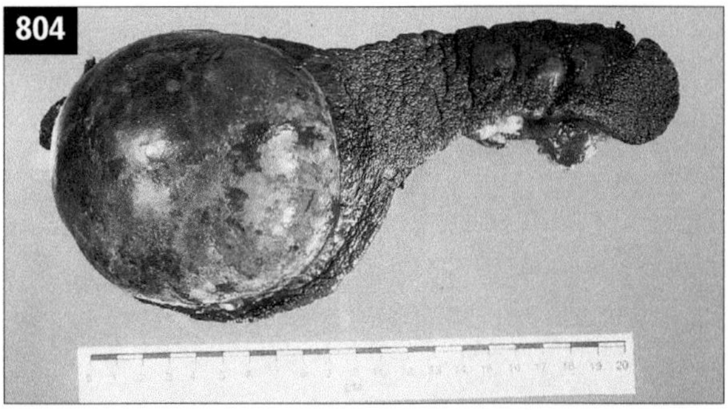

- Feline hypereosinophilic syndrome (see Chapter 7, p. 216).

Nodular splenomegaly may arise due to:

- Lymphoma, leukaemia, myeloma or myeloproliferative disease (see Chapter 13, p 342).
- Other tumours arising from, or metastatic to, the spleen (804, 805).
- Nodular hyperplasia; irregular areas of lymphoid or macrophage proliferation with foci of congestion (806). These lesions have recently

805
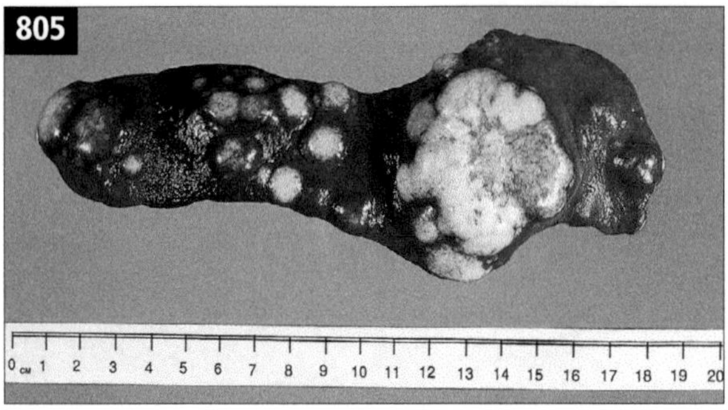

804, 805 Splenic neoplasia. A range of primary tumours may arise in the spleen, and this organ is often a site for metastasis of other neoplasms. (**804**) Spleen from an 11-year-old Irish Terrier with a well-circumscribed splenic lipoma. (From Day MJ, Lucke VM, Pearson H (1995) A review of pathological diagnoses made from 87 canine splenic biopsies. *Journal of Small Animal Practice* **36:**426–433, with permission.) (**805**) Spleen from a ten-year-old English Cocker Spaniel with pancreatic adenocarcinoma that had metastasized to lymph nodes, liver, spleen and lung.

806
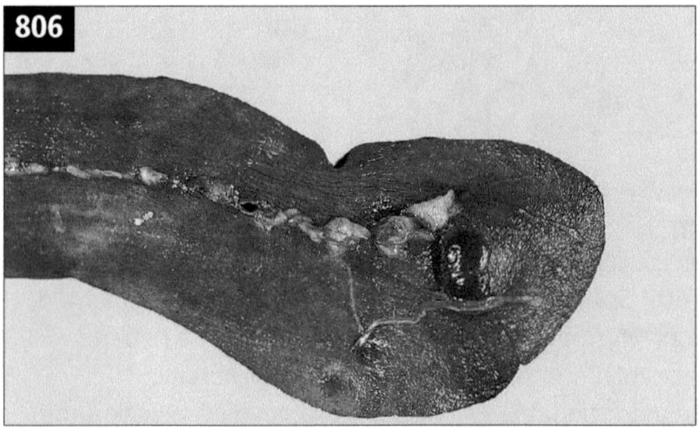

807
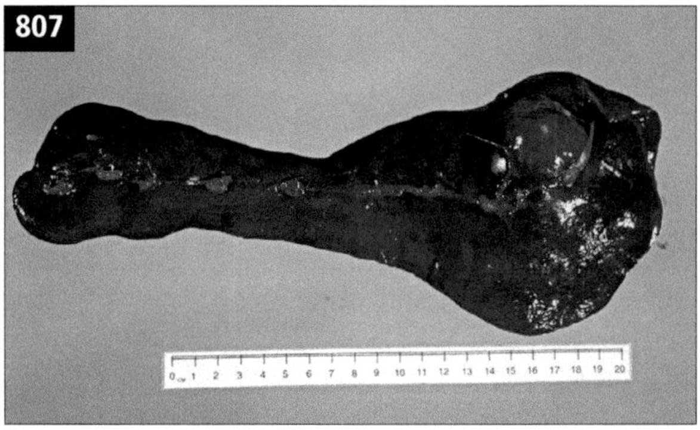

808
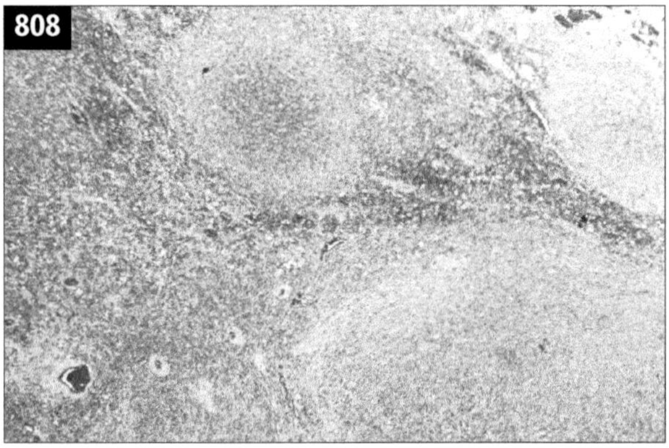

809
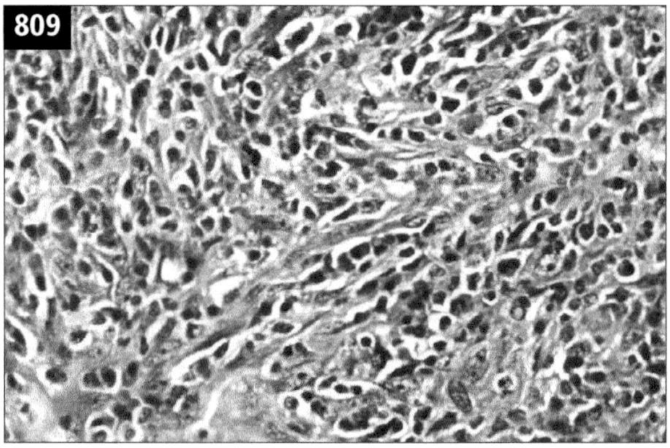

806 Splenic nodular hyperplasia. Single focus of nodular hyperplasia of the spleen, identified as an incidental necropsy finding in an old dog.

807–809 Splenic fibrohistiocytic nodule. (**807**) Spleen from a six-year-old crossbred dog with a discrete, raised, cream nodular mass within the ventral pole. (**808**) At lower power magnification this comprises nodular expansions, with narrow intervening zones of normal splenic red pulp. (**809**) High power magnification reveals these expanded areas to comprise admixed spindle cells, macrophages, plasma cells and lymphocytes.

been re-evaluated by pathologists and a spectrum of change defined. The 'fibrohistiocytic nodules' of the spleen are generally considered benign lesions that may have a dominant spindle cell (fibroblastic) or macrophage (histiocytic) content (807–809). However, at the more malignant end of this spectrum of lesion are the group of histiocytic sarcomas described in Chapter 13.

- Splenic infarction (e.g. following splenic or gastrosplenic torsion) due to occlusion of the arterial supply (810, 811).
- Abscessation or chronic infectious disease (812).
- Splenic haematoma (813, 814).

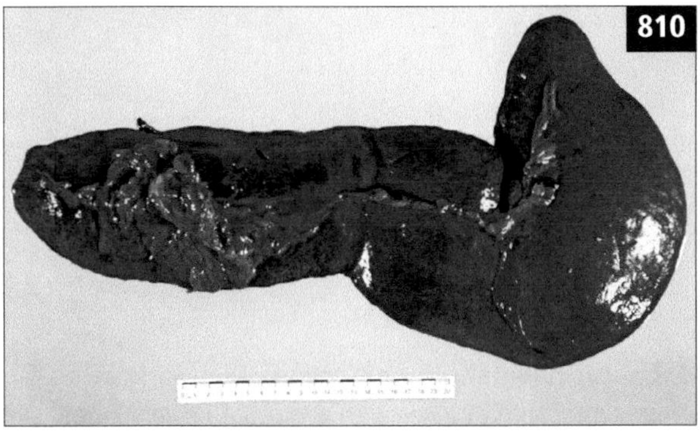
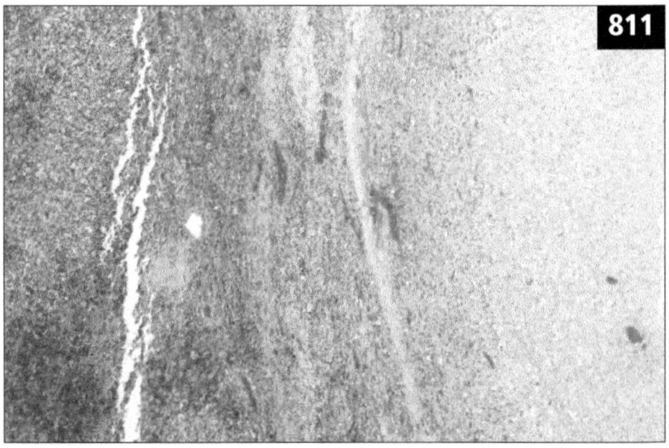

810, 811 Splenic infarction. (**810**) Markedly enlarged spleen removed from a four-year-old Great Dane. The entire organ is infarcted and this is a sequela to previous torsion, with occlusion of vascular supply. (**811**) Histological section of spleen from an 11-year-old Boxer with a more focal region of infarction. The junction between viable and infarcted tissue is shown.

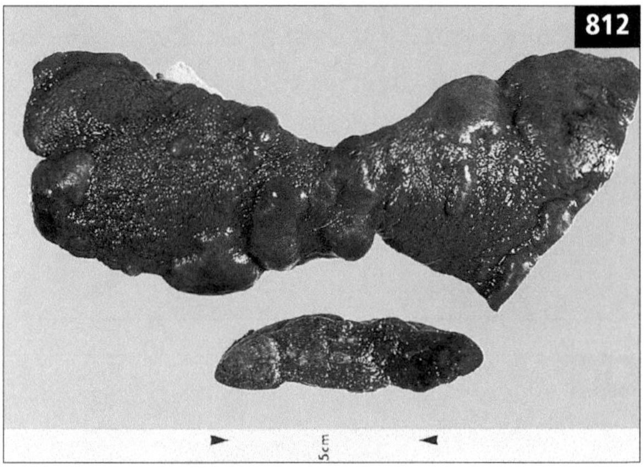

812 Splenic granulomata. Spleen from a GSD with disseminated aspergillosis (see Chapter 12, p. 304). There is multinodular enlargement of the organ, and microscopic examination confirms the presence of coalescing granulomata centred upon hyphal elements of *Aspergillus terreus*. (Photograph courtesy Pathology Unit, Murdoch University.)

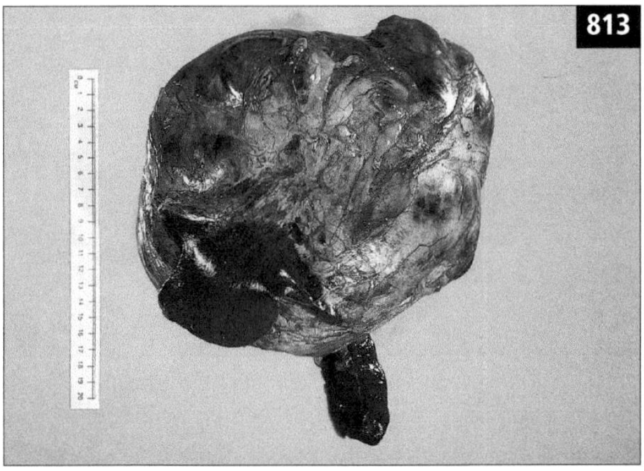
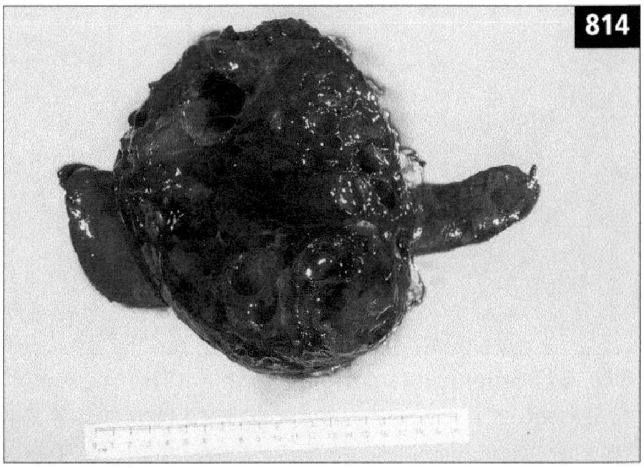

813, 814 Splenic haematoma. (**813**) Spleen surgically removed from a ten-year-old crossbred dog. A large splenic haematoma arises from the mid-portion of the organ. (**814**) On cut surface the haematoma has extensive areas of haemorrhage and necrosis and microscopic examination confirms the presence of deposition of fibrous connective tissue (organising haematoma).

- Splenic haemangioma (**815**).
- Splenic haemangiosarcoma; a malignant tumour of vascular endothelium, which is particularly common in GSDs (**816, 817**). The spleen is a common primary site for this tumour (also the right atrium of the heart, liver or skin), which may metastasize widely (**818–823**). The tumour cells will express factor VIII-related antigen on immunohistochemical labelling.

Senile atrophy of the spleen occurs in dogs and focal capsular encrustation due to deposition of iron and calcium (siderofibrotic plaque) is common. The diagnosis of splenic disease relies on imaging examination (radiography, ultrasonography and magnetic resonance imaging), often followed by exploratory laparotomy and diagnostic splenectomy. In recent years, ultrasound-guided fine needle aspiration of splenic lesions has also

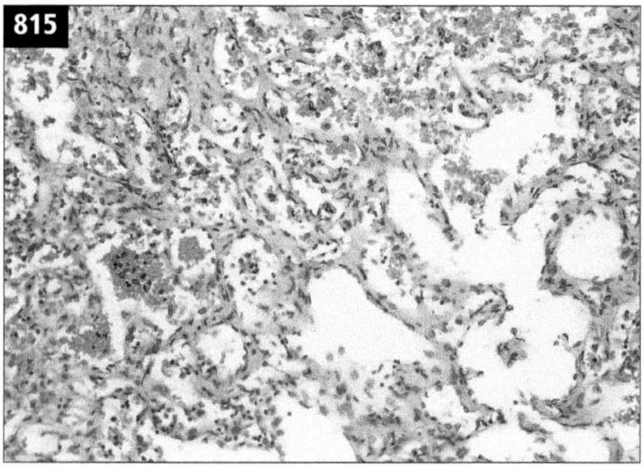

815 Splenic haemangioma. Section of spleen from a 14-year-old Labrador Retriever with a ruptured splenic mass and abdominal haemorrhage. There is a network of vascular channels lined by endothelial cells of normal microscopic appearance.

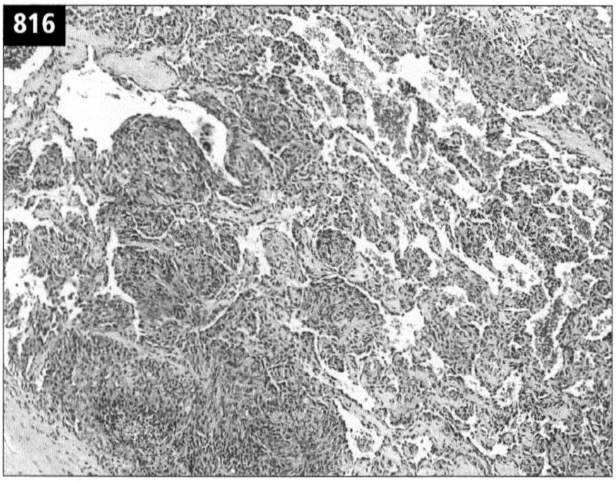

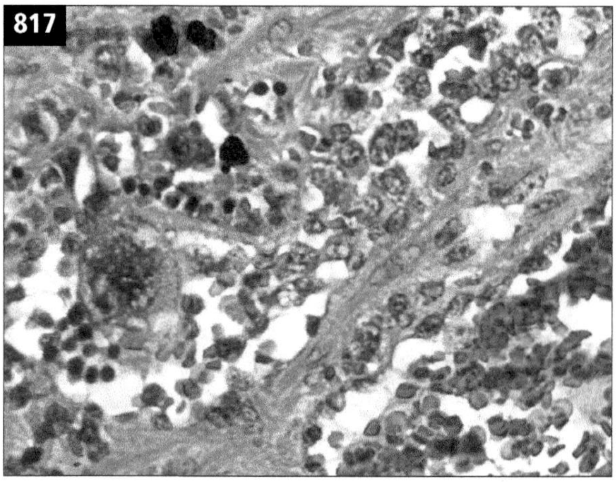

816, 817 Splenic haemangiosarcoma. (**816**) Section of spleen from a dog with haemangiosarcoma. The tumour is composed of pleomorphic and mitotic spindle cells that form irregular vascular channels. (**817**) High power field of canine splenic haemangiosarcoma showing plump spindle cells lining a vascular structure, with occasional binucleate and one large multinucleate cell.

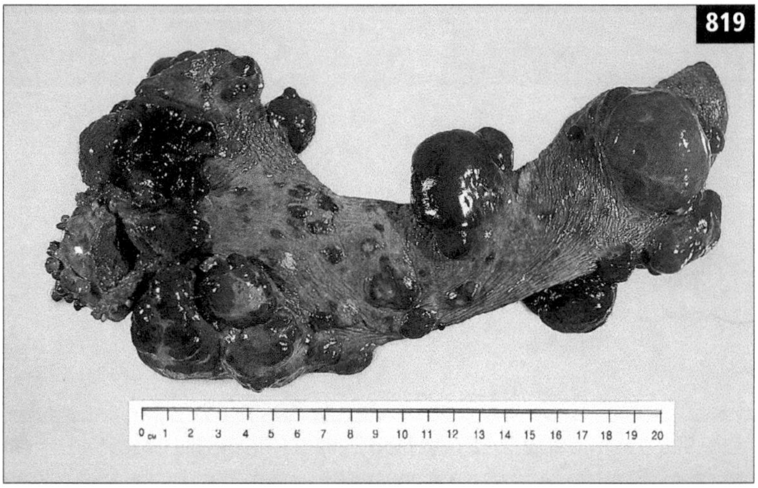

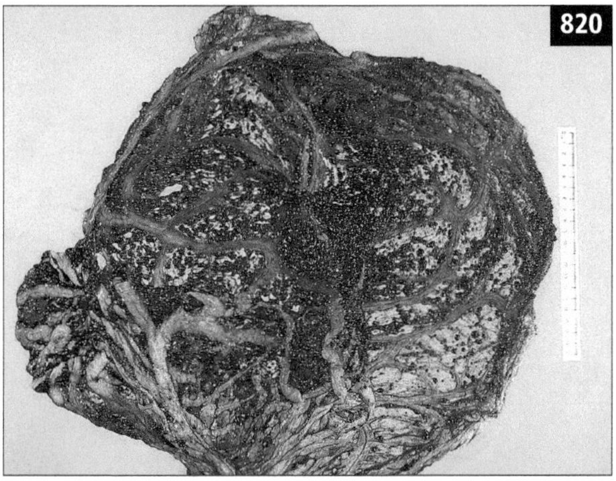

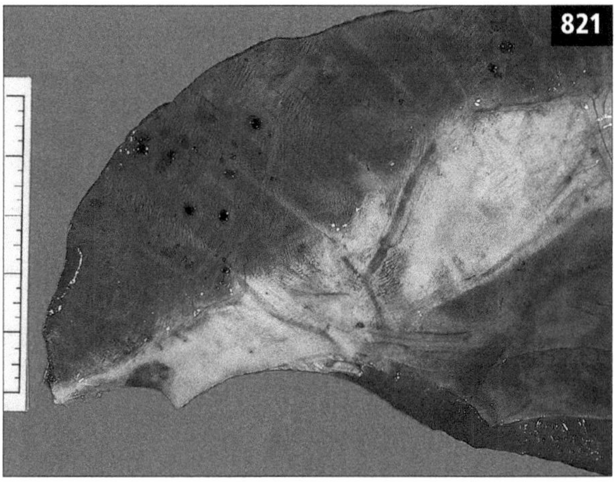

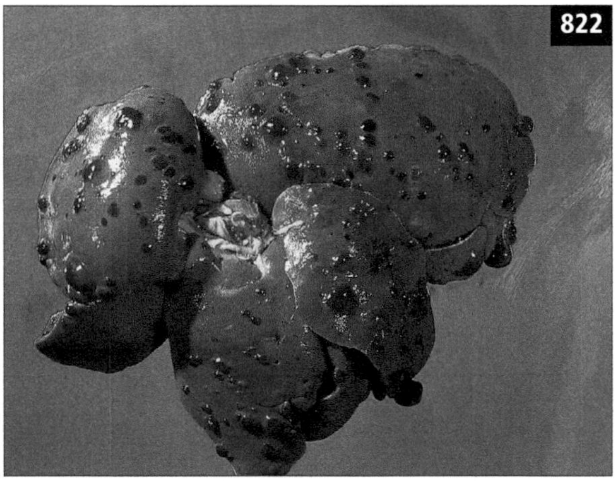

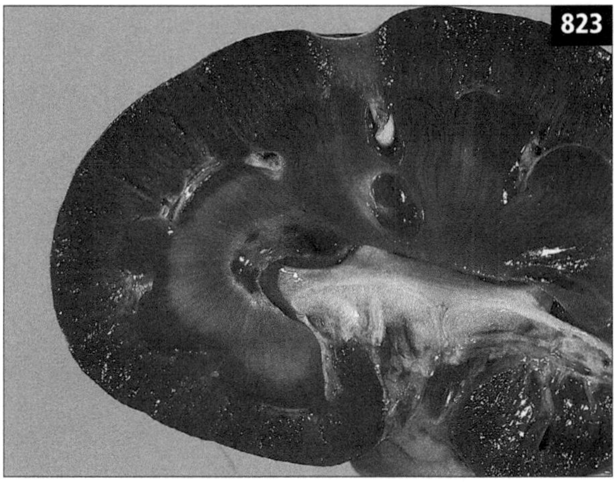

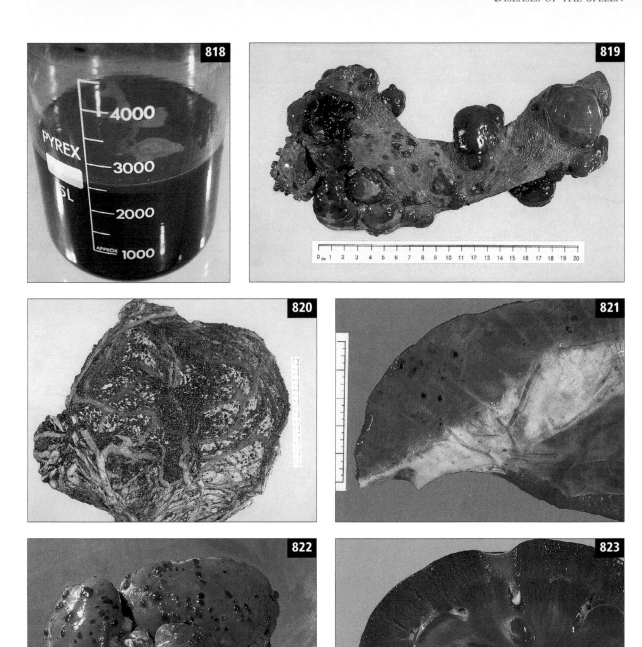

818–823 Splenic haemangiosarcoma. Necropsy specimens from a nine-year-old GSD with primary splenic haemangiosarcoma. (**818**) The abdominal cavity contained approximately 2.5 litres of bloody fluid. (**819**) There was multinodular enlargement of the spleen, with rupture of some nodules.(**820**) The tumour had seeded throughout the omentum and onto the abdominal surface of the diaphragm (**821**). Small foci of tumour were scattered throughout the liver (**822**), and an area of renal infarction (**823**) was associated with metastatic haemangiosarcoma.

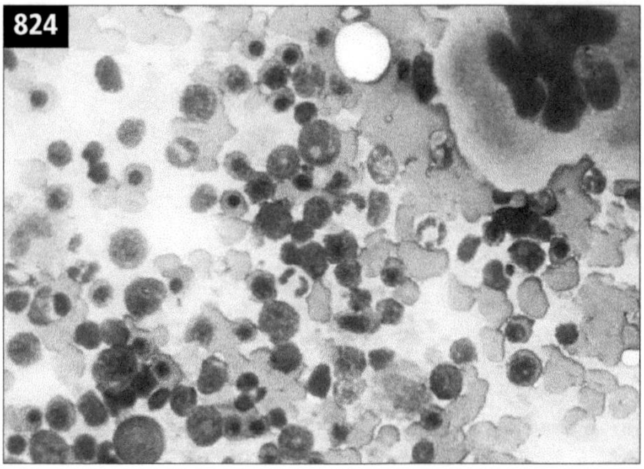

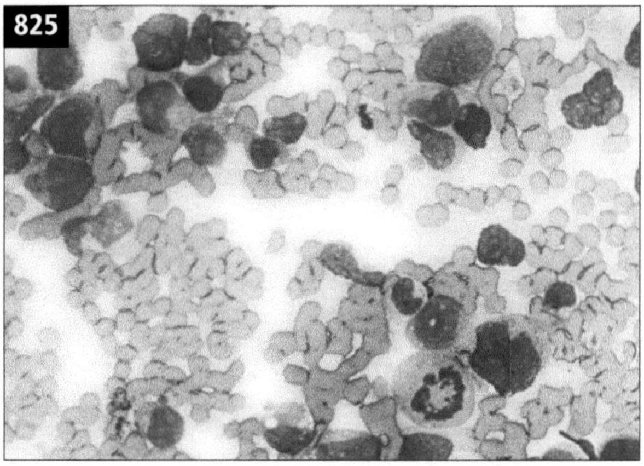

824, 825 Splenic aspiration cytology. (**824**) Fine needle aspiration cytology from the spleen of a four-year-old Bernese Mountain Dog with a regenerative anaemia and splenomegaly. There is prominent evidence of extramedullary haematopoiesis, with a range of erythroid and myeloid precursors and a single megakaryocyte. Additionally, there are several mature plasma cells and scattered lymphoblasts consistent with B cell reactivity. (**825**) Fine needle aspiration cytology from the spleen of a cat. There are numerous irregular lymphoblastic cells, with evidence of mitotic activity present; the appearance is consistent with splenic lymphoma.

become widely utilized. These samples are, however, often non-diagnostic due to the haemodilution that may be expected of a splenic aspirate (**824, 825**), although one recent study has reported that 87% of such aspirate samples were of diagnostic quality. Many authors describe the risks of splenic aspiration (e.g. rupture of haemangiosarcoma, seeding of tumour cells along the path of needle insertion), but in reality these complications are rarely reported. Similarly, impaired coagulation or thrombocytopenia is not necessarily a contraindication for splenic aspiration.

FURTHER READING

Ballegeer EA, Forrest LJ, Dickinson RM *et al.* (2007) Correlation of ultrasonographic appearance of lesions and cytologic and histologic diagnoses in splenic aspirates from dogs and cats: 32 cases (2002–2005). *Journal of the American Veterinary Medical Association* **230**:690–696.

Christopher MM (2003) Cytology of the spleen. *Veterinary Clinics of North America Small Animal Practice* **33**:135–152.

Christensen NI, Canfield PJ, Martin PA *et al.* (2009) Cytopathological and histopathological diagnosis of canine splenic disorders. *Australian Veterinary Journal* **87**:175–181.

Kull PA, Hess RS, Craig LE *et al.* (2001) Clinical, clinicopathologic, radiographic, and ultrasonographic characteristics of intestinal lymphangiectasia in dogs: 17 cases (1996–1998). *Journal of the American Veterinary Medical Association* **219**:197–202.

Laurenson MP, Hopper K, Herrera MA *et al.* (2010) Concurrent diseases and conditions in dogs with splenic vein thrombosis. *Journal of Veterinary Internal Medicine* **24**:1298–1304.

LeBlanc CJ, Head LL, Fry MM (2009) Comparison of aspiration and nonaspiration techniques for obtaining cytologic samples from the canine and feline spleen. *Veterinary Clinical Pathology* **38**:242–246.

Ploeman J-PHTM, Ravesloot WTM, van Esch E (2003) The incidence of thymic B lymphoid follicles in healthy Beagle dogs. *Toxicologic Pathology* **31**:214–219.

16 IMMUNOTHERAPY

Michael J. Day

INTRODUCTION

The most exciting area of contemporary immunology is that concerned with the development of novel immunotherapeutic agents. Many products are now in the stage of human clinical trials, but their development required detailed knowledge of disease pathogenesis (e.g. identification of immunodominant peptide sequences of allergens or autoantigens). Similar information must be obtained for dogs and cats before such methodology can be applied to treatment of disease in these species. Nevertheless, the potential for immunotherapeutic modulation of small animal disease is great, and several biotechnology companies are investigating the application of particular approaches to veterinary medicine.

This chapter considers the traditional methods of pharmacological immunomodulation used currently in the treatment of immune-mediated disease, and presents examples of immunological manipulations of disease in man or laboratory animal models that may be applicable to dogs and cats. The field of transplantation surgery as it applies to the dog and cat is reviewed.

IMMUNOMODULATORY DRUGS

The treatment of many of the diseases discussed in this book currently involves the use of immunomodulatory drugs. These may either non-specifically suppress a deleterious immune response such as autoimmunity or allergy (anti-inflammatory or immunosuppressive drugs) or enhance a protective immune response, or alter the balance of immunoregulation to provide a favourable clinical effect (immunopotentiating drugs). The blanket effects of such drugs on the immune system may be associated with complications; for example, the occurrence of opportunist infection during immunosuppression. A brief review of these drugs is given below. Therapeutic regimes for specific disorders are given elsewhere in this book.

Immunosuppressive or anti-inflammatory drugs

Glucocorticoids

The drugs most commonly used in the therapy of immune-mediated diseases of the dog and cat are glucocorticoids. These have a range of anti-inflammatory and immunosuppressive potency (*Table 35*), but in most instances prednisolone or

Table 35: Relative anti-inflammatory potency of glucocorticoids. The anti-inflammatory potency and duration of action of the most commonly utilized glucocorticoids are presented relative to hydrocortisone, which is assigned a value of 1.0.

Drug	Anti-inflammatory potency	Duration of action
Cortisone	0.8	Short acting
Hydrocortisone	1.0	Short acting
Prednisolone, prednisone	4.0	Intermediate
Methylprednisolone	5.0	Intermediate
Triamcinolone	5.0	Intermediate to long acting
Flumethasone	15.0	Long acting
Dexamethasone	30.0	Long acting
Betamethasone	35.0	Long acting

Short acting <12 hours; intermediate 12–36 hours; long acting >48 hours.

prednisone are selected and may be used in combination with other immunosuppressive agents. Despite the fact that glucocorticoids are one of the most commonly prescribed medicines in small animal practice, there has been limited study of the pharmacokinetics and immunological effects of these agents in the dog and cat. The long-standing immunosuppressive dosage regime used in these species is largely derived from human protocols that have been empirically applied to companion animals (*Table 36*). The use of immunosuppressive doses of glucocorticoids for prolonged periods is commonly associated with a range of side-effects in the dog. The two most significant syndromes are iatrogenic hyperadrenocorticism (i.e. 'steroid hepatopathy', hyperglycaemia with secondary diabetes mellitus, atrophic dermatopathy, secondary infection, polyuria, polydipsia, polyphagia and weight gain) and adrenal insufficiency after sudden withdrawal of therapy (**826, 827**). The risk of inducing these side-effects may be reduced by determining the minimal

Table 36: Immunosuppressive protocol for oral prednisolone in the dog. This example is based on a dog receiving an induction dose of 1.0 mg/kg q12h. The induction immunosuppressive dose of oral prednisolone ranges from 1.0–2.0 mg/kg q12h for a dog and from 2.2–6.6 mg/kg q 12h for a cat. Treatment should never be withdrawn abruptly, but may be eventually withdrawn after a tapering regime. However, in some dogs, lifelong low dose maintenance therapy may be required.

Dose	Duration (based on clinical effect)
1.0 mg/kg q12h	10–28 days
0.75 mg/kg q12h	10–28 days
0.5 mg/kg q12h	10–28 days
0.25 mg/kg q12h	10–28 days
0.25 mg/kg q24h	10–28 days
0.25–0.5 mg/kg every other day	At least 21 days
0.25–0.5 mg/kg every third day	At least 21 days

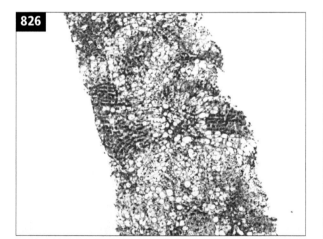

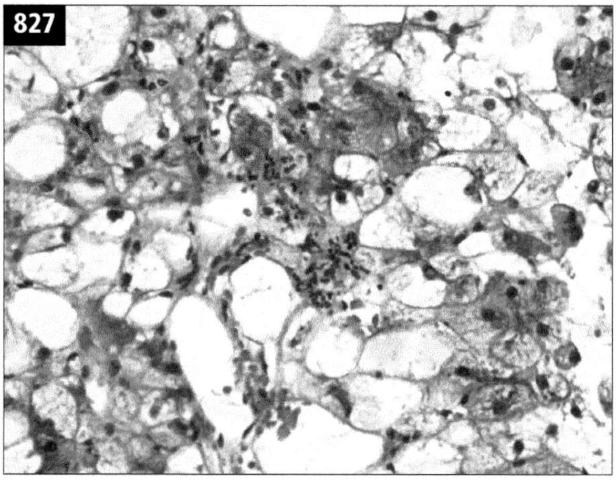

826, 827 Steroid hepatopathy. Low (**826**) and high (**827**) power appearance of a needle core biopsy of liver taken from an eight-year-old Cocker Spaniel that had been treated with immunosuppressive doses of oral prednisolone for IMTP. The irregular zones of macrovesicular hepatocyte vacuolation reflect lipid or glycogen accumulation and are characteristic of 'steroid hepatopathy'.

maintenance dose, given on alternate days if possible, and by using a glucocorticoid with an intermediate duration of action (e.g. prednisolone). However, individual patients do often require long-term therapy to prevent recurrence of disease. The cat is relatively less sensitive to glucocorticoid immunosuppression and higher doses are required in this species. This may reflect the reduced expression of receptors for glucocorticoid (dexamethasone) that has been documented in the tissues (skin and liver) of cats. Similarly, the cat is also less likely to suffer adverse effects of glucocorticotherapy, which chiefly manifest as polyuria, polydipsia, polyphagia and weight gain in this species.

The mode of action of glucocorticoids (828) is pleotropic and these agents are both anti-inflammatory and immunosuppressive. There is controversy over the effects attributed to the drugs, but their effects on the immune system may include:

- Decreased extravasation of white cells.
- Decreased macrophage FcR expression, phagocytosis, antigen presentation and IL-1 production.
- Decreased number of circulating lymphocytes, with reduced T cell function and production of T cell cytokines. B lymphocytes are generally regarded as being more resistant to glucocorticoids, so any effect on antibody production (reduced serum immunoglobulin concentrations) is considered indirect via inhibition of T cell help.
- Inhibition of complement pathways (reduced serum C3).
- Inhibition of the passage of immune complexes through basement membranes.
- Decreased neutrophil margination and migration, although in the dog prednisolone has been shown to increase the chemotactic response and phagocytic function of neutrophils.

Most of these effects are simply presumed to occur in companion animals based on extrapolation from human and experimental rodent studies; there has been very limited study of the immunological effects of glucocorticoids in the dog and cat. One recent abstract has reported the effect of administration of oral prednisolone (10 mg total dose q24h) on immune function in normal cats. These animals had reduced percentages of T and B cells in peripheral blood, reduced response to mitogen stimulation and increased transcription of the IL-10 gene. In contrast, there was no significant effect on serum IgG or IgA concentration or on expression of genes encoding IL-2, IL-4 or IFNγ. A further study has examined the effect of culturing feline blood lymphocytes in the presence of dexamethasone. Contrary to the predicted effect, this led to an elevation in proliferation of both $CD4^+$ and $CD8^+$ T lymphocytes, consistent with studies in murine systems, suggesting that glucocorticoids may have a more selective immunomodulatory effect than often assumed and may in fact enhance some Th2-mediated immune effects. In the same study, culture with combined glucocorticoid and ciclosporin led to reduced lymphocyte proliferation, significantly greater than observed with ciclosporin alone.

In the dog, oral administration of prednisone (2 mg/kg q24h) for a two-week period resulted in reduced concentrations of serum IgG, IgM and IgA

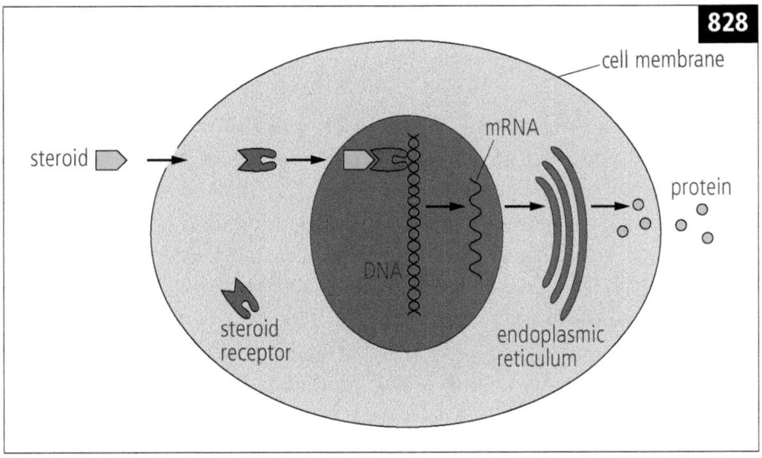

828 Action of glucocorticoids. Steroids pass through the cell membrane and bind to intracytoplasmic receptors. The complex of steroid and receptor then passes to the nucleus and associates with DNA to alter gene transcription and, ultimately, the production of proteins that alter cell function.

in addition to lowered percentage of $CD4^+$ and $CD8^+$ T cells and B cells. These data are inconsistent with B cell 'resistance' to glucocorticoid and highlight potential species differences in the immune effects of these drugs. One further recent study investigated the effect of administration of a short (three-day) course of oral prednisone (approximately 2 mg/kg) on the phenotype of lymphocytes aspirated from the popliteal lymph node for a 38-day period post treatment. There was depression in the proportion of $CD3^+$ T cells within these aspirates, with a more marked reduction in $CD4^+$ than $CD8^+$ subsets.

Cytotoxic drugs

The second group of immunosuppressive agents are the cytotoxic drugs used in the treatment of refractory autoimmune disease or cancer. As adjunct immunosuppressives, these agents are generally used in combination with glucocorticoids, and such combination usually allows for lower doses of glucocorticoid to be used in the maintenance phase of therapy. These drugs have severe side-effects involving bone marrow (myelosuppression) and the gastrointestinal tract.

The alkylating agents include **cyclophosphamide** and **chlorambucil**, which alkylate DNA, causing breaks or cross-linkage between or within the strands. This interferes with DNA replication and RNA transcription, thereby affecting both dividing and intermitotic cells (cell cycle non-specific) (**829**).

The thiopurines include **azathioprine**, which acts on the S phase of the cell cycle, competing with adenine in nucleic acid synthesis and leading to substitution with 'nonsense' bases. Azathioprine is considered predominantly to affect T lymphocytes and cell-mediated immunity, with only indirect effects on antibody production by removal of T cell help. The azathioprine-like drug mycophenolate mofetil has enhanced safety and is currently being evaluated as an adjunct immunosuppressive.

The vinca alkaloids (e.g. **vincristine**) bind tubulin and disrupt the mitotic spindle, arresting the cell cycle in M phase. However, the major use of vincristine in the management of immune-mediated disease is as an adjunct thrombopoietic treatment in canine IMTP (see Chapter 4, p. 112) rather than as an immunosuppressive.

As for glucocorticoids, the use of these agents in veterinary medicine is not well-founded in basic pharmacokinetic and immunological studies. There are, for example, suggested to be species differences in tolerance to azathioprine; cats appear to have lower levels of thiopurine methyltransferase (TPMT), which is an enzyme involved in the conversion of the active form of azathioprine (6-mercaptopurine) to inactive metabolites, and in both dogs and cats expression of TPMT is under genetic control, with a range of activities recognized amongst individuals within a population.

Ciclosporin

Ciclosporin has been available for a number of years in a topical ophthalmic form for the treatment of canine KCS (see Chapter 11, p. 272), or as a systemic human formulation, but it is now also licensed as an orally administered microemulsion formulation for the treatment of canine AD (see Chapter 5, p. 133). Ciclosporin has been shown to have clear benefit in the medical therapy of anal furunculosis (see Chapter 7, p. 219). The mode of action of ciclosporin suggests that it should be of benefit in the treatment of numerous other immune-mediated diseases, but to date the efficacy of this drug in the management of conditions such as IMHA, IMTP or IBD has been equivocal. In the context of treatment for this range of immune-mediated disease, ciclosporin has been used in

829

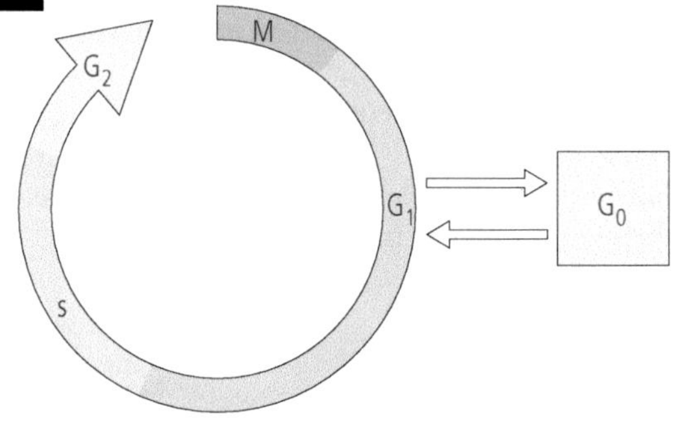

829 The cell cycle. Cytotoxic drugs may affect the cell cycle in a phase-specific or non-specific manner. The cell cycle is initiated by mitosis that is followed by the gap 1 (G1) phase in which there is RNA and protein synthesis. The length of the G1 phase varies between tissues and may extend for days or weeks. From G1, cells may enter a resting state in which they may remain for long periods, or return to G1 to proceed with the cell cycle. During the S phase (usually approximately two hours) there is DNA synthesis, and this is followed by the G2 phase (6–8 hours) during which there is further RNA and protein synthesis.

combination with oral prednisolone as an adjunct therapeutic. The microemulsion formulation of ciclosporin has greater bioavailability and less variation in pharmacokinetics, thus leading to more stable blood concentrations. This latter property means that the frequent monitoring of blood concentrations of ciclosporin recommended for the original form of the drug may not be required for the microemulsion.

Ciclosporin inhibits clonal expansion of T cells by blocking the synthesis of IL-2 and a range of other cytokines. It binds to a cytoplasmic molecule (cyclophilin) and this complex in turn binds to and inhibits the cytoplasmic phosphatase calcineurin, which would normally be activated by increased intracellular calcium to activate the 'nuclear factor of activated T cells' (NFAT) that migrates to the nucleus and binds the transcription factor AP-1. The NFAT and AP-1 complex in turn induces transcription of genes involved in T cell activation, in particular the IL-2 gene. Ciclosporin therefore reduces clonal proliferation of T cells in addition to inhibiting production of IL-2, IL-3, IL-4, G-CSF and TNFα. T cell inhibition results in indirect suppression of B cell function and ciclosporin also has an indirect influence on the activity of granulocytes, macrophages, NK cells, eosinophils and mast cells. Ciclosporin may enhance production of TGFβ, which further increases the immunosuppressive effects of the drug. Much of the preceding information is derived from human medicine or experimental studies and there are few data regarding the immunological effects of ciclosporin in companion animals. One investigation examined the effect of incorporating this agent into cultures of canine blood lymphocytes stimulated with the mitogen PHA. Ciclosporin led to a reduction in transcription of genes encoding IL-2, IL-4 and IFNγ, but did not down-regulate TNFα gene expression.

The related drug **tacrolimus** also acts on this pathway, preventing IL-2 production, and another agent, **rapamycin**, blocks the signalling pathway that is activated after IL-2, IL-4 or IL-6 binds the appropriate membrane receptor. These drugs may be used in combination to prevent both IL-2 production and function. The use of systemic tacrolimus and rapamycin in dogs and cats is currently restricted to experimental studies of transplantation. There is also a topical formulation of tacrolimus, which is effective when applied to the lesions of AD or anal furunculosis. There are numerous potential side-effects from the use of ciclosporin including anorexia, nausea, vomiting, diarrhoea, weight loss, gingival hyperplasia, papillomatosis, hirsuitism, hair shedding, transient lameness and involuntary shaking. Systemic administration of ciclosporin is cost prohibitive and concurrent administration of ketoconazole or grapefruit juice enables reduced dosage because these agents antagonize cytochrome P450 (which metabolizes ciclosporin), thus increasing the bioavailability of ciclosporin.

Leflunomide

The drug leflunomide inhibits pyrimidine synthesis and tyrosine kinase activity and has been used successfully in combination with ciclosporin to induce immunosuppression for transplant surgery. Preliminary studies have shown that leflunomide is effective in the treatment of glucocorticoid-refractory autoimmune diseases (AIHA, AITP, polymyositis, polyarthritis, pemphigus) and systemic histiocytosis in dogs.

Gold salts

Gold salts (chrysotherapy) have been used in the treatment of immune-mediated diseases such as polyarthritis (see Chapter 6, p. 180) and the autoimmune skin disorders (see Chapter 5, p. 148) as either orally administered or injectable agents. They are largely anti-inflammatory in effect, decreasing macrophage function and the production of inflammatory mediators (e.g. leukotrienes), and scavenging oxygen radicals. Immunological effects may include inhibition of T cell function, antibody production and complement C1 activity. Gold salts have a prolonged onset of action and therapy is generally given over several months. These drugs are expensive and associated with a range of side-effects (diarrhoea, cytopenias, muco-cutaneous drug eruption, encephalitis, neuritis, hepatotoxicity or renal disease, the latter particularly in cats). Regular monitoring of haematological and renal parameters is indicated.

Human immunoglobulin

The use of high dose, intravenous human immunoglobulin in the therapy of canine IMHA, IMTP and some forms of immune-mediated skin disease (e.g. EM, TEN) has been described in Chapters 4 and 5. The mode of action of this therapy in IMHA and IMTP largely relates to blockade of macrophage FcRs and inhibition of extravascular phagocytosis of antibody-coated erythrocytes or platelets. The efficacy of this agent in the treatment of diseases of the EM–TEN spectrum is likely due to the interaction of the human immunoglobulin with lymphocyte surface molecules, and specifically interference with the interaction of the Fas–Fas ligand (CD95–CD95L) combination (830).

Summary

Although the range of immunosuppressive medicines described above is widely used, there have been limited attempts to evaluate the optimum protocols for treatment of companion animal immune-mediated disease through well-designed, multicentre, placebo-controlled, blinded studies. There has recently been some attempt to examine combination immunosuppressive protocols through retrospective analysis of case series at individual institutions, and this has led to some re-evaluation of the protocols used. The best example of this has been several publications reviewing therapy of canine IMHA, where the use of combination prednisone and cyclophosphamide has been shown to be associated with a worse clinical outcome, and the use of prednisone plus ciclosporin has not been shown to have benefit over prednisone alone.

Immunopotentiating drugs

A range of non-specific immunopotentiating agents has historically been used in the dog and cat. For example, in canine staphylococcal pyoderma, a killed suspension of *Proprionobacterium acnes* (Immunoregulin™) has been used in addition to staphylococcal antigen preparations (Staphage Lysate™, Staphoid A-B™). An extract of aloe vera (Acemanan™) has been given by intralesional injection into canine and feline cutaneous fibrosarcomas and a range of other tumours. This agent has also been used as adjunct therapy for cats with FeLV or FIV infection and is purported to influence macrophage function and pro-inflammatory cytokine production. Similar effects on macrophages are claimed for an extract of *Serratia marcescens* and products derived from the cell wall of *Mycobacterium* (Regressin-V™; muramyl tripeptide), which have been used as adjunct agents in animals receiving chemotherapy for neoplasia. The immunological effects of such agents are poorly characterized and none is a licensed veterinary product.

One exception to this group of microbial immune stimulants is the formulation of inactivated *Parapoxvirus ovis* (previously Baypamune™, now Zylexis™; currently US licensed only for horses), which is used as adjunct therapy for a range of infectious or stress-related disorders in dogs, cats, horses, pigs and cattle. There is evidence that this agent is able to enhance aspects of innate immunity, particularly related to the action of APCs and activation of T lymphocytes. Stimulation of the production of antiviral interferons and cytokines such as IL-6, IL-12, TNFα and IFNγ has been demonstrated in several species (including man). This product is given by subcutaneous injection on three occasions during the course of disease. It has been most widely applied to the management of FCV infection and canine respiratory disease.

Levamisole was once popular as an immunostimulant on the basis that this drug supposedly enhanced the function of T and B lymphocytes, monocytes and neutrophils, possibly via effects on the metabolism of cyclic nucleotides (c-AMP, c-GMP). Levamisole has also been used in the treatment of canine SLE (see Chapter 14, p. 361). Despite this clinical application, the

830

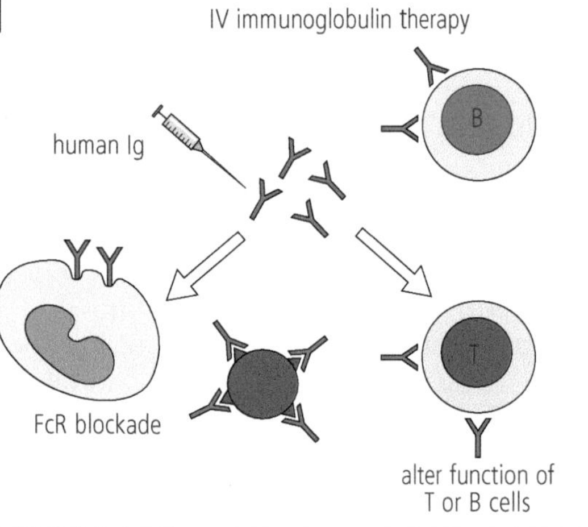

830 Human immunoglobulin therapy. Intravenous administration of a high dose of human immunoglobulin has proven effective in the treatment of canine IMHA, IMTP and skin diseases of the EM–TEN group. The major mechanism of action in IMHA and IMTP is blockade of macrophage FcRs, thereby inhibiting the uptake and extravascular removal of antibody-coated red cells or platelets. In the skin diseases, the effect most likely relates to the binding of lymphocyte surface molecules by human immunoglobulin with modulation of the effector function of these cells. In particular, interference with the CD95–CD95L interaction may block the induction of apoptosis within target cells of a cytotoxic reaction.

immunological effects of levamisole were never seriously evaluated in the dog and use of the drug was associated with a relatively high risk of cutaneous drug eruption. Levamisole can no longer be recommended for this indication.

In human medicine the most promising current means of immunopotentiation involves the use of recombinant cytokines, and there are now numerous such products licensed for human use. The development of such products, and their clinical application, is well-founded in fundamental immunological knowledge of the interplay between the various effector and regulatory T lymphocyte subsets described in Chapter 1 (e.g. Th1, Th2, Th17 and Treg cells). Recombinant cytokines may be administered to modulate or augment an immune response, particularly those to tumours or infectious agents. The nature of the immune response made to such an antigenic stimulus can be manipulated by altering the 'cytokine milieu' in which antigen processing and presentation occurs. The use of recombinant cytokines has been widely shown to be able to manipulate the outcome of experimentally induced disease in rodent models. For example, in murine models of infectious disease, recombinant cytokines such as IL-12, IL-18 or IFNγ are a potent means of inducing protective Th1 immunity (**831**). Recombinant IFNγ has also been used to inhibit type 2 responses and reduce the severity of AD and asthma; for example, delivery of a plasmid containing the IFNγ gene in a liposome carrier directly into the lung of allergen-sensitized mice results in local IFNγ production and inhibition of type 2 pathology. Recombinant IL-4 or IL-13 has been used to prevent the onset of Th1-mediated autoimmune disease (experimental allergic encephalomyelitis) in rodent models.

Similar clinical effects may be predicted with the use of recombinant cytokines in human medicine. The most widely used approach involves the systemic administration of rHuIFNγ in patients with chronic infection, cancer or immunodeficiency disease. Local intralesional injection of rHuIFNγ may also be of benefit in the treatment of human lepromatous leprosy or leishmaniosis. rHu-IL-10 has been used to effect to treat patients with Crohn's disease or psoriasis by down-regulating the pathogenic Th1 effector cells that underlie these conditions. Such cytokine therapy may induce side-effects such as pyrexia or malaise and long-term use may be associated with development of autoimmune disease.

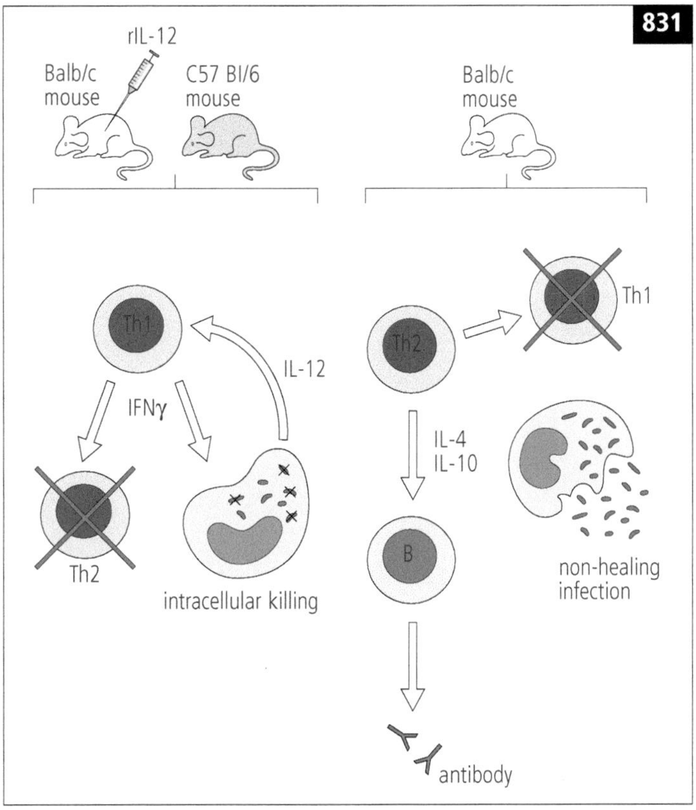

831 Recombinant IL-12 induces cell-mediated immunity. The presence of IL-12 during T cell priming selectively induces a type 1 immune response with IFNγ production and cell-mediated effects. In the murine model of leishmaniosis, C57Bl/6 mice develop a self-healing localized infection (resistant), whereas Balb/c mice develop a non-healing fatal infection (susceptible). This reflects the preferential activation of Th1 versus Th2 CD4+ T cells in each strain. In a type 1 response (C57Bl/6), IFNγ enables intracellular killing of amastigotes within infected macrophages, while suppressing activation of the Th2 population. In a type 2 response (Balb/c), release of Th2-derived IL-4 and IL-10 inhibits activity of the Th1 population, while driving production of specific antibody. Treating susceptible Balb/c mice with recombinant IL-12 results in cure and resistance to infection, with decreased IL-4 production and increased IFNγ synthesis by CD4+ T cells isolated from lymph node.

In human cancer therapy, blood mononuclear cells, or T cells extracted from tumour sites, have been activated by *in vitro* culture with IL-2 (lymphokine activated killer [LAK] cells) and then re-infused into the patient. Approaches such as targeting these cells to the tumour using bi-specific monoclonal antibodies, or transfecting the cytotoxic cells with cytokine genes, have also been studied.

Few clinical studies of recombinant cytokine therapy have been carried out in dogs and cats. LAK cells have been generated from dogs with neoplasia, and recombinant human TNFα and IL-2 have been administered to dogs with mast cell tumour, altering the kinetics of mitogen stimulation of blood lymphocytes in some cases. Recombinant human G-CSF is able to raise neutrophil counts in the dog and cat, but antibodies to the human molecule are produced and may cross-react with endogenous G-CSF, eventually leading to recurrence of the neutropenic state. Such antibodies appear not to develop when human G-CSF is administered during intensive chemotherapy to reverse the neutropenia induced by chemotherapy. Recombinant canine G-CSF and canine stem cell factor have been produced, and canine G-CSF has been used successfully to treat cyclic haematopoiesis and to reverse myelosuppression associated with chemotherapy and parvovirus-induced neutropenia in the dog. Recombinant canine GM-CSF can also elevate neutrophil counts in dogs. Recombinant forms of feline IFNγ, IL-12 and IL-18 have been produced and assessed as potential vaccine adjuvants (see Chapter 17, p. 416), and a recent report suggests that administration of recombinant canine IFNγ to dogs with AD may have therapeutic benefit (Chapter 5) (**832**).

In feline medicine the practice of treating cats affected with chronic viral disease (FeLV, FIV, FIP, FCV-associated chronic gingivostomatitis, FHV-associated keratitis) with adjunct type I interferon has been used for many years. A number of recombinant human IFNα products have been administered either systemically or orally to cats for their antiviral and immunopotentiating effects, but with repeated systemic use an anti-human cytokine immune response will be made as described above. Recently, the first licensed companion animal recombinant cytokine product has become available (Virvagen Omega™). This recombinant feline type I interferon (interferon omega) was initially licensed for the adjunct therapy of dogs with parvoviral enteritis and subsequently for the support of cats with retroviral infection. The use of recombinant cytokine therapy in animals may also be associated with side-effects. For example, in dogs the use of recombinant feline interferon omega may be associated with transient pyrexia, vomiting and pancytopenia and there is a possible theoretical risk of the induction of autoimmunity with long-term use.

832

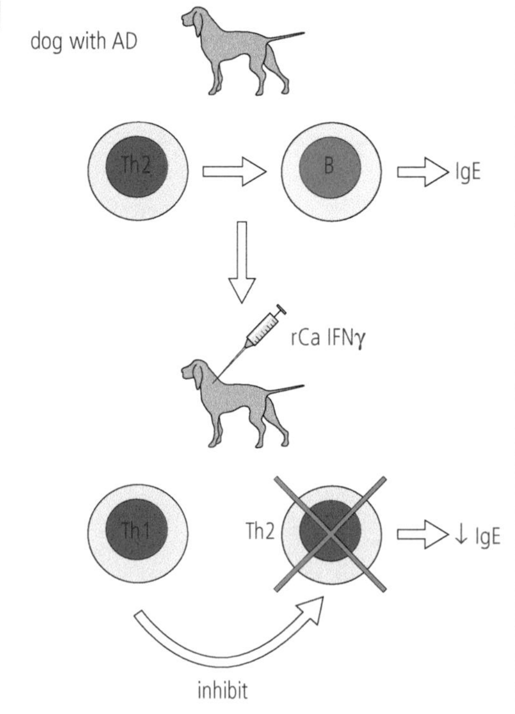

832 Recombinant cytokine therapy for canine atopic dermatitis. In canine AD the immune response is dominated by Th2 regulatory cells, which drive the production of allergen-specific IgE. Administration of recombinant canine IFNγ likely inhibits the function of Th2 cells and may also enhance the activity of the allergen-specific Th1 population.

MONOCLONAL ANTIBODIES IN IMMUNOTHERAPY

Many novel immunotherapies rely on the use of monoclonal antibodies. Monoclonal antibody technology involves the *in vitro* production of antibody of a single specificity (from a single B cell clone) in virtually unlimited quantity (**833**). Most monoclonal antibodies are of mouse or rat origin, but other species, including human or dog, can be a source of immunized cells, and a canine heterohybridoma secreting, nematode-specific IgE has been produced by fusion of canine lymphocytes with a mouse myeloma line.

A major application of monoclonal antibody therapy has been for the management of neoplastic disease. Monoclonal antibodies designed to recognize 'tumour antigens' will selectively target neoplastic cells when injected into a patient. They may be used as carriers of various toxic agents or act to optimize immune attack on the neoplastic population (**834**). There are numerous examples of the ability of monoclonal antibodies to alter the outcome of disease in experimental rodent models by targeting specific immunological molecules and interfering with their function. In these models the antibodies are generally administered systemically by intraperitoneal or intravenous injection.

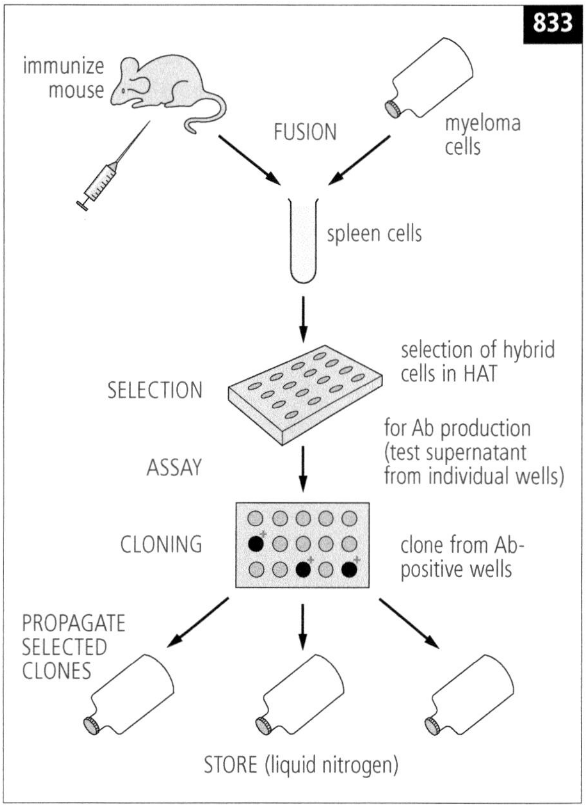

833 Monoclonal antibody production. A mouse is immunized with the antigen of interest and when serum antibody is detected, the spleen is removed and a suspension of splenocytes prepared. Polyethylene glycol is used to fuse the splenocytes to a myeloma cell line, and the resulting hybridoma cells are selected by growth in HAT medium. Unfused splenocytes will die in culture, and myeloma cells lack an enzyme of the purine salvage pathway and so are sensitive to HAT and also die. In contrast, hybrid cells are HAT resistant and grow in culture (i.e. have properties of both fusion partners). The hybrid colonies may contain a number of different cell clones and produce antibodies of several specificities, so the process of cloning by limiting dilution gives rise to new colonies that are derived from a single B cell hybrid. The monospecific clone can now be propagated in large vessels and the monoclonal antibody is secreted into the tissue culture supernatant. The monoclonal antibody may be concentrated or, alternatively, the hybridoma cells can be inoculated intraperitoneally into a mouse. The hybrid cells grow *in vivo* and release monoclonal antibody into ascites fluid. Aliquots of the cell line are stored frozen in liquid nitrogen.

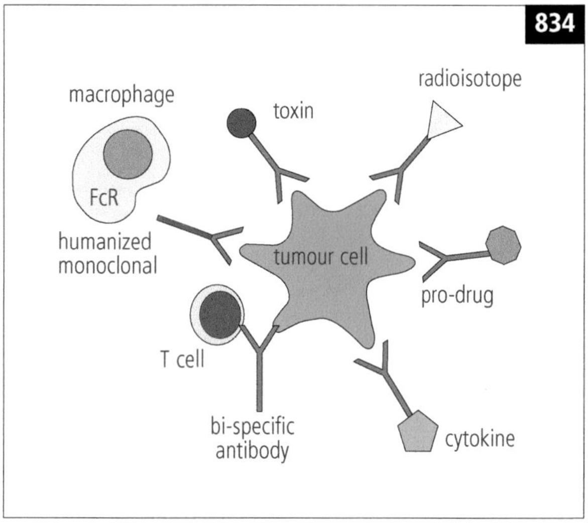

834 Use of monoclonal antibodies in oncology. Genetically engineered monoclonal antibodies with a human immunoglobulin framework and murine antigen binding sites have been produced to reduce the antigenicity of foreign monoclonal antibodies in a human recipient. Such antibodies have the benefit of potentially interacting with human FcRs in the elimination of target (e.g. tumour) cells. Bi-specific monoclonal antibodies have been produced that have one Fab able to bind to tumour antigens and a second Fab specific for T cell or NK cell surface molecules. Monoclonal antibodies specific for tumour antigens may be conjugated to toxins (e.g. ricin), cytotoxic drugs or radioisotopes, enzymes able to activate pro-drugs, or cytokines (immunocytokines). These will all be selectively delivered to the site of the tumour.

Examples of these applications include:

- Monoclonal antibodies binding to specific lymphocyte populations (via surface molecules such as CD4, CD8, CD3, TCR) and 'depleting' these cells (via complement-mediated cytotoxicity) or down-regulating the target molecule, thus rendering the cell functionally inactive. This approach has been used to prevent a range of experimental autoimmune diseases (**835**) or to deplete alloreactive T cells and prevent graft rejection.
- Monoclonal antibodies may be used to inhibit the interactions of MHC class II, TCR and co-stimulatory molecules (**836**).
- Monoclonal antibodies specific for adhesion molecules may prevent the egress of cells into inflammatory sites (**837**).
- Monoclonal antibodies may be used to neutralize cytokines *in vivo* and prevent or cure disease (**838**).

Monoclonal antibodies have also been applied to the treatment of infectious disease (for example by targeting and blocking receptor molecules used by microorganisms).

Monoclonal antibody therapy is now commonplace in human medicine, where an increasing range of licensed products is available for treatment of specific disorders. The most successful of these products have been monoclonal antibodies specific for the T cell surface molecule CD52 (Campath-1™) and for the cytokine TNFα (Infliximab™; Remicade™). Campath-1 has been successfully employed in

835

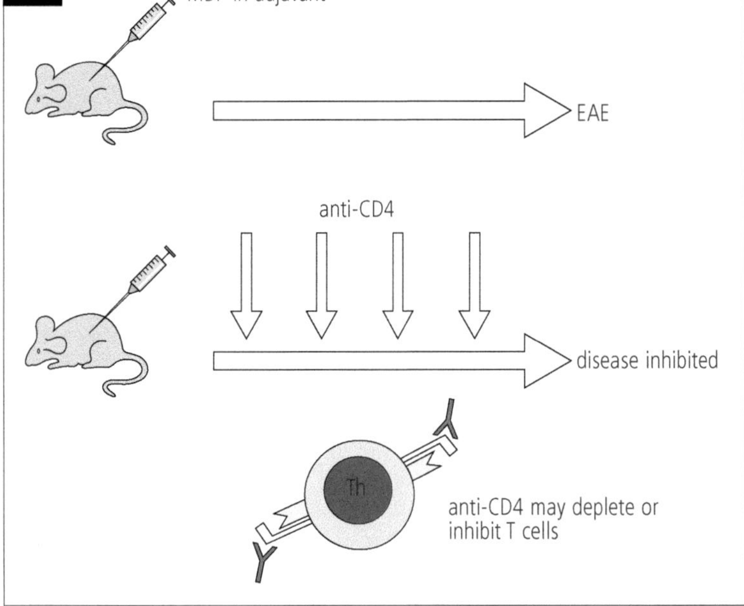

835 Therapeutic use of T cell-specific monoclonal antibodies. Organ-specific autoimmune disease may be induced in particular strains of mice or rats by immunization with autoantigen in adjuvant. For example, lymphocytic thyroiditis may be induced by injection of thyroglobulin or EAE (a model for multiple sclerosis) by injection of myelin basic protein (see **166**). If T cells (particularly $CD4^+$ T cells) are depleted or made functionally inactive by repeated administration of monoclonal antibody, T cell priming does not occur and the animals do not develop autoimmune disease. The blanket suppression of $CD4^+$ T cells will non-specifically influence other (protective) immune responses.

836

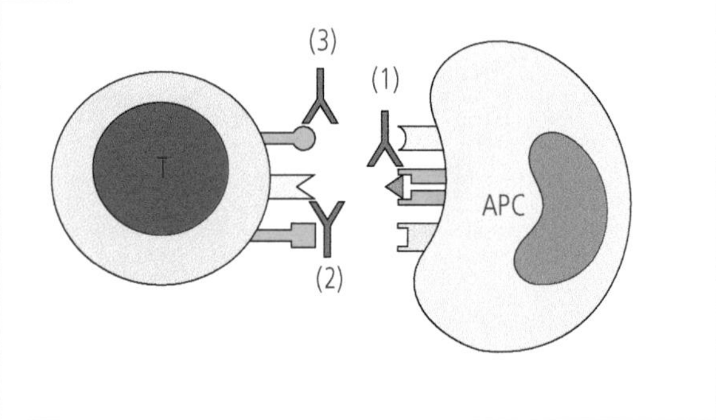

836 Therapeutic use of anti-class II monoclonal antibody. (1) Monoclonal antibody specific for MHC class II will bind to these histocompatibility molecules and interfere with the binding of the TCR. This approach has been used to prevent the onset of EAE (see **835**). The monoclonal antibody will non-specifically suppress all other immune responses that rely on MHC class II restricted antigen presentation. Similarly, monoclonal antibodies specific for (2) the TCR or (3) co-stimulatory molecules will also suppress such responses.

patients with RA and multiple sclerosis, and used in the immunosuppression of transplant patients. Infliximab^{TM} has a beneficial effect in patients with RA, Crohn's disease and psoriasis. However, the *in vivo* use of monoclonal antibodies in humans has not been without problems. In order to achieve the desired effects, antibodies must be given in relatively high doses over a long period of time. The antibody itself is a foreign protein and the recipient may make antibody to the rodent Ig, leading to formation of CICs. This problem has been reduced in man by methods including the creation of 'humanized' monoclonal antibodies with human heavy chain and murine antigen-binding site. Even so, some patients treated with monoclonal antibodies have gone on to develop a 'serum sickness'-like syndrome, secondary infection or autoimmune disease. Examples of other human monoclonal antibody products include anti-IgE (Omalizumab^{TM}), which is used to complex free IgE and prevent binding to mast cells or basophils in patients with allergic asthma; anti-IL-5 or anti-eotaxin, which is used in allergic patients to reduce eosinophil infiltration of tissues; and anti-α_4 (Natalizumab^{TM}), which is used to block the interaction between the $\alpha_4\beta_7$ molecule on the surface of circulating T cells with the vascular addressin MAdCAM-1, thus preventing egress of

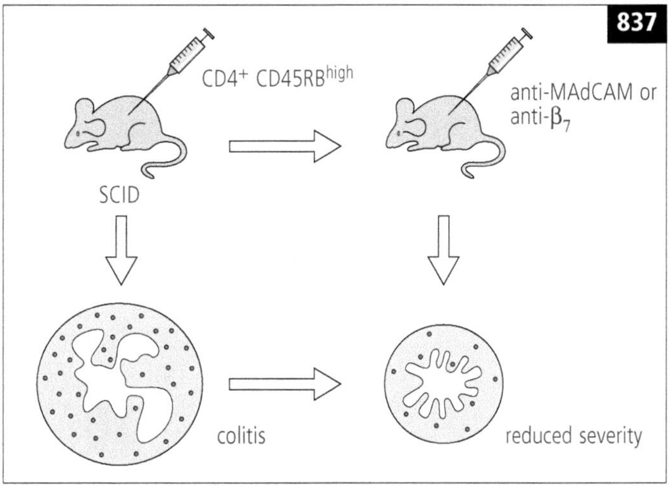

837 Therapeutic use of monoclonal antibodies specific for adhesion molecules. The specific homing of activated lymphocytes and other leukocytes to a tissue underlies many immune-mediated diseases. For example, when SCID mice (that lack normal populations of T and B lymphocytes) are injected with normal mouse CD4$^+$ T cells enriched for the CD45RB^{high} subpopulation, the cells are recruited to the colon and induce severe inflammatory disease. If mice destined to develop chronic colitis are treated by injection of monoclonal antibody specific for mucosal endothelial addressin (MAdCAM-1) or the T cell ligand for this molecule (β_7 integrin), the egress of T cells is prevented and the severity of the colitis reduced. (Data from Picarella D, Hurlbut P, Rottman J *et al.* [1997] Monoclonal antibodies specific for β_7 integrin and mucosal addressin cell adhesion molecule-1 reduce inflammation in the colon of SCID mice reconstituted with CD45RB^{high} CD4$^+$ T cells. *Journal of Immunology* **158:**2099–2106.)

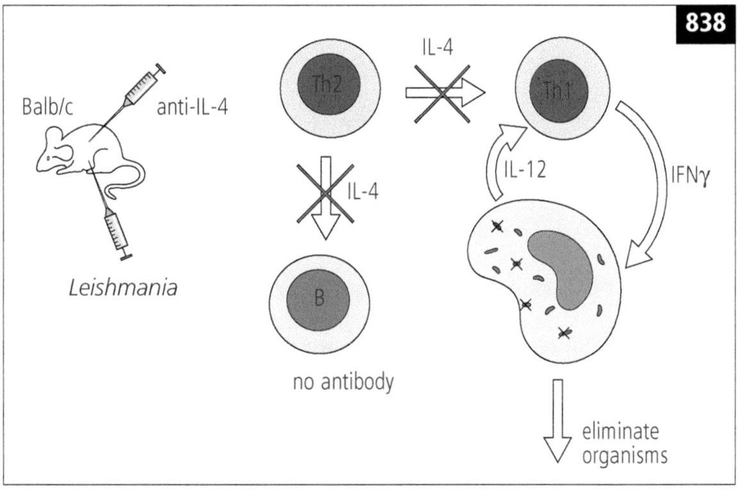

838 Therapeutic use of monoclonal antibody to cytokine. The outcome of disease in the murine model of leishmaniosis described in **831** can also be manipulated by the use of monoclonal antibodies specific for cytokines. For example, administration of monoclonal antibody to IL-4 can enable Balb/c (susceptible) mice to mount a type 1 response and eliminate intracellular amastigotes to recover from infection.

lymphocytes from blood into intestinal lamina propria in patients with inflammatory bowel disease.

An alternative to the use of monoclonal antibodies for neutralization of cytokines *in vivo* is the use of a 'cytokine trap' such as a soluble, recombinant form of the cytokine receptor. The efficacy of these molecules can be greatly enhanced by forming complexes of cytokine receptor and immunoglobulin Fc, and this type of complex also reduces the likelihood of the patient forming neutralizing antibodies to the cytokine receptor molecule. Yet another possibility is blockade of cytokine receptors by the use of monoclonal antibodies specific for these molecules, or cytokine analogues that compete with endogenous cytokines for available receptor sites.

A similar approach has been the use of antagonist molecules to interfere with other key immunological molecular interactions. For example, a recombinant LFA-3 fused to human immunoglobulin Fc (Alefacept^{TM}) binds to CD2 on the surface of T cells, thus preventing the natural engagement of this molecule by endogenous LFA-3 expressed by the APC. Similarly, a construct of recombinant CTLA-4 with human Fc binds the

839

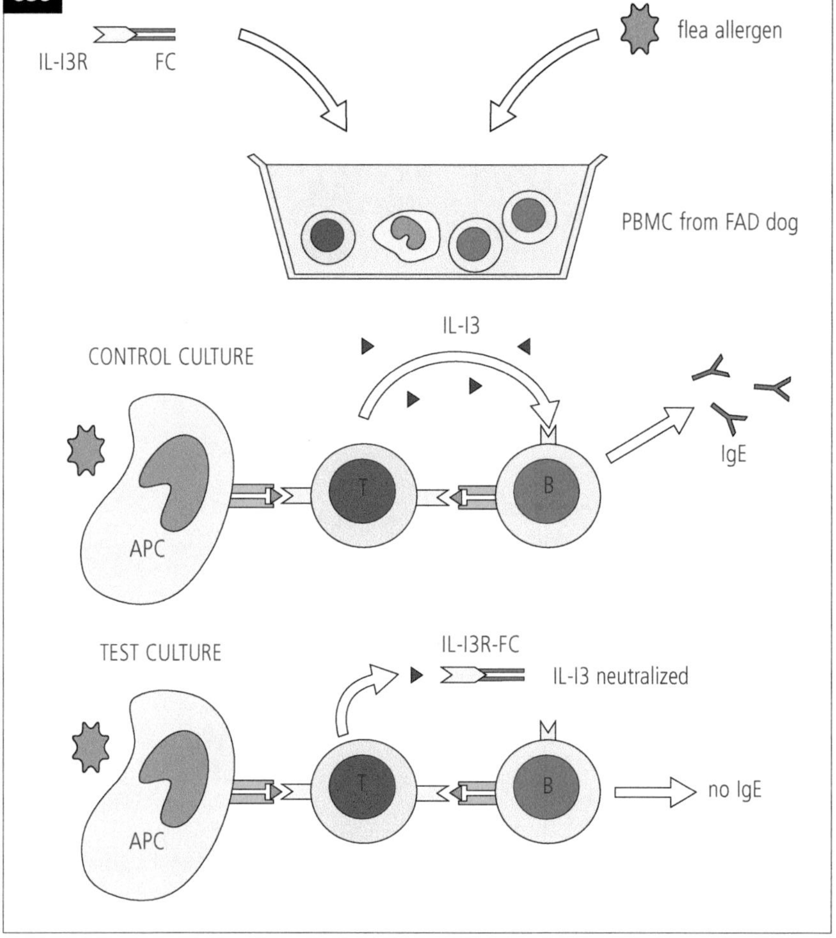

839 Cytokine 'trap' therapy. Cytokine function may be neutralized by the use of cytokine receptor 'traps', which compete with endogenous cytokine receptor for cytokine. In this study a construct of canine IL-13R 'protected' by complexing with canine Fc was used to neutralize IL-13 produced by antigen-specific T cells from dogs with flea allergy dermatitis (FAD) stimulated *in vitro*. Neutralization of the cytokine prevented activation of flea allergen-specific B cells and, therefore, the production of allergen-specific IgE within the culture system. A similar effect may be predicted to occur *in vivo*. (Data from Tang L, Boroughs KL, Morales T *et al*. [2001] Recombinant canine IL-13 receptor α_2-Fc fusion protein inhibits canine allergen-specific IgE production *in vitro* by peripheral blood mononuclear cells from allergic dogs. *Veterinary Immunology and Immunopathology* **83:**115–122.)

natural CTLA-4 ligand (CD80/86) expressed by APCs. This prevents this ligand from engaging the T cell surface molecule CD28, which would result in T cell activation (see Chapter 1, p. 57).

To date, there has been limited study of monoclonal antibody therapy in companion animal medicine, although a monoclonal antibody specific for canine IFNγ has been used to prolong the life of experimental kidney allografts in this species and an anti-human TNFα product has been evaluated for treatment of CLE in the German Shorthaired Pointer (Chapter 5). A recent advance is the construction of the canine IL-13 receptor linked to canine Fc, which has been shown to neutralize canine IL-13 by inhibiting *in vitro* proliferation and IgE production by antigen-stimulated blood mononuclear cells from flea-allergic dogs (**839**).

ANTIGEN-SPECIFIC IMMUNOTHERAPY

Antigen-specific immunotherapy involves identification of specific peptide sequences of an antigen and administration of them (or sometimes of entire antigen) in a manner that induces an immune response different to that which occurs when antigen enters the body by the naturally occurring (pathogenic) route. This approach is essentially based on the induction of immunological tolerance (see Chapter 1, p. 58), which most likely involves the induction of IL-10 producing Treg cells. The major benefit of antigen-specific immunotherapy lies in selective targeting of antigen-relevant pathogenic lymphocytes, without affecting the entire immune system in a 'blanket' fashion, thus reducing the likelihood of secondary infection.

Autoantigens (or peptides derived from them) may be delivered orally to modulate the onset or clinical course of autoimmune disease. This method has been used to prevent or ameliorate autoimmune disease in rodent models (**840**, **841**), and in human trials there has been some success in individual patients fed antigens for the treatment of multiple sclerosis, RA, uveitis or type 1 diabetes. The mechanism of tolerance may involve a switch from a Th1 to a Th2 dominated response or induction of regulatory cells (e.g. Th3 cells), and it appears to be dose dependent. The switch may be potentiated by conjugation of antigen to 'mucosal adjuvants' such as cholera toxin or the B-subunit of *E. coli* heat-labile enterotoxin.

A similar approach involves intranasal administration of autoantigen or allergen to prevent or ameliorate autoimmunity or type I

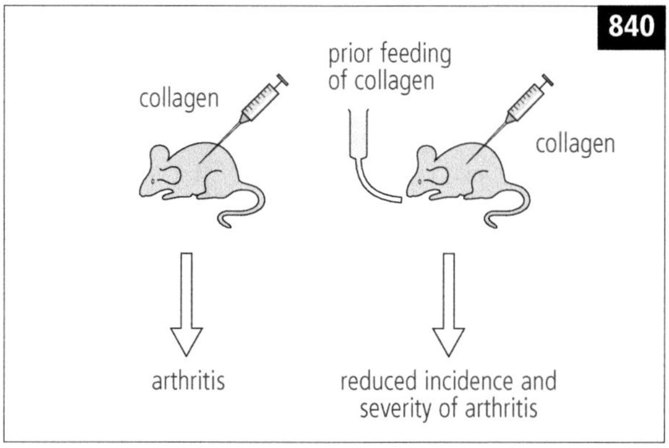

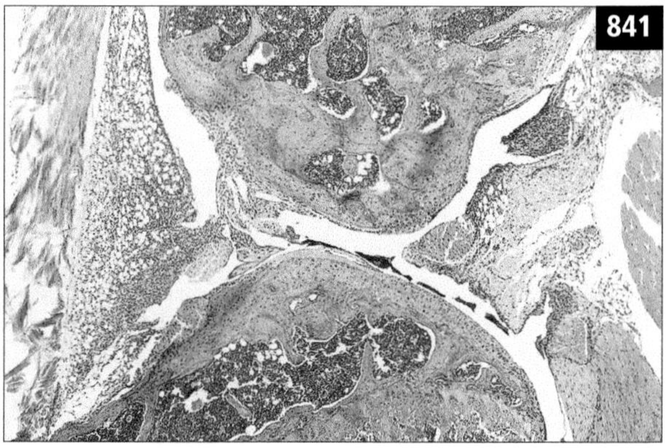

840, 841 Feeding autoantigen prevents experimental autoimmune disease. In experimental models of autoimmune disease induced by immunizing with specific autoantigen, prior feeding of the autoantigen may prevent the pathology and clinical signs of disease. The mechanism underlying this approach is poorly characterized, but may reflect an alteration in the balance of immunoregulatory cytokines. (**840**) The approach has been used effectively in a range of disease models including collagen-induced arthritis, which is a model of rheumatoid arthritis. (**841**) Section of stifle joint from a mouse with collagen-induced arthritis demonstrates marked infiltration of the synovium by neutrophils and macrophages, with articular erosions and pannus formation.

hypersensitivity (**842**). Intranasal peptide administration is more powerful than the use of the oral route, and exquisitely small doses of antigen have potent effects. Although one peptide is used in the treatment, there is intramolecular spreading of tolerance to all peptides in the antigen.

Coupling antigen to monoclonal antibody specific for IgD targets antigen for presentation by B lymphocytes and selective induction of a Th2 response (**843**).

Synthetic peptides may be designed that compete with endogenously derived self-peptides for MHC binding sites, but do not permit TCR interactions. These analogue peptides may also induce analogue-specific immune responses that cross-regulate those to the natural self-peptide. A recent study has described an immunotherapeutic vaccine for canine myasthenia gravis. Complementary peptides were designed to bind to autoantigenic peptides from the AchR acting as an antigen-receptor mimic. Injection of these peptides induces an antibody that can block T- or B-cell receptors

A number of immunotherapeutic approaches to AD are under investigation (**844–846**). There has been some application of antigen-specific

842

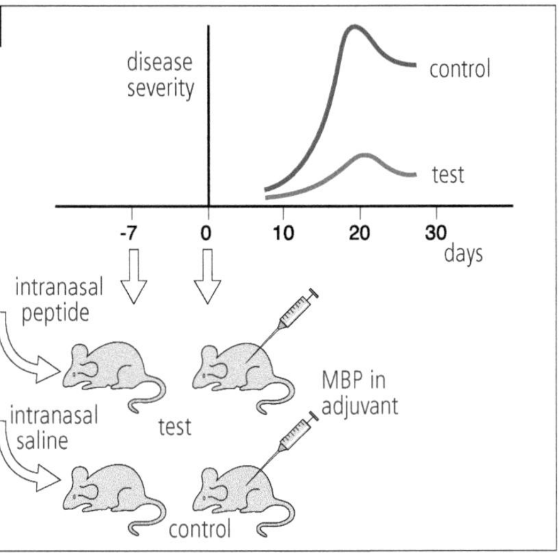

842 Intranasal peptide therapy. Intranasal administration of small doses of peptide derived from autoantigen or allergen prevents subsequent induction of a pathogenic immune response to the entire antigen. In addition, such treatment may ameliorate an ongoing pathogenic response if given later in the course of disease. In this example, mice were given a peptide (residues 1–11) derived from MBP by intranasal deposition, and seven days later immunized with entire MBP in adjuvant subcutaneously. The severity and incidence of disease (EAE) was markedly reduced relative to control animals that did not receive intranasal peptide.

843

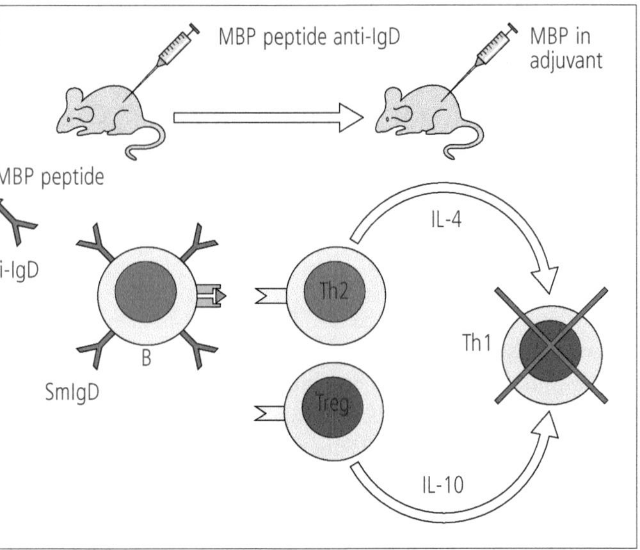

843 Therapeutic use of selective induction of type 2 responses. In the rat model of EAE, the encephalitogenic peptide of MBP was conjugated to a monoclonal antibody specific for rat IgD. When administered to rats, this effectively targeted the peptide for presentation by B lymphocytes and induction of a type 2 immune response. Subsequent administration of entire MBP in adjuvant failed to induce EAE of normal severity and incidence, as the pathogenic Th1 cells were down-regulated by the presence of Th2-derived IL-4 and Treg-derived IL-10.

844 IgE blockade in type I hypersensitivity. A conserved decapeptide sequence of IgE has been identified. When given to animals or man it induces formation of an antibody that can bind to this region of mast cell-associated IgE and prevent cross-linking of these molecules by allergen. This approach is effective in experimental rodents and human patients, and trials for canine flea allergy dermatitis are being undertaken.

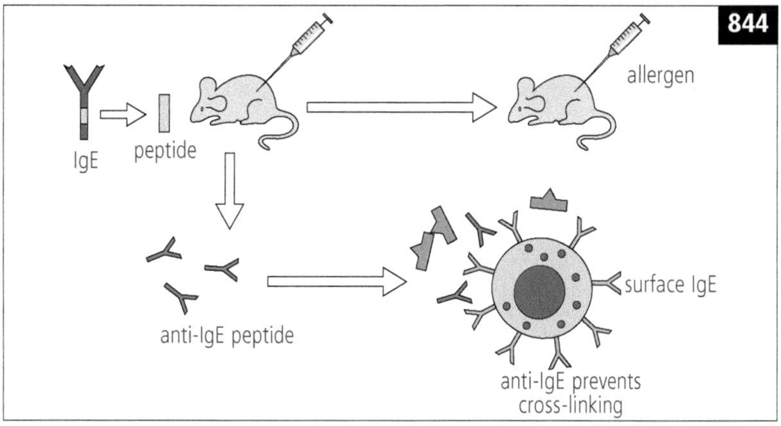

845 IgE blockade in type I hypersensitivity. In this study, a synthetic peptide was produced from the area of the IgE heavy chain that interacts with the high affinity FcεRI found on the surface of mast cells. The peptide was linked to a T cell epitope derived from the measles virus as a means of breaking the normal 'tolerance' towards endogenous IgE, such that an anti-IgE humoral immune response could be produced. Dogs vaccinated with this construct had reduced concentration of serum IgE. (Data from Wang CY, Walfield AM, Fang XD *et al.* [2003] Synthetic IgE peptide vaccine for immunotherapy of allergy. *Vaccine* **21:**1580–1590.)

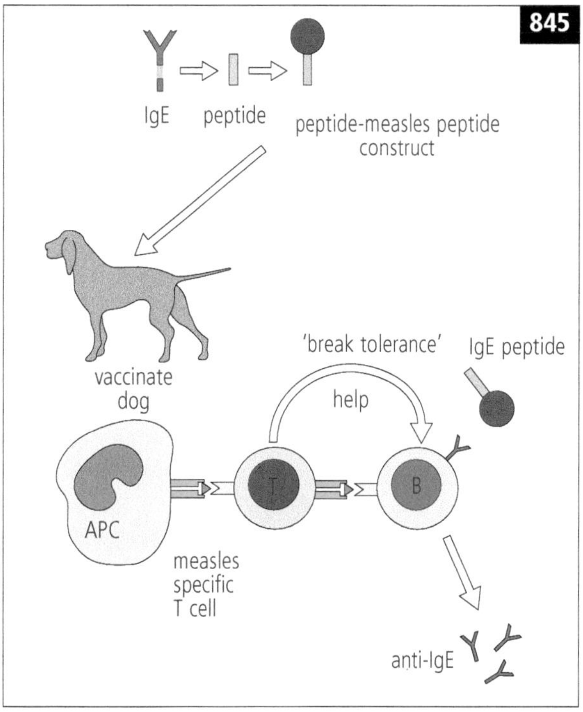

846 IgE blockade in type I hypersensitivity. In this study a recombinant protein was produced using a construct containing the canine $C_{\varepsilon3}$ gene flanked by the $C_{\varepsilon2}$ and $C_{\varepsilon4}$ genes from the opossum. When given to dogs by intramuscular injection in adjuvant, the foreign opossum portions of the recombinant protein induce loss of tolerance to the canine sequence, permitting the establishment of an anti-dog IgE response, which lowers serum IgE concentration in the vaccinated animals. (Data from Ledin A, Bergvall K, Hilbertz NS *et al.* [2006] Generation of therapeutic antibody responses against IgE in dogs, an animal species with exceptionally high plasma IgE levels. *Vaccine* **24:** 66–74.)

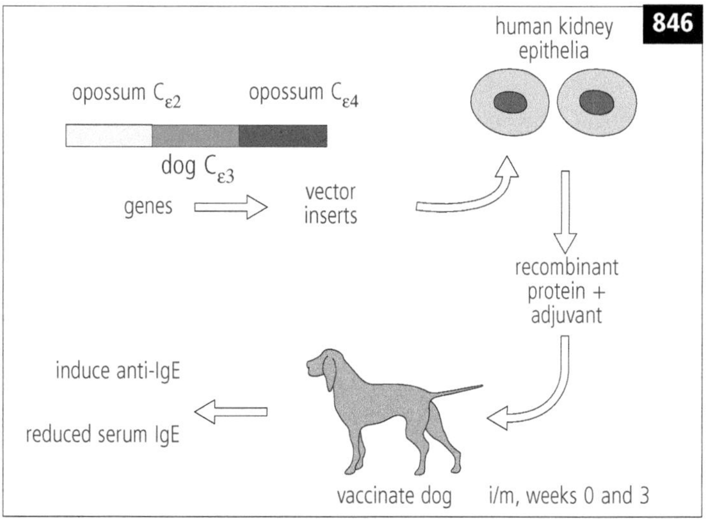

immunotherapy to canine immune-mediated disease. For example, allergen-specific immunotherapy is regularly used for AD (see Chapter 5, p. 133), autogenous vaccination with patient-derived staphylococcal preparations is used in the therapy of pyoderma, and oral tolerance may be experimentally induced in dogs (**847**). An unlicensed product is available that is based on the oral administration of collagen type II to dogs with arthritis in an attempt to ameliorate joint disease by

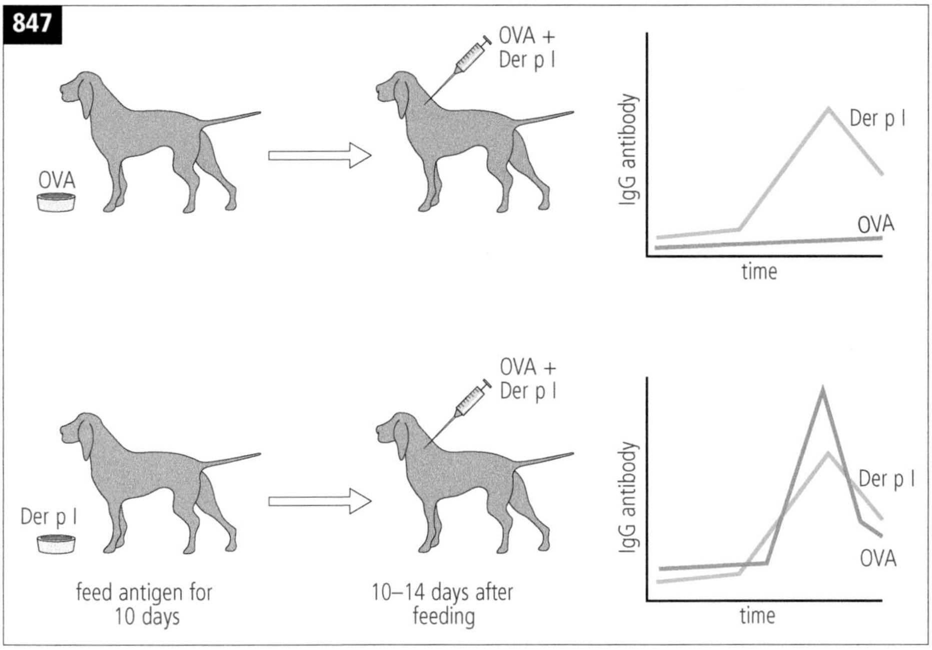

847 Induction of oral tolerance in the dog. Young dogs maintained in an animal house environment were fed the antigen ovalbumin (OVA) (10 g q24h for 10 days) and subsequently challenged with OVA (1 mg) and the house dust mite-derived antigen Der pI (400 μg) in adjuvant by subcutaneous injection. The antibody response obtained to the fed antigen (OVA) was markedly reduced relative to the response to Der p I. In the same experiment it was not possible to induce oral tolerance to Der pI, as an insufficient quantity of the recombinant molecule was available to provide an optimum oral dose. (Data from Deplazes P, Penhale WJ, Greene WK *et al.* [1995] Effect on humoral tolerance (IgG and IgE) in dogs by oral administration of ovalbumin and Der pI. *Veterinary Immunology and Immunopathology* **45:**361–367.)

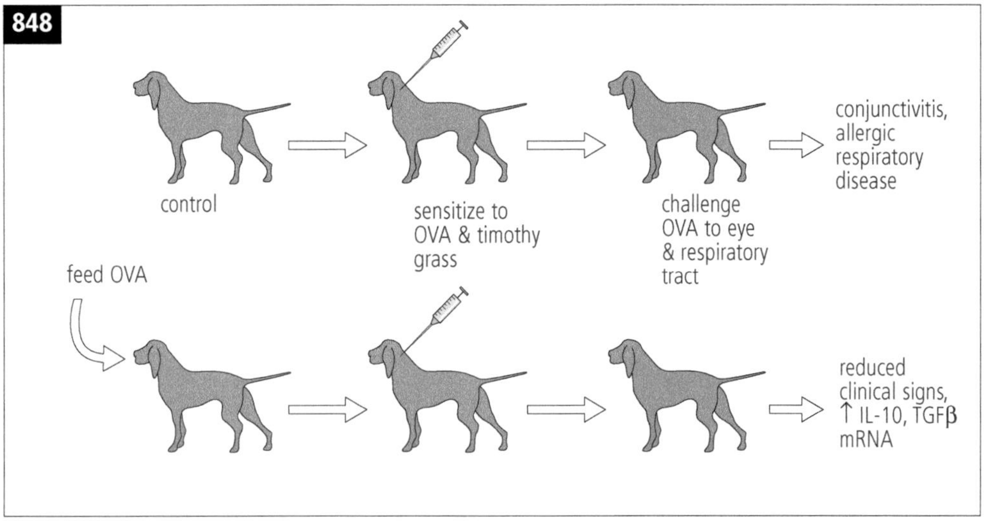

848 Therapeutic oral tolerance in the dog. One of two groups of experimental dogs was orally tolerized to OVA before both groups were sensitized to this antigen (and also Timothy grass). After sensitization, both groups were challenged by ocular (conjunctival) and respiratory tract (nebulization) exposure to OVA. Dogs that had been orally tolerized had less severe clinical reactions to allergen challenge and higher levels of mRNA encoding immunoregulatory cytokines (IL-10, TGFβ) in cells collected from BAL fluid.

restoring immunological tolerance to joint collagen. In a recent experimental study, high IgE responder Beagle dogs were orally tolerized to OVA and subsequently sensitized by repeated injection to both ovalbumin and recombinant Timothy grass pollen allergen. A control group was sensitized without prior oral tolerization. Tolerized dogs had reduced allergic conjunctivitis following ocular challenge with OVA, and reduced features of allergic airway disease following challenge by nebulization. These protective effects were associated with elevation of levels of mRNA expressing the regulatory cytokines IL-10 and TGFβ in cells derived from the bronchoalveolar lavage fluid (848).

GENE THERAPY

There are two broad applications of 'gene therapy' in the treatment of immune-mediated disease. The first involves the delivery of genes encoding immunoregulatory molecules to animals or humans with disease as an alternative to delivery of the recombinant protein form of the same molecule. Gene delivery may be achieved using a viral vector or, more directly, by incorporating the gene into a plasmid ('naked DNA'), which directly transfects host cells and leads to gene expression. Delivery of gene sequence may be a more potent means of manipulating an immune response than administration of recombinant protein with short half-life. This principle has now been well documented in experimental rodent models of disease. For example, the administration of vectored genes (IL-12 or IL-18) or 'naked DNA' by nebulization into the airways of allergen-sensitized animals can ameliorate the immune response following allergen challenge. In the context of manipulating immune responses towards a Th1-dominated outcome, the incorporation of 'molecular adjuvants' such as CpG motifs may further enhance the effect (see also Chapter 17). This approach has already been experimentally applied to the treatment of dogs with AD, in addition to the delivery of plasmids containing genes encoding the specific allergen that triggered the clinical disease (see Chapter 5, p. 135).

Other microbial derivatives are also recognized as potent immunomodulators capable of reversing the balance of T cell activity. For example, the B-subunit of *E. coli* heat-labile enterotoxin can switch the immune response from Th1 to Th2 and prevent the clinical signs and joint pathology in mice with adjuvant-induced arthritis. Intranasal administration of BCG from *Mycobacterium* can prevent the signs of allergic airway disease on challenging sensitized mice, suggesting in this case a switch from Th2 to Th1 immunity or induction of Treg cells. A single injection of heat-killed *M. vaccae* has recently been shown to be of benefit in the management of dogs with mild to moderate AD and, presumptively, it acts in this fashion. Delivery of cytokine-encoding genes (e.g. IL-4, IL-10) to the synovium of animals with immune-mediated arthritis, or intralesionally into neoplastic tissue (e.g. IL-2 or IFNγ), may have a similar beneficial outcome, and cytokine genes have also been used as vaccine adjuvants (see Chapter 17, p. 416).

The second application for 'gene therapy' is for the correction of monogenic defects that underlie primary metabolic or immunodeficiency disorders. In dogs and cats this is unlikely to become a widespread practice, as genetic counselling and elimination of affected breeding lines may be of greater relevance (see Chapter 12, p. 313), but preliminary studies have shown that gene therapy can be applied to the dog. Experimental gene transfer has been performed into haemopoietic progenitor cells of normal dogs and dogs with cyclic haematopoiesis, and viral vectors have been used successfully to transfer gene constructs to a range of canine cell types. An inbred line of dogs with haemophilia B were given a retroviral vector containing canine factor IX cDNA by infusion into the portal vasculature after partial hepatectomy. This procedure produced detectable plasma canine factor IX, with reduced clotting time for up to nine months after treatment. An alternative approach, using an adenovirus vector incorporating the gene and administered by intramuscular injection, was also successful until the treated dogs generated an immune response to the factor IX, which was essentially 'foreign' to their immune system. Recent studies of X-SCID dogs have reported intravenous administration of retrovirus vector incorporating the gene encoding the canine γ chain of the IL-2 receptor. In three of four treated dogs there was normalization of T cell number and function, followed by normalization of B cell number, serum IgG concentration and ability to seroconvert following CDV and CPV vaccination. Although such gene replacement therapy holds enormous promise, preliminary clinical trials in human patients revealed the potential for induction of unforeseen side-effects; for example, leukaemia in treated children.

TRANSPLANTATION AND STEM CELL THERAPY

Transplantation

Graft rejection is complex, but the major factor initiating rejection is recognition of MHC incompatibility between donor and recipient (alloreactivity) (**849**). Rejection may be hyperacute (minutes to hours) in recipients with pre-existing antibodies to donor antigens (MHC or blood group) following previous blood transfusion, transplantation or pregnancy. In this case there is complement-mediated endothelial damage, resulting in thrombosis and ischaemic necrosis of the graft. Acute rejection occurs due to primary (days to weeks) or secondary (days) T cell activation, with infiltration of the graft and destruction of vascular endothelium and parenchyma. Antibody may also have a role in acute rejection (**850**). Chronic (months to years) rejection is less well understood and may involve a range of mechanisms including low-grade cell-mediated processes or local immune complex deposition.

'Tissue typing' is performed to identify the closest match between donor and recipient and, due to the nature of inheritance of MHC, siblings or parents provide the best chance for compatible transplantation. Identification of tissue type was traditionally carried out serologically for class I products and by mixed leukocyte culture (MLC) for class II molecules. These procedures have now

849

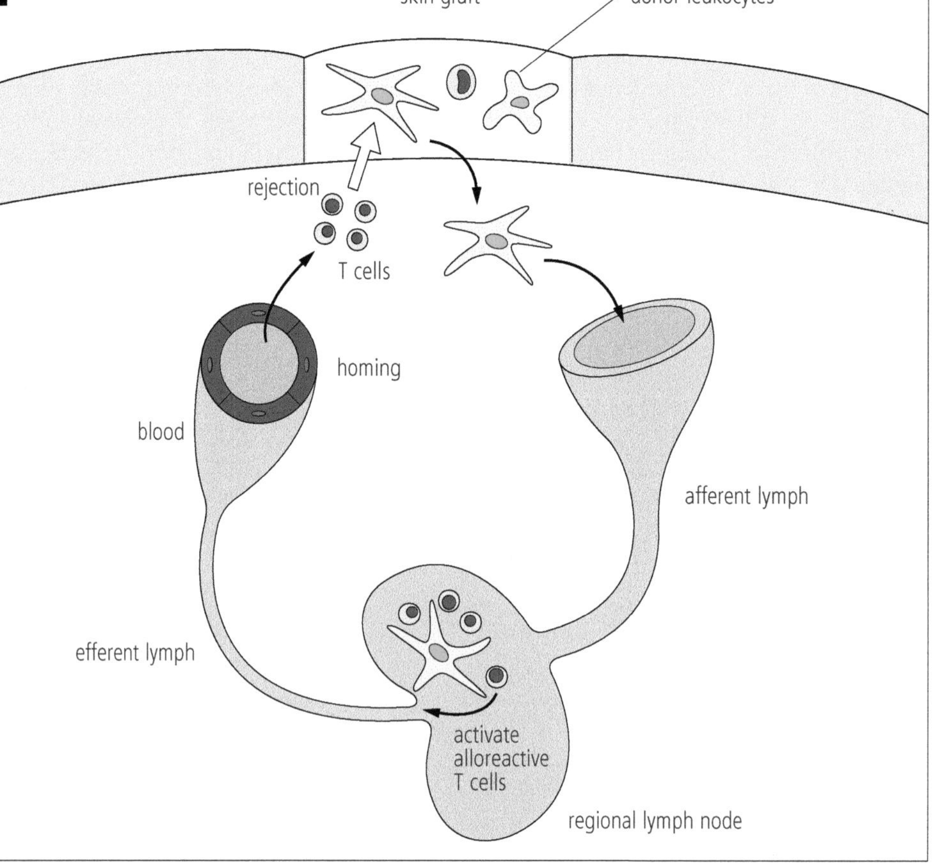

849 Alloreactive T cell activation in acute graft rejection. Grafted tissue contains donor 'passenger' leukocytes such as dendritic cells that migrate to the lymph node draining the graft, where they are exposed to recipient alloreactive T cells. Shed donor antigens may also be taken up by host APCs for T cell activation. Activated effector cells migrate to the graft via the vasculature and mediate cytotoxic destruction of the graft, but the mechanism by which donor APCs activate recipient T cells is poorly understood.

largely been superseded by molecular techniques involving:

- Amplification of specific genomic DNA by PCR and determination of sequence differences between individuals.
- The creation of oligonucleotide probes based on these areas of sequence difference and their use to screen genomic DNA by direct hybridization.

There is a vast literature on tissue (bone marrow) and organ (e.g. kidney, liver, heart/lung, pancreas, intestine) transplantation in the dog, as this species has been used experimentally in the development of transplantation science. The success of canine transplantation has been augmented by the administration of immunosuppressive drugs and anti-T cell (Thy-1, CD4, CD8) or anti-cytokine (IFNγ) monoclonal or polyclonal antibodies. Monoclonal antibodies can deplete lymphocyte subpopulations from donor bone marrow and prevent graft versus host disease on transfer of the marrow to mismatched, irradiated recipients. In graft versus host disease, leukocytes within a graft attack the tissues of an immunoincompetent or immunosuppressed recipient.

There are fewer reports of the use of cats in transplantation studies, and one potential problem that has been demonstrated in this species is the transmission of FeLV from infected donor to recipient. A feline allograft model using a gracillus musculocutaneous flap has been studied. Rejection of the flap involved vasculitis, with perivascular CD4 and CD8 infiltrating cells. Rejection was delayed with ciclosporin and prednisolone immunosuppression. Successful autologous and allogeneic bone marrow transplantation has recently been described in the cat.

There have been few reports of the application of these studies to clinical veterinary medicine. Bone marrow transplantation has been used successfully to treat a dog with cyclic haematopoiesis and four cats with Chediak-Higashi syndrome, and there are isolated reports of the clinical use of bone marrow transplantation. One cat with myeloid leukaemia

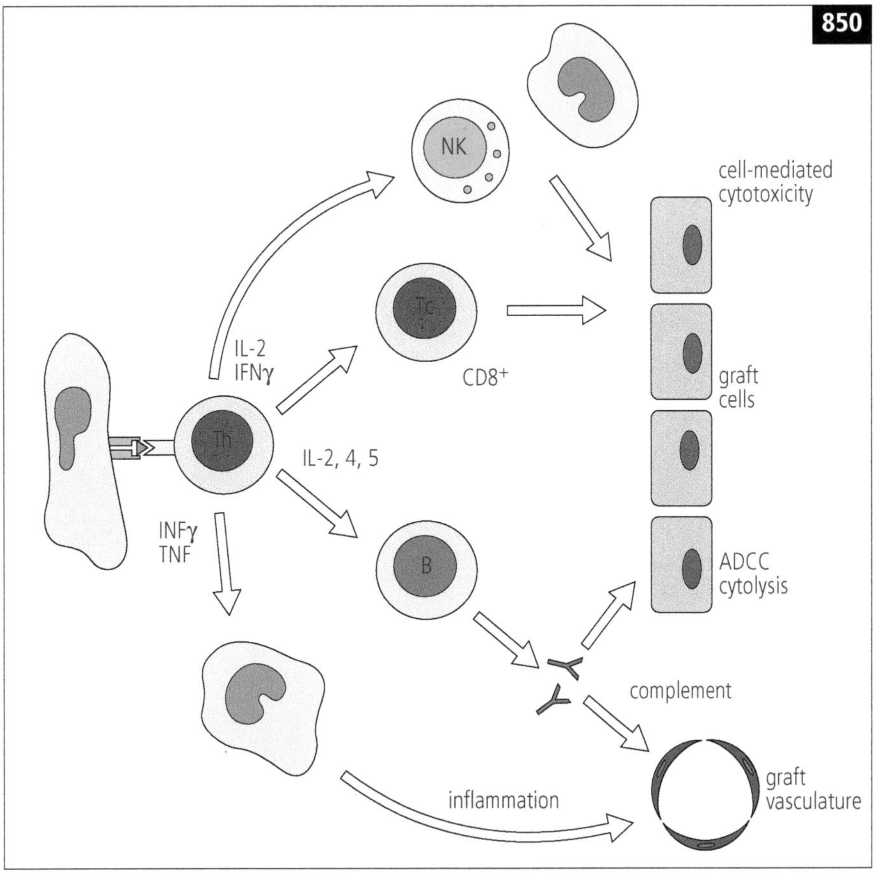

850 Graft rejection mechanisms. A range of immunological mechanisms is involved in the different forms of graft rejection; most are dependent upon the activation of alloreactive T cells by foreign MHC.

851

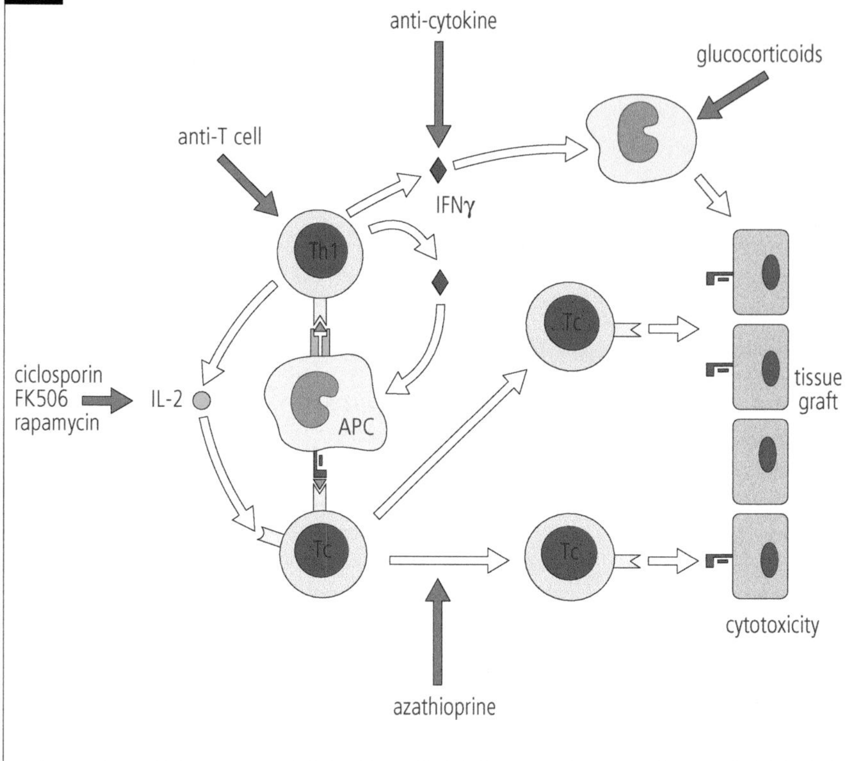

851 Immunosuppression in transplantation surgery. A range of pharmacological and immunological approaches has been taken to immunosuppress recipients in transplantation surgery, and combination modalities are designed to effect different points of the immune response. Administration of monoclonal antibodies to T cells may deplete or inhibit the alloreactive populations. Ciclosporin and tacrolimus prevent IL-2 production and T cell activation, whereas rapamycin inhibits the effect of any IL-2 that is produced. Azathioprine prevents division of activated cells. Glucocorticoids suppress inflammation and macrophage APC function. Anti-cytokine (e.g. anti-IFNγ) antibody counteracts the effect of released cytokine.

852

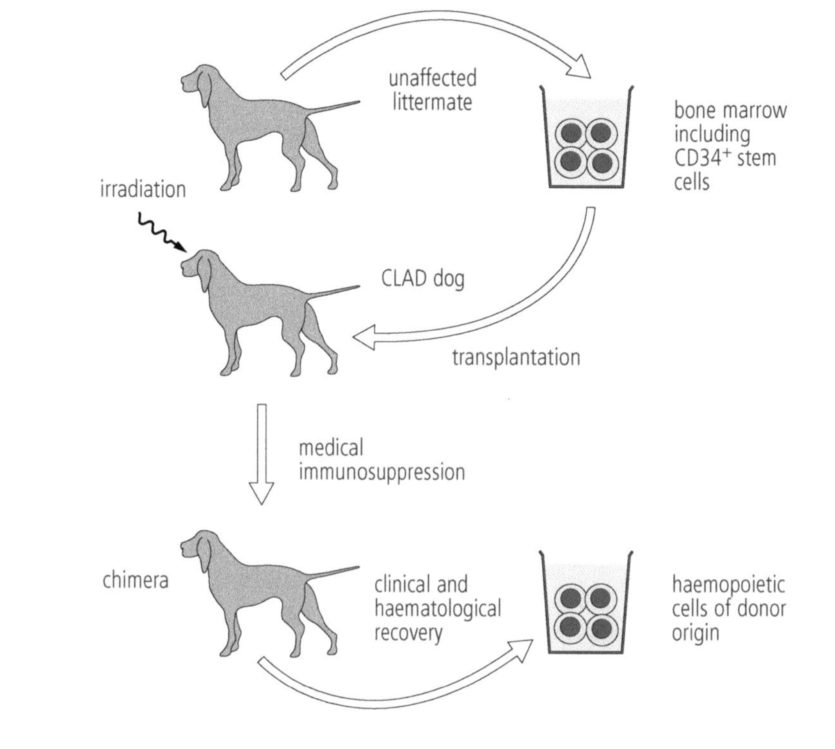

852 Stem cell therapy. An Irish Setter pup with canine leukocyte adhesion deficiency (CLAD) was irradiated and then transplanted with bone marrow cells (including stem cells) from an unaffected littermate. Following transplantation the recipient dog was maintained on immunosuppressive therapy. The donor stem cells repopulated the recipient with functionally normal leukocytes able to interact with endothelium and pass from blood into tissues. The recipient dog therefore made a clear clinical recovery from the manifestations of CLAD.

(FeLV and FIV negative) was successfully transplanted with bone marrow from a sibling and it remained healthy throughout the four-year follow-up period. In some countries and institutions, kidney transplantation in cats with chronic renal failure has now become a routinely available procedure; for example, a 2004 report from the University of California, Davis, documents 166 feline renal transplants performed since 1987. In general, these donor-recipient pairs are matched only for blood group and there has been no investigation of tissue type. Despite this the procedure may be successful, with no evidence of acute rejection, but occasional death occurs from other complications, in particular a range of infections including bacterial, viral, fungal and protozoal infections. Immunosuppression with ciclosporin and prednisolone is generally used. In a review of 66 transplanted cats, 19 died in the perioperative period, 28 of 47 cats that were discharged survived for a mean of 15 months post surgery, and 18 survived until the time of the report (mean 26 months post surgery). The donor cats remained healthy, with minimal abnormality on haematological or biochemical examination or urinalysis, for periods of up to five years after donation. The histopathology of feline renal graft rejection has now been examined and there are clear differences in reaction pattern to those described for human transplant patients. Acute cellular rejection of feline kidneys is most commonly represented by interstitial lymphocytic infiltration, and the presence of neutrophilic arteritis and glomerulitis suggests an antibody-mediated component to the rejection process. The vascular changes may also be linked to ciclosporin toxicity.

Kidney allografting for end-stage renal disease in the dog is also reported, and preliminary studies have indicated some success with an immunosuppressive regime including rabbit anti-dog T cell antiserum, prednisolone, ciclosporin, azathioprine and donor bone marrow infusion (**851**). The combination of leflunomide and ciclosporin has also proved successful in canine renal allografting studies. One recent study reviewed 15 canine renal transplants conducted on the basis of blood typing and cross-match only. Six of these dogs survived to at least 12 months after surgery, with two of the animals reported alive at 36 and 80 months respectively.

Stem cell therapy

Recently, much attention has been focussed on the potential for stem cell therapy as a means of replenishing or repairing damaged tissue. In equine medicine this procedure is already practised, with the injection of stromal stem cells into damaged tendons resulting in histological evidence of repair and clinical regaining of function. Bone marrow-derived stem cells ($CD34^+$) can be readily isolated from dogs and have recently been used to experimentally treat a dog with CLAD (see Chapter 12, p. 309) (**852**). This affected dog received sublethal whole body irradiation before transplantation of donor bone marrow containing stem cells. Post transplant, the dog was medically immunosuppressed, but it made remarkable clinical recovery with reduced leukocytosis and expression of CD18 on circulating leukocytes. Molecular studies were used to show that the recipient dog was a 'chimera' in which the haemopoietic cells were of donor origin. Other current experimental studies are examining the potential for purified $CD34^+$ canine stem cells to repair tissue lesions; for example, experimentally induced myocardial infarcts.

FURTHER READING

Ammersbach MAG, Kruth SA, Sears W *et al.* (2006) The effect of glucocorticoids on canine lymphocyte marker expression and apoptosis. *Journal of Veterinary Internal Medicine* **20**:1166–1171.

Colopy SA, Baker TA, Muir P (2010) Efficacy of leflunomide for treatment of immune-mediated polyarthritis in dogs: 14 cases (2006-2008). *Journal of the American Veterinary Medical Association* **236**:312–318.

Creevy KE, Bauer TR, Tuschong LM *et al.* (2003) Mixed chimeric haematopoietic stem cell transplant reverses the disease phenotype in canine leukocyte adhesion deficiency. *Veterinary Immunology and Immunopathology* **95**:113–121.

Day MJ (2005) Immunotherapy. In *Advances in Veterinary Dermatology, Volume 5.*

(eds A Hillier, AP Foster, KW Kwochka) Blackwell Publishing, Oxford, pp. 107–122.
De Cock HEV, Kyles AE, Griffey SM *et al.* (2004) Histopathologic findings and classification of feline renal transplants. *Veterinary Pathology* **41**:244–256.
deMari K, Maynard L, Sanquer A *et al.* (2004) Therapeutic effects of recombinant feline interferon-omega on feline leukemia virus (FeLV)-infected and FeLV/feline immunodeficiency virus (FIV)-coinfected symptomatic cats. *Journal of Veterinary Internal Medicine* **18**:77–482.
Deparle LA, Gupta RC, Canerdy TD *et al.* (2005) Efficacy and safety of glycoslyated undenatured type-II collagen (UC-II) in therapy of arthritic dogs. *Journal of Veterinary Pharmacology and Therapeutics* **28**:385–390.
Dewey CW, Cerda-Gonzalez S, Fletcher DJ *et al.* (2010) Mycophenolate mofetil treatment in dogs with serologically diagnosed acquired myasthenia gravis: 27 cases (1999-2008). *Journal of the American Veterinary Medical Association* **236**:664–668.
Fellman CL, Stokes JV, Archer TM *et al.* (2011) Cyclosporine A affects the *in vitro* expression of T cell activation-related molecules and cytokines in dogs. *Veterinary Immunology and Immunopathology* **140**:175–180.
Galin FS, Chrisman CL, Cook JR *et al.* (2007) Possible therapeutic vaccines for canine myasthenia gravis: implications for the human disease and associated fatigue. *Brain, Behavior, and Immunity* **21**:323–331.
Iwasaki T, Hasegawa A (2006) A randomized comparative clinical trial of recombinant canine interferon-γ (KT-100) in atopic dogs using antihistamine as control. *Veterinary Dermatology* **17**:195–200.
Kadar E, Sykes JE, Kass PH *et al.* (2005) Evaluation of the prevalence of infections in cats after renal transplantation: 169 cases (1987–2003). *Journal of the American Veterinary Medical Association* **227**:948–953.
Pressler BM (2010) Transplantation in small animals. *Veterinary Clinics of North America Small Animal Practice* **40**:495–505.
Ricklin Gutzwiller ME, Reist M *et al.* (2007) Intradermal injection of heat-killed *Mycobacterium vaccae* in dogs with atopic dermatitis: a multicentre pilot study. *Veterinary Dermatology* **18**:87–93.
Shimamura S, Kanayama K, Shimada T *et al.* (2010) Evaluation of the function of polymorphonuclear neutrophilic leukocytes in healthy dogs given a high dose of methylprednisolone sodium succinate. *American Journal of Veterinary Research* **71**:541–546.
Thacker EL (2010) Immunomodulators, immunostimulants, and immunotherapies in small animal veterinary medicine. *Veterinary Clinics of North America Small Animal Practice* **40**:473–483.
Ting-De Ravin SS, Kennedy DR, Naumann N *et al.* (2006) Correction of canine X-linked severe combined immunodeficiency by *in vivo* retroviral gene therapy. *Blood* **107**:3091–3097.
Whitley N, Day MJ (2011) Immunomodulatory drugs and their application to the management of canine immune-mediated disease. *Journal of Small Animal Practice* **52**:70–85.
Zemann B, Schwaerzier C, Griot–Wenk M *et al.* (2003) Oral administration of specific antigens to allergy-prone infant dogs induces IL-10 and TGF-β expression and prevents allergy in adult life. *Journal of Allergy and Clinical Immunology* **111**:1069–1075.

17 VACCINATION

Michael J. Day

INTRODUCTION

In the western world vaccination has been widely used for over 200 years, ever since the pivotal work of Edward Jenner, who is widely accredited with the introduction of this procedure following his demonstration that vaccinia virus can be used to protect against human smallpox. It is little known that similar experiments were conducted some 20 years before those of Jenner by the Dorset farmer Benjamin Jesty. In companion animal medicine, vaccination has been most widely employed in the past four decades, although in the majority of western countries there is only a moderate uptake of pet vaccination (approximately 30–50% of the target population). The nature of the vaccines that are currently administered to animals has not changed dramatically over this time. Although occasional new products are introduced in response to newly arising infectious diseases (e.g. canine parvovirus, FeLV, FIV), current vaccine technology (with some exceptions) is firmly rooted in the 1960s. This chapter will review the fundamentals of vaccinology, the types of veterinary vaccine, the regulatory means by which vaccines are licensed for use, and current vaccine guidelines that have arisen from debate over the adverse consequences of vaccination.

THE AIM OF VACCINATION

The aim of vaccination is to create a level of protective immunity to infection in an animal. As such, vaccination should mimic the natural response of the immune system to field challenge with a virulent form of the organism under consideration. Vaccination involves the induction of an immune response, as for any other foreign antigen and as described in Chapter 1. One of the most pivotal events with respect to vaccination is the induction of immunological memory.

BASIC REQUIREMENTS OF A VACCINE

In practical terms the ideal vaccine would be cheap to produce and administer in order to maximize uptake amongst a population. The product would be stable for ease of use in the field (i.e. have a long shelf life without requiring a cold chain), and would lack any side-effects. Immunologically, the ideal vaccine would induce a potent memory immune response that would persist over a long period of time (long duration of immunity and duration of protection). Moreover, the nature of the immune response induced would be appropriate for the infectious agent (i.e. would induce either or both humoral and cell-mediated immunity where required and therefore be of a type that was able to protect the animal from challenge with virulent organism). In terms of basic immunological mechanisms, an ideal vaccine would:

- Be administered via a route that mimicked that for natural exposure to the organism.
- Be readily taken up by APCs for antigen processing and presentation.
- Be able to stimulate functionally appropriate populations of antigen-specific T and B lymphocytes specific for a range of protective epitopes.
- Be capable of inducing persisting memory.

TYPES OF VACCINE

Vaccines designed to protect from infectious disease now come in a range of different forms. The application of molecular biology to vaccine production has resulted in a new generation of products that are now routinely used in veterinary practice.

Live organisms

Live organisms incorporated into vaccines may be virulent (rarely, and not in companion animals), attenuated or heterologous. The most common form of companion animal live organism vaccine involves attenuation such that the organism has reduced virulence and cannot cause overt disease. There are a variety of means of achieving attenuation, including:

- Heating to below thermal death point.
- Exposure to sublethal concentration of chemicals.

- Adaptation of the organism to growth in unusual conditions, or growth in cells or a species to which it is not normally adapted.

The best example of the use of antigenically-related 'heterologous' organisms to induce protective immunity is the use of measles virus to protect dogs from distemper, although this practice is now rarely undertaken. It is important that the organisms incorporated into vaccines remain relevant to the field strains that are currently present within a particular geographical area. This relies on knowledge of current field isolates and an active programme of regional disease surveillance. Unfortunately, there are limited such data for companion animal infections. Examples of the evolution of veterinary vaccines include the recent introduction of canine killed *Leptospira* vaccines including a greater number of serovars (in the US), and the change in canine parvovirus vaccines, which now contain biotypes that reflect the mutation of this virus since the original vaccines were formulated. There has been debate over the geographical relevance of the newly introduced FIV vaccine, which incorporates virus of clades A and D that may not be representative of those clades present in the field in some parts of the world. Against this, evidence has been produced to support cross-protection induced by the current vaccine against other isolates.

Live organism vaccines have numerous advantages over killed versions. These include:

- Live organisms should induce more potent immunity, as they infect cells and retain some replicative ability; also they are more likely to enter a range of cell types (including APCs) and spread to a range of anatomical sites and may be more readily delivered by a natural route of exposure.
- Live organisms should require fewer doses to achieve the desired response.
- Live organisms generally do not require adjuvant.

However, there are also particular disadvantages to live organisms, including:

- A theoretical possible greater risk of adverse events.
- A possibility of 'reversion to virulence' (i.e. loss of attenuation leading to overt disease).
- A greater possibility of contamination by other agents during production.
- A lower stability that generally requires cold chain storage.

Killed organisms

The alternative approach to live organism vaccination is to utilize a killed organism that is unable to infect, replicate or induce disease, but is antigenically intact and able to stimulate a host immune response. A range of means of killing organisms has been used, but most involve chemical inactivation with substances such as formaldehyde, alcohol or alkylating agents. The major advantage of killed organism vaccines is their stability and the fact that they are relatively economical to produce. However, for reasons outlined above, they are less potent and generally require multiple doses and to be given in adjuvant. Because of the nature of the adjuvants most widely used in vaccine production (e.g. aluminium based), such vaccines are more likely to induce a Th2 immune response characterized by antibody production rather than strong cell-mediated immunity. Adjuvant is also deemed as being less than desirable, as these substances may be associated with side-effects (e.g. potential role in the induction of feline injection site sarcoma).

Metabolic or structural products from organisms (subunit vaccines)

This type of vaccine contains specific metabolites or structural proteins from an organism rather than the entire microbial particle. Production of this type of vaccine necessitates knowledge of the most relevant antigenic epitopes carried by an organism that are likely to induce protective immunity. An example of such a product is the FeLV vaccine that contains FeLV glycoprotein isolated from cell culture.

Synthetic peptide antigens

Synthetic peptide vaccines take the subunit approach one step further and utilize synthetically produced epitopes rather than native molecules obtained by fractionating an entire organism. These vaccines generally require adjuvants and are often of low immunogenicity.

Genetically modified organisms

The molecular revolution has impacted on vaccine production in recent years, and there are several approaches to the use of such technology for vaccine production.

Modify microbial genes to attenuate the organism

Organisms may be attenuated by modification or deletion of specific genes that are involved in their virulence. For example, removal of the thymidine kinase gene from the herpesvirus causing swine pseudorabies has produced a virus that retains the ability to infect neurons but cannot replicate and cause disease. There are currently no examples of this approach for companion animal vaccines.

Recombinant viral antigens

Molecular techniques may be employed to manufacture large quantities of highly pure 'recombinant' proteins. This methodology involves identification of genes encoding relevant antigens and the incorporation of these (e.g. viral) genes into a plasmid that is subsequently placed into a bacterial, insect or mammalian cell line. The product of the gene is expressed and the recombinant protein secreted into the culture medium. Such recombinants generally require adjuvant for efficacy. An example of this type of product is the FeLV vaccine that is based on a recombinant form of FeLV gp70 (**853**).

Recombinant organisms

An even more novel and powerful approach involves taking the gene encoding antigenic molecules and inserting this into a harmless 'carrier organism' that is administered to the animal. A range of such carriers have been used; for example, vaccinia virus or attenuated *Salmonella* for oral delivery of vaccine. The recombinant organism expresses the molecule derived from the original infectious agent, and this is processed and presented to the immune system to induce an antigen-specific immune response. The canary pox

853 Genetic engineering in vaccine production. The RNA encoding a protective viral antigen (e.g. gp70 from FeLV) is reverse transcribed and the specific gene encoding the molecule excised from the DNA transcript with restriction endonucleases. The gene is inserted into an *E. coli* plasmid as a vector for expression of large quantities of pure recombinant molecule that can by utilized in vaccine production.

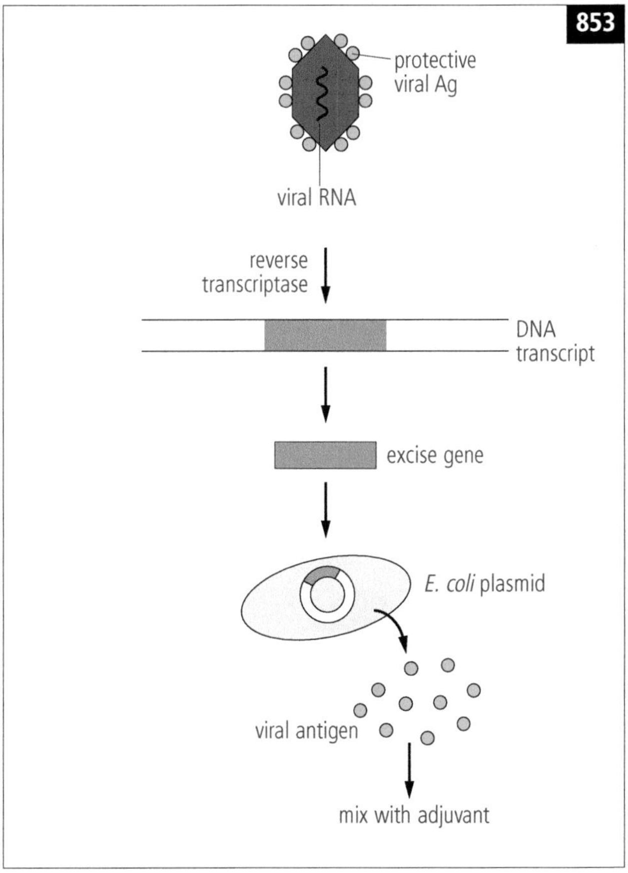

vector used for FeLV, rabies and distemper vaccines is an example of the use of this technology (**854**). The immune responses induced by this mechanism are strong, and this method has the added advantage that such vaccination may be effective in the face of maternal immunity (see below).

This type of technology lends itself to the development of further advances such as the use of molecular adjuvants. For example, the incorporation of genes encoding particular host species cytokines might direct that a specific functional type of immune response is made to the vaccine. Inclusion of genes encoding the cytokines IL-12, IL-18 or IFNγ might, for example, engender a strong cell-mediated (Th1) immune response. Although this latter approach is founded in good immunological theory, in reality such approaches may sometimes lead to unexpected outcomes. For example, an experimental DNA vaccine against FIP virus that incorporated the feline IL-12 gene led to adverse clinical effects rather than enhanced protection from infectious challenge.

Naked DNA vaccines

The final molecular development involves a similar approach to that described above, but without the use of carrier organisms. The plasmid DNA may be injected directly to the recipient animal via a number of routes including intramusularly, subcutaneously, percutaneously or orally (coupled to protective inert carrier). With naked DNA vaccines, the gene 'transfects' host cells, particularly APCs, resulting in peptide expression on the surface of the cell associated with histocompatibility complex molecules. These APCs migrate to regional lymphoid tissue to induce an immune response.

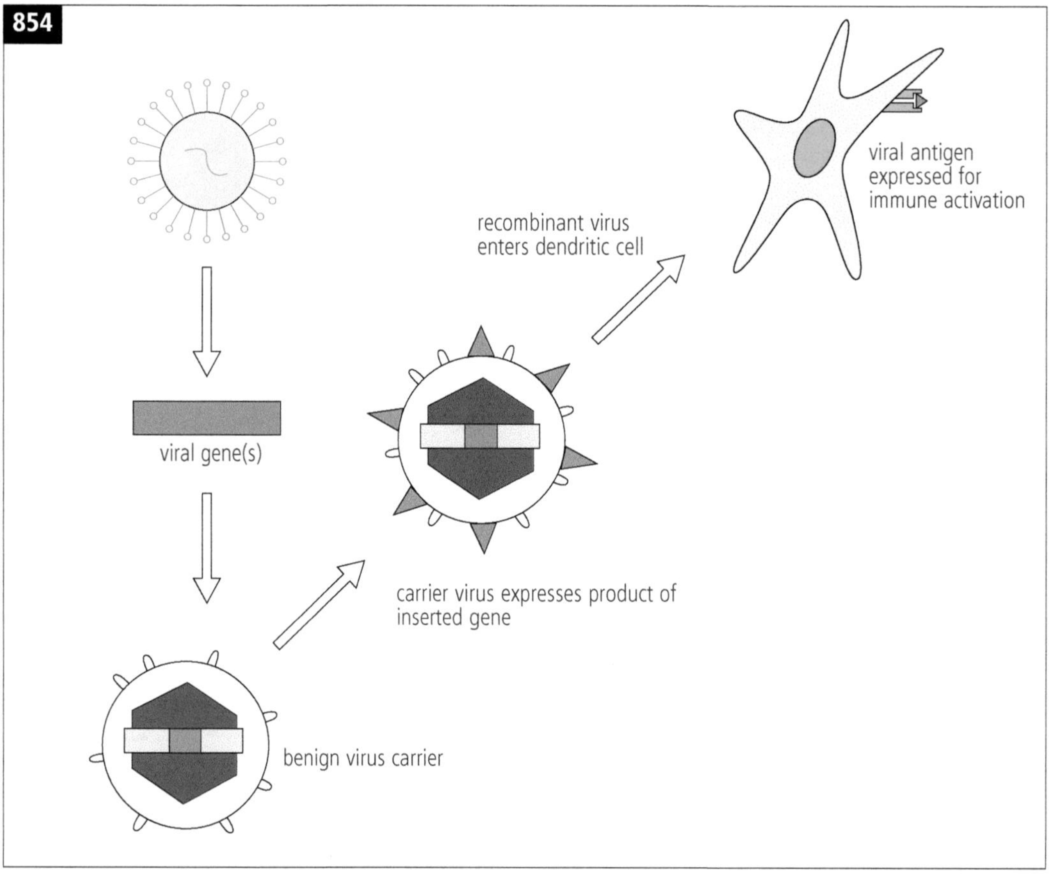

854 Recombinant virus vaccines. In this approach to vaccine production it is first necessary to identify genes in the target organism that encode key antigenic proteins that act as targets in a protective immune response. These genes are incorporated into a harmless 'carrier' organism (such as the canarypox virus) and become expressed so that the carrier organism displays these antigenic structures. After vaccination, the recombinant organism is taken up by APCs and the expressed proteins are processed and presented to the host immune system.

Naked DNA vaccination has been shown to be a particularly powerful means of inducing protective immunity, as both strong humoral and cell-mediated immune responses are made. Experimentally, naked DNA vaccination has been shown to work in dogs and cats with rabies, distemper and FIV viral genes. For example, a single intradermal injection of plasmid containing the gene encoding rabies glycoprotein G to the pinna of dogs induces protective immunity that prevents experimental challenge with virulent virus 12 months post vaccination. The approach might induce immunity in the face of maternal immunoglobulin, which has clear attraction for field use. Moreover, similar means of adjuvanting these vaccines by incorporation of cytokine genes or immunostimulatory bacterial CpG motifs into the plasmid have been tried. The first such product, designed for therapeutic use in dogs with malignant melanoma, has recently become available (see below).

Marker vaccines

Marker vaccines are a recent advance in vaccinology that enables a distinction to be made between an animal that is seropositive to a particular infectious agent because it has been vaccinated, and one that is seropositive because it has been infected with virulent field organism. There are numerous situations in which this distinction is crucial; for example, in the UK this was one reason why vaccination was not used in the 2001 outbreak of foot and mouth disease. A marker vaccine has recently been introduced to enable distinction of cattle vaccinated for infectious bovine rhinotracheitis. The vaccine is based on a glycoprotein E-negative mutant of the virus, so a cow that has serum antibody to this glycoprotein must have been naturally infected (**855**). The use of marker vaccines necessitates parallel development of appropriate diagnostic tests to enable the distinction to be made. In companion animal medicine there is a need for marker vaccines. For example, seropositivity to *Borrelia* in dogs might reflect vaccination rather than field exposure, although the use of western blotting can distinguish between these possibilities, as vaccinated animals make a strong antibody response to the OspA protein. Moreover, the Snap^{TM} 4Dx^{TM} diagnostic test utilizes an antigen that appears to be specific for field infection. Another example is the FIV vaccine, which induces serum antibody equivalent to field exposure, thus rendering ineffective the current range of serodiagnostic tests for this infection. A marker vaccine or PCR testing would help distinguish between these possibilities.

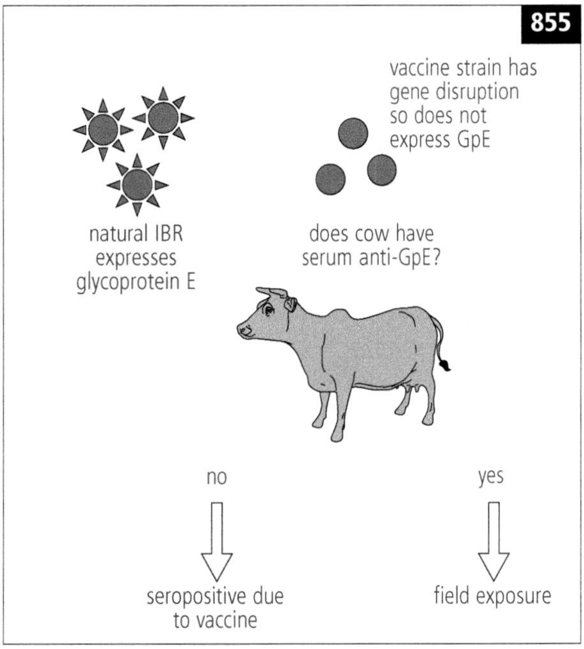

855 Marker vaccines. This approach to vaccine development permits the distinction to be made between animals that are seropositive due to vaccination, and those that are seropositive due to field exposure to the organism (infection). An example of such a product is the vaccine for bovine infectious rhinotracheitis, which is based on a virus that lacks the gene encoding glycoprotein E. Vaccinated animals will therefore not make an antibody response to glycoprotein E, whereas naturally infected cows will have antibody of this specificity.

VACCINES OF THE FUTURE

The future of vaccinology is immensely exciting and current experimental work in model systems has shown numerous new potential approaches. These include:

- The use of new technologies (e.g. direct immunization of dendritic cells or use of novel adjuvants such as bacterial CpG motifs, or cholera toxin/*Escherichia coli* enterotoxin B for mucosal delivery of vaccine).
- New routes of delivery (e.g. oral, percutaneous, intranasal, intranodal). There is already focus on percutaneous delivery for companion animal vaccines, with the recent introduction of 'needle free vaccination'. This entails the use of an apparatus developed for the administration of human medicines (e.g. insulin, growth hormone). It is a multiuse, high pressure system that can accurately deliver small volumes across the epidermal barrier and target this antigen to epidermal and dermal dendritic cells (**856**).
- New vehicles (e.g. plant delivery for edible vaccines, which has enormous potential for human vaccination in the third world; such an approach has been taken in the development of modern poultry vaccines).
- New protocols. For example, the 'prime-boost' method, which involves initially priming the immune response with one type of vaccine (e.g. DNA vaccine) and subsequently boosting the response with an alternative form (e.g. protein vaccine).
- The development of vaccination for a spectrum of diseases other than infectious diseases (e.g. allergy, autoimmunity and cancer). The first licensed vaccine for canine neoplasia has recently been introduced. This product is a DNA vaccine that incorporates the gene encoding human tyrosinase, a target tumour antigen in canine malignant melanoma. Repeated administration of the product induces an anti-tumour immune response that is of clinical benefit to affected patients (**857**). Vaccines to other than viral or bacterial infectious agents are already commercially produced (e.g. canine *Babesia* or *Leishmania* vaccines) and products aimed at control of nematode parasites have been proven efficacious in research trials. An immunocontraceptive vaccine based on administration of leuteinizing hormone releasing hormone peptide (a B cell epitope) coupled to a peptide derived from the fusion protein of CDV (a Th epitope) has been tested in the dog (**858**).
- The development of vaccines tailored for specific types or breed, or even individual animals of a particular genetic background. Exciting new research is correlating the serological response to vaccine with MHC genotype in dogs and cats, and this knowledge could form the basis for such products. Already

856

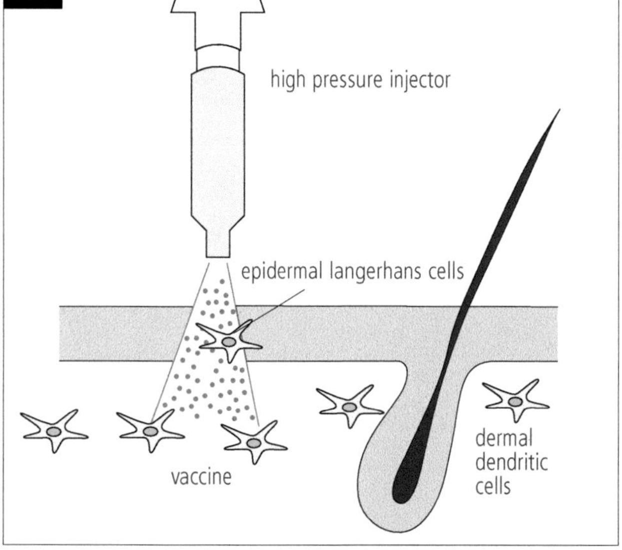

856 Needle-free vaccination. There are numerous approaches to the delivery of vaccines other than by needle injection. One novel delivery mechanism that has recently been licensed in the US for delivery of FeLV vaccine to cats involves the use of a multiuse, high pressure apparatus (Vetject^{TM}) that forces vaccine across the epidermal barrier such that it has very efficient contact with epidermal and dermal dendritic cells. Targeting dendritic cells in this way leads to a very efficient means of initiating the regional immune response and a reduced does of vaccine antigen may be used.

there are examples of breed differences in responsiveness, with small breed dogs often making a superior serological response than larger dogs, an effect that may be related to dosage. Coupled with observations of a higher incidence of immediate hypersensitivity reactions to vaccination in small breeds (see below), there is logic to suggesting that manufacturers should look to producing a specific low-dose vaccine formulation for small breeds. This is contrary to the long-held belief that 'one size fits all' for canine vaccination, based on the suggestion that although body size may vary, the immune repertoire of a Great Dane and Chihuahua are similar (**859**). These studies have also confirmed that some canine breeds (e.g. the Rottweiler) make

857

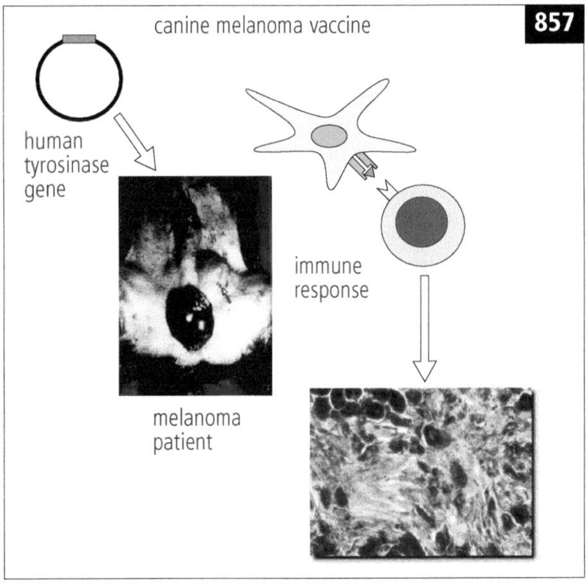

857 Melanoma vaccine. A molecular vaccine for the management of dogs with oral melanoma received conditional license in the US in 2006. This vaccine incorporates the gene encoding human tyrosinase, a molecule that serves as a target for the tumour-specific immune response. Expression of this gene within antigen presenting cells leads to presentation of tyrosinase peptides and amplification of tumour immunity.

858

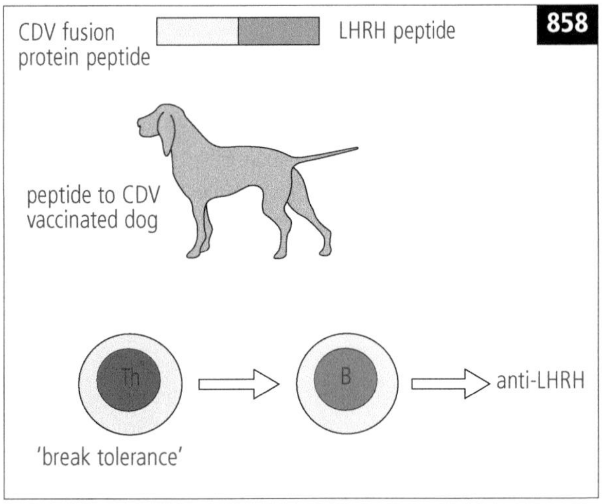

858 Immunocontraceptive vaccine. In this novel approach to vaccination a construct is prepared that comprises linked peptides from the canine distemper virus and the leuteinizing hormone releasing hormone (LHRH). When injected into dogs, the CDV peptide is recognized as a foreign antigen and induces a Th response. These Th cells inappropriately stimulate LHRH peptide specific B cells, which present the CDV antigenic component of the construct. This has the effect of breaking immunological tolerance to the LHRH and the ensuing antibody production interferes with the hormonal pathway.

859

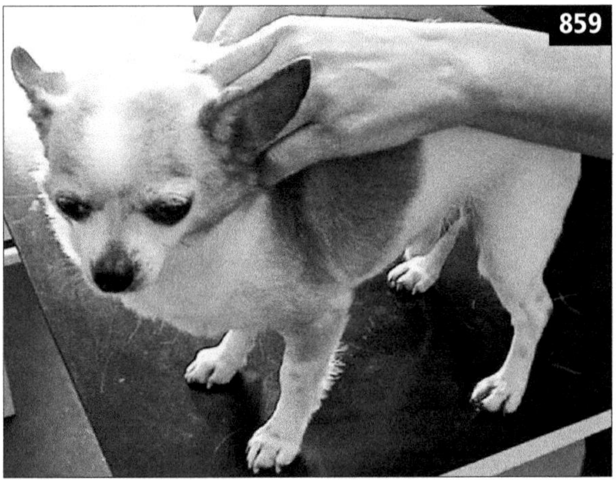

859 Breed response to vaccination. This Chihuahua is receiving the same dose of vaccine as would be given to a Great Dane as both dogs have an equivalent antigen-specific T and B cell repertoire. However, emerging evidence suggests that small breed dogs make a stronger serological response to vaccination than large breed dogs and, concurrently, have a higher risk of adverse hypersensitivity reactions post vaccination.

860

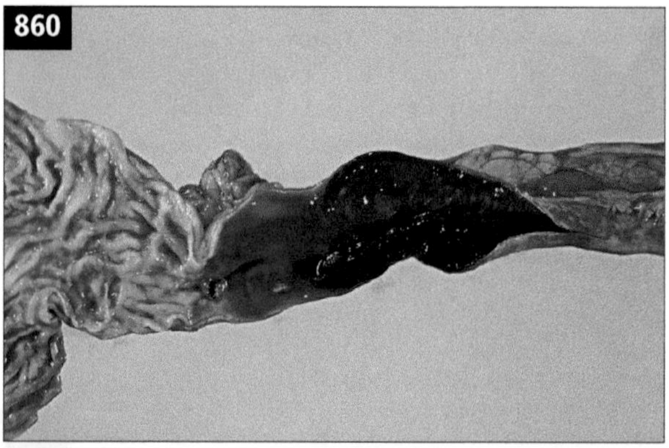

861

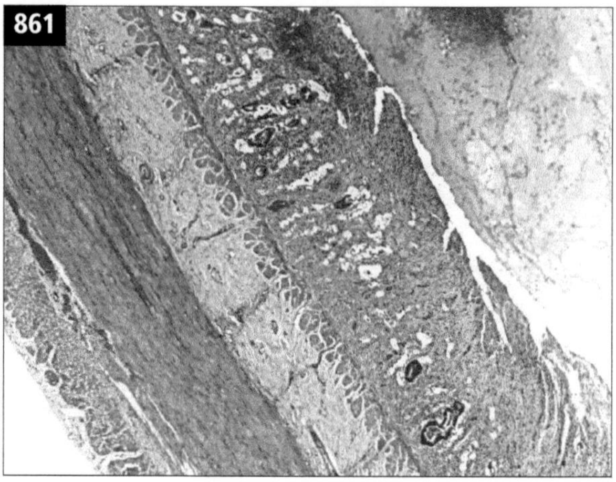

860, 861 Breed response to vaccination. Particular breeds of dog are known to respond differently to vaccines. For example, it has long been recognised that Rottweiler dogs apparently respond poorly to parvovirus vaccination and may remain susceptible to this infection. Shown are gross (**860**) and microscopic (**861**) images of the small intestine of a seven-month-old Rottweiler that died from parvovirus infection (confirmed by PCR). The dog had been vaccinated at eight and ten weeks of age using an 'early finish' product.

generally poor serological response to vaccination, and may explain the prevalence of parvovirus infection in vaccinated dogs of this breed (**860, 861**).

Although these all sound to be of great potential benefit, one should caution that the road to development, licensing and marketing of new vaccines is long and expensive. In reality, the veterinary market place is relatively small and it is likely to be many years before products are widely available that will replace the current generation of modified live, multicomponent vaccines.

DURATION OF IMMUNITY

As stated above, the aim of administering a vaccine to an animal is to induce protective immunity. This antigen-specific immune response may be measured in the vaccinated individual in the same fashion as any other response to antigen exposure. The most readily determined measure of responsiveness is the amount of specific IgG antibody present within serum post vaccination. Although there are several means of testing for the presence of cell-mediated immunity, these procedures are technically more demanding and more expensive to undertake. Consequently, although many of the vaccines that are administered to companion animals will induce both types of immune response, it is generally the antibody response that is measured. This provides a potential pitfall when serological response is used to determine whether an animal is 'protected' following vaccination. For most vaccine components (e.g. CDV, CAV, CPV, FPV, FCV, rabies) there is proven correlation between seropositivity and protection, but for others (e.g. FHV) the correlation is weak and protection is more likely associated with the cell-mediated immune response. For this reason, an animal that is seropositive is likely to have protective immunity (depending on the antigen involved), but a vaccinated animal that is seronegative is not necessarily unprotected, as there may be a strong protective cell-mediated response in the absence of serum antibody. For example, rabies vaccination might induce an acceptable antibody response only transiently, but the animal might still have protective cellular immunity.

There are further problems with the manner in which the serological response to a vaccine is currently assessed. Although serological testing is the 'gold standard', there is no standardization in methodology or interpretation between testing laboratories. What is deemed as a protective titre by one laboratory might not be considered so by another. Current WSAVA Guidelines (see later) suggest that any detectable titre (for core vaccines) indicates protection. In-practice test kits are now marketed for confirmation of protective titre. Antibody has a finite half-life (approximately 14 days in dogs and cats) and so will degrade and eventually become undetectable in the circulation in the absence of continued antigenic stimulation. Therefore, after administration of a puppy or kitten course of vaccine, or after administration of an adult booster vaccine, the serum antibody produced will theoretically eventually degrade and disappear, as there is no prolonged antigenic stimulus to maintain its production. The time taken for antibody to reduce significantly in concentration in companion animals following vaccination depends upon a number of factors:

- **The type of vaccine.** Some vaccines will preferentially induce a strong humoral immune response that will persist for longer periods than other vaccines. For example, dogs vaccinated against canine distemper virus will generally have lifelong seropositivity, even in the absence of repeated boosting. This may in part relate to the nature of the vaccine. The duration of an immune response to a vaccine antigen might be extended by simply providing more prolonged exposure to antigen; for example, via the 'depot' effect of some adjuvants, which slowly release antigen to maintain immune stimulation.
- **The retention of vaccine antigen.** One of the theories underlying immunological memory is that the immune system is capable of retaining small quantities of all foreign antigens to which it is exposed, possibly associated with dendritic cells that remain in lymphoid tissue. Periodic re-expression of this stored antigen might help maintain immunological memory and seropositivity by allowing low level division of memory lymphocytes.
- **Field exposure.** In the case of some vaccines, it is possible for a vaccinated animal to have the vaccine-specific immune response engendered by the vaccine restimulated by field exposure to the microbe contained within the vaccine. Alternatively, a related microbe sharing antigenic epitopes ('cross-reactive') might stimulate an antibody response that appears vaccine antigen-specific in serological testing. It is known that these processes are possible, as on occasion unvaccinated adult animals are seropositive to vaccine antigens.
- **The individual animal.** There is variation in the immune response to vaccination in individuals because of their breed (genetic background), nutritional or disease status, or stress level; therefore, one vaccine given to two different dogs might produce a different duration of serological response. Again, this is widely known, as serosurveys of populations of dogs that have not been vaccinated for some time reveal that some individuals will have a protective titre and others will not. Although the age of a vaccinated animal might be expected to influence outcome, one recent study has compared the response to vaccination in young and old adult dogs and shown no impairment in serological response in the older animals.

Although vaccinal antibody titres may decline, there will hopefully be persistence of immunological memory.

What are duration of immunity and duration of protection?

Duration of immunity (DOI) and duration of protection (DOP) are two regulatory terms related to vaccine efficacy. They are often used interchangeably, but in fact have distinct meaning. DOI refers to the period of time following administration of vaccine when a vaccine-specific immune response can be detected in that individual. DOI is most often measured by testing the serological response to vaccination (i.e. the presence of serum antibody as detected via ELISA, haemagglutination inhibition or virus neutralization assays). In contrast, DOP refers to the length of time following vaccination during which an animal is actually protected from challenge with virulent infectious agent. As discussed above, DOI might therefore correlate with DOP and act as an *in vitro* correlate of protection, but the two intervals technically need not be identical.

As part of the data generated for the licensing of vaccines, manufacturers must determine a DOP that will define the revaccination interval recommended for the product (see below). Because of the duration, expense and welfare implications of such experimental studies, most challenges in DOP trials have traditionally been performed at an arbitrary period of 12 months post vaccination.

Table 37: Vaccine seropositivity in the canine population.

Study	CDV	CAV-2	CPV
McCaw *et al.*, 1998 USA (1)	79% protective titre (n = 122)	NT	73% protective titre (n = 122)
Twark and Dodds, 2000 USA (2)	97.6% protective titre (n = 1441)	NT	95.1% protective titre (n = 1441)
Mouzin *et al.*, 2004 USA (3)	99.2% protective titre (n = 119 dogs vaccinated 12–18 months previously) 94.7% protective titre (n = 19 dogs vaccinated >48 months previously)	99.2% protective titre (n = 119 dogs vaccinated 12–18 months previously) 100% protective titre (n = 19 dogs vaccinated >48 months previously)	98.3% protective titre (n = 119 dogs vaccinated 12–18 months previously) 100% protective titre (n = 19 dogs vaccinated >48 months previously)
Böhm *et al.*, 2004 UK (4)	71.5% protective titre (n = 144 adult dogs vaccinated ≥3 years previously)	82% protective titre (n = 144 adult dogs vaccinated ≥3 years previously)	94.4% protective titre (n = 143 adult dogs vaccinated ≥3 years previously)

(1) McCaw DL, Thompson M, Tate D *et al.* (1998) Serum distemper virus and parvovirus antibody titers among dogs brought to a veterinary hospital for revaccination. *Journal of the American Veterinary Medical Association* **213:**72–75.
(2) Twark L, Dodds WJ (2000) Clinical application of serum parvovirus and distemper virus antibody titers for determining revaccination strategies in healthy dogs. *Journal of the American Veterinary Medical Association* **217:**1021–1024.
(3) Mouzin DE, Lorenzen MJ, Haworth JD *et al.* (2004) Duration of serologic response to five viral antigens in dogs. *Journal of the American Veterinary Medical Association* **224:**55–60.
(4) M. Böhm H, Thompson A, Weir AM *et al.* (2004) Serum antibody titres to canine parvovirus, adenovirus and distemper virus in dogs in the UK which had not been vaccinated for at least three years. *Veterinary Record* **154:**457–463.

Table 38: Vaccine seropositivity in the feline population.

Study	FPV	FCV	FHV
Mouzin *et al.* 2004 USA	96.3% protective titre (n = 108 adult cats vaccinated 12–18 months previously) 93.9% protective titre (n = 33 adult cats vaccinated >48 months previously)	99.1% protective titre (n = 108 adult cats vaccinated 12–18 months previously) 100% protective titre (n = 33 adult cats vaccinated >48 months previously)	84.3% protective titre (n = 108 adult cats vaccinated 12–18 months previously) 84.8% protective titre (n = 33 adult cats vaccinated >48 months previously)

Mouzin DE, Lorenzen MJ, Haworth JD *et al.* (2004) Duration of serologic response to three viral antigens in cats. *Journal of the American Veterinary Medical Association* **224:**61–66.

This means that most veterinary vaccines were licensed with a 12 month DOI/DOP, as scientific evidence was only provided to support that length of effect. The problem with this approach is that most core vaccines are capable of inducing a much longer-lived protective immune response, but the scientific proof for this was not generated, as the experiment was terminated after 12 months. The licensing of vaccine products with 'extended duration of immunity' of three or four years is now occurring. This simply means that the manufacturer has produced experimental data to demonstrate that a vaccinated animal will have a persisting, protective immune response for this extended period of time. In fact, for some vaccines the real duration of protective immunity (maximum DOI) is likely much longer than even a three-year period, but the evidence for this has not been formally generated in an experimental setting. Again, the extremes of DOI will vary between individuals, but a vaccine with a claim for a three-year DOI should induce protective titres of antibody in the vast majority of animals for that period of time.

To further support the concept of long-lived protection afforded by companion animal vaccines, there have been several recently published 'field' serological studies that have examined the presence of 'protective' titres of antibody specific for vaccine antigens in dogs and cats in the clinic setting (*Tables 37, 38*). These studies suggest that seropositivity persists for periods much greater than 12 months in previously vaccinated animals that have not received a booster vaccine, and they support the experimental studies that show that some of the live attenuated core viral vaccines that are currently administered have a DOI/DOP of between three and nine years. Moreover, in some studies, animals that have never been vaccinated may have protective antibody titres, presumably acquired by field exposure to naturally occurring or vaccinal antigen. However, these population studies also show that a proportion of animals with a previous vaccination history do not have a serum antibody titre that would be considered 'protective', and this suggests that on an individual animal basis, vaccination according to data sheet recommendations is still appropriate. The availability of prolonged DOI products goes some way towards helping to resolve the conflict between recommendations for extending revaccination intervals and the risk that an individual might not be protected without regular revaccination. Serological testing is not used routinely in pet animals as a basis for determining protection and the need for revaccination, but it may be recommended to determine whether an individual puppy or kitten has responded adequately to the primary vaccine course.

VACCINE LICENSING

All vaccines licensed for use in animals undergo a rigorous assessment by the relevant national or regional licensing authority before being approved for release to market. The generation of data used to support any application is a prolonged and costly exercise for the vaccine manufacturers, and a list of specific requirements must be met in order for any application to be successful. As for all licensed veterinary therapeutics, assessment of vaccines focuses on the three key areas of quality, safety and efficacy.

The **quality assessment** of a vaccine examines in detail the source and purity of the constituents of the product (including the antigenic components and any preservatives or adjuvant) and the production process by which the vaccine is formulated. A key element in vaccine production is the consistency of various batches of the final product. The major measure of this consistency is the 'potency' of the vaccine and this relates to the antigenic content and its ability to induce a protective immune response. Many potency tests are still performed *in vivo* by challenging animals vaccinated with each batch of product with virulent organisms in order to determine protection; however, where the serum antibody response to vaccine provides a good correlate with protection, a serological test of potency may be permitted. The quality assessment also determines the sterility and shelf life under proposed storage conditions of each vaccine.

Studies of the **safety of a vaccine** must be conducted with batches of maximum potency. The safety in the target animal species is determined using animals of the minimum age for which the vaccine is to be used (e.g. pups and kittens). The clinical, laboratory and histological effects of administration of vaccine by the proposed protocol (and protocols giving up to a ten times overdose of the product) are determined. These studies provide information on any potential adverse effects of vaccination, which is then listed on the data sheet that accompanies the product. For most products, the 'operator safety' of the person administering the vaccine will be assessed. In addition, where relevant, the effects of the vaccine on the environment (e.g. by shedding or secreting vaccine) will be determined. This is particularly true of vectored organism vaccines, where the potential for reversion to virulence or recombination of the genetically modified organism with field strains of wild-type organism must be considered.

The data generated concerning the **efficacy of the vaccine** are used to formulate the 'claim' for the product. Efficacy studies are performed using batches of vaccine of minimum potency. This provides a more rigorous test of the protective effect of the vaccine. For companion animal vaccines, the most significant efficacy studies are experimental. These involve challenge experiments, where a requisite number of animals are vaccinated and an equal number of controls remain unvaccinated. Subsequently, both groups are challenged with virulent organism (ideally of a different strain to that incorporated into the vaccine). For most regulatory bodies the vaccine must provide protection to at least 80% of vaccinates, whereas at least 80% of controls must develop clinical or pathological signs of infection. It is worth noting that in many such studies the vaccines administered are not 100% efficacious (i.e. they do not protect all of the vaccinated animals). For multivalent vaccines, there must be experimental challenge with the virulent form of each microbial component and the DOP of the entire vaccine is related to the component for which there is the shortest DOP.

In parallel with such experimental studies, the vaccine must be trialled in a field situation. Field studies generally utilize vaccine at the intended 'release potency'. For companion animal products this is somewhat less relevant than vaccines designed for production animals, as there is little chance of exposure to natural 'field infection' due to the success of vaccination in controlling the target diseases. Such studies do, however, provide further safety information about use of the vaccine in the intended clinical setting.

The efficacy package will also address the effect of maternally-derived antibody (MDA) in order to determine the minimum age at which vaccination may be successfully instigated, together with the DOI and DOP as described above. The compatibility with other vaccine products that are administered concurrently (generally from the same manufacturer) will also be examined, to prove that there is no inhibition of the effectiveness of individual components within a combination protocol.

The various efficacy studies support the specific wording that is used in the 'claim' for the vaccine. A series of standard phrases are used to describe the protective effects of a vaccine and these should be carefully considered by the veterinary users of these products. A vaccine may be licensed with a claim of being able to 'prevent infection' if challenged vaccinates never become infected. In contrast, some vaccines may claim to 'reduce infection', but not entirely prevent it. A similar claim would be to 'prevent mortality and/or clinical signs and/or pathological lesions', which implies that infection may occur but does not lead to disease. The weakest claim is one of 'reduction of mortality and/or clinical signs and/or pathological lesions', implying that infection may occur and result in a mild form of disease.

All of these data on quality, safety and efficacy are encapsulated in the 'summary of product characteristics' (SPC), which forms the basis for the data sheet or package insert that accompanies the vaccine. Veterinarians should study these sheets carefully so as to become fully conversant with the products they are recommending.

ADVERSE EFFECTS OF VACCINATION

In recent years much attention has been focused on the potential for the vaccines administered to companion animals to induce adverse side-effects. This focus has driven widespread debate within the veterinary profession and amongst the general public and the media, particularly concerning the practice of annual administration of booster vaccines, which is perceived as increasing the risk of such adverse effects occurring.

A wide range of adverse consequences of vaccination has been documented in companion animals. Probably the most common of these is transient post-vaccinal non-specific illness (e.g. pyrexia, lethargy and anorexia, regional lymphadenopathy for some days post vaccination), which likely directly relates to the activation of immune and inflammatory pathways by the process of needle vaccination (**862**).

It has long been suggested that vaccination might also lead to transient immunosuppression in dogs and cats, and some studies have investigated this phenomenon. One recent report clearly documented elevation in humoral immunity, but depression in cellular and innate immunity, in GSDs two weeks post vaccination, although post-vaccinal immunosuppression had not been a consistent observation between studies. Vaccination-induced immunosuppression may on occasion be sufficient to permit the development of severe disease in animals that are carrying subclinical opportunist pathogens, as has been described for an outbreak of salmonellosis in a group of vaccinated kittens.

As discussed in Chapter 12 (p. 306), it seems likely that the multisystemic infectious/inflammatory disorder of young Weimaraner dogs with poorly characterized immune deficiency may also be triggered by vaccination.

Local injection site reactions are rarely documented in companion animals, although it is clear that tissue inflammation does occur at sites of vaccination, particularly with the use of adjuvanted products (**863, 864**). The most visible of local reactions are the range of aggressive feline sarcomas for which the working hypothesis suggests that adjuvant-induced chronic inflammation might

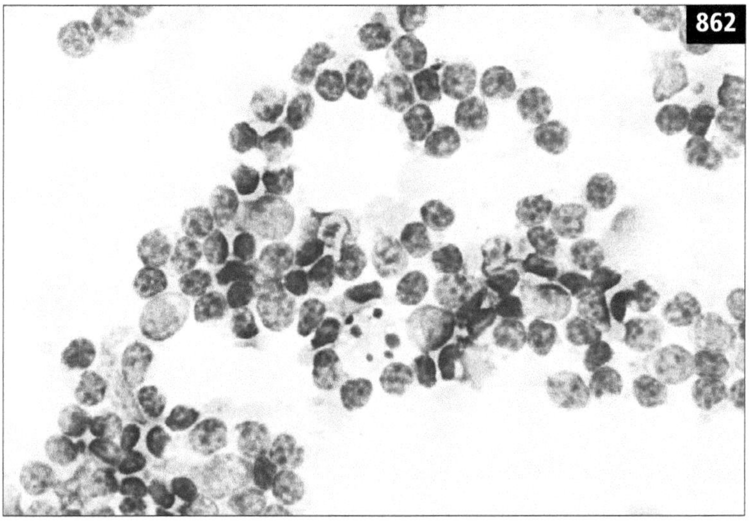

862 Regional lymph node hyperplasia secondary to vaccination. A pup developed palpable enlargement of a lymph node draining the site of vaccine administration. Fine needle aspiration of this node revealed an expanded population of lymphoblasts consistent with reactive hyperplasia secondary to antigenic stimulation.

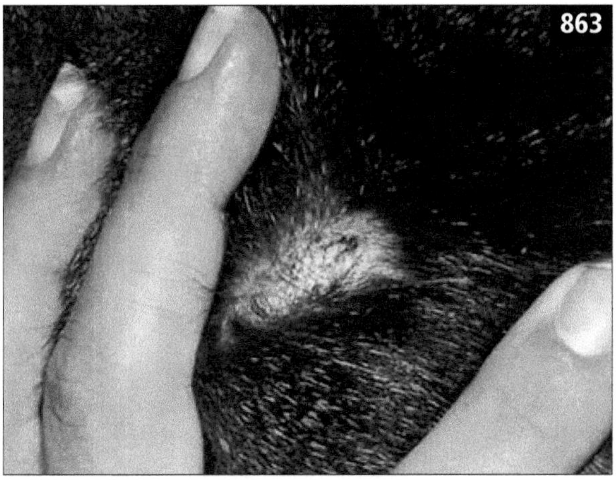

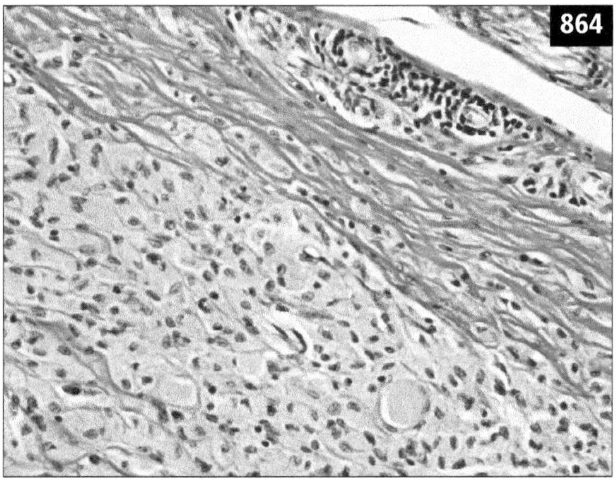

863, 864 Local reactions to vaccination. (**863**) A small focus of alopecia, superficial crusting and dermal thickening at the site of recent vaccine administration in a cat. It is possible that such minor inflammatory reactions may act as triggers for neoplastic transformation of stromal cells. (**864**) Section taken from the subcutis of a cat receiving alum adjuvanted vaccine reveals an accumulation of blue-grey adjuvant within the cytoplasm of macrophages.

trigger the genetic changes that underlie neoplasia (**865–867**). Numerous research studies have now been published that address potential molecular and immunological mechanisms in induction of this neoplasm, and studies have incriminated adjuvanted rabies and feline leukaemia vaccines as particularly linked to tumour induction. The development of alternative, non-adjuvanted products may go some way towards reducing the incidence of this pathology; however, these tumours still present a major clinical problem in many parts of the world.

Another distinct class of adverse effects are the spectrum of allergic (hypersensitivity) and autoimmune reactions. Acute reactions with a proposed type I hypersensitivity mechanism (e.g. angioedema, anaphylaxis) are one of the most frequently documented adverse consequences of vaccination, although it is of note that these may occur following administration of primary vaccine, raising the question of how immunological sensitization has occurred (possibly via maternal

865
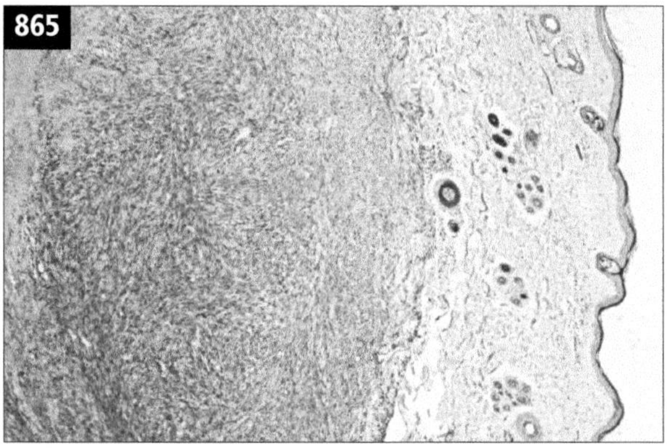

866
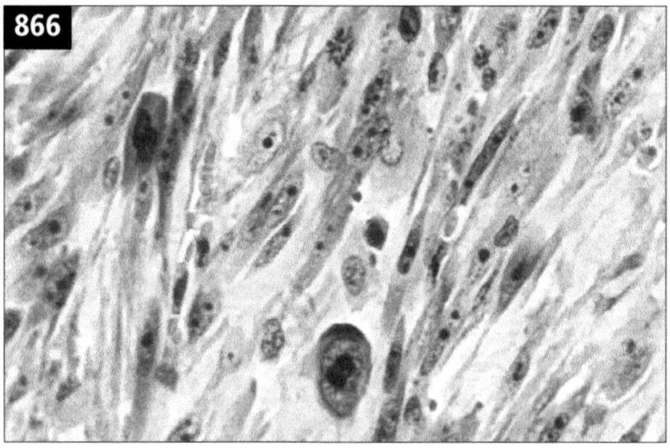

867
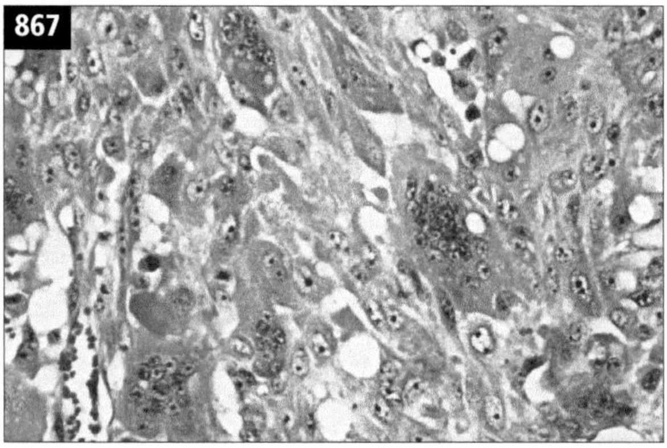

865–867 Feline injection site sarcoma.
Low (**865**) and high (**866**) power views of a sarcoma excised from the site of previous vaccination in a 13-year-old neutered male DSH cat. This is an aggressive and pleomorphic population of spindle cells. A multinucleate cell and a cell with a giant nucleus is present in this field, together with evidence of mitotic activity. (**867**) In this further example there is much greater cellular pleomorphism, with a prominent multinucleated cell component.

868
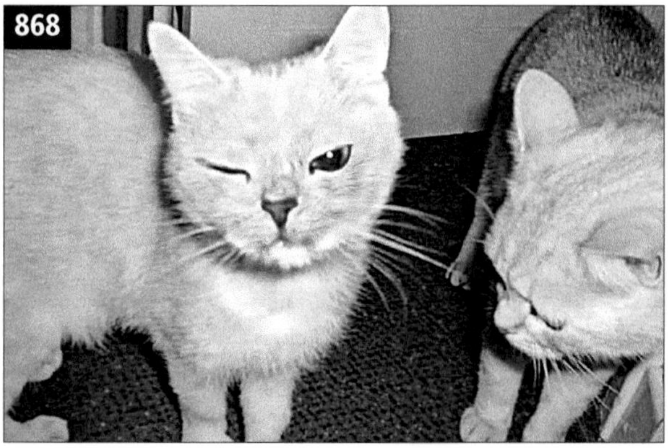

868 Immediate hypersensitivity vaccine reaction.
These two cats have just been vaccinated, but within 15 minutes post vaccination the cat on the left developed marked facial oedema. Such reactions are likely to reflect an immediate (type I) hypersensitivity pathogenesis involving IgE antibody. These reactions are generally transient, but may recur on subsequent vaccination.

transfer) (**218**, **868**). Recent experimental and clinical canine studies have shown that vaccinated dogs make an IgG and IgE antibody response to a range of bovine proteins (e.g. bovine serum albumin, fibronectin) that are incorporated into vaccines as residue from fetal calf serum used in cell culture for vaccine production. Canine vaccines also have a relatively high antigenic content of bovine serum albumin and bovine IgG, many orders of magnitude greater than the level recommended by the World Health Organisation for human products. It has been suggested that these IgE responses might act as a risk factor for the subsequent development of atopic disease or dietary hypersensitivity and mimic the proposed role of vaccines in the induction of human allergy, although limited evidence exists for this hypothesis at this time both in veterinary and human medicine.

Vaccination is linked to a range of autoimmune disorders (primarily in the dog) including IMHA, IMTP, polyneuritis and polyarthritis (see Chapters 3, 4 and 6). Although these associations are generally accepted, there are virtually no data that define the mechanisms underlying them. A number of possibilities (e.g. disturbance of immunoregulation by vaccination; non-specific immune activation via adjuvants or microbe-derived 'superantigens'; exposure to cross-reactive tissue protein incorporated into vaccines; molecular mimicry between autoantigens and vaccinal microbes) have been proposed and these are discussed in Chapter 3. Some studies have shown the development of IgG anti-bovine and autoantibodies specific for a range of proteins post vaccination. For example, vaccinated dogs develop thyroglobulin autoantibody in addition to anti-bovine thyroglobulin antibodies, but this is not linked with clinical hypothyroidism. Similarly, proteins from the Crandall Rees feline kidney cell line are incorporated into feline virus vaccines and are able to induce autoantibody to feline renal extract. At this stage, however, there is no evidence to suggest that these antibodies induce significant clinical, histological or ultrastructural renal disease in vaccinated cats.

Reactions involving type III (immune complex) hypersensitivity are also reported; for example, the cutaneous vasculopathy that may follow rabies virus vaccination, in which immunohistochemical studies have demonstrated vascular deposition of rabies virus antigen and complement (**152–155**). The pathogenesis of adenoviral-related 'blue eye' in dogs is also well defined (see Chapter 11, p. 275 and **534**).

A different category of adverse outcome to vaccination is lack of efficacy. Failure of vaccine to adequately protect from infectious disease is clearly a serious problem; however, it is more often due to inappropriate administration or administration to immunosuppressed or immunodeficient individuals, than to batches of subnormal efficacy. Moreover, it is important to remember that no currently licensed vaccine can claim 100% efficacy on the basis of experimental challenge or field studies. As discussed above, some breeds of dog (e.g. Rottweiler) may be more susceptible to this problem, perhaps due to a genetically-mediated suboptimal response to vaccination. There is currently concern over reports of suspected lack of efficacy related to the so-called 'early finish' canine vaccines (**860**, **861**). These products were developed to provide protective immunity, with the second of two puppy vaccines being administered at ten weeks of age. The advantage of this approach is that the vaccinated pup is then able to attend socialization classes, which have significant benefit for behavioural development. However, although experimental data confirms the protective capacity of these products, the effect of MDA in the field may be more prolonged and current guidelines suggest that the timing of puppy vaccination should in fact be extended to a 16 week finish.

Other rare complications of vaccination include residual virulence of attenuated vaccine strains of microbe or batch contamination during manufacture. Finally, a recent adverse effect that has received much attention in the US and Australia is the interference of the newly released FIV vaccine with current serological diagnostic methods for this infection, a situation that has not yet been completely resolved by the availability of alternative molecular diagnostic tests.

Scientific basis of adverse reactions

Although there is little doubt that adverse reactions to vaccines occur, they are probably rare occurrences and are extremely poorly characterized mechanistically. Accurate surveillance data of sufficient quantity and quality for meaningful analysis of the prevalence of companion animal vaccine reactions simply do not exist. Moreover, the reports of adverse reactions are generally anecdotal clinical descriptions, and the 'association' between clinical event and vaccination is often a temporal link, whereby vaccination preceded the onset of the event by an arbitrary period of time, which is generally accepted as four weeks. As discussed above, there are minimal clear scientific data that explain mechanistically how the majority of vaccine reactions occur. These problems are exemplified by feline injection site sarcoma where, despite extensive research, the pathogenesis of the lesion remains hypothetical and the precise incidence of the condition is far from well-established in most geographical areas. A recent study suggested that feline vaccine-associated sarcoma in the US may be far less widespread (0.63 sarcomas/10,000 cats vaccinated) than previously thought. A further example lies in the purported link between vaccination and IMHA in the dog. Since this association was first flagged in 1996, there have been numerous retrospective case series published; however, in none of these has a significant association been found, other than possibly in low numbers of individual cases. It is of note that the evidence base for vaccine associations with disease in human medicine is also very limited.

Recent epidemiological research has begun to address the incidence of adverse effects in the canine and feline population. The electronic medical records for a large, multicentre veterinary hospital group have been searched for incidents of adverse reaction, providing information on over one million vaccinated dogs. In this study, acute onset hypersensitivity within three days of vaccination was recorded in 0.38% of vaccinated dogs. Affected animals were more likely to be of small breed and to have received multiple components in the vaccination protocol. Similar studies involving almost 500,000 vaccinated cats reported adverse reactions in 0.51% of vaccinates over the 30 day period post vaccination.

Table 39: Suspected adverse reactions to canine and feline vaccines in the UK, 2010.

	Dog	Cat
Total reports of reactions to all veterinary products	751	468
Inactivated vaccine	41	83
Mixed vaccine	186	10
Live vaccine	147	110
Vector vaccine	0	20
All vaccines	374	223
Percentage of total reactions	(50%)	(48%)

Data from the Veterinary Medicines Directorate (Dyer F, Diesel G, Cooles S, Tait A (2011) Suspected adverse reactions, 2010. *Veterinary Record* **168**:610–613)

Pharmacovigilance

Over many years, data on adverse reactions to companion animal vaccines have been collected by manufacturers and licensing authorities. The single best example of such an adverse reactions reporting scheme is the computerized 'suspect adverse reaction surveillance scheme' (SARSS), which has been run since 1984 by the UK licensing authority, the Veterinary Medicines Directorate (VMD). Similar monitoring schemes do not exist, or are at best rudimentary, in other countries. Recently, even one of the independent reporting routes for adverse events in the US was closed. The SARSS figures are published annually in the UK in the *Veterinary Record* and they provide an indication of the prevalence of adverse reactions to vaccination in companion animals (*Table 39*). A spectrum of clinical events is reported in association with these reactions. Despite the success of SARSS, it is believed that only a small proportion of adverse reactions are actually reported, as the scheme is 'passive' in nature and requires that owners or veterinary surgeons voluntarily report each occurrence.

The SARSS database was recently analysed by a working group of the Veterinary Products Committee (VPC), which is an independent scientific advisory committee to the UK government. SARSS data from 1985–1999 recorded 1,190 suspected vaccine adverse reactions to feline vaccines and 1,133 to canine vaccines. The figures for the period 1995–1999 were related to company sales data, which provide an indication of the number of vaccines sold (and presumptively administered) over that time. In that period, the mean incidence for feline reactions was 0.61 per 10,000 doses sold and for the dog 0.21 per 10,000 doses sold. These low incidence rates are in accord with the limited published data and reinforce the relative rarity of adverse reactions to vaccination in these species.

An analysis was also made comparing animals with vaccine-related suspected adverse reactions with non-vaccine-related suspected adverse reactions. Relevant features of this analysis included identification of significant associations with male dogs and cats, pedigree cats, toy and utility dog breeds and animals of less than six months of age. The incidence per 10,000 doses of specific types of vaccine reaction were also recorded for the period 1995–99, and included data for anaphylactic reactions (0.026 dog, 0.018 cat), injection site reactions (0.099 cat, 0.012 dog, perhaps reflecting the more widespread usage of adjuvanted vaccines in the cat), IMHA (0.001 dog), IMTP (0.002 dog), canine 'blue eye' (0.002) and polyarthropathy (0.044 cat, 0.006 dog).

The report suggested that there was an increasing incidence of feline injection site sarcoma in the UK, with an incidence of 0.21 per 10,000 doses sold between 1995 and 1999. These were predominantly older (mean 7.91 years), non-pedigree cats, and sarcomas more frequently arose in animals receiving FeLV vaccine or alum-adjuvanted vaccines.

A more recent analysis of the SARSS database (2005–2010) recorded a figure of 1.85 reactions per 10,000 doses of vaccine sold during that period.

An epidemiological study into canine vaccine reactions in the UK was recently initiated by the National Office for Animal Health (NOAH). This study specifically addressed the question of whether there was an increased prevalence of ill-health in dogs in the three-month period following vaccination. The study was performed by questionnaire to pet owners registered at 28 veterinary practices. A total of 3,966 useable questionnaires were obtained from 9055 issued. The main finding of the survey was that 16.4% of dogs vaccinated within the previous three months had an episode of illness in the two-week period preceding completion of the questionnaire, whereas 18.8% of dogs that last received a vaccine more than three months previously had an episode of illness within the same time frame. This suggests that vaccination does not increase the prevalence of illness within the immediate three-month post-vaccination period.

VACCINATION GUIDELINES

The major question that emerged from the companion animal vaccine debate described above was whether the prevalence of adverse reactions reflected the frequency of administration of vaccines to animals. Within the veterinary profession, those in the US were notably pro-active in addressing this question and clear guidelines on vaccination schedules have been produced and recently updated by the American Association of Feline Practitioners and the Academy of Feline Medicine, the American Veterinary Medical Association and the American Animal Hospital Association. The World Small Animal Veterinary Association has also convened a working group to address vaccination guidelines internationally. The fundamental concepts enshrined in these various guidelines include:

- The concept of 'core' versus 'non-core' vaccines (*Table 40*). This recognizes that some vaccines are essential for dogs and cats to receive in order to maintain protection in those individuals and in the general population from serious infectious disease. Other vaccines are considered 'core' by virtue of a legal requirement for their administration (e.g. rabies). However, there are other vaccines that are not essential because they may not be relevant to a particular geographical area or the lifestyle of the individual animal, or may be of limited proven efficacy.
- The extension of revaccination intervals to reduce vaccine load on individual animals. There is increasing availability of core products licensed with three year duration of immunity, which now makes this concept achievable and removes any legal concerns that might arise when vaccines are used contrary to data sheet recommendations. Even in the absence of such licensing, it is appropriate for a

Table 40: Core versus non-core vaccines for dogs and cats.

	Dog	Cat
Core	CDV	FPV
	CAV	FHV
	CPV	FCV
	Rabies (legal)	Rabies (legal)
Non-core	*Bordetella*	*Bordetella*
	Borrelia	*Chlamydophila*
	CPi	FeLV
	Leptospira	FIV

Recommendations for core versus non-core vaccines as given in various guidelines. Note that rabies vaccination is considered core where there is a legal requirement for its use.

veterinarian to use any core vaccine in this way following appropriate risk-benefit analysis and obtaining informed client consent for such usage. There is growing awareness of legal issues surrounding vaccination and the potential for litigation if vaccination fails to afford protection.

- The use of single component products to enable the application of vaccine protocols, whereby some components may be administered every three years, but others may be given annually.
- The administration of feline vaccines linked to fibrosarcoma to specific anatomical sites to minimize surgical complexity in tumour removal. Current WSAVA guidelines recommend vaccination of cats into the skin of the lateral abdomen.
- The avoidance of adjuvanted vaccines, particularly in cats.
- The development of tailored vaccine programmes for individual animals based on lifestyle and predicted disease exposure or for breeds of dog perceived to be 'at risk' from adverse reactions to vaccines. Similarly, specific guidelines for animals in a high risk (of exposure to infectious agents) shelter environment have been formulated.
- The fundamental shift in attitude by practising veterinarians and clients from the view that an animal visits the surgery every year for an 'annual vaccine booster', towards the concept that there is an annual (or even twice yearly) 'wellness examination' at which vaccination requirements will be reviewed and discussed, even if vaccination is not performed on that occasion.

Underlying this entire debate has been clear recognition of the essential benefits of vaccination for human and animal health. Vaccination has been extraordinarily successful in controlling (and sometimes eliminating) infectious disease, and there are clear epidemiological data that show recurrence of disease during periods of 'vaccine breakdown'. The most frequently cited example of this is the re-emergence of canine distemper virus infection in Finland, which followed a period of reduced vaccine uptake. The outcome of the vaccine debate has been a focus on 'risk assessment' for populations and individual animals with respect to the balance between the likelihood of adverse reaction compared with the risk of infectious disease.

FURTHER READING

Bergman PJ, McKnight J, Novosad A *et al.* (2003) Long-term survival of dogs with advanced malignant melanoma after DNA vaccination with xenogeneic human tyrosinase: a phase I trial. *Clinical Cancer Research* **9**:1284–1290.

Bohm M, Thompson H, Weir A *et al.* (2004) Serum antibody titres to canine parvovirus, adenovirus and distemper virus in dogs in the UK which had not been vaccinated for at least three years. *Veterinary Record* **154**:457–463.

Day MJ (2006) Vaccine side-effects: fact and fiction. *Veterinary Microbiology* **117**:51–58.

Day MJ, Schoon H-A, Magnol J-P *et al.* (2007) A kinetic study of histopathological changes in the subcutis of cats injected with non-adjuvanted and adjuvanted multi-component vaccines. *Vaccine* **25**:4073–4084.

Day MJ (2007) Vaccine safety in the neonatal period. *Journal of Comparative Pathology* **137**:S51–S56.

Day MJ, Horzinek M, Schultz RD (2010) Guidelines for the vaccination of dogs and cats. *Journal of Small Animal Practice* **51**:338–356.

Frana TS, Clough NE, Gatewood DM *et al.* (2008) Postmarketing surveillance of rabies vaccines for dogs to evaluate safety and efficacy. *Journal of the American Veterinary Medical Association* **232**:1000–1002.

Goubier A, Fuhrmann L, Forest L *et al.* (2008) Superiority of needle-free transdermal plasmid delivery for the induction of antigen-specific IFNγ T cell responses in the dog. *Vaccine* **26**:2186–2190.

Hosie MJ, Beatty JA (2007) Vaccine protection against feline immunodeficiency virus: setting the challenge. *Australian Veterinary Journal* **85**:5–12.

Kennedy LJ, Lunt M, Barnes A *et al.* (2007) Factors influencing the antibody response of dogs vaccinated against rabies. *Vaccine* **35**:8500–8507.

Lappin MR, Jensen WA, Jensen TD *et al.* (2005) Investigation of the induction of antibodies against Crandall–Rees feline kidney cell lysates and feline renal cell lysates after parenteral administration of vaccines against feline viral rhinotracheitis, calicivirus, and panleukopenia in cats. *American Journal of Veterinary Research* **66**:506–511.

Lodmell DL, Ewalt LC, Parnell MJ *et al.* (2006) One-time intradermal DNA vaccination in ear pinnae one year prior to infection protects dogs against rabies virus. *Vaccine* **24**:412–416.

Moore GE, Guptill LF, Ward MP *et al.* (2005) Adverse events diagnosed within three days of vaccine administration in dogs. *Journal of the American Veterinary Medical Association* **227**:1102–1108.

Moore GE, DeSantis-Kerr AC, Guptill LF *et al.* (2007) Adverse events after vaccine administration in cats: 2,560 cases (2002–2005). *Journal of the American Veterinary Medical Association* **231**:94–100.

Mouzin DE, Lorenzen MJ, Haworth JD *et al.* (2004) Duration of serologic response to five viral antigens in dogs. *Journal of the American Veterinary Medical Association* **224**:55–60.

Mouzin DE, Lorenzen MJ, Haworth JD *et al.* (2004) Duration of serologic response to three viral antigens in cats. *Journal of the American Veterinary Medical Association* **224**:61–66.

Norris JM, Krockenberger MB, Baird AA *et al.* (2006) Canine distemper: re-emergence of an old enemy. *Australian Veterinary Journal* **84**:362–363.

Ohmori K, Masuda K, Maeda S *et al.* (2005) IgE reactivity to vaccine components in dogs that developed immediate-type allergic reactions after vaccination. *Veterinary Immunology and Immunopathology* **104**:249–256.

Ohmori K, Masuda K, DeBoer DJ *et al.* (2007) Immunoblot analysis for IgE-reactive components of fetal calf serum in dogs that developed allergic reactions after non-rabies vaccination. *Veterinary Immunology and Immunopathology* **115**:166–171.

Patel JR, Heldens JGM (2009) Review of companion animal viral diseases and immunoprophylaxis. *Vaccine* **27**:491–504.

Paul MA, Carmichael LE, Childers H *et al.* (2006) AAHA canine vaccine guidelines. *Journal of the American Animal Hospital Association* **42**:80–89.

Ren J, Sun L, Yang L *et al.* (2010) A novel canine favored CpG oligodeoxynucleotide capable of enhancing the efficacy of an inactivated aluminium-adjuvanted rabies vaccine of dog use. *Vaccine* **28**:2458–2464.

Richards JR, Starr RM, Childers HE *et al.* (2005) The current understanding and management of vaccine-associated sarcomas in cats. *Journal of the American Veterinary Medical Association* **226**:1821–1842.

Richards JR, Elston TH, Ford RB *et al.* (2006) The 2006 American Association of Feline Practitioners feline vaccine advisory panel report. *Journal of the American Veterinary Medical Association* **229**:1405–1441.

Schultz RD, Thiel B, Mukhtar E *et al.* (2010) Age and long-term protective immunity in dogs and cats. *Journal of Comparative Pathology* **142**:S102–S108.

Shaw SC, Kent MS, Gordon IK *et al.* (2009) Temporal changes in characteristics of injection-site sarcomas in cats: 392 cases (1990-2006). *Journal of the American Veterinary Medical Association* **234**:376–380.

Strasser A, May B, Teltscher A *et al.* (2003) Immune modulation following immunization with polyvalent vaccines in dogs. *Veterinary Immunology and Immunopathology* **94**:113–121.

Wang C, Johnson CM, Ahluwalia SK *et al.* (2010) Dual-emission fluorescence resonance energy transfer (FRET) real-time PCR differentiates feline immunodeficiency virus subtypes and discriminates infected from vaccinated cats. *Journal of Clinical Microbiology* **48**:1667–1672.

Whittemore JC, Hawley JR, Jensen WA *et al.* (2010) Antibodies against Crandell Rees feline kidney (CRFK) cell line antigens, α-enolase, and annexin A2 in vaccinated and CRFK hyperinoculated cats. *Journal of Veterinary Internal Medicine* **24**:306–313.

GLOSSARY

Acanthocyte A discohesive epidermal keratinocyte. Typically, found within the pustule of an animal with pemphigus.

Acantholysis The process of breakdown of intercellular adhesion molecules between epidermal keratinocytes, leading to the formation of an intraepidermal vesicle/pustule.

Acute phase proteins A group of proteins found in the blood during the early stages of an infectious/inflammatory response.

Adaptive That form of immunity that is specifically stimulated by antigen, resulting in clonal selection of antigen-relevant lymphocytes. This provides a more potent immune response to support nonspecific innate immunity. The adaptive immune response generates immunological memory. Also 'acquired immunity'.

Adenitis Inflammation of a gland (e.g. sebaceous adenitis).

Adhesion molecules Mediate the binding of cell to cell, or cells to matrix proteins.

Adjuvant A substance that enhances the immune response. Traditional adjuvants are nonspecific in their effect, or they may have a 'depot effect' and cause sustained release of antigen. Modern adjuvants may have a more targeted effect on the immune response (e.g. cytokine adjuvants, CpG motifs).

Adult tolerance Induction of tolerance to an antigen in an adult animal.

Aeroallergen An airborne allergen that can be inhaled or absorbed across the skin.

Affinity Strength of binding of one molecule to another; specifically, the binding of a single antigenic epitope to a single Fab binding site within an immunoglobulin.

Agglutination Aggregation of particulate antigens by antibodies, in particular multivalent antibodies such as IgA and IgM.

Allele Two or more alternative forms of a gene.

Allergen An antigen that induces an allergic or hypersensitivity reaction.

Allergen-specific immunotherapy See 'hyposensitization'.

Allergy See 'hypersensitivity'.

Alloantigen A tissue antigen derived from a genetically dissimilar individual of the same species. Typically stimulates an immune response following incompatible grafting of tissue or cells.

Allograft Transplant of tissue or organ between genetically dissimilar individuals of the same species.

Alopecia Loss of hair coat by failure to grow, or interference with the hair cycle after growth.

Alopecia areata Immune-mediated destruction of the hair bulb, leading to alopecia.

Alum Adjuvant based on the use of aluminium phosphate or hydroxide.

Amastigote Stage of protozoal life cycle. That form of *Leishmania* found within tissue macrophages.

Amino acid The building block of protein.

Amyloid Polymerized protein forming a fibrillar structure arranged as a β-pleated sheet. AA amyloid is 'inflammatory', whereas AL amyloid is 'immunological'.

Amyloidosis Disease caused by tissue deposition of amyloid.

Anal furunculosis Disease primarily affecting German Shepherd Dogs and characterized by extensive ulceration and sinus tract formation within the perianal skin.

Anaphylaxis A systemic type I hypersensitivity reaction.

Anaphylotoxin A substance capable of directly degranulating a mast cell; typically, C3a and C5a of the complement pathway.

Anergy Failure of an immune response to a presented antigen due to lack of co-stimulation by the antigen presenting cell. Patients are 'anergic' when they fail to respond to an antigen by mounting a delayed-type hypersensitivity response.

Angioedema The sudden occurrence of large areas of subcutaneous oedema following a type I hypersensitivity reaction.

Anterior chamber-associated immune deviation An alteration in the nature of the systemic immune response to an antigen inoculated into the anterior chamber of the eye.

Antibiotic responsive diarrhoea Chronic diarrhoea that responds clinically to antibiotic therapy.

Antibody A protein that binds specifically to an antigen. Antibodies are secreted by plasma cells and can bind to pathogens to target them for removal. Each antibody has a unique antigen-binding capacity, but shares its structure with other antibodies or immunoglobulins.

Antibody-dependent cell-mediated cytotoxicity Cytotoxic destruction of a target cell coated by antibody that is recognized by an Fc receptor on the surface of the cytotoxic cell.

Antigen A substance that initiates an immune response; technically, a molecule that can bind to specific antibody, as some antigens do not elicit antibodies as part of the immune response.

Antinuclear antibody Autoantibody specific for one or more constituents of the cellular nucleus. May be present in many autoimmune diseases, but required in high titre for a diagnosis of systemic lupus erythematosus.

Antigen presentation Expression of small peptide fragments derived from an antigen (by antigen processing) on the surface of an antigen presenting cell within the binding groove of an MHC class I or II molecule.

Antigen processing Breakdown of antigen to small peptide components within the cytoplasm of an antigen presenting cell via either the endogenous or exogenous pathway.

Antiserum Serum collected from an individual following exposure to an antigen; contains antibodies that can be utilized in serological assays. A polyclonal antiserum contains multiple antibodies specific for different epitopes of the antigen. A monoclonal antiserum contains antibody of a single type that recognizes a single epitope.

Apoptosis Cell death resulting from activation of an 'internal death programme' within the cell, leading to DNA degradation, nuclear degeneration and condensation and phagocytosis of the cell remains. Also 'programmed cell death'.

Arthus reaction Local tissue type III hypersensitivity reaction involving immune complex formation in a sensitized individual following local exposure to antigen.

Asthma Respiratory disease that may have several causes,

one of which is type I hypersensitivity to aeroallergens.

Atopic dermatitis Skin disease that may have several causes, one of which is type I hypersensitivity to aeroallergens that are percutaneously absorbed. Likely has a genetic basis.

Atrophy Reduction in size of an adult tissue once normal size has been attained (e.g. lymph node atrophy in senile dogs).

Attenuation The reduction in virulence of an infectious agent so that it retains antigenic structure and limited replicative capacity, but cannot produce disease.

Auricular Of the ear (e.g. auricular cartilage).

Autoantigen An antigen derived from self-tissue that stimulates an autoimmune response.

Autoimmunity Generation of an immune response to self-tissue antigen, resulting in tissue pathology and autoimmune disease.

Avidity Strength of overall binding of two molecules that contact at multiple sites; specifically, the binding of multiple antigenic epitopes by multiple Fab binding sites within an immunoglobulin.

Azotaemia The presence of nitrogen-containing compounds in the blood (e.g. urea, creatinine and other end products of protein and amino acid metabolism). Also referred to as 'uraemia'.

Bence-Jones protein Free immunoglobulin light chains that may be produced in multiple myeloma and pass through the glomerular filter into the urine (Bence-Jones proteinuria).

Biclonal gammopathy Paraprotein produced by two clones of neoplastic plasma cells concurrently; presents as a double 'spike' on serum protein electrophoresis.

Blepharitis Inflammation of the eyelids.

Blepharospasm Spasm of the orbicular muscle of the eyelid.

Bronchiolar-associated lymphoid tissue Unencapsulated mucosal lymphoid aggregate associated with the bronchial mucosa.

Bronchoconstriction Narrowing of the diameter of a bronchus following contraction of the bronchial smooth muscle. May be mediated by mast cell or basophil contents in a type I hypersensitivity reaction.

Bystander suppression Nonspecific suppression of a local immune response not directly related to that being controlled by a suppressor lymphocyte.

C3b receptor Cell surface receptor that binds the third component (b subfragment) of complement.

Canine leukocyte adhesion deficiency Genetic mutation resulting in failure to express leukocyte adhesion molecules involved in the migration of leukocytes (in particular neutrophils) from blood to tissue. Occurs in Irish Setters.

Carcinogen The aetiological agent of neoplasia.

Cell-mediated immunity That type of immune response mediated by lymphocytes and typically involving cytotoxic destruction of target cells (e.g. infected cells, neoplastic cells, incompatible graft cells).

CH_{50} An *in vitro* test of the function of the classical and terminal pathways of complement.

Chediak–Higashi syndrome Abnormal granulation in the cytoplasm of neutrophils of blue smoke Persian cats. May be associated with functional impairment of these cells.

Chemokine A soluble protein released from a cell to form a chemotactic gradient responsible for the chemoattraction of specific leukocytes (e.g. into tissue from the circulation).

Chemosis Oedema of the conjunctiva.

Chemotaxis Migration of a leukocyte along a chemotactic gradient of increasing concentration of a chemoattractant.

Chorioretinitis Inflammation of the choroid and retina.

Chromatin The substance of the chromosomes within the cell nucleus; includes DNA and histone proteins.

Chronic hepatitis Portal inflammatory disease of the liver; thought to have an immune-mediated aetiology.

Chrysotherapy Treatment with gold salts.

Chylothorax Accumulation of chylous fluid within the pleural cavity secondary to thoracic duct trauma or a developmental defect, mediastinal neoplasia, etc. Lymphatic fluid contains triglyceride and small lymphocytes and has a characteristic milky white appearance.

Ciliary dyskinesia An ultrastructural abnormality of cilia, predisposing to infection of (for example) the respiratory tract.

Clonal deletion Removal by apoptosis of autoreactive lymphocytes bearing receptors specific for self-antigens. May occur within the thymus or bone marrow for T and B cells respectively (central deletion), or may occur within secondary lymphoid tissue (peripheral deletion).

Clonal differentiation Following activation of a lymphocyte by antigen, there are repeated rounds of cell division (clonal proliferation), during which the cells may acquire specific functional or effector characteristics.

Clonal proliferation Exponential expansion of a clone of lymphocytes following activation by antigen.

Clonal selection Selection (for activation) of antigen-relevant lymphocytes from the entire repertoire on exposure to antigen.

Cluster of differentiation Nomenclature used to define immune cell surface molecules.

Complement A series of plasma proteins, which, when activated, interact sequentially, forming a self-assembling enzymatic cascade and generating biologically active molecules mediating a range of end processes.

Conformation Three dimensional tertiary structure of a molecule.

Constant region That portion of an immunological molecule in which there is conserved amino acid sequence in the polypeptide chains of different molecules.

Contact allergy Type IV hypersensitivity reaction to percutaneously absorbed allergen.

Coombs test An agglutination test used to detect the presence of immunoglobulin and/or complement on the surface of erythrocytes in IMHA.

Core (vaccine) A vaccine that all animals should receive, as it protects from a serious infectious disease that is prevalent in that geographical location.

Cortex Outer zone of an organ; in immunology, specifically of the lymph node and thymus.

Co-stimulation Co-stimulatory signals are required to fully activate a lymphocyte following recognition of antigen. Co-stimulatory signals may be delivered by molecular interaction between lymphocyte and antigen presenting cell, or by cytokine released from the antigen presenting cell and binding cytokine receptor on the lymphocyte.

CpG motif A sequence of bacterial DNA rich in cytosine and guanidine nucleotides that is a potent stimulus for Th1 immune responses.

Cross-link Join together (i.e. cross-linkage of two mast cell surface Fcε receptors by allergen binding two individual receptor-bound IgE molecules).

Cross-reactive Two antigens may share common or similar

epitopes, enabling recognition by more than one antigen receptor (immunoglobulin or T cell receptor).

Cross-regulation Regulation of the function of one cell by another; typically, the mutually antagonistic effects of Th1 and Th2 lymphocytes.

Crust An amalgam of fibrin, degenerate inflammatory cells and epithelial cells that forms over the surface of inflamed or ulcerated skin.

Cryoglobulinaemia The presence of an abnormal immunoglobulin in serum that precipitates or gels at temperatures lower than 37°C.

Cryotherapy Therapeutic use of cold (e.g. to destroy a skin lesion by freezing).

Crypt abscess Lesion of the intestinal mucosa involving dilation of an individual crypt that becomes filled with necrotic debris and degenerate inflammatory cells.

Cyclic haematopoiesis Genetic mutation in grey coated Collie dogs, resulting in cyclic cytopenia and susceptibility to infectious/inflammatory disease.

Cytokine A soluble protein secreted by one cell that binds to a specific cytokine receptor expressed by another cell, leading to a change in function of this target cell. Cytokines are considered intercellular messengers of the immune system. Cytokine is a generic term for molecules including interleukins, monokines and lymphokines.

Cytotoxicity Destruction of a target cell by a cytotoxic effector cell.

D region A gene segment that links the joining and constant regions of immunoglobulin heavy chain and T cell receptor β chain loci.

Degranulation Release of cytoplasmic granules containing biological mediators following activation of a mast cell or basophil.

Delayed-type hypersensitivity A type IV hypersensitivity reaction involving activation of mononuclear cells and production of cytokine in a sensitized individual re-exposed to antigen. Takes 24–72 hours to become clinically manifest.

Dermatomyositis Immune-mediated disease involving both the skin and skeletal muscle. Most often occurs in Collies and Shetland Sheepdogs.

Dermatouveitis Immune-mediated disease involving both the skin and uveal tract. Most often occurs in Japanese Akitas. (See also uveodermatological syndrome.)

Desmoglein A molecule involved in the adhesion of epidermal keratinocytes and a target autoantigen in pemphigus.

Desmosome A group of molecules that forms the intercellular adhesion between epithelial cells.

Determinant See epitope.

Diapedesis A leukocyte squeezing between endothelial cells to enter tissue from a blood vessel.

Dietary hypersensitivity Hypersensitivity to food-derived allergen. (See also 'food allergy'.) Presents as cutaneous or alimentary disease. Most likely a type I hypersensitivity reaction.

Dimer A complex of two individual units (i.e. an IgA dimer).

Domain A conformational region of a polypeptide that may have a specific function (e.g. the domain structure of the immunoglobulin molecule).

Down-regulation Suppression.

Duration of immunity The period after vaccination in which an immune response to vaccine can be detected (usually serologically).

Duration of protection The period after vaccination for which the animal is protected from challenge with virulent organism.

Ectoparasite A parasite of the external surface of the body.

Effector cell One that actively participates in an immune response (e.g. by producing antibody or destroying a target cell via cytotoxicity).

Efficacy (vaccine) A measure of how well a vaccine works, by preventing infection and/or the tissue pathology and clinical signs of disease. Determined experimentally by challenge of vaccinated *versus* unvaccinated animals with virulent organism. May also be studied in the field where there is natural exposure to the organism.

Endogenous antigen Antigen produced within the cytoplasm of an antigen presenting cell (i.e. a self-antigen or viral antigen).

Endoparasite A parasite that lives within the body of the host.

Endophthalmitis Inflammation of the ocular cavities and adjacent structures.

Endoplasmic reticulum Folded membrane sheets within the cytoplasm that are sites of protein synthesis. Site of interaction between endogenous peptide and MHC class I in antigen processing.

Enterocyte Epithelial cell lining the intestinal tract.

Enzyme-linked immunosorbent assay An *in vitro* serological test used to determine the concentration of either antigen or antibody. Based on detection by an enzyme-conjugated secondary antiserum, which is demonstrated by providing an appropriate substrate that leads to a colour change that may be measured spectrophotometrically.

Eosinophilic bronchopneumopathy An asthma-like disease of the dog characterized by eosinophilic infiltration of the respiratory mucosa.

Eosinophilic enteritis Inflammation of the small intestine characterized by infiltration of the lamina propria by eosinophils.

Eosinophilic granuloma complex A group of three distinct feline cutaneous entities characterized by eosinophil infiltration into affected tissue. Considered to be manifestations of type I hypersensitivity in the cat.

Eotaxin A chemokine that attracts eosinophils into tissue. Includes eotaxin, eotaxin-2 and eotaxin-3.

Epiphenomenon An immunological change that occurs concurrently with, but is not integral to, a disease process (e.g. the occurrence of some autoantibodies may be a consequence of cell damage (with release of autoantigen) rather than an initiating cause of such damage).

Epiphora Overflow of tears down the face due to blockage of the nasolacrimal duct.

Episcleritis Inflammation of the episclera.

Episclerokeratitis Inflammation of the episclera and cornea.

Epitheliotropic lymphoma Lymphoma of skin or mucosae where the neoplastic lymphocytes specifically infiltrate the overlying epithelium. Also known as 'mycosis fungoides'.

Epitope A site on an antigen that may be recognised by an antibody or T cell receptor. The nature of epitopes bound by these two types of receptor is different. Also called an antigenic 'determinant'.

Epitope spreading Spreading of the immune response to other epitopes within an antigen (generally an autoantigen) after the response is initiated by presentation of one epitope.

Erythema Redness of the skin due to increased blood flow. One of the cardinal signs of inflammation.

Erythema multiforme Immune-mediated skin disease involving lymphocytic infiltration of the epidermis with keratinocyte apoptosis. Most often secondary to drug administration or underlying neoplasia.

Exclusion diet Used for the diagnosis and management of dietary hypersensitivity. Comprises a protein and carbohydrate source novel to the individual animal.

Exocrine pancreatic insufficiency Failure of the exocrine pancreas to produce appropriate levels of digestive enzymes.

Exogenous antigen External antigen taken up by the antigen presenting cell.

Exon The nucleotide sequence of a gene that is represented in the mRNA.

Extramedullary haematopoiesis Generation of haemopoietic cells within the spleen, liver or lung when demand for such cells exceeds the ability of the bone marrow to supply them.

Fc receptor Cell surface receptor that binds immunoglobulin.

Flea allergy dermatitis Type I hypersensitivity to antigens within flea saliva.

Fluorescence Colour emitted by a fluorochrome when activated by light of a specific wavelength (usually ultraviolet). Fluorochromes such as fluorescein isothiocyanate (FITC) may be coupled to antibodies to detect molecules within tissue (immunofluorescence) or on the surface of cells (by flow cytometry).

Follicle Area of lymphoid tissue within which B lymphocytes reside. Follicles are found within lymph nodes, spleen and mucosal lymphoid tissue. Primary follicles are inactive, whereas secondary follicles with a germinal centre and mantle zone reflect activation of the immune system by antigen.

Folliculitis Inflammation of the hair follicle. Generally involves a perifollicular infiltrate that extends into the external root sheath of the follicle (mural folliculitis).

Food allergy An immunological reaction to dietary antigens. Most often considered to be a type I hypersensitivity reaction. (See also 'dietary hypersensitivity'.)

Food intolerance A nonimmunological reaction to food.

Fragment antigen binding (Fab) Refers to the antigen-binding site at the N terminal end of the immunoglobulin molecule.

Fragment crystalizable (Fc) Refers to the heavy chains at the C terminal end of the immunoglobulin molecule.

Furunculosis Extensive inflammation of the hair follicle leads to rupture of the follicle. Exposure of hair and keratin causes amplification of the inflammatory response with destruction of the follicular structure.

Gammopathy An abnormality (generally an increase) in serum gammaglobulins; may be polyclonal or monoclonal depending on the source of the immunoglobulin involved.

Gastrointestinal-associated lymphoid tissue Unencapsulated lymphoid tissue associated with the alimentary mucosa. Includes tonsils, gastric lymphoid follicles, Peyer's patches and colonic lymphoid aggregates, in addition to more diffuse mucosal lymphoid tissue.

Genome The entire complement of genetic material contained within a haploid set of chromosomes.

Germinal centre Central region of a secondary lymphoid follicle where antigen-activated B lymphocytes divide.

Germline repertoire The theoretical number of different immunoglobulin or T cell receptor molecules that can be generated from the multiple gene segments encoding variable domains inherited by an individual. The repertoire can be further expanded by variable recombination or somatic mutation.

Giant cell An aggregate of macrophages formed during a chronic inflammatory (granulomatous) response.

Glycosylation The formation of linkages with glycosyl groups; the linkage of carbohydrate residues to a protein molecule.

Golgi apparatus A cytoplasmic organelle consisting of flattened sacs (cisternae) and vesicles involved in protein synthesis. Thought to have a role in the processing and presentation of endogenous antigen. Plasma cells have a distinct cytoplasmic 'Golgi zone'.

Granuloma A distinct arrangement of inflammatory cells forming in response to an infectious agent. Typically, a necrotic centre, surrounded by concentric layers of macrophages, then lymphocytes and plasma cells.

Granulomatous A type of inflammation dominated by macrophages.

Grave's disease Human autoimmune disease involving binding of autoantibody to thyroid stimulating hormone receptor and leading to uncontrolled thyroid activation and hyperthyroidism.

Grenz zone A narrow area of unaffected dermal tissue immediately beneath the epidermis in dermal lymphoma.

Haemangioma (sarcoma) Neoplasm of the endothelial lining cells of blood vessels.

Haematopoiesis (haemopoiesis) Generation of haemopoietic cells, normally in the bone marrow.

Haplotype A linked set of genes associated with one haploid genome. Used to describe a set of linked major histocompatibility complex genes inherited as a haplotype from one parent.

Hapten A small chemical group which, by itself, cannot elicit an immune response but, when bound to a 'carrier protein', is capable of generating an antibody or T cell response.

Hassall's corpuscle An epithelial structure found in the medulla of a thymic lobule.

Heat shock protein A molecule highly conserved across nature. Heat shock proteins serve as 'molecular chaperones', particularly in stressed (e.g. heat shocked) cells.

Heavy chain One of two large polypeptides making up the immunoglobulin molecule.

Hemidesmosome A half desmosome. Typically anchors basal epithelial cells into the underlying matrix.

Heterologous (vaccine) Use of an antigenically similar, related infectious agent that lacks virulence to cross-protect against another more virulent pathogen.

High endothelial venule A structural modification of the endothelial cells lining a venule such that they take on a cuboidal morphology, thus creating local turbulent flow to maximize the chance of interaction with leukocytes.

Hinge region That portion of an immunoglobulin molecule between Fab and Fc that permits movement of the 'arms' of the Y-shaped structure.

Histiocyte A tissue macrophage.

Histiocytic ulcerative colitis Disease of Boxers characterized by granulomatous inflammation of the colonic lamina propria.

Histiocytic sarcoma A malignant proliferation of histiocytic cells (dendritic cells in this context), which may be either localized or disseminated.

Histiocytoma A benign cutaneous neoplasm of epidermal Langerhans cells in the dog.

Histiocytosis A reactive proliferation of histiocytes (dendritic cells in this context) within tissue. May be either cutaneous or systemic.

Histocompatibility Immunological similarity between individuals. Determined by the cellular expression of histocompatibility molecules and forms the basis of tissue matching before transplantation.

Homing receptor Molecule expressed by leukocytes that enables interaction with specific endothelial vascular addressins to allow that leukocyte to enter tissue at particular anatomical locations.

Humanized monoclonal antibody A genetically engineered monoclonal antibody with human Fc region and murine antigen-binding region. Avoids development of anti-murine responses when used therapeutically in humans.

Humoral immunity Immunity mediated by antibodies.

Hydropic degeneration Swelling of a cell secondary to intracellular oedema following cell damage.

Hygiene hypothesis States that the western lifestyle with high sanitation and reduced exposure to microbes underlies susceptibility to allergic and autoimmune disease in humans.

Hypereosinophilic syndrome Characterized by eosinophilia and eosinophilic infiltration of a range of body tissues. A rare disorder, most frequently documented in the cat.

Hypergammaglobulinaemia An elevation in the concentration of serum gamma globulin.

Hyperplasia Increase in size of a tissue or organ due to an increase in the number of constituent cells (e.g. reactive hyperplasia of a lymph node due to antigenic stimulation of the lymphoid cells in that node).

Hypersensitivity A state of immunological sensitization to an innocuous antigen that leads to an excessive (symptomatic) immune response on re-exposure to the antigen. (See also 'allergy'.)

Hypervariable That portion of an antigen-binding molecule with the greatest variability in amino acid sequence. Typically forms the contact residues with antigen. Found in antibodies, T cell receptors and histocompatibility molecules.

Hyperviscosity syndrome A collection of clinical effects that may result from the presence in serum of macroglobulin or cryoglobulin.

Hypoallergenic diet A diet with reduced content of potential food allergens that is used in the diagnosis and management of allergic disease.

Hypogammaglobulinaemia A decrease in the concentration of serum gammaglobulin.

Hypoplasia (e.g. thymic) Reduced size of an organ or tissue from birth (i.e. a congenital defect due to incomplete development).

Hyposensitization Repeated injection of gradually increasing quantities of antigen to which an individual is sensitized diminishes the immune response on subsequent natural exposure to antigen. Used in the management of atopic dermatitis. (See also 'allergen-specific immunotherapy'.)

Idiopathic inflammatory bowel disease Chronic diarrhoea of unknown aetiology that responds to immunosuppressive therapy.

Idiotype A unique structure found within an antigen receptor (immunoglobulin or T cell receptor) that is itself antigenic and can be recognized by other receptors with anti-idiotypic specificity.

IgA deficiency Lack of IgA in serum and at mucosal surfaces, with resulting predisposition to infectious and immune-mediated disease. In man and dogs, IgA deficiency is a relative, rather than absolute, deficiency and it does not involve genetic mutation of genes encoding the IgA molecule.

Immediate hypersensitivity Occurs in a sensitized individual within minutes of re-exposure to antigen. Involves type I hypersensitivity.

Immune adherence Adherence of complement C3b-coated particles to macrophages bearing C3b receptors. A mechanism for clearance of circulating antigen within the bloodstream. C3b-coated particles are bound by C3bR onto erythrocytes and are subsequently removed from the red blood cells by macrophages within the spleen.

Immune complex Complex of antigen and antibody, with or without complement. Aggregated immunoglobulin can also form an immune complex in the absence of antigen.

Immune deviation Polarization of the immune response to a specific antigen such that the response is predominantly regulated by Th1 (CMI) or Th2 (humoral) cells.

Immune surveillance Surveillance of the entire body by the immune system for encounter with potential pathogens.

Immunodominant Those epitopes within an antigen that are most likely to engender an immune response.

Immunofluorescence See fluorescence.

Immunogen A substance that induces an adaptive immune response following injection into an individual.

Immunoglobulin A general term for all antibody molecules. There are five classes of immunoglobulin: IgD, IgM, IgG, IgA and IgE.

Immunoglobulin class switch Commitment of an antigen-activated B lymphocyte to express a single immunoglobulin class (IgA, IgG, IgM or IgE) instead of the combination of IgM and IgD that characterises the naïve B cell.

Immunoglobulin superfamily Relatedness of a series of immunological molecules that likely arose through gene duplication during evolution. There are conserved regions of structure between immunoglobulins, T cell receptors, major histocompatibility complex antigens and other cluster of differentiation molecules.

Immunohistochemistry Use of antibodies to probe a tissue section for the presence of a specific molecule. The binding of antigen and antibody is visualized by conjugating the antibody to either a fluorochrome (immunofluorescence) or enzyme (immunoperoxidase). Multiple layers of reagents can be used to amplify the signal intensity.

Immunological ignorance Tolerance of a lymphocyte due to failure to present the cognate antigen.

Immunopathogenesis The cellular and molecular reactions by which immunopathology develops.

Immunopathology Tissue pathology caused by an immune response. The hypersensitivity reactions may also be considered immunopathological mechanisms.

Immunoperoxidase A type of immunohistochemistry involving conjugation of the enzyme peroxidase to an antibody used to probe tissue sections for the presence of a specific molecule. On subsequent incubation with hydrogen peroxide and a chromogenic substrate there is colour deposition (usually brown) within the tissue section at the site of the reaction.

Immunoregulation Control of the immune response; may be a positive effect (up-regulation) or suppressive effect (down-regulation).

Immunosuppression Damping down or switching off an active immune response.
Induced suppressor (cell) A suppressor T cell induced as part of an immune response.
Innate That form of more primitive immunity that is evolutionarily older and provides continuous protection of body surfaces.
Interferon A type of cytokine. The type I interferons (e.g. IFNα, IFNβ) are antiviral molecules, whereas type II interferon (IFNγ) is a key immunological molecule.
Interleukin A type of cytokine secreted by one leukocyte that binds a receptor expressed by another leukocyte.
Intradermal (skin) test Intradermal injection of a small quantity of antigen to which an individual is sensitized. Formation of a local area of erythema and oedema (wheal) within minutes after injection is consistent with a type I hypersensitivity response. A local area of erythema and induration that arises 48–72 hours post injection suggests a delayed (type IV) hypersensitivity response. The procedure is used diagnostically to determine causative allergens in allergic disease.
Intron The portion of DNA that does not code for protein. The intervening sequence of nucleotides between coding sequences (exons).
Isosthenuria Maintenance of a constant urine osmolality despite changes in the osmotic pressure of the blood.

J chain Joining chain that links together monomers of IgA or IgM via their heavy chains.
Joining region A gene segment that links the variable and constant regions of an immunoglobulin or T cell receptor locus.

Keratitis Inflammation of the cornea.
Keratoconjunctivitis Inflammation of the cornea and conjunctiva. Chronic superficial keratitis/kerato-conjunctivitis (also known as 'pannus' or 'Uberreiter's syndrome') occurs in German Shepherd Dogs.
Keratoconjunctivitis sicca Lymphocytic destruction of the lacrimal glands leading to reduced production of tears and 'dry eye'.
Keratomalacia Softening and necrosis of the cornea.
Killed vaccine A vaccine containing an organism that has been killed but retains antigenic structure.
Kinetics The evolution of an immune response over time.

Langerhans cell A type of dendritic antigen presenting cell located within the epidermis of the skin.
Late phase response Occurs 24 hours after an immediate hypersensitivity reaction and involves the infiltration of eosinophils into affected tissue.
Lethal acrodermatitis Putative immunodeficiency disease affecting Bull Terrier dogs.
Leukaemic lymphoma Shedding of neoplastic lymphocytes into the circulating blood in the terminal stages of solid visceral lymphoma.
Lichenoid band Descriptive term for an infiltrate of mononuclear cells that forms a closely-packed band of cells obscuring the basement membrane zone between the epidermis and dermis.
Ligand A molecule that binds to another (i.e. the ligand for a specific receptor).
Light chain One of two small polypeptides making up part of the immunoglobulin molecule.
Lupus erythematosus Used to describe a group of autoimmune diseases involving either the skin (e.g. cutaneous lupus erythematosus) or multiple body systems (systemic lupus erythematosus). Name derives from the facial cutaneous rash that characterizes human systemic lupus erythematosus (lupus = 'wolf like').
Lymphadenitis Inflammation of a lymph node.
Lymphadenomegaly Enlargement of lymph nodes.
Lymphadenopathy Pathological change in lymph nodes, often used to describe lymph node enlargement in a clinical setting.
Lymphangiectasia Dilation of the central lacteal within villi of the small intestine due to occlusion of the lymphatic drainage (generally by downstream inflammatory lesions). Leads to oedema of the villi, with protein losing enteropathy and loss of lymphocytes, and resulting in hypoproteinaemia and lymphopenia.
Lymphangioma (sarcoma) Neoplasm of the endothelial lining cells of lymphatic vessels.
Lymphoblast Antigen-activated lymphocyte.
Lymphocytic–plasmacytic enteritis Inflammation of the small intestine characterized by infiltration of the lamina propria by lymphocytes and plasma cells.
Lymphoedema Oedema of a tissue due to occlusion of lymphatic drainage by pathology affecting the lymphatic vessel or lymph node. May be primary, congenital or secondary in nature.
Lymphoid leukaemia Neoplasia of lymphocytes that begins within the bone marrow, with subsequent release of neoplastic cells to the circulating blood.
Lymphoma Neoplasia of lymphocytes presenting as diffuse infiltration or mass lesions of the viscera.
Lymphomagenesis The pathogenesis of lymphoma.
Lymphomatoid granulomatosis A rare variant of lymphoma involving mixed populations of cells with an angiocentric and angioinvasive distribution.

Macroglobulinaemia The presence of an IgM paraprotein within serum.
Major histocompatibility complex A complex of genes encoding the molecules that mediate histocompatibility and the fundamental process of antigen presentation. These genes are highly polymorphic and are broadly divided into class I, II and III genes within the complex.
Mantle zone Outer region of a secondary lymphoid follicle; comprised of small lymphocytes.
Marker (vaccine) A vaccine containing a modified organism that induces a novel immune response that may be distinguished from the natural immune response to field strains of the organism.
Mastocytaemia Circulating neoplastic mast cells in mastocytosis.
Mastocytosis Systemic mast cell neoplasia.
Megaoesophagus Dilation and atony of the oesophagus; may occur as a localized form of myasthenia gravis in the dog.
Membrane attack complex The collection of terminal pathway complement components that form a channel through the membrane of a target cell, leading to osmotic lysis.
Memory The ability of the adaptive immune system to recall a previous encounter with an antigen and to make a more potent secondary immune response on re-encounter. Underlies the process of vaccination.
Meningoencephalitis Inflammation of both the meninges and parenchyma of the brain (e.g. granulomatous meningoencephalitis).
Microarray Molecular technique used to determine the gene expression profile in a tissue.
Microfold cell (M cell) Specialized cell found within the

epithelial surface of the 'dome' of an intestinal Peyer's patch. Thought to 'sample' antigen from the overlying intestinal lumen and transfer it to lymphoid cells below.

Mitogen A substance (often plant-derived) that can nonspecifically stimulate lymphocytes by binding to receptors other than the antigen-specific lymphocyte receptor.

Molecular adjuvant A gene (e.g. cytokine gene) or nucleotide sequence (e.g. CpG motif) incorporated into a molecular vaccine to enhance the immune response to the protein encoded by the vaccinal gene, or to direct the nature of the ensuing immune response (e.g. Th1 or Th2).

Molecular mimicry Shared structure or sequence of an epitope expressed by a pathogen and a self-molecule. Infection by such pathogens may give rise to autoimmunity.

Monoclonal An immune response specific for a single antigenic epitope, with activation of a single clone of lymphocytes.

Monoclonal antibody Antibody of a single specificity produced *in vitro* in large quantity for research, diagnostic or therapeutic purposes.

Monoclonal gammopathy A single species of immunoglobulin derived from neoplastic plasma cells in multiple myeloma (or rarely B cells in lymphoma) that presents as a 'spike' in the gamma globulin region on serum protein electrophoresis. May occasionally occur in some infectious diseases (e.g. monocytic ehrlichiosis or leishmaniosis).

Monomer A single unit (i.e. of antibody).

Mononuclear cells Leukocytes with a large round to oval nucleus (e.g. monocytic and lymphocytic cells). Often used to refer to these populations in the circulation (peripheral blood mononuclear cells).

Mucocutaneous junction The junction between haired skin and mucous membrane.

Mucosa-associated lymphoid tissue Unencapsulated lymphoid tissue associated with the mucosal surfaces of the body.

Mucosal Pertaining to surfaces of the body lined by a mucosa and in direct contact with the external environment; specifically, the conjunctiva, respiratory tract, alimentary tract, urogenital tract and mammary gland.

Mucosal adjuvant A substance that enhances the immune response to antigen delivered via a mucosal surface (e.g. cholera toxin). In some instances (depending upon dosage regime) the same adjuvant may enhance the development of mucosal tolerance to the antigen.

Multiple myeloma Malignant neoplasia of plasma cells. May target bone or soft tissue and is associated with paraproteinaemia.

Myasthenia gravis Autoimmune disease involving autoantibody binding the acetylcholine receptor at the neuromuscular junction. Inhibition of acetylcholine binding leads to muscle weakness.

Mydriatic Drug that causes pupillary dilation.

Myelodysplasia Dysplasia of the bone marrow; involves altered numbers, ratios and cytological appearance of haemopoietic cells, but is not overtly neoplastic. May be induced by FeLV in the cat.

Myeloid Of the bone marrow or referring to leukocytes of the myeloid series (granulocytes and monocytes).

Myelophthisis A 'space-occupying lesion' within the medullary cavity of bone that reduces the space available for normal haemopoietic tissue and may lead to pancytopenia.

Myeloproliferative disease Neoplasia of one or more haemopoietic lineages within the bone marrow. May lead to shedding of neoplastic cells into the circulating blood and seeding of these to viscera such as liver and spleen.

Myxoedema Accumulation of mucinous matrix within the dermis, resulting in thickened skin. Characteristic of canine hypothyroidism.

Naïve Pertaining to a lymphocyte that has not previously encountered the antigen that its receptor is programmed to recognize. (See also 'virgin lymphocyte').

Naked DNA (vaccine) Vaccination with plasmid containing a gene of interest leads to direct transfection of host antigen presenting cell, with expression of peptides derived from the protein encoded by the gene. This induces a powerful humoral and cell-mediated immune response in the recipient.

Nasal tolerance Induction of tolerance (systemic nonresponsiveness to antigen) by previous exposure of the antigen through the nasal mucosa. Akin to oral tolerance.

Natural killer (NK) cell Lymphoid cell with granular cytoplasm that mediates cytotoxicity of targets via the NK cell receptor or Fc receptor. (See also antibody-dependent cell-mediated cytotoxicity.)

Natural suppressor (cell) A suppressor cell naturally active in the body; important in controlling responses to self-antigens or allergens.

Needle-free vaccination Delivery of a vaccine other than by injection. Includes oral, intranasal and percutaneous administration. The latter may be via a purpose-designed apparatus that delivers vaccine under high pressure and which can pass through the epidermis to target dermal dendritic cells.

Negative selection Selection of those developing T lymphocytes within the thymus that bear a T cell receptor able to recognize self-antigen with high affinity. These cells are deleted by apoptosis within the thymus.

Neonatal tolerance Failure of immune response to an antigen in adult life due to exposure to that antigen *in utero* or during the early neonatal period.

Neovascularization Of the cornea as a sequela to inflammation. Extension of vessels into the cornea from the limbus.

Non-core (vaccine) Vaccine not recommended for every individual, perhaps because the vaccine has poor efficacy, the infection is not prevalent in the geographical area in which the individual lives, or the lifestyle of that individual is unlikely to bring him/her into contact with the infectious agent.

Nucleotide The building blocks of DNA: adenine, thymine, guanine, cytosine.

Oedema Accumulation of fluid within tissue; immunologically this generally follows vasodilation as part of an inflammatory response.

Oncofetal Inappropriate activation of a gene involved in fetal development within a neoplastic cell. May lead to expression of 'oncofetal proteins' by tumour cells.

Oncogene A gene encoding a molecule involved in regulation of cell growth and division. Mutation or inappropriate activation of such genes underlies neoplasia.

Oncogenesis The pathogenesis of neoplasia.

Opsonization The coating of a particle with antibody and/or complement to enhance the effectiveness of phagocytosis.

Optic neuritis Inflammation of the optic nerve.
Oral tolerance An experimental phenomenon. When an antigen is first fed to an animal and the same antigen is subsequently delivered systemically in an immunogenic dose, the immune system fails to respond to the antigen. The same effect can be induced by primary antigen exposure at other mucosal surfaces (e.g. nasal tolerance).

Pannus Granulation tissue that extends from the synovium to cover articular cartilage defects in rheumatoid arthritis. (See also 'keratoconjunctivitis'.)
Panuveitis Inflammation of all parts of the uveal tract.
Papule A focal, well-circumscribed firm elevation of the skin.
Paracortex Intermediate area of a lymph node that envelopes the cortical follicles. Area of the lymph node in which T lymphocytes reside.
Paraneoplastic effect A manifestation of neoplasia not directly related to the local or metastatic growth of tumour within the viscera (e.g. the secretion of abnormal immunoglobulin or parathyroid hormone-like peptide by neoplastic plasma cells in multiple myeloma).
Paraprotein An abnormal immunoglobulin secreted by neoplastic plasma cells (multiple myeloma) or, rarely, B cells. Results in a monoclonal gammopathy within serum.
Patch testing Application of allergen to the skin of a sensitized individual by close apposition of an allergen-impregnated patch. Development of a local skin reaction over 48–72 hours is indicative of type IV hypersensitivity.
Pathogen A microorganism that causes disease or tissue damage when it infects a host.
Pathogen-associated molecular pattern A conserved antigen expressed by pathogenic microbes, which is recognized by the pattern recognition receptor on the dendritic cell. Also known as 'Toll-like receptor'.
Pattern recognition receptor Receptor on the surface of dendritic cells that recognizes specific conserved antigens expressed by pathogenic microbes (pathogen-associated molecular pattern). (See also 'Toll-like receptor'.)
Pauciarthritis Inflammation of between two and five joints.
Pautrier's microabscess An intraepithelial cluster of neoplastic lymphocytes in epitheliotropic lymphoma.
Pelger–Huët anomaly Genetically mediated hyposegmentation of neutrophil nuclei of no apparent clinical significance.
Pemphigoid An autoimmune skin disease characterized by the formation of subepidermal vesicles/pustules (bullous pemphigoid).
Pemphigus A group of autoimmune blistering skin diseases characterized by the formation of vesicles/pustules within the epidermis.
Peptide Short stretch of amino acids.
Perforin A molecule released from a cytotoxic cell that polymerizes to form a pore within the cell membrane of the target cell, allowing the influx of other cytotoxic molecules, ions and water.
Periarteriolar lymphoid sheath Area of white pulp of the spleen in which T lymphocytes reside. Three dimensionally, the T cells form a cylindrical sheath that surrounds an arteriolar blood vessel.
Peribulbar Around the hair bulb (e.g. the inflammation in alopecia areata).
Peyer's patch Area of organized but unencapsulated lymphoid tissue within the small intestinal mucosa.
Phacoclastic uveitis Uveitis associated with rupture of the lens capsule and release of lens protein.
Phacolytic uveitis Uveitis associated with leakage of lens protein through the intact capsule of a resorbing cataract.
Phagocytosis Internalization of a particle by a phagocytic cell (e.g. neutrophil or macrophage).
Phagolysosome A digestive vacuole within the cytoplasm of a phagocytic cell formed by the fusion of the phagosome with the enzyme-rich lysosome.
Phagosome A membrane-bound vesicle within the cytoplasm of a phagocytic cell containing the phagocytozed material.
Phenotype The outward appearance; immunologically, the identity of a cell as determined by the expression of a range of surface molecules or cellular function.
Plaque An elevated area of skin that is generally firm in consistency.
Plasma cell Late stage of differentiation of a B lymphocyte. The cell that synthesizes and secretes immunoglobulin.
Plasmacytoid Having the appearance of a plasma cell.
Plasmacytoma A localized, benign tumour of plasma cells usually involving the skin or mucous membranes.
Plasmapheresis Process of removing whole blood from an animal, separating the cells and plasma, and returning the cellular content to the animal. Has the effect of reducing concentrations of antibody and immune complexes.
Plasmoma Lymphoplasmacytic inflammation of the anterior surface of the third eyelid. Also known as 'nictitans plasmacytic conjunctivitis'.
Pododermatitis Inflammation of the skin of the foot.
Polarization Of an immune response, where the response to a specific antigen may be dominated by antibody production or cell-mediated immunity.
Polyacrylamide gel electrophoresis Used to separate the components of a complex antigen on the basis of their molecular size.
Polyarteritis nodosa Inflammation and degeneration of the wall of several arterial blood vessels in different anatomical locations.
Polyarthritis Inflammation of several (usually > six) joints.
Polyclonal An immune response activating multiple clones of lymphocytes specific for numerous epitopes of an antigen.
Polymerase chain reaction An *in vitro* means of amplifying a particular portion of DNA.
Polymeric Ig receptor Receptor expressed at the basolateral surface of mucosal epithelial cells for the capture of IgA or IgM and transfer of these immunoglobulins across the mucosal barrier.
Polymorphic As related to genetic loci; many different possible alleles at any one locus.
Polymyositis Inflammation of several muscles.
Polyneuritis Inflammation of several peripheral nerves.
Positive selection Selection of those developing T lymphocytes within the thymus that bear a functional T cell receptor able to recognize antigen in the context of major histocompatibility complexes.
Potency (of vaccine) A measure of the strength of a vaccine and thus the ability of the vaccine to protect from infection or disease. Most tests of vaccine potency relate to how well the vaccine can protect a group of animals that are challenged with virulent organism following vaccination.
Primary immune response Immune response made by an individual on first encounter with a foreign antigen.
Pro-inflammatory Enhancing the inflammatory response (i.e. pro-inflammatory cytokines amplify inflammation).
Proliferative response Measure of the ability of lymphocytes to respond to antigen or mitogen *in vitro* by

dividing. Generally performed using mononuclear cells derived from the blood.
Proptosis Bulging of the eye (exophthalmos).
Proteinuria The presence of serum proteins in the urine. Used as an indicator of renal disease.
Pruritus Itching. A sign of a cutaneous type I hypersensitivity reaction, manifest in animals by scratching and self-trauma.
Pseudogene DNA sequence resembling a gene, but containing codons that prevent transcription into full length RNA.
Pseudopelade Autoimmune disease targeting the mid-level of the hair follicle.
Pustule An intraepidermal vesicle filled by inflammatory cells (neutrophils or eosinophils) and acanthocytes. May be sterile (e.g. in pemphigus) or caused by bacterial infection.

Radiotherapy The treatment of a lesion by targeted delivery of ionizing radiation.
Rearrangement (of DNA) The process of looping out and deleting introns via the action of recombinase enzymes.
Recirculation The movement of lymphocytes between interstitial tissue, lymphoid tissue, lymphatics and the vasculature. Allows lymphocytes wide access to areas of the body to maximize the chance of encounter with the antigen that they have been pre-programmed to recognize.
Recombinant (vaccine) A pure source of protein produced *in vitro* by inserting a gene into a vector (e.g. bacterial, insect or mammalian cell). The gene is expressed and the protein released from the cells into the culture medium. Such recombinant proteins can form the basis for vaccines.
Recombination In genetics, recombination of genes by crossing-over between chromosomes during cell division.
Recruitment Particular cell types may be recruited to tissue to participate in any immune response (e.g. eosinophils may be recruited into the site of a nematode infection for their antiparasitic action).
Regulation Regulation of an immune response may be either positive (to amplify the response) or negative (to switch the response off).
Repertoire Immunologically, the complete range of antigen-specific receptors than may be generated within an individual.
Reverse transcriptase (RT)-PCR A means of quantifying mRNA in a sample by extracting RNA and reverse transcribing it to cDNA for the PCR reaction.
Rheumatoid factor Typically an IgM autoantibody with specificity for IgG. Found in the serum and synovial fluid of patients with autoimmune polyarthropathies.

Satellitosis Clustering of cytotoxic lymphocytes around an apoptotic keratinocyte, typically in diseases such as erythema multiforme or toxic epidermal necrosis.
Scleritis Inflammation of the sclera.
Secondary immune response Immune response made by an individual on secondary re-encounter with antigen. The secondary immune response is typically induced more rapidly, is more powerful and persists for a longer period.
Secretory piece A portion of the polymeric Ig receptor that wraps around the Fc portion of an IgA molecule when it is released from a mucosal surface and protects the molecule from enzymatic degradation. Also called 'secretory chain' or 'secretory component'.
Sensitization Repeated exposure to an antigen over time. A sensitized individual may make a hypersensitivity response on re-exposure to the antigen.
Serosurvey Application of a serological test to a population of animals to determine the proportion of animals that have serum antibody to the target antigen. A serosurvey for infectious disease will determine the proportion of the population that has been infected (exposed) to the organism.
Serotype The classification of an infectious agent by its ability to react with particular antisera.
Severe combined immunodeficiency A genetic mutation resulting in lack of functional T and B lymphocytes and severe immune impairment. The causative mutation differs in the three canine breeds affected.
Single radial immunodiffusion A serological technique based on the principle of precipitation of antigen and antibody. Often used to measure the concentration of immunoglobulin in serum.
Sjögren's-like syndrome Combination of keratoconjunctivitis sicca and xerostomia caused by autoimmune lymphocytic destruction of the lacrimal and salivary glands.
Small intestinal bacterial overgrowth The presence of greater than normal numbers of bacteria within the lumen of the small intestine. May be primary or secondary. May be associated with chronic diarrhoea.
Somatic mutation Mutations that spontaneously arise in genes in somatic cells (e.g. nucleotide substitutions or deletions), giving rise to diversity in the encoded proteins.
Splenomegaly Enlargement of the spleen.
Subunit (vaccine) Vaccine containing an antigenic fragment of an organism rather than the entire organism itself.
Superantigen Molecules that can nonspecifically activate T or B cells by binding to their receptors in a non-antigen-specific fashion. Typically derived from microbes.
Suppressor cell A lymphocyte that functions to suppress the actions of other (effector) lymphocytes to switch off an immune response.
Sympathomimetic An agent that produces effects resembling those induced by postganglionic fibres of the sympathetic nervous system.
Synovitis Inflammation of the synovium of a joint.
Systemic lupus erythematosus Multisystemic autoimmune disease often involving the skin, joints, blood and renal glomerulus. Characterized by the presence of high-titred serum antinuclear antibody.

Tc A cytotoxic T cell, usually $CD8^+$, that mediates destruction of a specific target cell.
T cell receptor Two chain molecule (αβ or γδ chains) on the surface of a T lymphocyte that recognizes antigenic peptide combined with major histocompatibility complex molecule on the surface of the antigen presenting cell.
Th0 A $CD4^+$ helper T lymphocyte that is a precursor to mature Th1 and Th2 cells.
Th1 A $CD4^+$ helper T lymphocyte that preferentially produces IFNγ and mediates cellular immunity.
Th2 A $CD4^+$ helper T lymphocyte that preferentially produces IL-4, IL-5, IL-10 and IL-13 and mediates humoral immunity.
Th3 A $CD4^+$ T lymphocyte that preferentially produces TGFβ and may be important in mediating oral tolerance.
Th17 A $CD4^+$ T lymphocyte that preferentially produces IL-17 and has an important role in various immune-mediated diseases.
Thoracic duct The major lymphatic vessel of the body into which all lymphatics flow. The thoracic duct in turn

empties into the bloodstream to permit the recirculation of leukocytes within the body.

Thymic aplasia A congenital defect resulting in absence of the thymus. Often associated with hairlessness and results in impairment of T cell-mediated immunity.

Thymoma Neoplasm of thymic epithelial cells. Generally accompanied by a reactive proliferation of small lymphocytes. Can be associated with myasthenia gravis in the dog.

Titre A measure of the concentration of antibody produced in an immune response. In a serological test, the titre is the inverse of the last serum dilution, giving an unequivocally positive reaction in the test system.

Tolerance Failure of the immune system to respond to an antigen.

Toll-like receptor See pathogen-associated molecular pattern.

Toxic epidermal necrolysis Severe immune-mediated skin disease characterized by extensive full-thickness epidermal necrosis with loss of fluids and electrolytes.

Tr1 A $CD4^+$ T lymphocyte that preferentially produces IL-10 and mediates immunosuppression. (See also 'induced suppressor cell'.)

Transcription Synthesis of messenger RNA from a DNA template.

Transduction (of signal) Following occupation of a cell surface receptor, a positive or negative signal is delivered to the cell via cell membrane transduction molecules that activate cytoplasmic pathways leading to gene activation.

Transfection Insertion of small pieces of DNA into cells. The DNA may be expressed without integrating into the host cell DNA (transient transfection), or it may integrate into host cell DNA, thereby replicating whenever host cell DNA is replicated (stable transfection).

Translation Synthesis of polypeptide from the mRNA template.

Transmembrane A molecule on the surface of a cell that is anchored through the cell membrane into the cytoplasm.

Treg An IL-10 producing $CD4^+$ T lymphocyte that also expresses CD25 and mediates immunosuppression by direct contact with the target cell. (See also 'natural suppressor cell'.)

Triaditis The combination of inflammatory bowel disease, exocrine pancreatitis and portal hepatitis of cats. Thought to involve an ascending bacterial infection due to the commonality of the bile and pancreatic ducts in this species.

Trichohyalin Target autoantigen in alopecia areata.

Ulcer Localized loss of an epithelial surface.

Uraemia See also 'azotaemia'. Also used to describe the clinical syndrome that occurs due to end-stage renal failure.

Urticaria A cutaneous reaction characterized by the sudden appearance of erythematous and oedematous foci (wheals). Most often secondary to a type I hypersensitivity reaction.

Uveitis Inflammation of the uveal tract (i.e. the combination of iris, ciliary body and choroid).

Uveodermatological syndrome Immune-mediated disease affecting both the uveal tract and skin in Japanese Akitas.

Vaccination Induction of an adaptive immune response with immunological memory by deliberate exposure to an antigen. Typically, the antigen is an attenuated or killed pathogen and the process of vaccination induces an immune response that can protect the individual from field exposure to virulent pathogen.

Variable region That portion of an immunological molecule in which there is variability in amino acid sequence between the polypeptide chains of different molecules.

Vascular addressin Molecules expressed by high endothelial venules that are unique to the anatomical location of that venule. Only leukocytes bearing corresponding 'homing receptors' can interact with these endothelia and migrate into the local tissue.

Vasculitis Inflammation of the wall of a blood vessel leading to increased permeability of the vessel. Often induced by deposition of circulating immune complex within the wall.

Vasodilation Dilation of a blood vessel, with increased permeability between endothelial cells allowing egress of fluid, protein and cells into the surrounding tissue.

Vectored (vaccine) Insertion of a specific gene into a carrier organism (bacteria or virus) such that the organism expresses the protein encoded by the gene and thus acts as a 'vector' for transport of the protein. Such recombinant organisms have been used in vaccination.

Vesicle Fluid-filled space or blister (i.e. within the epidermis in immune-mediated skin disease).

Villous atrophy Feature of intestinal inflammation involving reduced height of the small intestinal villi.

Virulent The form of an infectious agent capable of producing tissue pathology and clinical disease.

Western blotting Serological technique used to determine the specific antigenic epitopes within an antigen to which antibody responses are made. Involves separation of epitopes by polyacrylamide gel electrophoresis and transfer to a membrane (e.g. nitrocellulose), which is then incubated with serum. Also called 'immunoblotting'.

Wheal A small raised, erythematous and oedematous focus within the skin. Most often associated with type I hypersensitivity reactions.

Xenoantigen A tissue antigen derived from another species. May induce an immune response following transplantation of an incompatible tissue xenograft.

Xerostomia Dry mouth. Occurs in Sjögren's-like syndrome due to destruction of the salivary gland tissue.

INDEX

Note: page numbers in *italics* refer to figures and tables

For Product Safety Concerns and Information please contact our EU representative GPSR@taylorandfrancis.com Taylor & Francis Verlag GmbH, Kaufingerstraße 24, 80331 München, Germany

* 9 7 8 1 8 4 0 7 6 1 7 1 9 *

T - #0190 - 090625 - C464 - 267/194/20 - PB - 9781840761719 - Gloss Lamination